KINESIOLOGY

KINES

7th edition

Kathryn Luttgens, Ph.D.

Professor
Boston-Bouvé College of Human Development Professions
Northeastern University

Katharine F. Wells, Ph.D.

Formerly Associate Professor
Wellesley College and Visiting Associate Professor
Mary Washington College

IOLOGY

Scientific Basis of Human Motion

SAUNDERS COLLEGE PUBLISHING

Philadelphia   New York   Chicago
San Francisco   Montreal   Toronto
London   Sydney   Tokyo   Mexico City
Rio de Janeiro   Madrid

Address orders to:
383 Madison Avenue
New York, NY 10017

Address editorial correspondence to:
West Washington Square
Philadelphia, PA 19105

This book was set in Melior by Graphic Arts Composition.
The editors were John Butler, Salena Kern, Lynne Gery, and Louise Robinson.
The art & design director was Richard L. Moore.
The text design was done by Larry Didona.
The cover design was done by Larry Didona.
The new artwork was drawn by Danmark & Michaels, Inc.
The production manager was Tom O'Connor.
This book was printed by Fairfield Graphics.

Library of Congress Cataloging in Publication Data

Luttgens, Kathryn, 1926–
    Kinesiology : scientific basis of human motion.

    Rev. ed. of: Kinesiology/Katharine F. Wells,
Kathryn Luttgens. 6th ed. 1976.
    Includes bibliographies and index.
    1. Kinesiology.   I. Wells, Katharine F.
II. Wells, Katharine F. Kinesiology.   III. Title.
QP303.L87 1982   612'.76   81-53074
ISBN 0-03-058358-6   AACR2

Kinesiology   ISBN 0-03-058358-6

234 144 98765432

CBS COLLEGE PUBLISHING
Saunders College Publishing
Holt, Rinehart and Winston
The Dryden Press

Preface to the Seventh Edition

Since the publication of the first edition of this text 32 years ago, courses in kinesiology have undergone many changes in both content and emphasis. Each subsequent edition has reflected these changes, and the seventh edition is no exception. The primary goals of this revision have been to update and expand the material where appropriate and to strengthen the textbook as a pedagogical tool. To this end, chapter outlines and objectives have been added. Several of the chapters have been reordered, expanded, or reorganized, and many new photographs and illustrations have been included. The resultant organization and content makes this a book ideally suited to help students achieve the course competencies specified in the Guidelines and Standards for Undergraduate Kinesiology, which were developed by the Kinesiology Academy and endorsed by the Executive Committee of the National Association of Sport and Physical Education in 1980.

The textbook is designed as a basic source to introduce the undergraduate student to the fundamentals of kinesiology. Because the fundamentals are presented without compromise of basic theory, this may be used as a basic (introductory) text. The book presents the subject in a fashion that presupposes little background in anatomy and physics, but does not shy away from presenting material that requires some theoretical foundations in these areas. Whatever background is needed for understanding the various applications is supplied, and numerous examples and exercises are provided. There is extensive discussion of both anatomical and mechanical fundamentals of human motion and the application of these fundamentals to the analysis of a wide variety of motor skills. For these reasons, the text is especially appropriate for use in courses with these objectives:

1. To provide information that will help students obtain an understanding of the anatomical and mechanical fundamentals of human motion.
2. To afford students the opportunity to learn a systematic approach to the analysis of human motion.
3. To provide the types of experiences that ask students to apply anatomical and mechanical analysis to the learning and improvement of a broad spectrum of movement activities.

The organization of the text is as follows:

Part One: Anatomical and Physiological Fundamentals of Human Motion

Part Two: Fundamentals of Biomechanics

Part Three: Motor Skills: Principles and Applications

Part One consists of eight chapters, all of which discuss the anatomical background essential for understanding human movement. The emphasis throughout is on the *relation of anatomical structure to function,* not on anatomy as such. Applications of the knowledge of structure to the analysis of motion are introduced early in the text so that the student can begin to put theory into practice immediately, rather than waiting until the knowledge base is more complete. Additional laboratory experiences have been added to assist with this practice.

Other changes in Part One include an expanded coverage on joint ranges of motion in Chapter 1, additional material on muscle mechanics in Chapter 2, and considerable revision of the material on the neuromuscular basis of human motion in Chapter 3. Chapters 4 through 8 have been reordered and updated according to the latest electromyographic information on muscle function. There is no longer a separate chapter on the thorax and respiration. That material has been incorporated into the chapter on the spinal column. Information on the pelvic girdle is now located in the chapter on the lower extremity and hip region.

Part Two presents the fundamentals of mechanics as they apply to human movement analysis. The first chapter introduces the student to terminology and to units of measure used when motion and the forces that cause it are studied. This chapter is followed by chapters in which motion and the forces that cause and modify it are described. The section concludes with a chapter on the center of gravity and stability.

Throughout Part Two efforts have been made to maintain an elementary approach to the material without oversimplifying to the point where misconceptions could occur. In many instances the student is shown the "proof" of a principle through experimental examples or mathematical derivation. This approach is used in the belief that greater understanding will result and that the reward will be greater comprehension of the reasons "why" optimum movement patterns occur as they do. It should be remembered, however, that the emphasis in a first undergraduate course in kinesiology should be on the development of the qualitative method of analysis and that the introduction of the quantitative method, if used, should be limited to understanding fundamental concepts and not for extensive application to analysis of movement patterns.

Part Three begins with a much enlarged chapter that discusses approaches to the kinesiological analysis of human movement, including a motor-skills classification system and an outline for a systematic approach to analysis inclusive of *description, evaluation, and prescription*. The motor-skills classification presented in this chapter forms the basis for the organization of the six chapters that follow. In each of these chapters the basic principles of anatomy and mechanics are identified and applied to specific motor skills. Sample analyses are also included.

Part Three continues with a chapter on exercises for special purposes, namely exercises for increasing range of motion, strengthening muscles, and correcting postural faults and weaknesses. The final summary chapter addresses the implications that a knowledge of kinesiology has for the teaching and learning of motor skills.

There are nine appendices. Those starred are partially or completely new to this edition:

The authors wish to express grateful appreciation to Gerry Schrader for photographs taken especially for this edition; to Marjorie Everett, Mary Huntington, and William Cargill for serving as subjects for those pictures; to Jack Grinold, Northeastern University Sports Information Director, for providing additional photographs; to John Clayton and Peter McGrain for critical review of certain chapters; and to Gail Ramsay for assistance in the typing of the revised mauscript.

Appreciation is also expressed to the authors and publishers who graciously gave permission to quote passages and reproduce illustrations from their publications. The authors also wish to acknowledge their indebtedness to the generations of students whose stimulus has been a vital reason for the existence of this book. Finally, they would like to express their sincere thanks to the editorial and production staffs of Saunders College Publishing for their helpfulness throughout the preparation of the edition.

KATHRYN LUTTGENS, *Wellesley, Massachusetts*
KATHARINE F. WELLS, *Needham, Massachusetts*

Preface to the First Edition
Abridged

This book is intended as a kinesiology text both for the teacher and for the student. It is believed that there is enough material to use it as a text for a full year's course yet, at the same time, by judicious selection of the subject matter, by omission of the supplementary material and by the substitution of classroom demonstrations for some of the laboratory exercises, the book should serve equally well as a text for a one semester course in kinesiology. It is left to the discretion of the instructor to select the material that meets his particular needs.

In its original form this textbook was an unpublished handbook-laboratory manual. It was used by the author in her kinesiology classes for three years before it was expanded to its present form. The original manual did not serve as an independent textbook. It was intended to be used as a companion book to a kinesiology or anatomy text. Since this limited its usefulness, however, it was decided to expand it to what is intended as a complete and independent textbook. For those who like to use a single textbook for a course it should suffice. To help the student (and the instructor) in his collateral reading, most chapters in this text contain a comprehensive bibliography. In many cases there is also a list of readings which are particularly recommended. These bibliographies and reading lists provide a rich source of information for the inquiring student.

In regard to the value of laboratory exercises and projects as a means of learning, James B. Stroud, in his book *Psychology in Education,* points out that "Effectiveness of instruction is not determined so much by what the teacher does, as by what he leads the pupils to do. . . ." Again, "Perhaps one of the most successful procedures for infusing learning with significance has been the [educational method known as] constructive activities. . . . The activity is thus a means of making learning meaningful and of giving it a purpose." In accord with this point of view numerous laboratory exercises are suggested. In conformity to the same principle, only a few complete analyses of skills are presented, for it is the writer's contention that the student will gain far more from making one complete analysis himself than from reading a dozen or more ready-made analyses.

As a further means of enriching the kinesiology course a number of the chapters include supplementary material in the form of brief descriptions of research projects in the field of anatomy and kinesiology. A few of these were carried out by the author, but the majority were conducted by other investigators and reported in the professional journals. The purpose of including this material is to broaden the instructor's background and to provide supplementary reading assignments for advanced students.

It has been the intention of the author to write simply and to use nontechnical terminology whenever this conveyed the meaning as clearly and specifically as technical terms. The latter have been used, however, whenever they served to avoid ambiguity. While it is desirable for the kinesiology student to enlarge his scientific vocabulary, a text which confronts him with a staggering list of new and strange words defeats its purpose. Textbooks should stimulate the curiosity of their readers, not frighten them with a forbidding vocabulary.

The author acknowledges her indebtedness to many individuals without whose help it is doubtful if this book could have been written. She wishes to express her grateful appreciation particularly to Professor C. H. McCloy of the State University of Iowa for his continued guidance, encouragement and criticism, also for his generous permission to use material from his course in The Mechanical Analysis of Motor Skills, and to the students in her kinesiology classes of the last three years who served patiently as "guinea pigs" and who made many constructive suggestions concerning the laboratory exercises.

For the illustrations, which add immeasurably to the usefulness of the text, grateful acknowledgment is made to Miss Mildred Codding, who made the anatomic drawings.

The author is under obligation to a number of individuals for the use of photographs and to several publishers for permission to reproduce copyrighted materials. To all writers and teachers from whom the author, either wittingly or unwittingly, has derived ideas which have provided the necessary background for the writing of this book she humbly acknowledges her indebtedness.

KATHARINE F. WELLS

Contents

Part One

Anatomical and Physiological Fundamentals of Human Motion

Part Two

Fundamentals of Biomechanics

Introduction to the Study of Kinesiology

Kinesiology, as it is known in physical education, orthopedics, and physical medicine, is the study of human movement from the point of view of the physical sciences. The study of the human body as a machine for the performance of work has its foundations in three major areas of study, namely, mechanics, anatomy, and physiology; more specifically, biomechanics, musculoskeletal anatomy, and neuromuscular physiology. The majority of courses in kinesiology are based primarily on the first two of these and a separate course, physiology of muscular activity, covers much of the third. There is some overlapping, however, as there are certain physiological concepts which even the most elementary course in kinesiology cannot afford to ignore.

In the early days of physical education, when few activities were taught other than gymnastics and the dance, the content of a course in kinesiology was confined chiefly to functional anatomy. Gradually, as sports and dance assumed a more important place in the curriculum, the concept of kinesiology was broadened to include the study of the mechanical principles which apply to the techniques used in sport and dance. The principles were applied not only to the movements of the body itself, but also to the movements of the implements, balls, and other equipment. In like manner, the development of the kinesiology course in schools of physical therapy and occupational therapy has kept pace with the development of their expanded curricula. Having started as "muscle reeducation," it has come to include the application of mechanical principles to postural adjustments, to the gait, to the use of tools and household implements, and to the modifications of vocational and homemaking activities necessitated by limitations in neuromuscular capacity and skeletal structure.

Some authorities refer to kinesiology as a science in its own right; others claim that it should be called a study rather than a true science because the principles on which it is based are derived from basic sciences such as anatomy, physiology, and physics. In any event, its unique contribution is that it selects from many sciences those principles which are pertinent to human motion and systematizes their application. However it may be categorized, to the inquiring student it is a door opening into a whole new world of discovery and appreciation. Human motion, which most of us have taken for granted all our lives, is seen through new eyes. One who gives it any thought whatever cannot help being impressed not only by the beauty of human motion, but also by its apparently infinite possibilities, its meaningfulness, its orderliness, its adaptability to the surrounding environment. Nothing is haphazard; nothing is left to chance. Every structure that participates in the movements of the body does so in obedience to physical and physiological principles. The student of kinesiology, like the student of anatomy, physiology, psychology, genetics, and other biological sciences, can only look with reverent wonder at the intricate mechanism of the body and, in the words of the psalmist, exclaim to the Creator, "I will praise thee, for I am fearfully and wonderfully made."

But kinesiology is not studied merely for the purpose of inciting our interest in a fascinating and mysterious subject. It has a useful purpose. We study kinesiology in order to learn how to analyze the movements of the human body and to discover their underlying principles. The study of kinesiology is an essential part of the educational experience of students of physical education, dance, sport, and physical medicine. For the first three it has a dual purpose: on the one hand, the purpose of perfecting performance in motor skills and, on the other, the purpose of perfecting the performer, himself. Kinesiology helps to prepare physical educators to teach effective performance in both fundamental and specialized motor skills. Furthermore, it enables them to evaluate exercises and activities from the point of view of their effect on the human structure. As Dr. William Skarstrom used to say to his kinesiology students, the human machine has this advantage over the manufactured machine: Whereas the latter wears out with use, the former improves with use (within limits), *provided it is used in accordance with the principles of efficient human motion*. The function of kinesiology, therefore, is to contribute not only to *successful participation* in various physical activities, but also to the *improvement* of the human structure through the intelligent selection of activities and the efficient use of the body.

For the physical therapist and the occupational therapist the purpose of studying kinesiology (whether called by that name or by some other) is not unlike that of the physical education teacher. The difference is in emphasis, rather than in purpose. The therapist is primarily concerned with the effect that exercises and other techniques of physical medicine have upon the body. He or she is concerned particularly with the restoration of impaired function and with methods of compensating for lost function. Effective performance is a goal for the therapist as it is for the physical educator, but to the therapist "effective performance" refers not so much to *skillful* performance in athletic activities as to *adequate* performance in the activities associated with daily living. Whereas the educator applies knowledge of kinesiology chiefly to the movements of the normal body, the therapist is concerned with the movements of a body which has suffered an impairment in function.

The educator and the therapist have at least one application in common in studying kinesiology. Both are concerned with posture and body mechanics of daily life skills, hence both are interested in discovering the anatomical and mechanical bases for training in this area. Both apply their knowledge of kinesiology to analyzing the postural needs of others, to the intelligent selection of posture exercises based on individual need and to the mechanically efficient methods of using the body in daily life skills.

The most satisfactory way of studying kinesiology is by supplementing book study with laboratory experimentation. It is a truism that we learn best by doing. Laboratory experiences should include two types of activity. The first type consists of experiments performed under controlled conditions. Activities in this category are selected to help the student gain insight into and understanding of the nature and complexity of human motion. Although the emphasis is primarily on qualitative analysis in the beginning course, some quantification of data is appropriate, as is the use of "laboratory"-type instruments. Especially helpful is the stop-action motion picture projector, whose use enables the careful and prolonged study of a very small moment in the performance of a technique and permits the observation of detail unavailable to the naked eye.

The second type of laboratory experience should consist of practice in analysis under the conditions that exist every day in the gymnasium or clinic. Only through practice under these conditions will the student learn how to apply a knowledge of kinesiology and develop the skills necessary for accurate diagnosis and treatment of faulty motor performance.

Whatever method of teaching or study is employed, it is well for the student to keep in mind the aims of a kinesiology course and the intended applications for what will be learned. It must be remembered that the analysis of motion is not an end in itself, but rather a means to the learning of new movement patterns and the improvement of old ones. This is as true for the physical therapist teaching amputees and paraplegics to walk again as it is for the physical educator teaching a sport technique. Finally, it must be remembered that the skill itself is of less importance than the one who practices it. Kinesiology serves only half its purpose when it provides the background for learning or teaching motor skills. It must also serve to lay the foundation for perfecting, repairing, and keeping in good condition that incomparable mechanism—the human body.

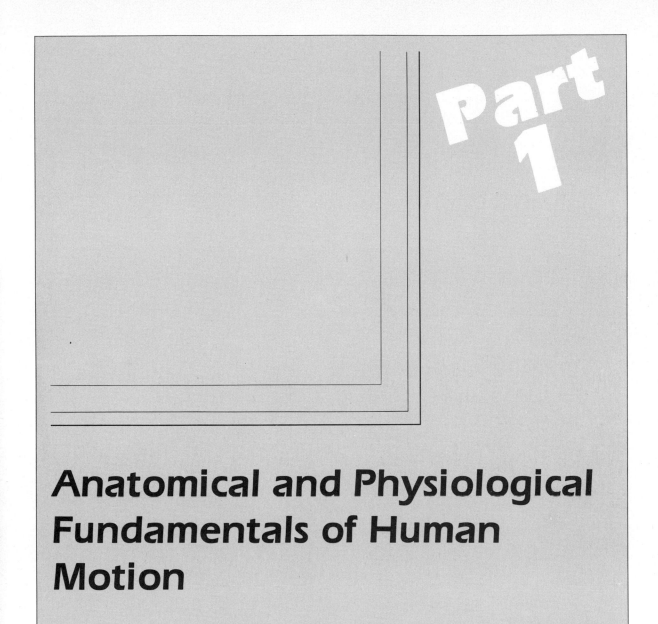

Part 1

Anatomical and Physiological Fundamentals of Human Motion

Introduction to Part 1

Where does anatomy end and kinesiology begin? This is a question frequently argued by kinesiologists. Yet, in truth, there is no answer because the question itself is not a valid one. One might as well ask, "Where does the study of words end and the writing of compositions (or articles, or books) begin?" Or, "Where does the study of building materials end and the designing and erecting of buildings begin?" Just as words are the elements used in all writing, whether creative, factual, or expository, and just as bricks, wood, cement, metal, and glass are some of the elements used in building, so bones, joints, muscles, connective tissue, blood vessels, and nerves are the vital elements of human motion. They are the essential elements used in batting a baseball, passing and carrying a football, shooting a basketball into the basket—in fact, in all running, walking, jumping, throwing, striking, catching, and swimming; likewise, one finds them in typewriting, manual labor, picture painting, sewing, knitting, and so forth, almost without end.

One aim of Part One is to prepare students of human motion, whether they are in physical education, athletic training, physical therapy, corrective therapy, occupational therapy, or other related professions, to analyze human movements in terms of muscles and joints, and to apply the knowledge provided to improve performance in motor skills. This section should not be looked upon merely as a review of anatomy but as the very foundation for analysis of human motion. It demonstrates the close relationships between anatomical structure and function, and it provides a body of knowledge that can be utilized in the learning and perfecting of various motor skills. It aims to demonstrate how the bones, joints, and muscles serve as elements in anatomical levers, which act in accord with the laws of mechanics. It also aims to make clear the influences of gravitational and other external forces on muscular actions. For instance, under certain circumstances, these forces may cause an action to be the exact opposite from what one would expect in view of the movement that is being performed. It should be obvious, therefore, that memorizing the actions of muscles will not prepare the student for making accurate analyses. Rather, a true understanding of all the conditions that influence the functions of the muscles is necessary.

A second aim of Part One is to equip the future physical education instructor, coach, trainer, or therapist with the anatomical knowledge essential for understanding the nature of common athletic injuries and their prevention. For this reason considerable emphasis is placed upon the structure of each joint, the factors that contribute to its stability, and the factors that influence the range of motion of each joint. One factor of which many seem to be in ignorance is the timetable of ages at which the epiphyseal cartilages become ossified. It should be of interest because it marks the turning point between the period of bone growth and the period of bone maturity. Because of the significance of this information a schedule of the maturation age of each bone that participates in common activities has been included in the first chapter.

There are eight chapters in Part One—two on the musculoskeletal system and its movements, one on the neuromuscular aspects of motion, and five on the anatomy and fundamental movements of specific segments of the body. The order in which these chapters are studied is entirely optional. The authors appreciate the fact that the students who use this text may differ widely in their educational backgrounds. Some may already have completed courses in anatomy, possibly even including the experience of human dissection. Others may have had only brief courses and will feel the need of receiving more detailed information. Still others may have had no anatomical instruction whatsoever and may expect none other than what is included in the kinesiology course. This situation obviously leaves authors of kinesiology texts with a dilemma. In an attempt to meet the needs of all students, whatever their backgrounds, the authors of this text have presented in Part One what they consider to be a fairly complete coverage of the aspects of anatomy that relate to movement and, at the same time, have omitted details whose relation to movement seems less significant. Hence, specific muscle attachments are not included in the main body of the text but may be found in chart form in an appendix at the end of the book for those who want to refer to them. On the other hand, the muscle's line of pull and its relation to the joint at which the motion is occurring are emphasized, since these are considered essential elements of movement.

In the light of the aforementioned aims of Part One—to provide the student of human motion with the knowledge necessary for analyzing human motion and applying such an analysis to the improvement of performance in motor skills, and to equip the instructor, therapist, or coach with the anatomical background for understanding the nature of athletic injuries and their prevention—it might seem that the student should wait until the entire anatomical section has been completed before attempting to analyze movement. On the contrary, the earlier the application of knowledge begins, the better. In fact, attempting to analyze basic movements as soon as possible serves as a stimulus to the study of anatomy. An example of this situation is given below.

Let us consider starting with the arm in its anatomical position and flexing the forearm at the elbow against the stabilized upper arm. Note that we have already defined the starting position and the movement. We could be even more specific if we wished and state whether the movement was executed quickly or slowly, and whether the movement was performed against resistance as though lifting a weight.

The next step would be to consider the joint itself. The structure of the elbow joint should be reviewed. Since it was stipulated that the movement was made from the anatomical position, it would be advisable to review the radioulnar articulations also, especially the proximal joint because of its close relationship to the elbow joint. It would be helpful to refer to Chapter 2 or Appendix D to check on the types and characteristics of these joints.

The muscles performing the movement should be considered next and an attempt made to answer such questions as the following: What muscles flex the elbow joint?

How are they affected by the starting position and the position of the forearm throughout the movement? Try to discover whether the amount of resistance to this movement affects the participating muscles, but do not overstress this point. Include all of the muscles that unquestionably contribute to flexion in this position without being overly concerned at this time as to whether they are "principal" or "assistant" contributors. Review the section on the coordination of the muscular system (see page 42) and try to identify those muscles serving in the capacity of stabilizers or of neutralizers.

Following the above procedure throughout the study of Part One will pave the way for the later analysis of more complex movements. Procedural steps for analyzing fitness exercises, sport skills, and other physical activities are presented in Appendix E. For the present, however, it is suggested that the student make simple joint and muscle analyses until the process is thoroughly familiar.

The Musculoskeletal System
I. The Skeletal Framework and its Movements

Objectives

At the conclusion of this chapter, the student should be able to:

1. Classify joints according to structure, and explain the relationship that exists between a joint structure and its capacity for movement.
2. Explain how the schedule of ossification of epiphyseal cartilage is related to the nature of sports suitable for different age groups.
3. Name the factors which contribute to joint range of motion and stability, and explain the relationship that exists between range of motion and stability.
4. Assess a joint's range of motion, evaluate the range, and describe desirable procedures for changing it when indicated.
5. Name and define the orientation positions and planes of the body and the axes of motion.
6. Demonstrate and name fundamental movement patterns using correct movement terminology.
7. Isolate and name single joint actions that are part of complex movements.

It is customary—especially for students of human movement and exercise—to begin the study of anatomy with a detailed study of the bones, then to proceed to the joints, and then to the muscles. This path of investigation sometimes dampens the enthusiasm of the students, whose chief focus of interest is movement. Therefore, the first two chapters of this text emphasize the concept of the total musculoskeletal system as a mechanism for motion. It is hoped that by using this concept the student will find the study of the structural elements of this system to be more meaningful.

The musculoskeletal framework, as the phrase implies, is an arrangement of bones and muscles. Adjacent bones are attached to one another by joints, which provide for the motion of the articulating bones, and the muscles that span the joints provide the force for moving the bones to which they are attached. Mechanically speaking, the total bone-joint-muscle structure is an intricate combination of levers that makes possible a great number of coordinated movements, ranging from the small hand and finger motions used in assembling a television set or playing the piano to the total body movements of a swimmer or a pole vaulter. Any single one of the levers involved in such movements is relatively simple. Physics tells us that a lever is defined as a rigid bar that turns about a fulcrum (fixed axis or pivot) when force is applied to it at some specific point. An anatomical lever, therefore, is simply a bone that engages in an angular or turning type of movement when a muscle attached to it contracts and thus applies force to it. This force is always a *pulling* force because muscles, being flexible, are unable to push; they can only pull.

The Bones

Although anatomy texts give the number of bones in the human skeleton as 206, only 177 of them engage in voluntary movement.* The skeleton consists of two major parts, the axial skeleton and the appendicular skeleton (Figure 1–1). The axial section comprises the skull, spinal column, sternum, and ribs, and the appendicular section includes the bones of the upper and lower extremities. The bones of the upper extremity include the scapula, clavicle, humerus, ulna, radius, carpal bones, metacarpals, and phalanges, and those of the lower extremity include the three fused bones of the pelvis, the femur, tibia, fibula, tarsal bones, metatarsals, and phalanges. Although the pelvis may be classified with either the axial or the appendicular skeleton, it is actually a link between the axial skeleton and the lower extremity branch of the appendicular skeleton and is functionally as important to one as to the other.

Types of Bones   In spite of the great variety of shapes and sizes of bones, there are only four major categories of them—namely, long, short, flat, and irregular.

LONG BONES   Characterized by a cylindrical shaft with relatively broad, knobby ends. The shaft or body has thick walls and contains a central cavity known as a medullary canal. The bones belonging in this category are the clavicle, humerus, ulna, radius, metacarpals, and phalanges of the upper extremity, and the femur, tibia, fibula, metatarsals, and phalanges of the lower extremity.

SHORT BONES   Relatively small, chunky, solid bones. The carpals and tarsals (wrist and ankle bones) belong to this category.

FLAT BONES   These include the sternum, scapulae, ribs, pelvic bones, and patellas.

IRREGULAR BONES   The bones of the spinal column—the 24 vertebrae, the sacrum, and the coccyx—are found in this category.

---

*The bones not included are the hyoid, the coccyx (the sacrum and coccyx are treated as a single bone since there is no voluntary motion of one on the other), 6 ossicles, and 21 skull bones, the skull being treated as a single bone with reference to the spinal column.

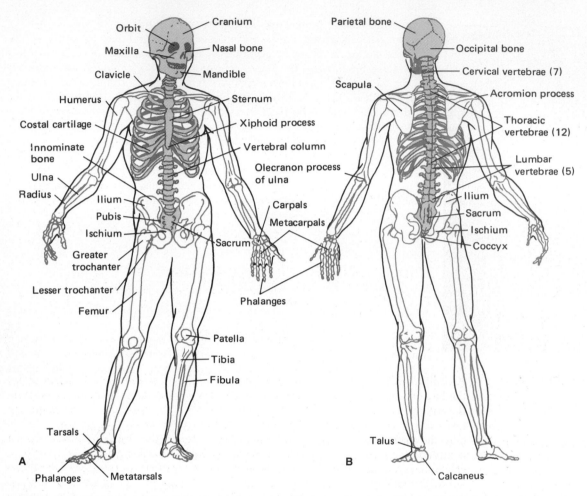

Figure 1–1   Skeleton. Axial skeleton is snaded; appendicular system is unshaded. *A,* Anterior view. *B,* Posterior view. (Adapted from Anthony, C. P., and Thibodeau, G. A.: *Textbook of anatomy and physiology.* 10th ed. St. Louis, C. V. Mosby, 1979.)

Mechanical Axis of a Bone

It has already been stated that bones serve as levers. When the mechanical analysis of muscular action is undertaken, one must know what is meant by the mechanical axis of the bone, or the body segment, that is serving as the lever. The student will find it advantageous, therefore, to learn what this term is now while studying the bones. *The mechanical axis of a bone or segment is a straight line that connects the midpoint of the joint at one end with the midpoint of the joint at the other end or, in the case of a terminal segment, with the midpoint of its distal end.* This axis does not necessarily pass lengthwise through the shaft of the bony lever. If the shaft is curved or if the articulating process projects at an angle from the shaft, the greater part of the axis may lie outside of the shaft, as in the case of the femur (Figure 1–2).

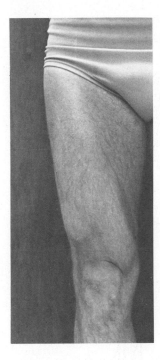

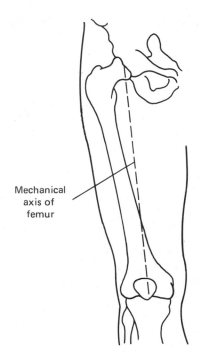

Mechanical
axis of
femur

Figure 1–2   Mechanical axis of femur.

The Epiphyses

An epiphysis is a layer of cartilage whose presence in the bone is an indication that the bone has not completed its growth. In the long bones the shaft is separated from the ends and from articulating knobs by epiphyseal cartilages. This is where growth takes place. As growth ceases, the cartilages gradually become ossified and, when closure is complete, no more growth can occur. Surprisingly, several epiphyses do not completely ossify until the twentieth, or even the twenty-fifth, year. Hence, most high school boys and many college men are engaging in vigorous sports before their bones are fully matured. Physical education instructors, trainers, and coaches need to be aware of this fact. Although this is not usually harmful in the case of noncontact sports, in violent contact sports like football and boxing the consequences may be extremely serious (Larsen and McMahan, 1966). Protective devices are helpful, but many of those in current use have been judged inadequate. High standards for these devices must be insisted upon. Even more important, coaches, especially those of young adolescents, must be both knowledgeable and conscientious. They must accept their responsibility for the health and safety of each individual player as being of far greater importance than the development of a winning team. The coach who tells a high school boy to aim the top of his helmet at the numeral on his opponent's shirt and run full force into him (known as "sticking") is either grossly ignorant or callously indifferent.

There is also danger to elementary and junior high school youngsters who are permitted to bear weights that are too heavy for them. "Husky-looking" boys and girls are often mistakenly permitted to form the base of a pyramid because they give the impression of being strong. If they are on their hands and knees supporting a second and perhaps a third row of youngsters, the weight may be too much for them. This is especially likely to be the case if the individuals in the upper rows are careless about

TABLE 1–1 Approximate Ages of Epiphyseal Closures*

	AGE
SPINAL COLUMN	
Vertebrae and sacrum	25
THORAX	
Sternum	25
Ribs	25
UPPER EXTREMITY	
Clavicle	25
Scapula	15–17
Humerus	
Head fused with shaft	20
Lateral epicondyle	16–17
Medial epicondyle	18
Ulna	
Olecranon	16
Lower end	20
Radius	
Head and shaft	18–19
Lower end to shaft	20
LOWER EXTREMITY	
Pelvic bone	
Inferior rami of pubis and ischium (almost complete)	7–8
Acetabulum	20–25
Femur	
Greater and lesser trochanters	18
Head	18
Lower end	20
Tibia	
Upper end	20
Lower end	18
Fibula	
Upper end	25
Lower end	20

*Listed by body section.

where they place their hands and knees. If these are not placed in line with the supporting individuals' arms and thighs, the vertebrae and possibly the arms and thighs will be subjected to rotatory stress, which may result in serious injury to the epiphyses of these bones. Dr. Charles L. Lowman was a pioneer in warning of such dangers. In spite of the early dates of their publication, his writings are strongly recommended to today's instructors and coaches (Lowman, 1947).

The approximate ages at which the ossification of the epiphyseal cartilages is completed are presented in Tables 1–1 and 1–2 (Goss, 1973).

Articulations

The structure and function of joints are so interrelated that it is difficult to discuss them separately. Hence, in the discussion of structure there is much that relates to function and, conversely, much that relates to structure when function is discussed. Careful inspection of the joints depicted in Figure 1–3 will give an idea of the

TABLE 1–2 Approximate Ages of Epiphyseal Closures*

APPROXIMATE AGE
7–8
    Inferior rami of pubis and ischium almost complete
15–17
    Upper extremity: scapula, lateral epicondyle of humerus, olecranon process of ulna
18–19
    Upper extremity: medial epicondyle of humerus, head and shaft of radius
    Lower extremity: femoral head and greater and lesser trochanters, lower end of tibia
About 20
    Upper extremity: humeral head, lower ends of radius and ulna
    Lower extremity: lower ends of femur and fibula, upper end of tibia
20–25
    Lower extremity: acetabulum in pelvis
25
    Spine: vertebrae and sacrum
    Upper extremity: clavicle
    Lower extremity: upper end of fibula
    Thorax: sternum and ribs

*Listed by age.

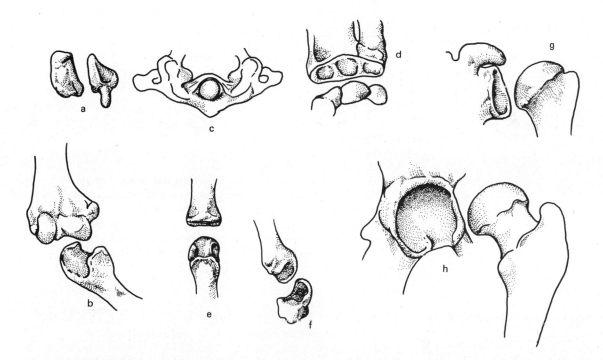

Figure 1–3 Major types of diarthrodial joints. *a,* Plane (intercarpal). *b,* Hinge (elbow or humeroulnar). *c,* Pivot (atlantoaxial). *d,* Condyloid (radiocarpal). *e,* Condyloid (metacarpophalangeal). *f,* Saddle (thumb or carpometacarpal). *g,* Ball-and-socket (shoulder). *h,* Ball-and-socket (hip). (Adapted from Hollinshead, W. H., and Jenkins, D. B.: *Functional anatomy of the limbs and back.* 5th ed. Philadelphia: W. B. Saunders, 1981.)

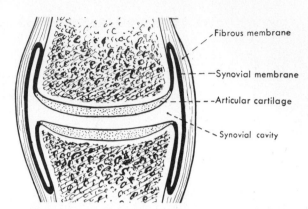

Figure 1–4   Frontal section of a diarthrodial joint. (From Hollinshead, W. H., and Jenkins, D. B.: *Functional anatomy of the limbs and back.* 5th ed. Philadelphia: W. B. Saunders, 1981.)

relationship between the shape of the joint and the movements that it permits. In much the same way that railroad tracks determine the route available to the train, the configuration of the bones that form an articulation, together with the reinforcing ligaments, both determine and limit the movements that the involved segment can make.

Structural Classification

There are many different patterns of joint structure, and these form the basis for their classification. The classifications in two well-known anatomy texts (Goss, 1973; Schaeffer, 1953), are based on the presence or absence of a joint cavity—i.e., a space between the articulating surfaces of the bones. Each type of joint is further classified either according to shape or according to the nature of the tissues which connect the bones. These classifications, with their subdivisions, may be grasped more readily if presented in outline form.

I.   Diarthrosis (from the Greek, meaning a joint in which there is a separation or articular cavity) (Figures 1–3, 1–4, and 1–5)
  A. Characteristics
    1.   An articular cavity is present.
    2.   The joint is encased within a sleevelike ligamentous capsule.
    3.   The capsule is lined with synovial membrane that secretes synovial fluid for lubricating the joint.
    4.   The articular surfaces are smooth.
    5.   The articular surfaces are covered with cartilage, usually hyaline, but occasionally fibrocartilage.

  B. Classification*
    1.   Irregular (arthrodial; plane). The joint surfaces are irregularly shaped, usually flat or slightly curved. The only movement permitted is of a gliding nature, hence it is nonaxial. Example: the carpal joints (Figure 1–3A) and articulations of the vertebral arches (Figure 8–5).
    2.   Hinge (ginglymus). One surface is spool-like; the other is concave. The concave surface fits over the spool-like process and glides partially around it in a hinge type of movement. This constitutes movement in

---

*This classification is based on the one in *Morris' human anatomy* (Schaeffer, 1953).

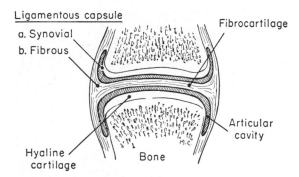

Ligamentous capsule
a. Synovial
b. Fibrous

Fibrocartilage

Figure 1–5   Frontal section of a diarthrodial joint having fibrocartilage.

Articular cavity

Hyaline cartilage

Bone

one plane about a single axis of motion; hence it is uniaxial. The movements that occur are flexion and extension. Example: elbow joint (Figure 5–1).

3.   Pivot (trochoid; screw). This kind of joint may be characterized by a peglike pivot, as in the joint between atlas and axis, or by two long bones fitting against each other near each end in such a way that one bone can roll around the other one, as do the radius and ulna of the forearm. In the latter type a small concave notch on one bone fits against the rounded surface of the other. The rounded surface may be either the edge of a disk (like the head of the radius) or a rounded knob (like the head of the ulna). The only movement permitted in either kind of pivot joint is rotation. It is a movement in one plane about a single axis; hence the joint is uniaxial. Examples: atlantoaxial (Figures 1–3C and 8–9) and radioulnar joints (Figure 5–1).

4.   Condyloid (ovoid; ellipsoidal). An oval or egg-shaped convex surface fits into a reciprocally shaped concave surface. Movement can occur in two planes, forward and backward, and from side to side. The former movement is flexion and extension, and the latter abduction and adduction or lateral flexion. The joint is biaxial. When these movements are performed sequentially, they constitute circumduction. Example: wrist joint (Figures 1–3 and 5–12) and metacarpophalangeal joints (Figures 1–3 and 5–13).

5.   Saddle (sellar; reciprocal reception). This may be thought of as a modification of a condyloid joint. Both ends of the convex surface are tipped up, making the surface concave in the other direction, like a western saddle. Fitting over this is a reciprocally concave-convex surface. Like the condyloid joint, this is a biaxial joint, permitting flexion and extension, abduction and adduction, and circumduction. The difference between the two is that the saddle joint has greater freedom of motion. Example: carpometacarpal joint of thumb (Figures 1–3F and 5–13).

6.   Ball-and-socket (spheroidal; enarthrodial). In this type of joint the spherical head of one bone fits into the cup or saucerlike cavity of the other bone (Figures 1–3, 4–1, 4–2, 6–1, and 6–2). It is very like the swivel joint on top of a camera tripod. It permits flexion and extension, abduction and adduction, circumduction (the sequential combination of the preceding), horizontal flexion and extension, and rotation. It is a triaxial joint since it permits movements about three axes.

C. Summary classification of diarthrodial joints:

Number of Axes:	0	1	2	3
	Nonaxial	Uniaxial	Biaxial	Triaxial
Classification:	Irregular	Hinge Pivot	Condyloid Saddle	Ball-and- socket

(See Appendix B for a more complete chart of diarthrodial joints and their motions.)

II. Synarthrosis (from the Greek, meaning literally "with joint" or, according to our usage, a joint in which there is no separation or articular cavity)

A. Characteristics
  1. In two of the types (cartilaginous and fibrous) the two bones are united by means of an intervening substance, such as cartilage or fibrous tissue, which is continuous with the joint surfaces.
  2. The third type (ligamentous) is not a true joint but is a ligamentous connection between two bones, which may or may not be contiguous.
  3. There is no articular cavity, hence no capsule, synovial membrane, or synovial fluid.

B. Classification
  1. Cartilaginous (synchondrosis; from the Greek, meaning "with cartilage"). Only the joints that are united by fibrocartilage permit motion of a bending and twisting nature. Example of fibrocartilaginous type: articulations between the bodies of the vertebrae (Figure 8–2).* Those united by hyaline cartilage permit only a slight compression. Example of hyaline type: epiphyseal unions.
  2. Fibrous (suture, from the Latin word for "seam"). The edges of bone are united by means of a thin layer of fibrous tissue, which is continuous with the periosteum. No movements are permitted. Only example: the sutures of the skull.
  3. Ligamentous (syndesmosis; from the Greek, meaning "with ligament"). Two bodies, which may be adjacent or may be quite widely separated, are tied together by one or more ligaments. These ligaments may be in the form of cords, bands, or flat sheets. The movement that occurs is usually limited and of no specific type. Examples: coracoacromial union (Figure 4–3); midunion of radius and ulna (Figures 5–2 and 5–3).

C. Summary
  The synarthrodial joints of greatest concern to the kinesiologist are those of the vertebral bodies. Owing to the thickness of the intervertebral disks, these permit a moderate amount of motion simulating that of ball-and-socket joints. The movements are flexion and extension, lateral flexion, circumduction, and rotation.

Suggestions for Studying Joint Structure

In order to understand thoroughly the structure of a joint and especially the relation of structure to function, the student should supplement book study with firsthand study of a skeleton or of the disarticulated bones that enter into the formation of each major joint. Following this preliminary study, the student may find it helpful to "construct"

---

*In some anatomy texts these are classified in a separate major category as amphiarthrodial joints.

a joint by taking the two bones (in some cases, three) and fastening them together with pieces of adhesive or masking tape, carefully placed to represent the specific ligaments of the joint. Pieces of thick felt, cut in the proper shape, may be used to represent the fibrocartilage. This technique is particularly helpful for studying the knee, hip, and shoulder joints.

The movements of each joint should be studied both on the skeleton and on the living subject. When using the latter method, it is important to consider all the joints involved in the movement in question. For instance, in studying the movements of the elbow joint, the articulation between the humerus and radius must not be overlooked. The close relationship that exists between certain joints should be noted as, for example, the relationship between the elbow joint and proximal radioulnar articulation. The tilting of the pelvis that accompanies many movements of the lower extremity and lumbar spine should be recognized, as should the movements of the shoulder girdle that accompany those of the shoulder joint. There is a particular pitfall awaiting those who study the movements of the shoulder joint only by observing the living subject. If not forewarned, students may overlook the part played by the shoulder girdle. Its movements may be detected by palpating the scapula and clavicle in all movements of the upper arm. To follow the movements of the scapula the thumb should be placed at the inferior angle, one finger on the root of the scapular spine and another on the acromion process. Firm contact should be maintained as the scapula moves.

X-ray analysis also affords a valuable tool for studying the structure and function of the joints. Of even greater value would be the x-ray motion picture or possibly the fluoroscope, if readily available for such purposes.

Joint Stability

The function of the joints is obviously to provide the bones with a means of moving or, rather, of being moved. But, because such provisions bring with them a threat of instability, the joints have what might be called a secondary function of providing for stability without interfering with the desired motions.

All the joints of the body do not have the same degree of strength or stability. Some, such as the hip or elbow, are fairly stable. Others, such as the shoulder or knee, are less stable and therefore more easily injured. The strength or degree of freedom of joints follows Emerson's law: "For everything that is given, something is taken." In the shoulder, movement is gained at the expense of stability, while in the hip, movement is sacrificed for stability.

By joint stability we mean resistance to displacement. Steindler uses the term *cohesion* and suggests four factors that are responsible for this stability: the joint ligaments such as the lateral ligaments of hinge joints, muscle tension (see stabilizing components of muscular force), fascia, and atmospheric pressure (Steindler, 1970). The latter is particularly effective at the hip joint. A fifth factor is suggested here—namely, the shape of the bony structure.

SHAPE OF BONY STRUCTURE   This may refer to the kind of joint, such as hinge, condyloid, or ball-and-socket, but it is even more likely to refer to specific characteristics of the particular joint in question. The shoulder and the hip joints, for instance, are both ball-and-socket joints, yet they differ markedly in their stability. The depth of the cuplike acetabulum of the hip joint, in contrast to the small size and shallowness of the glenoid fossa of the shoulder joint, is a case in point. The bony structure of the hip joint obviously gives greater protection against displacement.

LIGAMENTOUS ARRANGEMENT   Ligaments are strong, flexible, stress-resistant, somewhat elastic, fibrous tissues that may be in the form of straplike bands or round cords. They attach the ends of the bones that form a movable joint and help to maintain them in the right relationship to each other. They also check the movement when it reaches its normal limits, and they resist movements for which the joint is not constructed. For instance, the collateral ligaments of the knee help to prevent any tendency there might be for this joint to ab- or adduct. Likewise the ulnar and radial collateral ligaments of the elbow prevent ab- and adduction. The ligaments do not always succeed in preventing abnormal or excessive movements because collisions and violent motions may cause them to be torn. Also, if they are subjected to prolonged periods of stress, they become abnormally stretched. Because they are not very elastic, ligaments take a long time to recover from a stretch. If overstretched, they may never regain their normal length. Ligaments stretched and damaged in joint injuries should be given plenty of time to heal before being subjected to strenuous activity and strain. As long as the ligaments remain undamaged they are an important factor in contributing to joint stability but, once stretched, their usefulness is permanently affected and stability is diminished.

MUSCULAR ARRANGEMENT   The muscles and muscle tendons that span the joint also play a part in the stability of joints, especially in those joints whose bony structure contributes little to stability. The shoulder joint is a notable example, getting its greatest strength from the shoulder and arm muscles which cross it. Of the six muscles that act on the shoulder joint, four of them, known as the rotator cuff (subscapularis, supraspinatus, infraspinatus, and teres minor) are particularly important as stabilizers of this joint. One of their chief functions is protection of the shoulder joint and prevention of displacement of the humeral head. Figure 4–6 shows that all four of these muscles have a strong inward pull on the humeral head toward the glenoid fossa. Likewise, the knee joint is greatly dependent upon the tendons of the quadriceps femoris and hamstring muscles for its strength. A most important defense against joint injury is an increase in the strength of the muscles that support the joint. Chapter 2 discusses in greater detail the role of muscles as stabilizers as opposed to that of movers or neutralizers.

FASCIA AND SKIN   Fascia consists of fibrous connective tissue that forms sheaths for individual muscles, partitions that lie between muscles, and smaller partitions that separate bundles of muscle fibers within a single muscle. According to their location and function they may vary in structure from thin membranes to tough fibrous sheets. In composition they are similar to ligaments in that they are flexible and elastic, within limits, but are susceptible to permanent stretch if subjected to too intense or too prolonged stress. The iliotibial tract of the fascia lata and the thick skin covering the knee joint are examples of fascia and skin serving to help stabilize a joint.

ATMOSPHERIC PRESSURE   The importance of atmospheric pressure as a factor in resisting dislocation of a joint was demonstrated many years ago in a unique experiment. First, all of the muscles and then the ligaments of a hip joint (including the teres femoris ligament) were severed, but surprisingly the head of the femur remained in place. Then a hole was drilled through the acetabulum of another hip joint whose ligaments were intact, and immediately thereafter the femoral head separated from the socket (Steindler, 1970).

Factors Affecting the Range of Motion

The simplest way to limit motion is to put an obstacle in the path of the moving object. An obstacle limiting joint motion may be of soft or rigid tissue or both. Consequently, all joints in the same individual do not have the same amount of movement, and the same joints in different individuals do not have the same amount or range of motion (ROM). The ROM is dependent upon several factors. Three factors that affect the stability of a joint are also related to its range of motion. These are the shape of the articular surfaces, the restraining effect of the ligaments, and the controlling action of the muscles.

Muscles and their tendons are undoubtedly the single most important factor in maintaining both the stability and degree of movement in joints. The tightness of the hamstring tendons (behind the knees) is often felt when someone attempts to touch the floor without bending the knees. Many have also discovered that continued practice will stretch these tendons and improve the joint's range of motion appreciably. It is important to remember that flexibility should not exceed the muscles' ability to maintain the integrity of the joints. Exercising the muscles on all sides of a joint can contribute to both flexibility and strength. The apposition of bulky tissue also affects the degree of movement in a joint. Well-developed musculature or excessive fatty tissue will restrict motion. Bulky arm muscles restrict flexion of the forearm at the elbow, and large deposits of abdominal fat limit trunk flexion. Additional factors in the range of motion include sex, body build (both the mesomorph and the ectomorph usually have greater flexibility than the endomorph), heredity (in addition to the body-build factor), occupation, personal exercise habits, current state of physical fitness, and age.

Methods of Assessing a Joint's Range of Motion

The usual way of assessing a joint's range of motion is to measure the number of degrees from the starting position of the segment to its position at the end of its maximal movement. This is the way to measure flexion; extension is usually measured as the return movement from flexion. If the movement continues beyond the starting position, that constitutes hyperextension. Abduction and adduction are either measured separately from the starting position or, if desired, the total range from maximal abduction to maximal adduction is measured.

There are various ways of measuring ROM, depending upon the joint that is measured. The instrument most commonly used is the double-armed goniometer, with one arm stationary and the other movable (Figure 1–6). The pin or axis of the movable arm is placed directly over the center of the joint at which the motion occurs. The stationary arm is held in line with the stationary segment and the movable arm is either held against the segment as it moves or placed in line with the segment after its limit of motion has been reached. At the completion of the movement, the indicator shows the number of degrees through which the segment has moved. When the

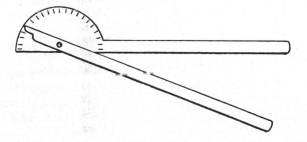

Figure 1–6 Double-armed goniometer.

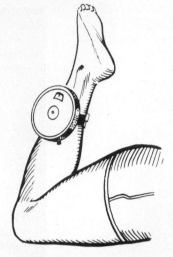

Figure 1–7   Measuring knee flexion with a Leighton flexometer.

anatomical landmarks are well defined, and the examiner has identified the joint center properly, the use of the goniometer may be considered accurate, but when the bony landmarks are not well defined because of excess soft tissue coverage or other causes, or the goniometer axis is not properly placed over the joint axis, the goniometer may provide inaccurate information.

Another instrument frequently used is the Leighton flexometer. This is a highly accurate 360-degree gravity-type goniometer that is strapped to the moving segment (Figure 1–7) (Leighton, 1955). An electronic instrument for the continuous recording

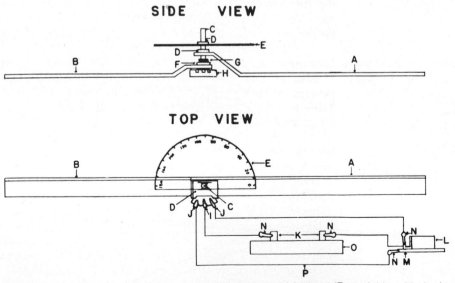

Figure 1–8   Laboratory elgon with protractor, meter, and battery. (From Adrian, M. J.: An introduction to electrogoniometry. In *Kinesiology review 1968*. Washington, D.C.: American Association for Health, Physical Education and Recreation, 1968.)

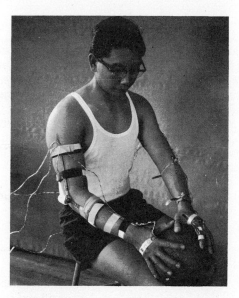

Figure 1–9   Elbow and wrist elgons on right arm; index finger and forearm elgons on left arm. (From Adrian, M. J.: An introduction to electrogoniometry. In *Kinesiology review 1968*. Washington, D.C.: American Association for Health, Physical Education and Recreation, 1968.)

of the movements of body segments, known as an electrogoniometer or "elgon," was developed by Karpovich and his associates (Figures 1–8 and 1–9) (Adrian, 1968). This instrument is most often used in laboratory and research settings.

Measurements of ROM using the double-armed goniometer, flexometer, and elgon are all performed directly on the subject. The fourth method makes use of film. Before filming the subject, joint centers are marked so as to be visible in the picture prints. Joint angles can then be obtained from the film images. The range of motion is the difference between the joint angles of two pictures, one taken at the start of the movement and the other at its completion (Figure 1–10). When this method is used, the segment action must occur in the picture plane (i.e., at a right angle to the camera).

Average Ranges of Joint Motion

Because of the many factors that affect range of motion, patterns vary and it is difficult to establish norms. Where the extremities are concerned, the individual's opposite is perhaps the best norm. Some averages that may be used as a guide are presented in Table 1–3. Illustrations showing joint range of motion for most fundamental movements are found in Appendix C.

Techniques for Increasing Joint Flexibility

Joint flexibility or range of motion is increased through the judicious use of force to stretch the restrictive tissue crossing the joint. The source of this force may be external, such as gravity or another person, or it may be internal muscular force. The stretching is called passive when the force for stretching is externally applied, and active when it is self-administered. When the force is applied so that the body tissues to be stretched are held without movement in a lengthened position, the method is *static stretching*. *Ballistic stretching* occurs when repeated rhythmic movements or body segments produce a rebound stretch of the affected tissues.

Hanging by the hands in order to stretch the pectoral muscles as well as the anterior shoulder joint ligaments and fascia is an example of passive static stretching using gravity as the force. Sitting with the legs extended while grasping the feet or ankles with the hands and repeatedly pulling the head toward the knees in a bobbing fashion is an example of active ballistic stretching of the lower back, posterior hip, and thigh tissues, using momentum and muscular force. Pulling the head toward the knees in one sustained and held pull is an example of active static stretching with muscle as the internal force. These same tissues could also be stretched either ballistically or statically using the force of another person pushing steadily (static) or rhythmically (ballistic) on the subject's back. In both of these instances, the stretching would be passive rather than active.

All the procedures for stretching, active or passive, static or ballistic, are effective in increasing joint range of motion, but *static, active stretching,* in which the agonists are used to stretch antagonists, appears to be the most desirable method. There is less chance of damaging tissues through overstretching, there is less muscle soreness (de Vries, 1962) and less energy consumed, and, because of the use of reciprocal innervation, there is less antagonistic muscle activity to impede optimal stretching (Jacobs, 1976).

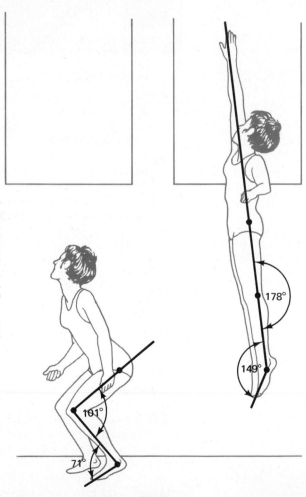

Figure 1–10 The range of motion at a joint can be determined using film tracings of the joint action. The angles at the knee and ankle joints were measured at the point of greatest flexion (*A*) and at the peak of the jump (*B*). The difference between the two measures (*B* minus *A*) is the range of motion (ROM) for the given joint. The ROM at the knee joint was 177° and at the ankle joint was 78°.

A

B

TABLE 1–3 Average Ranges of Joint Motion*

JOINT	SOURCES				AVERAGES
	1	2	3	4	
Elbow					
Flexion	150	135	150	150	146
Hyperextension	0	0	0	0	0
Forearm					
Pronation	80	75	50	80	71
Supination	80	85	90	80	84
Wrist					
Extension	60	65	90	70	71
Flexion	70	70		80	73
Radial flexion	20	20	30	30	33
Ulnar flexion	30	4	15	20	19
Shoulder					
Flexion	150	170	130	180	158
Hyperextension	40	30	80	60	53
Abduction	150	170	180	180	170
Horizontal flexion				135	135
Horizontal extension	40	30	80	60	53
Shoulder					
Rotation (arm in abduction)					
Inward				70	70
Outward				90	90
Hip					
Flexion	100	110	120	120	113
Hyperextension	30	30	20	30	28
Abduction	40	50	55	45	48
Rotation (in extension)					
Inward	40	35	20	45	35
Outward	50	50	45	45	48
Knee					
Flexion	120	135	145	135	134
Ankle					
Plantar flexion	40	50	50	50	48
Dorsiflexion	20	15	15	20	18
Spine (thoracic and lumbar)					
Flexion	90			80 (4″)	85 (4″)
Hyperextension	30			20–30	30
Lateral flexion	20			35	28
Rotation	30			45	38

Sources: 1. Committee on Medical Rating of Physical Impairment, AMA.
2. Committee of California Medical Association and Industrial Accident Commission of State of California.
3. William A. Clarke, Mayo Clinic.
4. Committee on Joint Motion, American Academy of Orthopaedic Surgeons.

*Adapted from table presented in *Joint motion: Method of measuring and recording,* a manual published by the American Academy of Orthopaedic Surgeons (1965).

Movements of the Skeletal Units

In preparation for defining the fundamental movements of the major segments of the body and for the analysis of these movements, certain orientation concepts and points of reference need to be established. The essential ones are the center of gravity, the line of gravity, the orientation planes of the body and axes of motion, and the standard starting positions from which the fundamental movements are made.

The Center of Gravity

The center of gravity is defined as "an imaginary point representing the weight center of an object"; it is also "that point in a body about which all the parts exactly balance each other," and can be viewed as "the point at which the entire weight of the body may be considered as concentrated." In a perfect sphere or cube the weight center coincides with the geometric center. Its precise location in the human body depends upon the individual's anatomical structure, habitual standing posture, current position, and whether external weights are being supported. In a person of average build standing erect with the arms hanging at the sides, the center of gravity is located in the pelvis in front of the upper part of the sacrum. It is usually lower in women than in men because of their heavier pelves and thighs and shorter legs. (See Chapter 13 for a more detailed discussion of the center of gravity and related concepts.)

The Line of Gravity

The line of gravity is an imaginary vertical line that, by definition, passes through the center of gravity. Hence, its location depends upon the position of the center of gravity, which changes with every shift of the body's position.

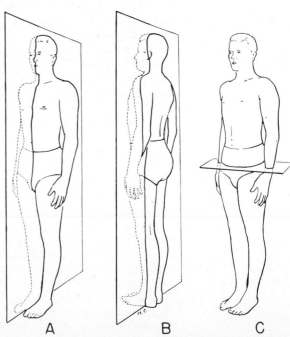

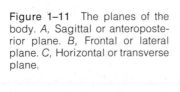

Figure 1–11 The planes of the body. *A,* Sagittal or anteroposterior plane. *B,* Frontal or lateral plane. *C,* Horizontal or transverse plane.

Orientation Planes of the Body and Axes of Motion

There are three traditional planes corresponding to the three dimensions of space. Each plane is perpendicular to each of the other two. There are likewise three axes of motion, each perpendicular to the plane in which the motion occurs. The planes and axes of the body are defined as follows (Figure 1–11A, B, and C):

Planes
1. The sagittal, anteroposterior, or median plane is a vertical plane passing through the body from front to back, dividing it into right and left halves.
2. The frontal, lateral, or coronal plane is a vertical plane passing through the body from side to side, dividing it into anterior and posterior halves.
3. The transverse or horizontal plane is a horizontal plane which passes through the body, dividing it into upper and lower halves.

Since each plane bisects the body, it follows that each plane must pass through the center of gravity. Hence the center of gravity may be defined as the point at which the three planes of the body intersect one another, and the line of gravity as the vertical line at which the two vertical planes intersect each other. When describing a movement in terms of a plane, such as "a movement of the forearm in the sagittal plane," we mean that the movement occurs in a plane parallel to the sagittal plane. It does not necessarily imply that the movement occurs in a plane passing through the center of gravity. If the latter is intended, the term "cardinal plane" is used. Thus nodding the head is a movement occurring in the cardinal sagittal plane.

Axes
1. The frontal-horizontal (lateral) axis passes horizontally from side to side.
2. The sagittal-horizontal (anteroposterior) axis passes horizontally from front to back.
3. The vertical axis is perpendicular to the ground.

A rotary (axial, angular) movement of a segment of the body occurs *in* a plane and *around* an axis. The axis around which the movement takes place is always at right angles to the plane in which it occurs. Forward lifting of the leg (flexion) occurs in the sagittal plane about a frontal-horizontal axis, sideward raising of the arm (abduction) occurs in the frontal plane about a sagittal-horizontal axis, and turning the head to the side (lateral rotation) is movement in the transverse plane about a vertical axis.

Nonaxial Movements

Movements permitted at any diarthrodial joint except the arthrodial or plane joint are rotary movements and occur in a plane about an axis. Movements in plane joints are nonaxial. An example is the gliding movement that occurs between the articular facets of the spinal column. Nonaxial movements may also occur when body segments are moved as the result of rotatory action of adjacent segments. In a pushing action the hand moves linearly forward in the sagittal plane because of the axial movements of arm segments at the shoulder, elbow, and wrist joints. Similarly, in a deep knee bend, the trunk and head move linearly because of the rotatory actions of the leg segments.

Standard Starting Positions

FUNDAMENTAL STANDING POSITION In this position the individual stands erect with the feet slightly separated and parallel, the arms hanging easily at the sides with palms facing the body (Figure 1–12A). This is the position usually accepted as the point of reference for analyzing all the movements of the body's segments, *except those of the forearm.*

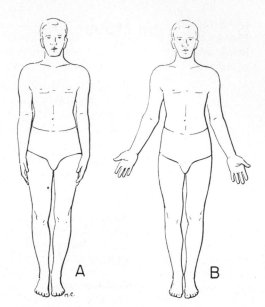

Figure 1–12 Standing positions. *A*, Fundamental standing position. *B*, Anatomical standing position.

ANATOMICAL STANDING POSITION   This is the position usually depicted in anatomy textbooks. The individual is erect with the elbows fully extended and the palms facing forward. The legs and feet are the same as for the fundamental standing position (Figure 1–12B). It is usually accepted as the point of reference for the movements of the forearm, hand, and fingers.

Figure 1–13 Movements of the body in three planes. *A*, Movement of the forearm in the sagittal plane around a frontal-horizontal axis. *B*, Movement of the trunk in the frontal plane around a sagittal-horizontal axis. *C*, Movement of the head in the horizontal plane around a vertical axis.

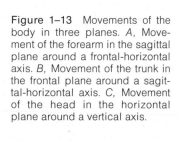
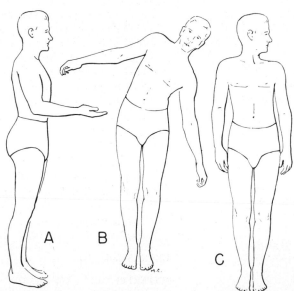

Fundamental Movements of the Major Segments of the Body

Being a multijointed structure, the human body consists of many movable segments. When we watch a skillful acrobat, dancer, or basketball player, it might seem like a hopeless task to try to organize their movements into a meaningful classification. The task is greatly simplified, however, when we consider one segment at a time and visualize each movement as though it were performed from the anatomical standing position. This may take a bit of imagination, but knowing ahead of time the movements of which each joint in the body is capable is nine-tenths of the battle. These are described in Chapters 4 through 9 in the systematic discussions of the regions of the body. The information given below is basic to understanding the movements of specific joints and segments. *Note:* The anatomical standing position is the point of reference for these movements.

Movements in the Sagittal Plane About a Frontal-Horizontal Lateral Axis (Figure 1–13A)

Viewed from the side.

FLEXION   The angle at the joint diminishes.
Examples:

1. The forward and backward tipping of the head.
2. Lifting the foot and leg backward from the knee.
3. Raising the entire lower extremity forward-upward as though kicking.
4. With the upper arm remaining at the side, raising the forearm straight forward (Figure 1–13A).
5. With the elbow straight, raising the entire upper extremity forward-upward. The "diminishing angle" is hard to see in this movement until one views the raising of the arm from the shoulder in the same way that the raising of the thigh from the hip joint is viewed. In the latter, one automatically notices the angle that appears between the top of the thigh (i.e., the anterior surface) and the trunk, or the part of the body that lies above the hip joint. Similarly, when raising the arm, the angle to look for is the angle between the top of the arm and the neck-head segment, not the angle between the underside of the raised arm and the trunk. It is necessary to train oneself to view the sagittal plane movements of the arm at the shoulder as being similar to those of the thigh at the hip joint.

    For general purposes the upper arm may be considered fully flexed when it has reached the overhead vertical position. Later, when the role of the shoulder girdle in arm movements has been studied, it will be seen that the elevation of the arm does not take place solely at the shoulder joint. The movements of the scapula and clavicle are an important part of the total arm movement. Strictly speaking, the shoulder joint is in a fully flexed position when the humerus is raised until it is parallel with the long axis of the scapula (i.e., when it is in the same plane as the scapula). For the present, however, the upper arm will be considered fully flexed when it has been raised forward-upward until it has reached the vertical position and hyperflexed when it passes beyond this.

EXTENSION   The return movement from flexion.

HYPERFLEXION   This term refers only to the movement of the upper arm. When the arm is flexed beyond the vertical, it is considered to be hyperflexed. In other joints of the body flexion is terminated by contact of the moving segment with another part of the body—e.g., the forearm against the upper arm, the lower leg against the thigh, or by structural limitations of the joints themselves (e.g., flexion of the thoracic and lumbar spine).

HYPEREXTENSION   The continuation of extension beyond the starting position or beyond the straight line.

Examples:

1.   Hyperextension of the upper arm is said to occur when the arm is extended backward beyond the body.
2.   The forearm is considered to be hyperextended when the angle at the elbow joint has exceeded 180 degrees.

REDUCTION OF HYPEREXTENSION   Return movement from hyperextension. This could also be called flexion to the starting position—i.e., the fundamental or the anatomical starting position, as the case may be.

Movements in the Frontal Plane About a Sagittal-Horizontal (Antero-posterior) Axis (Figure 1–13B)

Viewed from the front or back.

ABDUCTION   Sideward movement away from the midline or sagittal plane or, in the case of the fingers, away from the midline of the hand. This term is used most commonly for sideward movements of the upper arm away from the trunk—in other words, sideward elevation of the arm—and for sideward elevation of the lower extremity. The jumping-jack exercise involves both of these.

ADDUCTION   The return movement from abduction.

LATERAL FLEXION   This refers to the lateral bending of the head or trunk. It may also be used for sideward movements of the middle finger, but the more specific terms, radial or ulnar flexion, are usually used for these.

HYPERABDUCTION   Like hyperflexion, this term usually refers to the upper arm when the latter is abducted beyond the vertical, as seen from the front or back.

HYPERADDUCTION   The trunk blocks hyperadduction of the upper extremity and the presence of the supporting lower extremity blocks hyperadduction of the other lower extremity. By combining slight flexion with hyperadduction, the upper extremities can move across the front of the body, and one lower extremity can move across in front of the supporting one.

REDUCTION OF HYPERADDUCTION   The return movement from hyperadduction.

REDUCTION OF LATERAL FLEXION   The return movement from lateral flexion.

Movements in the Transverse Plane About a Vertical Axis (Figure 1–13C)

Viewed or visualized from overhead or from directly beneath—e.g., through a glass platform. The point of reference for all rotations of the upper extremities is the midposition as in the fundamental (not anatomical) standing position.

ROTATION LEFT AND RIGHT   Applies to rotation of the head or neck in such a way that the anterior aspect turns respectively to the left or right.

OUTWARD (LATERAL) AND INWARD (MEDIAL) ROTATION   Applies to rotation of the thigh, the upper arm, or the upper or lower extremity as a whole in such a way that the anterior aspect of the segment turns laterally or medially.

SUPINATION AND PRONATION   Apply respectively to outward (lateral) and inward (medial) rotation of the forearm.

REDUCTION OF OUTWARD ROTATION, INWARD ROTATION, SUPINATION, OR PRONA-TION   Rotation of the segment back to the midposition.

Movements in an Oblique Plane About an Oblique Axis

Many movements take place in planes between the sagittal and frontal planes, the sagittal and transverse planes, and the frontal and transverse planes. These are oblique (diagonal) planes, and the axes about which the movements occur are oblique (diagonal) axes. Whatever the degree of obliquity of the plane, the axis for a movement in that plane is always perpendicular to it. Although it is possible to define the obliquity precisely in terms of the number of degrees that it deviates from the fundamental planes, descriptive terms are adequate for general purposes (Logan and McKinney, 1970).

A familiar example of an oblique plane movement is raising the arm between the straight forward and straight sideward directions. A golf swing and a tennis serve are also examples of arm movements that take place in oblique planes. Lower extremity examples include the breast-stroke kick in swimming and a deep knee bend performed with the heels together and the knees separated.

CIRCUMDUCTION   An orderly sequence of the movements that occur in the sagittal, frontal, and intermediate oblique planes so that the segment as a whole describes a cone is known as *circumduction*. It consists of an axial movement that may occur in any plane. The movement may occur at biaxial or triaxial joints. Arm circling and trunk circling are also examples of circumduction.

Laboratory Experiences

1. By studying a skeleton and observing a living subject, classify the following joints without referring to a textbook: hip, elbow, knee, ankle, wrist, radioulnar, metacarpophalangeal joint of finger, shoulder joint. (Do not confuse the motion at the elbow or wrist joints with that of the radioulnar joints.)

2. Take turns with a partner performing simple movements of the head, trunk, upper extremity, and lower extremity and identify the planes and axes concerned.

3. Construct a simple device to illustrate the planes and axes in relation to the human body.

4. Study the tracing of the soccer throw-in (Figure 5–2 in Appendix I). The action between A and B represents the "force phase" and between B and C the "follow-through phase." Following the example given for the right metatarsophalangeal joint, complete the table on the next page for the "force phase." Repeat for the "follow-through."

5. Measure the joint ranges of motion on 10 to 15 subjects for the movements indicated, using either a goniometer or flexometer. Compare the results obtained with the averages given in Table 1–3. Explain why you think the differences among individuals exist. (The figure numbers refer to Appendix C.)

    a. Elbow flexion and hyperextension (Figure C–1)

    b. Shoulder flexion and hyperextension (Figure C–4B).

    c. Shoulder rotation (Figure C–5).

    d. Lateral flexion of trunk (Figure C–11B).

    e. Hip flexion (Figure C–7).

    f. Medial and lateral hip rotation (Figure C–8B).

    g. Plantar flexion and dorsiflexion (Figure C–10).

Name of Joint	Type of Joint	Starting Position	Observed Joint Action	Plane of Motion	Axis of Motion
R. metatarso-phalangeal	ellipsoid	sl. hyper-extension	hyper-extension	sagittal	frontal horizontal
R. ankle					
R. knee					
R. hip					
Lumbar spine					
R. shoulder					
R. elbow					
R. wrist					
R. fingers					

6. Select one or two joint actions (e.g., shoulder flexion and hip flexion). Perform a comparison study of the range of motion for the actions selected using two groups of people, such as:
   a. Males vs. females.
   b. Varsity athletes from different sports (swimming vs. basketball or wrestling vs. gymnastics).
   c. Different age groups (20–30 vs. 50–60).
   d. Joggers vs. sedentary people.
   Subjects in each group should be matched on the basis of age and sex. Are there any "group" differences apparent? Explain your results.

7. Measure the degree of motion in one ankle. Tape the ankle and repeat the measurements immediately and then following 10 to 15 minutes of exercise during which the ankle is used (e.g., jogging, basketball, handball). Record your results and compare the differences. What effect, if any, did the tape have on range of motion for plantar and dorsiflexion? inversion and eversion? Using the results of your measurements as the basis, discuss the value of taping as a means of preventing ankle injuries.

8. Measure the ranges of motion at the hip and knee joints during the back somersault depicted in Figure 5–6 in Appendix I.
   a. On each tracing, mark the location of the right hip, knee, and ankle joints with a dot. Also place a dot at the midpoint of the waist. Connect the dots with straight lines so as to make a stick figure of the leg.
   b. Using a protractor, measure and record the angles between the trunk and thigh, and the thigh and lower leg, on each tracing.
   c. Determine the range of motion for each joint action from start to end of takeoff (A to C) and from peak to touchdown (B to E).
   d. What effect does range of motion in these joints have on skillful performance of this technique? As a coach or trainer, what specific training techniques would you include in the program of the performer to improve the range of motion where needed?

References

Adrian, M. J. 1968. An introduction to electrogoniometry. In *Kinesiology review 1968,* pp. 12–17. Washington, D.C.: American Association of Health, Physical Education and Recreation.

American Academy of Orthopaedic Surgeons. 1965. *Joint motion: Method of measuring and recording.* Chicago: The Academy.

deVries, H. A. 1962. Evaluation of static stretching procedures for improvement of flexibility. *Res. Q. Am. Assoc. Health Phys. Educ.* 33:223–29.

Goss, C. M., ed. 1973. *Gray's anatomy of the human body.* 29th ed. Philadelphia: Lea & Febiger.

Harris, M. L. 1969. Flexibility (review of the literature). *J. Am. Physiol. Assoc.* 49:591–601.

Holland, G. J. 1968. The physiology of flexibility; a review of the literature. In *Kinesiology Review 1968*, pp. 49–62. Washington, D.C.: American Association of Health, Physical Education and Recreation.

Jacobs, M. 1976. Neurophysiological implications of slow active stretching. *Am. Correct. Ther. J.* 30:151–54.

Kraus, H., and Eisenmenger-Weber, S. 1945. Evaluation of posture based on structural and functional measurements. *Physiother. Rev.* 25:267–71.

Larson, R. L., and McMahan, R. D. 1966. The epiphyses and the childhood athlete. J.A.M.A. 196:607.

Leighton, J. R. 1955. An instrument and technic for the measurement of range of joint motion. *Arch. Phys. Med. Rehabil.* 36:571–78.

Logan, G. A., and McKinney, W. C. 1970. *Kinesiology.* Dubuque, Iowa: William C. Brown.

Lowman, C. L. 1947. The vulnerable age. *J. Health Phys. Educ.* 18:635–36, 693.

Schaeffer, J. P., ed. 1953. *Morris' human anatomy.* 11th ed. New York: McGraw Hill.

Sobotta, J. 1967. *Atlas of human anatomy.* Translated by E. Uhlenhuth. New York: Hafner Publishing.

Steindler, A. 1970. *Kinesiology of the human body.* Springfield, Ill.: Charles C Thomas.

The Musculoskeletal System
II. The Musculature

Objectives

At the conclusion of this chapter, the student should be able to:

1. Describe the structure and properties of the whole muscle, red and white muscle fiber, and the myofibril.
2. Explain how the relationship of the muscle's line of pull to the joint axis affects the movement produced by the muscle.
3. Describe the relationship between the skeletal muscle's fiber arrangement and its function.
4. Define the roles a muscle may play (agonist, antagonist, stabilizer, and neutralizer), and explain the cooperative action of muscles in controlling joint actions by naming and explaining the muscle roles in a specified movement.
5. Define the types of muscular contraction (concentric, eccentric, and static), and name and demonstrate each type of action.
6. Demonstrate an understanding of the influence of gravity and other external forces on muscular action by correctly analyzing several movement patterns in which these forces influence the muscular action.
7. Describe the various methods of studying muscle action, citing the advantages and disadvantages of each method.
8. State the force-velocity and length-tension relationships of muscular contraction, and explain the significance of these relationships in static and dynamic movements.

Body parts are moved by external or internal forces. The internal force responsible for the movement and positioning of the bony segments of the body is the action of skeletal muscles. These muscles are able to serve this function because they can contract, they are attached to the body segments, and they cross a joint. In addition, they are constructed of bundles of striated muscle fibers, which differ in both structure and function from the highly specialized cardiac muscle and from the smooth muscle of blood vessels, digestive organs, and urogenital organs.

Skeletal Muscle Structure

Properties of Muscular Tissue

The properties of striated muscle tissue are extensibility, elasticity, and contractility. The first two enable a muscle to be stretched like an elastic band and, when the stretching force is discontinued, to return again to its normal resting length. Tendons, which are simply continuations of the muscle's connective tissue, also possess these properties. The unique property of contractility is possessed by muscle tissue alone. Experiments have shown that the average muscle fiber can shorten to approximately one-half its resting length (Arkin, 1941; Steindler, 1970). It can also be stretched until it is approximately one-half again as long as its resting length. The range between the maximal and minimal lengths of a muscle fiber is known as the amplitude of its action. The elongation varies proportionately with the length of the fiber and inversely with its cross section.

The Muscle Fiber

A single muscle cell is a threadlike fiber about one to three inches in length. Microscopic examination has revealed that the fiber consists of many myofibrils embedded in sarcoplasm, held together by a delicate membrane known as sarcolemma (Figure 2–1). Each fiber is enclosed within a thin connective tissue sheath called *endomysium*. The microscopic myofibrils, which are the contractile elements, are arranged in parallel formation within the fiber, and are made up of alternating dark and light bands which give the muscle fibers their striated appearance. The electron microscope has revealed the striations to be a repeating pattern of bands and lines due to an interdigitating arrangement of two sets of filaments. It has been postulated that these are filaments of the contractile proteins, mainly actin and myosin and that, when stimulated, they slide past each other (Edington and Edgerton, 1976). The myofibril is divided into a series of several *sarcomeres*, with each sarcomere consisting of the portion of the myofibril between two Z lines (Figure 2–2). The sarcomere is considered to be the functional contractile unit of skeletal muscle. This explanation is a condensed and highly simplified one of contraction, a function that is the unique property of muscle tissue.

The muscle fibers are bound into bundles within bundles (Figure 2–1). Each individual bundle of muscle fibers is enclosed in a fibrous tissue sheath called *perimysium;* the group of bundles that constitutes a complete muscle is in turn encased within a tougher connective tissue sheath called *epimysium.* In long muscles whose fibers run parallel to the long axis of the muscle, the bundles form "chains," which function as though the individual fibers ran the entire length of the muscle.

Slow and Fast Twitch Fibers

There are at least two types of skeletal muscle fibers in humans, the fast twitch and the slow twitch. Most muscles contain some of each, but the proportions vary among both muscles and individuals. Fast twitch fibers are large and pale, while slow twitch

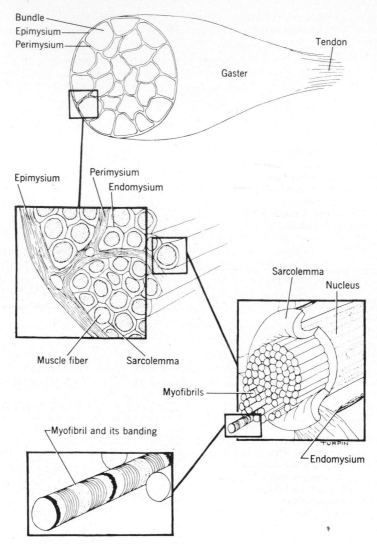

Figure 2–1   The architecture of a skeletal muscle and its fibers. (From Torrey, T. W.: *Morphogenesis of the vertebrates.* New York: John Wiley & Sons, 1962.)

fibers are small and red. The red color of slow twitch fibers is due to their rich supply of myoglobin (hemoglobin). They tend to be more plentiful in the muscles that are responsible for low-tension activities, such as the leg muscles of endurance runners or cyclists, and also in muscles, such as the diaphragm, that participate in regularly repeated contractions. They are slow-fatiguing fibers and are thus important in any activity requiring endurance. Fast twitch (white) fibers, on the other hand, tend to predominate in muscles used for heavy-strength activities. They are fast-contracting, powerful, fast-fatiguing fibers, more evident in the muscles of athletes who engage in high-power, short-endurance events (Edington and Edgerton, 1976; Hill, 1970).

A. Magnification of single muscle fiber showing smaller fibers—myofibrils—in its sarcoplasm.

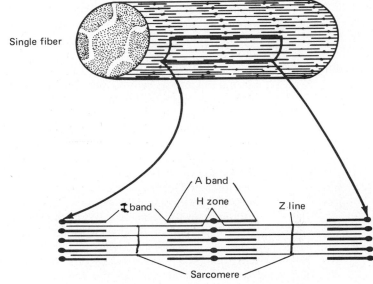

Single fiber

B. Myofibril magnified further to show thick and thin filaments composing it and producing its cross-striated appearance; dark A (anisotropic) bands alternate with light 1 (isotropic) bands; H zones, less dense midsections of A bands; Z lines, more dense midlines of I bands.

C. Molecular structure of myofibril; thick filaments, myosin molecules; thin filaments, actin molecules.

D. Scheme to show how myosin interacts with actin to shorten muscle fibers. The cross bridges of a single myosin fiber are believed to point at 60-degree angles at six actin filaments. The cross bridges bond to the actin filaments and slide them toward the center of the sarcomere.

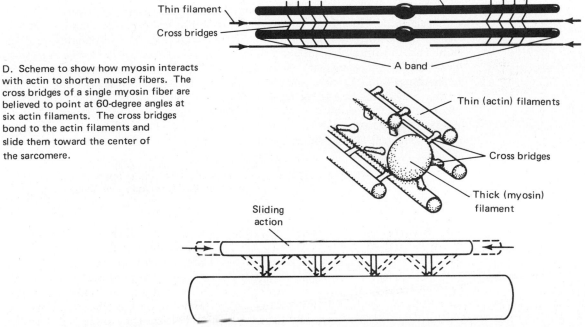

Figure 2–2   The single muscle fiber and its myofibrils. (Adapted from Anthony, C. P., and Thibodeau, G. A.: *Textbook of anatomy and physiology.* St. Louis: C. V. Mosby, 1979.)

Whether training or heredity is responsible for the differences in proportion of slow and fast twitch muscle fibers has not been well established at this time. A world-class marathon runner may be such because of being blessed genetically with a large proportion of fast twitch fibers. On the other hand, the runner's success may be due to a training regimen that either capitalized on the runner's innate characteristics or actually caused a modification in the proportion of red and white fibers.

Muscular Attachments

Muscles are attached to bone by means of their connective tissue, which continues beyond the muscle belly in the form either of a tendon (a round cord or a flat band) or of an aponeurosis (a fibrous sheet). It is customary for anatomy texts to designate the attachments of the two ends of a muscle as "origin" and "insertion." The origin is usually characterized by stability and closeness of the muscle fibers to the bone. It is usually the more proximal of the two attachments. The insertion, on the other hand, is usually the distal attachment; it frequently involves a relatively long tendon, and the bone into which the muscle's tendon inserts is ordinarily the one that moves. It should be understood, however, that the muscle does not pull in one direction or the other. When it contracts it exerts equal force on the two attachments and attempts to pull them toward each other. Which bone is to remain stationary and which one is to move depends upon the purpose of the movement. A muscle spanning the inside of a hinge joint, for instance, tends to draw the two bones toward one another. However, most precision movements require that the proximal bone be stabilized while the distal bone performs the movement. The stabilization of the proximal bone is achieved by the action of other muscles. Sometimes the greater weight or the more limited mobility of the proximal structure is sufficient to stabilize it against the pull of the contracting muscles.

Students often receive the impression that there is some physiological reason for a muscle to pull in a single direction. They fail to grasp the concept of a muscle merely contracting, and do not realize that it cannot pull in a predetermined direction. This misconception makes it difficult for them to understand seeming exceptions. Actually there are many movements in which the insertion or distal attachment of the muscle is stationary and the origin or proximal attachment is the one that moves. Such is the case in the familiar act of chinning oneself. The movement of the elbow joint is flexion, but it is the upper arm that moves toward the forearm, just the reverse of what happens when one lifts a book from the table. The grasp of the hands on the bar serves to immobilize the forearm and thus it provides a stable base for the

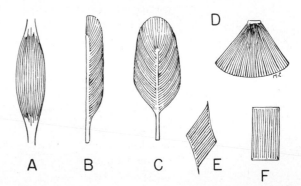

Figure 2–3 Examples of muscles of different shapes and internal structure. *A*, Fusiform or spindle. *B*, Penniform. *C*, Bipenniform. *D*, Triangular or fanshaped. *E*, Rhomboidal. *F*, Rectangular.

contracting muscles. In order to avoid the erroneous idea of a muscle always pulling from its insertion toward its origin the following terminology for muscular attachments is used in this text.

TERMINOLOGY FOR MUSCULAR ATTACHMENTS

Attachments of muscles of the extremities:
Proximal attachment.
Distal attachment.

Attachments of muscles of the head, neck, and trunk:
Upper attachment
} for muscles whose line of pull is more or less vertical—that is, parallel with the long axis of the body.
Lower attachment
Medial attachment
} for muscles whose line of pull is more or less horizontal.
Lateral attachment

Attachments of the diaphragm:
Peripheral attachment.
Central attachment.

Structural Classification of Muscles on the Basis of Fiber Arrangement

The arrangement of the fibers and the method of attachment vary considerably among the different muscles. These structural variations form the basis for a classification of the skeletal muscles.

LONGITUDINAL   This is a long straplike muscle whose fibers lie parallel to its long axis. Two examples are the rectus abdominis on the front of the abdomen, and the sartorius, which slants across the front of the thigh.

QUADRATE OR QUADRILATERAL (Figure 2–3E and F)   Muscles of this type are four-sided and are usually flat. They consist of parallel fibers. Examples include the pronator quadratus on the front of the wrist and the rhomboid muscle between the spine and the scapula.

TRIANGULAR OR FAN-SHAPED (Figure 2–3D)   This is a relatively flat type of muscle whose fibers radiate from a narrow attachment at one end to a broad attachment at the other. The pectoralis major on the front of the chest is an excellent example.

FUSIFORM OR SPINDLE-SHAPED (Figure 2–3A)   This is usually a rounded muscle which tapers at either end. It may be long or short, large or small. Good examples are the brachialis and the brachioradialis muscles of the upper extremity.

UNIPENNIFORM (Figure 2–3B)   In this type of muscle a series of short, parallel, featherlike fibers extends diagonally from the side of a long tendon, giving the muscle as a whole the appearance of a wing feather. Examples: extensor digitorum longus and tibialis posterior muscles of the leg.

BIPENNIFORM (Figure 2–3C)   This is a double penniform muscle. It is characterized by a long central tendon with the fibers extending diagonally in pairs from either side of the tendon. It resembles a symmetrical tail feather. Examples: flexor hallucis longus and rectus femoris of the leg and thigh, respectively.

MULTIPENNIFORM   In this type of muscle there are several tendons present, with the muscle fibers running diagonally between them. The middle portion of the deltoid muscle of the shoulder and upper arm is a prime example of a multipenniform muscle (see Figures 4–5 and 4–8).

Effect of Muscle Structure on Force and Range of Motion

The force a muscle can exert is proportional to its physiological cross section, a measure that accounts for the diameter of every fiber and whose size depends upon the number and thickness of the fibers. A broad, thick, longitudinal muscle will exert more force than a thin one, but a pennate muscle of the same thickness as a longitudinal muscle is capable of exerting greater force. The oblique arrangement of the fibers in the various classifications of penniform muscle allows for a larger number of fibers and thus a larger physiological cross section than in comparable sizes of the other classifications (see pp. 309–310 and Figure 11–1). Pennate muscles are the most common type of skeletal muscle and predominate when forceful movements are needed.

The range through which a muscle shortens depends upon the length of its fibers, with the average muscle fiber capable of shortening to one-half its resting length. Those long muscles with fibers longitudinally arranged along the long axis of the msucle, such as the sartorius, can exert force over a longer distance than muscles with shorter fibers. Muscles of the pennate type, with their oblique fiber arrangement and short fiber length, can exert their superior force through only a short range.

Skeletal Muscle Function

The basis for all muscle function is the ability of muscular tissue to contract. This should be kept in mind as various aspects of muscular function are considered.

Relation of the Muscle's Line of Pull to the Joint Structure

The movement that the contracting muscle produces—flexion, extension, abduction, adduction, or rotation—is determined by two factors: the type of joint that it spans and the relation of the muscle's line of pull to the joint. For instance, the contraction of a muscle whose line of pull is directly anterior to the knee joint may cause the joint to extend, whereas a muscle whose line of pull is anterior to the elbow joint may cause this joint to flex. The possible axes of motion are of course determined by the structure of the joint itself. It will be recalled that hinge joints have only a frontal horizontal axis and condyloid (ovoid) joints both a frontal horizontal and a sagittal horizontal axis; ball-and-socket joints have three axes, frontal and sagittal horizontal and vertical, while pivot joints have a vertical axis only. A muscle whose line of pull is lateral to the hip joint is a potential abductor of the thigh, but muscles whose lines of pull are lateral to the elbow joint cannot cause abduction of the forearm because the construction of the elbow joint is such that no provision is made for ab- or adduction. Because it is a hinge joint its only axis of motion is a frontal horizontal one, and the only movements possible are flexion and extension.

The importance of the relation of a muscle's action line to the joint's axis of motion is especially seen in some of the muscles that act on triaxial joints. Occasionally it happens that a muscle's line of pull for one of its secondary movements shifts from one side of the joint's center of motion to the other during the course of the movement. For instance, the clavicular portion of the pectoralis major is primarily a

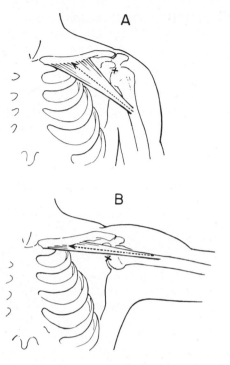

Figure 2–4 The clavicular portion of the pectoralis major muscle reversing its customary function. *A*, The line of pull is below the center of the shoulder joint. *B*, The line of pull is above the center of the shoulder joint.

flexor, but it also adducts the humerus. When the arm is elevated sideward to a position slightly above shoulder level, however, the line of pull of some of the fibers of the clavicular portion shifts from below to above the sagittal horizontal axis of the shoulder joint (Figure 2–4). Contraction of these fibers in this position contributes to abduction of the humerus, rather than to adduction. Similarly, several muscles or parts of muscles of the hip joint appear to reverse their customary function. Steindler (1970) has pointed out that as the adductor longus adducts the hip joint it also flexes it until the flexion exceeds 70 degrees. Beyond this point the adductor longus helps to extend the hip.

Table 2–1 presents muscle classification based on joint structure. It is not uncommon to classify and name muscles according to the relation of their line of pull to the joint structure. In other words, muscles whose line of pull is such that, when they shorten, the resultant joint action is flexion, are called flexors, and those in a position to cause extension are extensors. Similarly there would also be abductors, adductors, and rotators. The difficulty with this type of classification is that it may mislead the student into believing that the muscle is responsible for the related joint action under all circumstances when in reality this is not the case. The biceps brachii muscle, for instance, is usually listed as a flexor and supinator of the forearm, when in fact the results of electromyographic studies have established that the biceps plays little if any part in flexion of the prone forearm or supination of the extended forearm unless the movements are resisted (Basmajian, 1979). This example is not unusual. There are many situations in which the presence or absence of resistance governs a muscle's participation in a joint action. Other factors, such as the starting position for the joint action, the direction of the movement, and the speed of the movement may also alter a

TABLE 2–1 Muscle Classification Based on Joint Structure

DIARTHRODIAL AXIAL JOINTS	MUSCLES
Uniaxial	
Hinge	Flexors and extensors.
Pivot	Rotators.
Biaxial	
Condyloid (ovoid)	Flexors; extensors; abductors; adductors.
Saddle	Same as for condyloid joints.
Triaxial*	
Ball-and-socket	Flexors; extensors; abductors; adductors; rotators.

*Although the joints between the bodies of the vertebrae are cartilaginous synarthrodial joints and those between the articular processes of the vertebrae are nonaxial diarthrodial joints, the movements of the spinal column resemble those of triaxial joints. This is because of the ball-and-socket nature of the nucleus pulposus in the intervertebral disks.

muscle's involvement in the joint action. Therefore charts that classify muscles according to general function based on location should be used with the realization that there may be many exceptions to or conditions for a named muscle action. Knowing the general location of a muscle with respect to the joint axis—anterior, superior, lateral, or medial—and knowing the line of pull of the muscle is important information for deducing *possible* muscle participation during a body movement, but confirmation of those muscle actions must rely on the evidence of electromyography.

Types of Contraction

Because the word *contract* literally means to "draw together" or to shorten, the nature of muscular contraction may cause some initial confusion. A muscle contraction occurs whenever the muscle fibers generate tension in themselves, a situation that may exist when the muscle is actually *shortening, remaining the same length, or lengthening.*

CONCENTRIC OR SHORTENING CONTRACTION *Concentric* (toward the middle) contraction occurs when the tension generated by the muscle is sufficient to overcome a resistance and to move the body segment of one attachment toward the segment of its other attachment. As the arm is raised sideward the abductor shoulder muscles shorten to overcome the resistance of the arm. The muscle actually shortens and, when one end is stabilized, the other pulls the bone to which it is attached and turns it about the joint axis.

ECCENTRIC OR LENGTHENING CONTRACTION When a muscle slowly lengthens as it gives in to an external force which is greater than the contractile force it is exerting, it is in *eccentric* (away from the middle) contraction. The term "lengthening" is misleading, since in most instances the muscle does not actually lengthen. It merely returns from its shortened condition to its normal resting length (Figure 2–5A). The abductor shoulder muscles are in eccentric contraction when the arm is slowly lowered from an abducted position. In most instances in which muscles contract eccentrically the muscles are acting as a "brake" or resistive force against the moving force of gravity or other external forces. When the muscles contract in this manner they are said to perform negative work.

ISOMETRIC OR STATIC CONTRACTION   Isometric means "equal length." Tension of the muscle in partial or complete contraction without any appreciable change in length is *isometric* contraction. There are two different conditions under which this type of contraction is likely to occur.

1.   Muscles that are antagonistic to each other contract with equal strength, thus balancing or counteracting each other. The part affected is held tensely in place without moving. Tensing the biceps to show off its bulge is an example of this. The contraction of the triceps prevents the elbow from further flexing.
2.   A muscle is held in either partial or maximal contraction against another force such as the pull of gravity or an external mechanical or muscular force. Examples of this are holding a book with outstretched arm, a tug of war between two equally matched opponents, and attempting to move an object that is too heavy to move.

ISOTONIC CONTRACTION   Isotonic means "equal tension." Isotonic contraction is a contraction in which the tension remains constant as the muscle shortens or lengthens. It is commonly, although erroneously, used as a synonym for either eccentric or concentric contraction. The latter terms, however, do not indicate the degree of tension; they merely indicate an increase or decrease in length.

PHASIC AND TONIC CONTRACTION   These terms are used less now than formerly. They appear to have been replaced by isotonic and isometric, although they are not exactly comparable. In general, the term "phasic" appears to be used for shortening contraction, but there are instances in the literature in which it seems to mean any change in length, either shortening or lengthening. The term "tonic contraction" appears to have exactly the same meaning as "static contraction." Inasmuch as the use of these terms seems to be waning, the student need not be too concerned about their exact meanings.

The Influence of Gravity and Other External Forces on Muscular Action

Movements of the body or its segments may be in the direction of gravitational forces (downward), opposing gravity (upward), or perpendicular to gravity (horizontal). It is essential to consider the direction and speed of the movement when identifying the nature of the muscular involvement of any movement. The muscles may be contracting, either to provide the force for a movement or the force to resist and control the movement, or they may be completely relaxed (Figure 2–5). It may surprise the student to learn that the same muscles are used when placing a book on a low table or a suitcase on the floor as are used for lifting it. They are used in a different way, however. When the book or suitcase is lifted the muscles provide the force, and the weight of the object (gravity) is the resistance. In this case the muscles shorten in concentric contraction. When the object is slowly lowered, however, the muscles lengthen in eccentric contraction as they resist, but gradually give in to, the force of gravity. Without the muscular resistance, the force of gravity would lower the object at a far more rapid rate! Another example of the influence of gravity on muscular action is the action of the lower extremity muscles when one lowers the body weight by bending the knees to assume a squat or semisquat position, and then returns to the erect position. As the body is lowered the extensor muscles of the hips and knees are undergoing eccentric contraction. They are indeed lengthening in this instance, yet their tension is increasing as they assume the burden of the body weight and gradual-

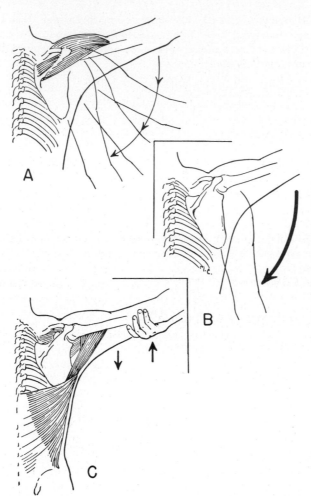

Figure 2–5 Influence of gravitational force on muscular action in sideward depression of the arm (adduction of the humerus). *A,* Eccentric contraction of the abductors in slow lowering of the arm. *B,* Absence of muscular action when the arm is dropped to the side. *C,* Concentric contraction of the adductors when the movement is performed against resistance.

ly lower it in a controlled manner. When the joint action is reversed and the body weight is lifted, the extensor muscles are contracting concentrically until the hips and knees are straight and the body is erect.

As has been demonstrated, any slow, controlled movement in the downward direction of gravity's force uses the same muscles in eccentric contraction that it uses in concentric contraction to perform the opposite upward movement (against gravity). Slow lowering of the forearm from a flexed position to one of extension is controlled by eccentric contraction of the elbow flexors, the same muscles that, by contracting concentrically, cause flexion. A forceful movement downward does not follow this pattern, however. When done forcefully, as in pounding the table, the same movement of elbow extension uses the elbow extensors in concentric contraction.

Muscular involvement in movements performed horizontally is not affected by gravity in the manner just described. Regardless of the force or speed of the movement, the muscle force for extension of the forearm at the elbow is provided by the elbow extensors. The only exception to this is seen when one is opposing an external force other than gravity, and it proves to be too strong. In a tug of war, for instance, the weaker opponents will find their elbows being pulled out straight in spite of themselves. The elbow flexor muscles are in eccentric contraction as they attempt to resist the force causing the extension at the elbow.

Finally, there are times when movement of the body or its segments occurs without muscular action. In these instances the external force causing the movement is not resisted by eccentric muscle action. Examples are allowing the force of gravity to cause the arm to drop to the side from a flexed or abducted position (Figure 2–5B) and the passive moving of a body segment by another person.

Length-Tension Relationship

There is an optimum length at which a muscle, when stimulated, can exert maximum tension. This length varies somewhat according to the muscle's structure but, as a general rule, it is slightly greater than the resting length of the muscle (de Vries, 1974). Lengths that are either greater or less produce less tension. This relationship applies for all three types of contraction, isometric, concentric, or eccentric. A typical length-tension curve is depicted in Figure 2–6. The maximum resting length occurs at 100. Curve 1 represents the tension generated when the muscle is passively stretched and Curve 2 represents the total tension generated in the muscle. The active tension of the muscle would thus be the difference between the passive and the total tension, Curve 2 minus Curve 1. This relationship suggests that when maximum force is desired, the muscle should be at or near resting length. However, other factors such as the muscle's angle of pull must be considered. It is rare for the angle of pull for optimum force application to occur when the muscle is in the resting position.

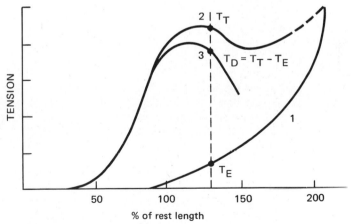

Figure 2–6 Tension-length curves for isolated muscle. Curve 1, passive elastic tension (T_E) in a muscle passively stretched to increasing lengths. Curve 2, total tension (T_T) exerted by muscle contracting actively from increasingly greater initial lengths. Curve 3, developed tension calculated by subtracting elastic tension values on Curve 1 from total tension values at equivalent lengths on Curve 2; i.e., $T_D = T_T - T_E$. (From Gowitzke, B., and Milner, M.: *Understanding the scientific bases of human movement.* 2d ed. Baltimore: Williams and Wilkins, 1980.)

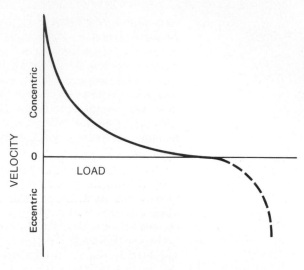

Figure 2–7 Force-velocity relationship. As the velocity of concentric contraction increases, the force that can be exerted decreases. When the velocity drops to zero, the contraction is isometric. In eccentric contraction, tension increases with the increased speed of lengthening.

Stored Elastic Capabilities

It has been established under controlled experimental conditions that when concentric contraction is preceded by a phase of active stretching, elastic energy, stored in the stretch phase, is available for use in the contractile phase. The work done by muscles shortening immediately after stretching was found to be greater than that done by those shortening from a resting state or from an isometric contraction. In addition, the differential increased with the speed of stretching and shortening. This research appears to provide experimental confirmation of the common sports pattern, which consists of a stretch before a counter concentric contraction. The backswings for a kick, tennis drive, or pitch not only provide more distance through which the foot, racket, or hand can develop speed, but also put the anterior hip and shoulder muscles on a stretch just prior to their contraction in the forward force phase (Cavagna et al., 1968).

Force-Velocity Relationship

As the speed of a muscular contraction increases, the force it is able to exert decreases (Edington and Edgerton, 1976). The velocity of contraction is maximal when the load is zero and the load is maximal when the velocity is zero (Figure 2–7). For any given load there is an optimum velocity that is somewhere between the slowest and fastest rate, and that differs for different activities and individuals. It is estimated to be 20 to 30 percent of maximum for muscle contractions under zero-load conditions. As the load increases the optimum rate decreases. Thus, if an activity requires the development of large forces, only a small amount of muscle shortening should be expected. If, on the other hand, high limb or implement velocities are needed, then little force should be expected from the contracting muscles.

The Coordination of the Muscular System

Roles of Muscles

An effective, purposeful movement of the body or any of its parts involves considerable muscular activity in addition to that of the muscles which are directly responsible for the movement itself. To begin with, the muscles causing the movement must have a stable base. This means that the bone (or bones) not engaged in the movement but providing attachment for one end of such muscles must be stabilized by other muscles. In some movements, such as those in which the hands are used at a high level, the upper arms may need to be maintained in an elevated position. This necessitates contraction of the shoulder muscles to support the weight of the arms. Many muscles, especially those of biaxial and triaxial joints, can cause moements involving more than one axis, yet it may be that only one of their actions is needed for the movement in question. A similar situation exists in regard to the muscles of the scapula. A muscle cannot voluntarily choose to effect one of its movements and not another; it must depend upon other muscls to contract and prevent the unwanted movement.

Thus even a simple movement such as threading a needle or hammering a nail may require the cooperative action of a relatively large number of muscles, each performing its own particular task in producing a single, well-coordinated movement. It may be noted, then, that muscles have various roles and that what their particular role is in a given movement depends upon the requirements of that movement. In summary, these roles are designated as movers, stabilizers, supporting muscles, and neutralizers. Furthermore, if one concedes that the negative function of remaining relaxed can be looked upon as a role, then the muscles that are antagonistic to the movers may also be included as participants in the total cooperative effort. The definitions of these roles are as follows:

MOVERS OR AGONISTS   A mover is a muscle that is directly responsible for effecting a movement. In the majority of movements there are several movers, some of them of greater importance than others. These are the principal movers. The muscles that help to perform the movement but seem to be of less importance, or contract only under certain circumstances, are the assistant movers. Muscles that help only when an extra amount of force is needed, as when a movement is performed against resistance, are sometimes called emergency muscles. This distinction between the various muscles that contribute to a movement is an arbitrary one. There may well be some difference of opinion as to whether a muscle is a principal or an assistant mover in a given movement.

FIXATOR, STABILIZING, AND SUPPORTING MUSCLES   This group includes the muscles that contract statically to steady or support some part of the body against the pull of the contracting muscles, against the pull of gravity, or against the effect of momentum and recoil in certain vigorous movements. One of the most common functions of these muscles is steadying or fixating the bone to which a contracting muscle is attached. It is only by the stabilizing of one of its attachments that the muscle is able to cause an effective movement of the bone at which it has its other attachment (Figure 2–8). The term "supporting" is used when a limb or the trunk must be supported against the pull of gravity while a distal segment such as the hand, foot, or head is engaging in the essential movement.

NEUTRALIZERS   A neutralizer is a muscle that acts to prevent an undesired action of one of the movers. Thus, if a muscle both flexes and abducts, but only flexion is desired in the movement, an adductor contracts to neutralize the abductory action of the mover.

Occasionally two of the movers have one action in common but can also perform second actions that are antagonistic to each other. For instance, one muscle may upward rotate and adduct while the other may downward rotate and adduct. When

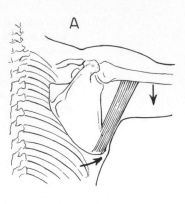

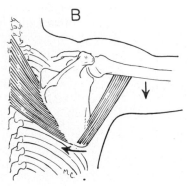

Figure 2–8   If the scapula were not stabilized, the teres major would increase the upward rotation of the scapula as it adducted the humerus. This dual action on the humerus and scapula is shown in A. In B, the scapula is stabilized by the scapular adductors and downward rotators. This permits the teres major to concentrate its force on the adduction of the humerus.

they contract together to cause adduction, their rotatory functions counteract each other (Figure 2–9). Muscles which behave this way in a movement are mutual neutralizers as well as movers. Some writers use the term "synergist" for muscles that have this neutralizing function (Watkins, 1974). The term is used by others for muscles that stabilize bones, and by still others for any muscles that work together to contribute to a movement, regardless of the specific function of each (Steindler, 1970). Because of this inconsistency, the use of the term has purposely been avoided in this text.

ANTAGONISTS   Muscles that have an opposite effect to movers or agonists are labeled as *antagonists*. Because they are located on the opposite side of the joint from the movers they are also called *contralateral* muscles. The elbow flexors, located on the anterior arm, are antagonistic to the elbow extensors located on the posterior arm. When the forearm is extended at the elbow, as in doing a push-up, the extensors are the movers and contract concentrically to provide the force for the movement. The flexors are the antagonists and are relaxed. In the return movement, the letdown, the joint action at the elbow is flexion but the flexors do not contract—they remain relaxed. The contracting muscles, once again, are the extensors, but now they are antagonists contracting eccentrically to resist gravity, and control the speed of the elbow flexion. When a body segment is moved by muscular effort, the contracting muscles are the movers in concentric contraction. When movement of a segment is effected by the force of gravity and resisted by muscle force, the contracting muscles are the antagonists in eccentric contraction.

Having stated the general rule, it is now necessary to describe what may at first appear to be a contradiction. If a movement performed with great force and rapidity is not checked, it will subject the ligamentous reinforcements of the joint to sudden strain. The tissues would probably be severely damaged. This is particularly true of quick movements of the arm or leg because of the tremendous momentum that can be developed in a long lever. To prevent such injury the muscles that are antagonistic to the movers contract momentarily to check the movement. As they contract, the movers relax, if indeed they have not already relaxed, allowing momentum to complete the movement. The situation is a little like taking the foot off the accelerator in order to put it on the brake. At the moment when the movement is being checked, the so-called antagonistic muscles are not truly antagonistic. In a vigorous movement, the antagonistic muscles may be said to perform two functions. Their first function is to relax in order to permit the movement to be made without hindrance; their second function is to act as a brake at the completion of the movement and, by doing so, to protect the joint.

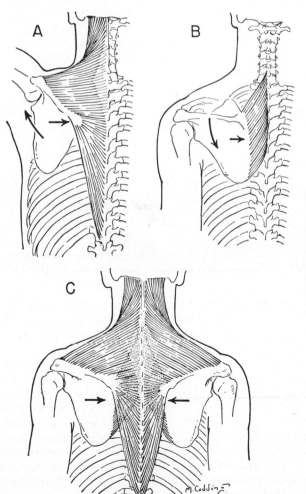

Figure 2–9 The trapezius and rhomboids as mutual movers and neutralizers. A, The trapezius alone adducts the scapula and rotates it upward. B, The rhomboids alone adduct the scapula and rotate it downward. C, Together the trapezius and rhomboids adduct the scapula without rotating it either upward or downward.

46   Kinesiology, Scientific Basis of Human Motion

 SUMMARY OF MUSCLE CLASSIFICATION BASED ON ROLE IN TOTAL MOVEMENT

Mover or agonist: A muscle that is directly responsible for effecting a movement.

Fixator, stabilizer, supporting muscle: Muscles that contract statically to steady or to support some part of the body against the pull of contracting muscles, the pull of gravity, or any other force that interferes with the desired movement.

Neutralizer: A muscle that acts to prevent an undesired action of one of the movers.

Antagonist: A muscle that causes the opposite movement from that of the movers.

EXAMPLE OF THE DIFFERENT ROLES OF MUSCLES IN A TOTAL MOVEMENT   Let us consider the movement of the right upper arm when playing shuffleboard (pushing a disk with a cue). The movement of the humerus at the shoulder joint is flexion, and this is accompanied by slight upward rotation and abduction of the scapula. The *movers of the humerus* are the anterior deltoid, the clavicular portion of the pectoralis major, and the coracobrachialis. (Look these up if you are not yet familiar with them.) The two former muscles are also inward (medial) rotators of the humerus, but since this movement is not desired, it must be prevented. The infraspinatus and the teres minor take care of this. Therefore, they are serving as *neutralizers* in this pushing action. Meanwhile, the scapula is rotating upward through the action of the serratus anterior and trapezius II and IV, which are serving as *shoulder girdle movers.* Trapezius II, which is an elevator as well as an upward rotator of the scapula, and trapezius IV, which is a depressor as well as an upward rotator, mutually neutralize each other with respect to elevation and depression while they are cooperating in rotating the scapula upward. Hence they are both *movers* and *mutual neutralizers.*

Consider the movers of the humerus once again, keeping in mind that muscles tend to pull both their distal and proximal ends toward each other. Note that the proximal attachments of both the anterior deltoid and the pectoralis major are side by side on the anterior border of the clavicle. As they contract they not only raise the humerus forward, but they also tend to pull the clavicle laterally, a movement which would put a strain on the sternoclavicular joint. They are prevented from doing this by the action of the subclavius muscle, which pulls the clavicle medially and thus serves as a *stabilizer.* So in this simple pushing movement we see that we have muscles acting as movers, neutralizers, and stabilizers, which, by their cooperative action, assure an efficient movement.

Cocontraction

This action of muscles is usually defined as the simultaneous contraction of movers and antagonists. This sounds simple and straightforward, but nevertheless it requires interpretation. In any given movement, even the simplest, several muscles other than the movers are likely to be involved. There are neutralizers and mutual neutralizers whose function it is to counteract an additional function of a mover that is not desired in the present movement (see Figure 2–9). There are also many movements that require the action of stabilizers. These may be for stabilizing a weight-bearing segment against gravity, or for the stabilization of a freely movable bone that provides for the proximal attachment of one of the movers (see Figure 2–8).

There are other situations that may be erroneously interpreted as examples of cocontraction, for instance in movements involving an interplay between movers and antagonists as a means of maintaining postural balance. Some believe that the alternation between contractions of these muscles may be so quick that the muscles appear to be contracting simultaneously and that there may actually be a slight amount of overlap, one muscle tapering off in eccentric contraction as the other begins. Even if this does happen it is not true cocontraction.

There is also the type of movement, exemplified by vigorous arm flinging, in which the opposing muscles come into quick action at the end of the movement, apparently for the protection of the ligaments and other tissues that would otherwise be subjected to violent stretching with possible tearing. This situation usually occurs in a ballistic-type movement. Basmajian (1979) cites an example of this type of movement, describing it as a whiplike motion in which there is a sudden burst of activity of the antagonists at the finish. He suggests that this motion serves the purpose of protecting the joint and preventing injury.

Genuine cocontraction means the simultaneous contraction of movers and their antagonists. Opinions differ concerning bona fide examples of cocontraction. Some believe that it occurs only in early attempts to master a difficult skill, especially one in which the emphasis is on accuracy rather than on speed. To those who hold this opinion cocontraction is characteristic of unskillful performance. Basmajian (1979) notes several electromyographic investigations that indicate that one effect of training is the progressive reduction of cocontraction.

Others are convinced that there are circumstances when cocontraction occurs apart from those related to early learning, lack of skill, stabilization of skeletal segments, or neutralization of unwanted functions of the mover muscles. Watkins, a defender of the latter point of view, bases her stand on original research concerning cocontraction and the relationship between opposing muscles (1974). Her findings suggest the need for further research to corroborate one position or the other.

Spurt and Shunt Muscles

These terms are used by MacConaill, a professor of anatomy from Ireland, to represent two opposing types of muscular action based on the relative distance of each attachment from the center of motion of the joint between them (Basmajian, 1979). Since the terms are not very meaningful to us in the United States it is best simply to learn his interpretation.

A *spurt muscle* is one in which the distance from its attachment to the stationary bone (usually the proximal attachment) to the joint is greater than the distance from its attachment to the moving bone (usually the distal attachment) to the joint. This means that the muscle's pull has a greater rotatory component than stabilizing component. The brachialis and biceps brachii are good examples of this (see Figures 5–5 and 5–7).

A *shunt muscle* is one in which the distance from its attachment to the moving bone (usually the distal attachment) to the joint is greater than the distance from its attachment to the stationary bone (usually the proximal attachment) to the joint. This means that the muscle's line of pull has a greater stabilizing component than rotatory component. The brachioradialis is a prime example (see Figure 5–8). Furthermore, it comes into action especially during quick movements which would otherwise have a centrifugal effect and would thus endanger the joint structure. (Rotatory and stabilizing components of force are discussed in Chapter 11 of this text.)

In other words, a spurt muscle is chiefly rotatory in its effect on the moving bone, since it provides the force that initiates and sustains the latter's movements. On the other hand, a shunt muscle is primarily stabilizing. By pulling lengthwise along the moving bone in the direction of the joint, it provides centripetal force which serves to protect the joint structures.

Tendon Action of Two-Joint Muscles

Another type of coordination of the muscular system may be seen in the so-called tendon action of the two-joint muscles—that is, the muscles which pass over and act upon two joints (Brunnstrom, 1972; Fenn, 1938; Rasch and Burke, 1978; Steindler, 1970). Examples of these are the hamstrings (the semitendinosus, the semimembranosus, and the biceps femoris), which flex the leg at the knee and extend the thigh at the hip; the rectus femoris, which flexes the thigh and extends the leg; the sartorius, which flexes both the thigh and the leg; the gastrocnemius, which helps to flex the leg in addition to its primary function of extending the foot; and the long flexors and extensors of the fingers. The latter are actually multijoint muscles, since they cross the wrist and at least two of the joints of the fingers. A characteristic of all these muscles, whether they act on joints that flex in the same direction, as in the case of the wrist and fingers, or in the opposite direction, as in the case of the knee and hip, is that they are not long enough to permit complete movement in both joints at the same time. This results in the tension of one muscle being transmitted to the other, in much the same manner that a downward pull on a rope which passes through an overhead pulley is transmitted in the form of a pull in the reverse direction to the rope on the other side of the pulley. Thus, if the hamstrings contract to help extend the hip, tension in the form of a stretch is placed on the rectus femoris, causing it to extend the knee. Or, if the rectus femoris contracts to help flex the hip, tension in the form of a stretch is placed on the hamstrings, causing them to flex the knee. This is a simplified version of what in actuality is a rather complex coordination.

When one-joint muscles contract, their shortening is accompanied by a corresponding loss of tension. In quick movements of the limbs, one-joint muscles rapidly lose their tension. The advantage of two-joint muscles is that they can continue to exert tension without shortening. The two-joint muscles have two different patterns of action. These have been described by Fenn (1938), Steindler (1970), and others as concurrent and countercurrent movements.

An example of concurrent movement is seen in the simultaneous extension of the hip and knee and also in the simultaneous flexion of these joints. As the muscles contract, they act on each other in such a way that they do not lose length; thus, their tension is retained. It is as though the pull traveled up one muscle and down the other in a continuous circuit. In simultaneous extension of the hip and knee, for instance, the rectus femoris's loss of tension at the distal or knee end is balanced by a gain in tension at the proximal or hip end. Similarly, the hamstrings, which are losing tension at their proximal end, are gaining it at their distal end.

The countercurrent pattern presents a different picture. In this type of movement, while one of the two-joint muscles shortens rapidly at both joints, its antagonist lengthens correspondingly and thereby gains tension at both ends. An example of this action is seen in the rapid loss of tension in the rectus femoris and corresponding gain of tension in the hamstrings when the hip is flexed and the knee is extended simultaneously. A vigorous kick is a dramatic illustration of this kind of muscle action. The backward swing of the lower extremity preparatory to kicking is a less spectacular but equally valid example. The forward swing in walking is another. In both patterns of movement the one- and two-joint muscles appear to supplement each other and thus, by their cooperative action, produce smooth, coordinated, efficient movements.

When a two-joint muscle contracts it acts on both joints it crosses. If action is desired in only one joint, the other joint must be stabilized by another muscle or by some external force. In such circumstances, Fujiwara and Basmajian (Basmajian,

1979) found, the rectus femoris shows maximum activity in hip flexion *or* knee extension and the medial hamstrings, similarly, are most active in hip extension *or* knee flexion. In the two-joint countercurrent movements of hip flexion and knee extension, the rectus femoris exhibited strong activity, as did the medial hamstrings during hip extension and knee flexion. When the motion was concurrent, however, the activity of the rectus femoris and hamstrings were inhibited when they were antagonists. This was especially true for the knee joint action. When the movement was concurrent hip flexion and knee flexion, the rectus femoris showed no activity but the hamstring did. Similarly, during knee extension and hip extension, the hamstrings were inhibited and the rectus femoris was active.

Types of Bodily Movements

Movements may be passive or active, and if active they may be slow or rapid. They may involve the constant application of force or, after the initial impetus has been given, they may continue without further muscular effort.

A *passive* movement requires no effort on the part of the person involved. It is performed by another person such as a therapist giving a treatment or an instructor or partner stretching tight ligaments, fascia, and muscles in an attempt to increase the range of motion of a particular joint. In some cases it is a movement that has been started by the subject's own effort but is continued by momentum. It might also be caused by the force of gravity if the subject remained relaxed and used no muscular effort to aid, restrain, or guide the moving part.

An *active* movement is effected by the subject's muscular activity. It is usually performed volitionally, but it may be a reflex reaction to an external or internal stimulus. It may be rapid or slow. In slow movements muscular tension is maintained throughout the range of motion. Pushing a heavy piece of furniture across the room is an example of this type of movement. In *rapid movements* tension could also be maintained throughout the range of motion, but this would be an inefficient way of performing them. For efficiency, rapid movements should be performed ballistically. The concept of *ballistic movement* was introduced a number of years ago by experimental psychologists. They used the term for movements that were initiated by vigorous muscular contraction and completed by momentum. This type of movement is characteristic of throwing, striking, and kicking. It is also seen in the finger movements used for typing and piano playing. When such movements are performed nonballistically—that is, with constant muscular contraction—they are uneconomical and hence not skillful. In fact, they are characteristic of the way in which beginners tend to attempt new coordinations, especially if they are concentrating on accuracy of aim rather than on a ballistic type of motion. They need to be encouraged in the early stages of learning a skill to concentrate on form rather than accuracy if they are to master the skill of moving ballistically.

Ballistic movements may be terminated by one of three methods: (1) by contracting antagonistic muscles, as in the forehand drive in tennis; (2) by allowing the moving part to reach the limit of motion, in which case it will be stopped by the passive resistance of ligaments, other tissues, or the braking action of antagonistic muscles, as in the case of the forceful overarm throw; or (3) by the interference of an obstacle, as when chopping wood.

In many movements found in both sports and skilled labor, three types of muscular action cooperate to produce a single act. This kind of cooperation is seen especially in striking activities that require the use of an implement, such as a tennis racket, golf club, or ax. Movements such as these involve (1) fixation to support the moving part and to maintain the necessary position, (2) ballistic movement of the active limb, and (3) fixation in the fingers as they grasp the implement.

Methods of Studying the Actions of Muscles

In addition to the obvious method of studying the actions of muscles in a textbook, there are a number of procedures that may be more meaningful to the student.

Conjecture and Reasoning

Using knowledge of the location and attachments of a muscle and the nature of the joint or joints it spans, one can deduce a great deal about a muscle's actions. Conjecture and reasoning is a method that is valuable to use in conjunction with other methods. Although the use of this method does not identify which muscles are actually contracting in a given action, a careful study of the muscles' attachments and line of pull (Figure 2–10) will enable one to see what movements a muscle is *capable* of causing.

Dissection

An excellent way of studying the location and attachments of a muscle and its relation to the joint it spans is dissection. This method provides a more meaningful basis for visualizing the muscle's potential movements, but it sometimes leads to misinterpretations and erroneous conclusions.

Inspection and Palpation

Even though its use is limited to superficial muscles, inspection and palpation of normal living subjects is a valuable method, as far as it goes. Much of the information in early anatomy textbooks was based on the combination of dissection of the cadaver and inspection and palpation of living subjects. Before the days of electromyography these were the chief methods of determining the actions of the muscles. There is a possibility of misinterpretation, however, against which students should be warned. When the force of a muscle contraction is weak, it is sometimes difficult to feel its contraction. If the subject repeats the action against greater resistance, the contraction

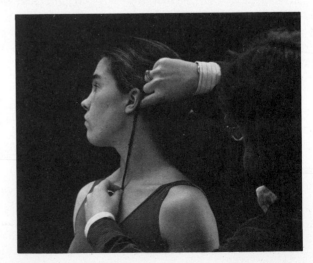

Figure 2–10 Locating a muscle's line of pull by placing ends of a string or elastic at the location of the muscle's attachment. The line of pull of the sternocleidomastoid is located using this procedure.

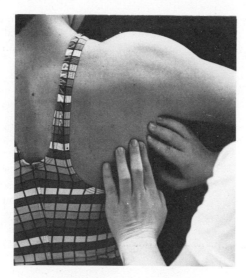

Figure 2–11   Palpation of a contracting muscle.

may be stronger and more easily felt (Figure 2–11). The conclusion may be drawn erroneously that the muscle is a major mover for the action involved when in fact it comes into action only as an *assistant* under conditions of heavy resistance.

Inspection and palpation of subjects, some of whose muscles are known to be paralyzed, has been used extensively by experienced investigators, such as Wilhelmine G. Wright and Signe Brunnstrom. Wright, who was an outstanding physical therapist and author during the 1920s, found that by observing with great care the movements that a patient was unable to perform, she could judge the normal action of the muscle that she knew was paralyzed. Written before the days of electromyography, her book is well worth reading because of her meticulous observations (Wright, 1962). The preface of her book, with its careful description of her technique of palpation, is especially helpful. Today's students who have the opportunity to work with subjects with paralyzed muscles may find this approach useful for the study of muscle actions.

Models and Gadgets

There are numerous devices, both commercial and homemade, that can be used for demonstrating and studying the actions of muscles. Probably the most commonly used device is the simplest of all—a long rubber band (or chain of short ones) held against the bones of a skeleton in such a way as to represent a single muscle. The movement is demonstrated by holding the elastic on a stretch with one end representing the proximal attachment and the other the distal attachment. The tendency of both bones to move toward each other can easily be demonstrated, as well as the necessity for stabilizing one bone for the muscle to be effective in moving the other bone.

Muscle Stimulation

To most kinesiologists the term "muscle stimulation" means G. B. Duchenne, the pioneer in the use of electrical stimulation as a means of studying the actions of the muscles and the author of *Physiologie des mouvements*. This classic work was translated into English and published in 1949. It made a tremendous contribution to the science of kinesiology, yet its limitations must be recognized. It demonstrates the contraction of individual muscles when they are stimulated electrically. Unfortunate-

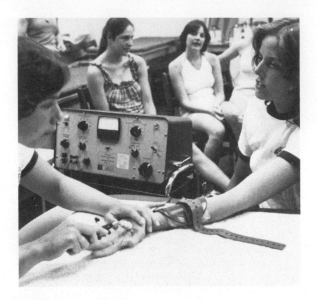

Figure 2–12 Using a muscle stimulator to determine muscle contraction.

ly, it cannot analyze the sequence of muscular actions that occur in an everyday act such as walking, lifting a package, or working with a common tool of workshop or kitchen. Neither can it reveal the complex combinations of muscular actions in ordinary sport techniques (Figure 2–12).

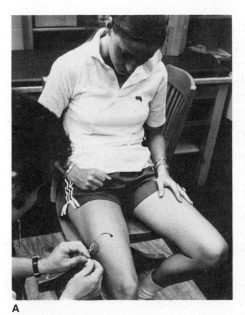
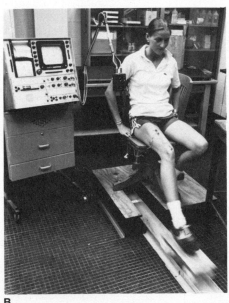

A   B

Figure 2–13 Electromyography is a valuable tool for studying muscle activity. *A,* Applying surface electrodes. *B,* Recording activity in the rectus femoris muscle during vigorous extension of the lower leg.

In spite of its limitations, muscle stimulation is being used in many modern kinesiology laboratories as a device for studying the responses of individual muscles to electrical stimulation. For those who are interested in knowing more about this technique two articles are recommended (Hoffman, 1968; Jokl, 1967).

Electromy-ography (EMG)   While not many undergraduate students may have the opportunity of personal experience with this technique, all may benefit by reading the reports of EMG investigations. A wealth of information concerning muscular action is available in such reports. Electromyography is based on the fact that contracting muscles generate electrical impulses. It is a technique of recording such impulses or action currents, as they are also called (Figure 2–13). It provides specific information about muscular actions that we have only been able to guess at in the past, information that has proved much of our guessing to be inaccurate. The unique advantages of EMG are that it reveals both the intensity and duration of a muscle's action and, in fact, discloses the precise time sequences of muscular activity in a movement. Furthermore, it reveals the actions not only of the agonists and antagonists but also of the muscles serving as stabilizers and neutralizers. Perhaps its greatest contribution to our knowledge of muscular action is its ability to record the impulses of deep as well as superficial muscles. Basmajian, the apostle of electromyography, says that it surpasses all the older methods of studying muscular action in that it reveals what the individual muscles are actually doing, not just what they "*can* do," or "*probably* do" (Basmajian, 1979; Waterland and Shambes, 1969).

Laboratory Experiences

1. Take two sticks that are joined at one end by a hinge. Attach a single piece of elastic or a long rubber band to the opposite ends of the two sticks.
    a. Separate the ends of the sticks as far as the elastic will permit and then demonstrate the way the elastic will pull both sticks together.
    b. Demonstrate the way in which the elastic will move only one of the sticks if the other one is stabilized.
    c. Repeat both *a* and *b,* using the arm of the skeleton instead of the sticks.
2. Get a subject to hold a heavy dumbbell in the right hand and slowly raise the arm sideward-upward without bending the elbow. Keep your fingers on the clavicular portion of the pectoralis major. Does it contract? If so, at what position of the arm does it begin?
3. Flex the fingers hard. Keep them flexed and flex the hand at the wrist as far as possible. What happens to the fingers? Explain.
4. Extend the fingers, and then hyperextend the hand at the wrist as far as possible. What happens to the fingers? Explain.
5. Get a subject to lie on the left side with the hip and knee in a partly flexed position and the right leg fully extended. The right thigh should now be flexed passively by an operator. The subject should attempt to keep the knee straight but not to the point of interfering with the hip flexion. What happens? Where does the subject feel discomfort? Explain.
6. Have the subject, in the same starting position as in 5, flex both the right thigh and right leg completely. The right thigh should now be passively extended by an operator, with the subject attempting to keep the leg flexed at the knee. As the thigh becomes fully extended, what

happens to the knee? Where does the subject feel discomfort? Explain. (Caution: Do not use an acrobat or acrobatic dancer as a subject for 5 or 6, or the experiments may not work. Why?)

7. Have a subject lie supine on a table with the knees at the edge and the lower legs hanging down. Ask the subject to extend one leg at the knee while you attempt to stop the motion by applying strong resistance at the front of the ankle. Note the amount of resistance you have to apply. Now ask the subject to flex the leg at the knee while you attempt to stop the movement by resisting at the rear of the ankle. Which action requires more resistance on your part?

Now ask the subject to sit up and flex the trunk well forward from the hips. Repeat the same two actions of knee flexion and extension against resistance. Which action requires more effort on your part this time? How does this compare with the first result? Explain.

It may help you to know that the rectus femoris crosses the front of the hip joint and the front of the knee joint. Hence it is a flexor of the hip and an extensor of the knee. The biceps femoris is located on the back of the thigh and therefore is an extensor of the hip and flexor of the knee.

Note: Laboratory exercises on the action of muscles as movers, stabilizers, and neutralizers are not included here because, in order to do them, it is necessary to know the individual muscles. They will be found in the laboratory sections of Chapters 4 through 8.

References

Arkin, A. M. 1941. Absolute muscle power: internal kinesiology of muscle. *Arch. Surg.* 42:395–410.

Basmajian, J. V. 1979. *Muscles alive.* 4th ed. Baltimore: Williams & Wilkins.

Brunnstrom, S. 1972. *Clinical kinesiology.* 3d ed. Philadelphia: F. A. Davis.

Cavagna, G. A., Dusman, B., and Margaria, R. G. 1968. Positive work done on a previously stretched muscle. *J. Appl. Physiol.* 24:21–31.

de Vries. H. A. 1974. *Physiology of exercise.* 2d ed. Dubuque, Iowa, William C. Brown.

Edington, D. W., and Edgerton, V. R. 1976. *The biology of physical activity.* Boston: Houghton Mifflin.

Fenn, W. O. 1938. The mechanics of muscular contraction in man. *J. Appl. Physics* 9:165–77.

Gowitzke, B., and Milner, M. 1980. *Understanding the scientific bases of human movement.* 2d ed. Baltimore: Williams & Wilkins.

Hill, A. V. 1970. *First and last experiments in muscle mechanics.* New York: Cambridge University Press.

Hoffman, F. P. 1968. *The use of electrical stimulation as a teaching aid in kinesiology. J. Health, Phys. Educ. Rec.* 39:79–82.

Hubbard, A. W. 1973. Homokinetics: muscular function in human movement. In *Science and medicine of exercise and sports,* 2d ed., ed. W. R. Johnson and E. Buskirk. Chapter 1. New York: Harper & Row.

Jokl, E. 1967. G. B. Duchenne's physiology of motion. *J. Health Phys. Educ. Rec.* 38:67–68.

Rasch, P. J., and Burke, R. K. 1978. *Kinesiology and applied anatomy.* 6th ed. Philadelphia: Lea & Febiger.

Steindler, A. 1970. *Kinesiology of the human body.* Springfield, Ill., Charles C Thomas.

Waterland, J. C., and Shambes, G. M. 1969. Electromyography: one link in the experimental chain of kinesiological research. *J. Am. Phys. Ther. Assoc.* 49:1351–56.

Watkins, M. P. 1974. Co-contraction and the relationship between opposing muscles. Master's thesis. Boston University, Sargent College of Allied Health Professions.

Wright, W. G. 1962. *Muscle function.* New York: Hafner Publishing. (Reprint of 1928 edition.)

The Neuromuscular Basis of Human Motion

Objectives

At the conclusion of this chapter, the student should be able to:

1. Name and describe the functions of the basic structures of the nervous system.
2. Explain how gradations in strength of muscle contraction and precision of movements occur.
3. Name and define the receptors important in musculoskeletal movement.
4. Explain how the various receptors function, and describe the effect each has on musculoskeletal movement.
5. Describe reflex action, and enumerate and differentiate among the reflexes which affect musculoskeletal action.
6. Demonstrate a basic understanding of volitional movement by describing the nature of the participation of the anatomical structures and mechanisms involved.

Introduction

The roles of the bones, joints and muscles in human movement were presented in the first two chapters. This chapter takes up the role of the nervous system in initiating, modifying, and coordinating muscular action.

Loofbourrow (1973) presents this topic so succinctly and vividly that his introductory paragraph is quoted here in full as an introduction to the present chapter:

The forces which move the supporting framework of the body are unleashed within skeletal muscles on receipt of signals by way of their motor nerves. In the absence of such signals, the muscles normally are relaxed. Movement is almost always the result of the combined action of a group of muscles which pull in somewhat different directions, so the control of movement involves a distribution of signals within the central nervous system (CNS) to appropriate motor nerves with precise timing and in appropriate number. In order for movements to be useful in making adjustments to external situations, it is necessary for the central nervous system to be appraised of these situations, which are continually changing. A means of providing this information promptly exists in a variety of receptors sensitive to changes in temperature, light, pressure, etc. These receptors are signal generators which dispatch signals (nerve impulses) to the CNS over afferent nerve fibers. The CNS receives these signals together with identical ones from within the muscles, joints, tendons, and other body structures and is led thereby to generate and distribute in fantastically orderly array myriads of signals to various muscles. This, despite the enormous complexity of the machinery involved, enables the individual to do one main thing at a time. This is integration. It is what Sir Charles Sherrington meant by "the integrative action of the nervous system."

The following discussion does not presume to be an exhaustive treatise on neuromuscular mechanisms. It attempts rather to present as simply as possible those mechanisms which are pertinent to the study of kinesiology. Because of the newer techniques made possible by electronic devices during the past two or three decades, great strides have been made in acquiring more accurate information concerning the intricacies of muscular function.

The Nervous System and Basic Nerve Structures

It is assumed that the kinesiology student is already familiar with the general plan of the nervous system; hence, it will not be described in full here. Only a brief outline of the major divisions will be presented, in order to give the reader a framework for the topics which have been selected for discussion.

I. Central nervous system
   A. Brain
   B. Spinal cord

II. Peripheral nervous system
   A. Cranial nerves (12 pairs)
   B. Spinal nerves (31 pairs)

III. Autonomic nervous system

The autonomic nervous system is not a distinct system based on structure and geographic location, as are the central and peripheral systems, but is rather a functional division that overlaps with those in specific areas. It includes those portions of the brain, spinal cord, and peripheral nervous system that supply cardiac muscle, smooth muscle, and gland cells.

Neurons

A neuron, the structural unit of the nervous system, is a single nerve cell consisting of a cell body and one or more projections. There are two kinds of neurons whose long fibers constitute the peripheral nervous system. These are sensory or afferent and motor or efferent (Figure 3–1). In addition to these there are numerous connector (internuncial) neurons within the central nervous system.

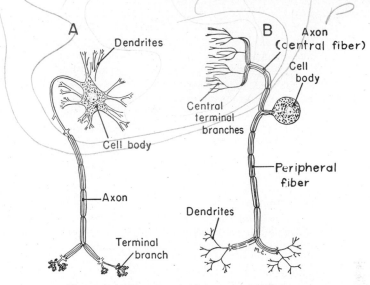

Figure 3–1   Neurons. *A,* Motor neuron. *B,* Sensory neuron.

The cell bodies of the majority of efferent or motor neurons are situated within the anterior horns of the spinal cord. (There are also some in the brain stem and sympathetic ganglia.) Many short threadlike extensions of the cell body, known as dendrites, make contact—i.e., synapse—with the axons of other cells, the latter being either sensory or connector neurons.

Each motor and connector neuron has a specialized process termed an axon. The axon of the motor neuron emerges from the spinal cord in a ventral root. It then travels by way of a peripheral nerve to the muscle that it helps to innervate. There it divides and subdivides into smaller and smaller branches, the most distal being known as the terminal branches. Each terminal branch ends within a single muscle fiber in the structure called the motor end-plate.

The cell body of a spinal afferent or sensory neuron, unlike that of a motor neuron, is situated in a dorsal root ganglion just outside of the spinal cord. (The cell bodies of cranial sensory neurons are in cranial nerve ganglia.) The neuron has a single short process that projects from the cell body and then bifurcates into two branches which go in opposite directions. One, the so-called central fiber, travels in the dorsal root of the nerve to the posterior horn of the spinal cord where it divides into numerous branches. It may terminate in the cord or it may ascend in the cord to the brain and terminate there. The other branch of the afferent neuron is the long peripheral fiber which comes from a receptor. It travels in a nerve trunk to the vicinity of the appropriate dorsal root ganglion where it unites with the cell body via the short stemlike process mentioned above (Figure 3–1B).

Authorities differ in their choice of nomenclature for the parts of a sensory neuron. Some apply the term "axon" to the short stemlike process; others apply this term to the central fiber—the branch that enters the spinal cord. This text adopts the latter use of the term, since it is in keeping with a commonly accepted definition, namely, that an axon is the fiber over which impulses are conducted *away from* the cell body, as opposed to dendrites, which convey impulses *toward* the cell body. When referring to a sensory neuron, the term dendrite is applied not to the long fiber that conveys impulses from peripheral regions to the cell body, but rather to its branches. The long sensory fiber itself is known simply as the peripheral fiber. Some authorities, however, do not designate any part of the sensory neuron as a dendrite, but say merely that the peripheral fiber and its branches *function like dendrites*.

It was noted above that the dendrites of efferent (motor) neurons make contact within the spinal cord, either with the terminal branches of afferent (sensory) neurons or with connector neurons. Connector neurons, also known as internuncial neurons, are a third type of nerve cell. They exist completely within the central nervous system and serve as connecting links. They may vary from a single small neuron, connecting a sensory neuron with a motor neuron, to an intricate system of neurons whereby a sensory impulse may be relayed to many motor cell bodies. We know from common experience that a complex motor act may result from a single sensory impulse. For instance, a sudden loud noise may cause us to jump, turn around, and tense nearly every muscle in our body. The connector neurons are responsible for this widespread response to the single sensory impulse. Thus there may be only one connector neuron participating in a movement, or there may be an intricate network making possible an almost limitless number of connections with other neurons.

Nerves

Just as an electric cable is an insulated bundle of wires for the transmission of electric currents, so a nerve is a bundle of fibers, enclosed within a connective tissue sheath, for the transmission of impulses from one part of the body to another. A nerve, or nerve trunk as it is frequently called, may consist entirely of outgoing fibers from the central nervous system to the muscles and other tissues, or it may consist only of incoming fibers from the sensory organs to the central nervous system. The typical spinal nerve, however, is mixed; that is, it contains both outgoing and incoming fibers. Each spinal nerve is attached to the spinal cord by a ventral (motor) root and a dorsal (sensory) root (Figure 3–2). The dorsal root bears a ganglion and it is just beyond the ganglion that the two roots unite to form the spinal nerve. Once outside the vertebral canal, each spinal nerve divides into an anterior and a posterior branch, each of which contains both motor and sensory fibers. The anterior branches supply the trunk and limbs, the posterior branches the back.

The Synapse

The connection between neurons in the central nervous system is known as a synapse (Figure 3–3). A synapse, and there may be thousands between any two neurons, is a contiguity of the membrane of an axon and the membrane of a dendrite or a cell body. There is no physical union between them. Conduction of impulses takes place in one

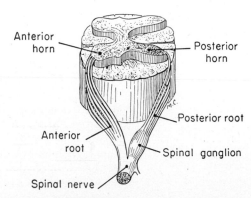

Figure 3–2 Section of the spinal cord showing the anterior and posterior roots of a spinal nerve.

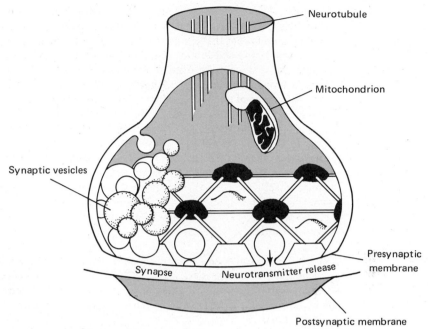

Figure 3–3 Nerve ending and synapse. (Adapted from Akert, K., Pfenninger, K., Sandri, C., and Moor, H.: Freeze etching and cytochemistry of vesicles and membrane complexes in synapses of the central nervous system. *In* Edington, D., and Edgerton, V.: *The biology of physical activity.* Boston: Houghton Mifflin, 1976, p. 86.)

direction only—from the axon of one neuron to the dendrites or cell body of another. The transmission of an impulse across a synapse depends upon the release of a chemical transmitter substance by the axon. This substance diffuses throughout the membranes, and an action potential is created in the postsynaptic neuron. The action potential may be excitatory or inhibitory. Synapses are influenced by use and disuse. The more often one is crossed, the easier it becomes for signals to pass through it.

The Motor Unit

To recapitulate, the structural units of the nervous and motor systems are, respectively, the neuron and the muscle fiber. Functionally, the two systems combine to form the neuromuscular system. The functional unit of the neuromuscular system is the *motor unit,* and it consists of a single motor neuron (Figure 3–1A), together with all of the muscle fibers that its axon supplies (Figure 3–4).

Motor units vary widely in the number of muscle fibers supplied by one motor neuron. In some motor units there may be as many as 2,000 or more muscle fibers; in others there may be fewer than 10. The number of motor units in a muscle depends in part upon the total number of fibers in the muscle and in part upon the number of fibers in a single motor unit (Gardner, 1975). A muscle which has a large number of motor units in relation to the total number of fibers—that is, a small ratio of muscle fibers to motor neurons—is capable of more precise movements than is the muscle with

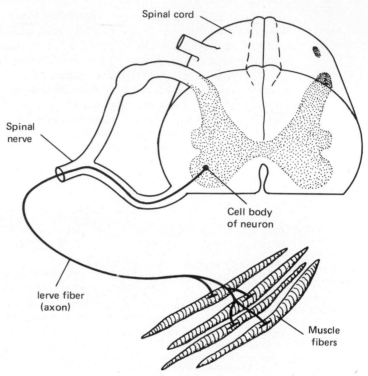

Figure 3–4   The organization of a motor unit. (Adapted from Basmajian, J. V.: *Muscles alive.* 4th ed. Baltimore: Williams and Wilkins, 1979.)

a small number of motor units for the same number of muscle fibers. Hence the ratio of muscle fibers to motor neurons has a direct bearing on the precision of the movements executed by the muscle. For example, the small muscles of the thumb and index finger are capable of effecting movements of great precision because their motor units have such a low ratio of muscle fibers to motor neurons or, to state it differently, such a large number of motor neurons per muscle. By way of contrast, the gluteus maximus has a relatively small number of motor neurons for its size, hence a large number of muscle fibers per neuron. It does not need to be pointed out that the movements for which the gluteus maximus is responsible can scarcely be described as precise.

Gradations in the Strength of Muscular Contractions

Common experience indicates that the same muscles contract with various gradations of strength according to the requirements of the task. The elbow flexors, for example, are able to contract just enough to enable the hand to lift a piece of paper from the desk; they can also contract forcefully enough to lift a 15-pound briefcase. How do they adjust to such extremes?

There are two major factors in the gradation of contraction. These are (1) the number of motor units which participate in the act, and (2) the frequency of stimulation. If the stimulus is of threshold value, all of the muscle fibers in the motor unit will contract maximally. If the stimulus is subliminal, in other words, below threshold value, none of the muscle fibers in the unit will contract at all. This characteristic is known as the *all-or-none principle of muscular contraction.* It must be emphasized that the principle applies only to individual motor units, not to entire muscles. To reiterate, if the stimulus is of threshold value, each muscle fiber in the participating unit will contract. Hence it follows that, other things being equal, the more motor units that contract, the greater will be the total strength developed.

If stimuli are discharged at low frequency the muscle fibers will partially relax between impulses, but if the stimuli are discharged at high frequency the fibers will have insufficient time to relax and the result is summation or maximal contraction. If these two factors are combined—that is, if the maximum number of fibers are stimulated with the impulses being discharged at high frequency—the resulting contraction is of maximal strength.

Receptors

Most activities of the nervous system begin with stimuli that activate sensory nerve terminals. These receptors are specialized cells or organs that are selective in their response to different types of stimuli. There are two major classifications, exteroceptors and interoceptors. Exteroceptors are located at or near a body surface and receive and transmit stimuli that come from outside the body, including the receptors of the familiar five senses: sight, hearing, smell, taste, and touch. Interoceptors include the receptors for other cutaneous sensations, such as heat, cold, pain, and pressure (Figure 3–5). The interoceptors may be subdivided into receptors that receive im-

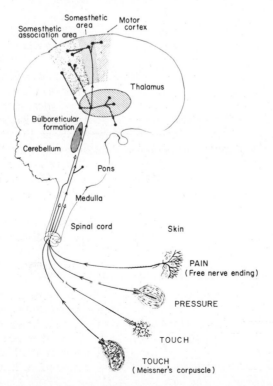

Figure 3–5 Transmission of exteroceptive sensation to the brain, showing the sensory receptors and the nerve pathways into the brain. (From Guyton, A. C.: *Function of the human body.* 4th ed. Philadelphia: W. B. Saunders, 1974.)

pulses from the viscera and those that receive impulses from the tissues directly concerned with musculoskeletal movements and positions. The former are known as visceroceptors, and the latter are called proprioceptors.

Proprioceptors

It is the proprioceptors in which students of motor activity and posture are especially interested, for these are the receptors that receive impulses that occur because of body movements or positions. They are located in the muscles, tendons, and joints, including the surrounding and protective tissues such as capsules, ligaments, and other fibrous membranes, and in the labyrinth of the inner ear. The proprioceptors are stimulated by motions of the body and in turn are responsible for transmitting a constant flow of information from these structures to the central nervous system. This information involves the appropriateness of the response in regard to the degree, direction, and rate of change of body movements. Without these sensory reports effective coordination in motor patterns would not occur. Information from the receptors is directed both to the conscious and unconscious levels and, in addition to giving us a sense of awareness of body and limb positions, provides us with automatic

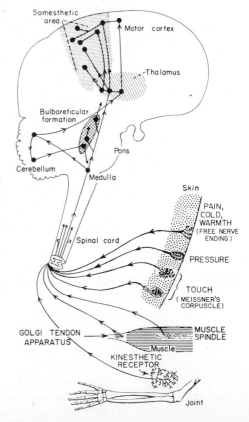

Figure 3–6 Transmission of proprioceptive sensations to the brain, showing the sensory receptors and the nerve pathways for transmitting these sensations into the brain. (From Guyton, A. C.: *Textbook of medical physiology.* 5th ed. Philadelphia: W. B. Saunders, 1976.)

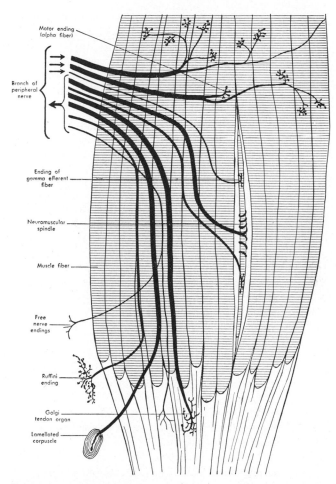

Motor ending
(alpha fiber)

Branch of
peripheral
nerve

Ending of
gamma efferent
fiber

Neuromuscular
spindle

Muscle fiber

Free
nerve
endings

Ruffini
ending

Golgi
tendon organ

Lamellated
corpuscle

Figure 3–7 Schematic representation of a muscle and its nerve supply. (From Gardner, E.: *Fundamentals of neurology.* 6th ed. Philadelphia: W. B. Saunders, 1975.)

reflexes. Proprioceptors are classified as muscle proprioceptors (muscle spindles and Golgi tendon organs), joint and skin proprioceptors (Ruffini endings and pacinian corpuscles), and labyrinthine and neck proprioceptors (Figures 3–6 and 3–7).

Muscle Proprio-ceptors

An abundance of these two types of receptors are located within muscles and tendons. Both are responsive to stretch tension. The muscle spindle detects relative muscle length and the Golgi tendon organ (GTO) detects muscle tension and active contraction.

MUSCLE SPINDLES The muscle spindles are scattered throughout the fleshy part of the muscle, lying between the muscle fibers and parallel with them. When the spindle is stretched a sensory nerve located in its center sends impulses to the CNS, which in turn activates the motor neurons innervating the muscle, thus causing it to contract. The muscle spindle is responsive to both length (tonic response) and rate of change in length (phasic response). A single spindle is a tiny capsule (about 1 mm long), filled with fluid and containing some specialized muscle fibers known as intrafusal fibers to distinguish them from the extrafusal or "regular" muscle fibers. There are two kinds of these fibers, *nuclear bag fibers* and *nuclear chain fibers* (Figure 3–8). They are similar in that they both have central noncontractile areas in which the nuclei are situated, and both have polar ends that are contractile. They differ in size and in the arrangement of the nuclei. The nuclear bag fiber is the larger of the two, and the nuclei appear crowded into the baglike central area, which gives the fiber its name. The small nuclear chain fiber is named for the single line, chainlike arrangement of the nuclei in its slim, noncontractile central portion. There are differences also in the intricate system of innervation.

Each spindle is supplied with one afferent neuron which has a characteristic ending known as the *primary* or *annulospiral* ending. This ending is divided into as many branches as there are intrafusal fibers, and each branch is coiled around the noncontractile midsection of the intrafusal fiber. The annulospiral (AS) ending is highly sensitive to changes in fiber length (phasic response), but only while the change is occurring. It also reacts to static (tonic) or length responses but with a sharp decline in frequency of impulse.

Most muscle spindles also have from one to five sensory endings which, because of their appearance, are given the picturesque name of *flower-spray (FS)* endings. Each FS ending has its own sensory fiber. The FS endings (also called *secondary* endings) are found at either end of the noncontractile midsection of the intrafusal fibers. They are believed to register static muscular length only (tonic response). The impulses transmitted by the FS endings increase almost directly in proportion to the amount of stretch, and continue for a prolonged period of time. The FS endings are less sensitive to muscle stretch than the AS endings, and therefore require a greater stimulus before responding. Since both the AS and FS endings innervate the nuclear chain fibers it is assumed that these fibers are responsible for the static response of both AS and FS endings. In contrast only the AS endings innervate the nuclear bag fibers. These fibers, then, must be responsible for the strong phasic response of the AS endings (Gowitzke and Milner, 1980).

Muscle spindles are also supplied with their own small efferent fibers. To differentiate these fibers from the motor neurons of the "regular" muscle fibers they are

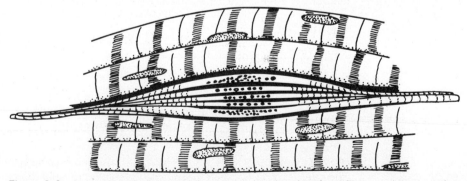

Figure 3–8   A muscle spindle containing two nuclear bag intrafusal fibers and three nuclear chain fibers, shown as it lies in parallel with the contractile (extrafusal) fibers of the muscle. Innervation is omitted. (From Gardner, E. B.: Proprioceptive reflexes and their participation in motor skills. *Quest* XII:4, 1969.)

termed *gamma fibers,* in contrast to the "regular" motor neurons whose axons are termed *alpha fibers* (Figure 3–7). As a group, the gamma fibers form a *gamma fiber system.* Impulses conveyed by gamma fibers (also called gamma efferents) cause the intrafusal muscle fibers to contract. This shortening of the spindle muscle fibers stretches their central noncontractile region where the AS endings are situated, and this stimulates them, causing their rate of firing to increase. Hence the effect of the gamma system is to increase the sensitivity of the spindle afferents. The AS endings can be caused to fire, not only by passive stretch of the muscle as a whole but also in the absence of such stretch by the function of the gamma system.

An exaggerated but familiar example of a single adjustment of this nature is seen when picking up an object that is thought to be heavy. When the opposite proves to be the case the correction in muscular effort is almost instantaneous. Less spectacular examples of this kind of coordination occur in all movements all the time. The gamma system provides a means of maintaining a position regardless of the tension put on it, and enables smooth rather than jerky muscle response (Guyton, 1976).

In summary, there are two different ways in which a muscle spindle can be stimulated: (1) by stretching the whole muscle, causing the spindle to stretch; and (2) by contracting the ends of the intrafusal fibers via the gamma efferent system, thus stretching the center receptor portion of the spindle. The muscle spindle response is *tonic* in reacting to a static length and *phasic* in reacting to a change in length. Primary (AS) endings are sensitive to both tonic and phasic stretches but secondary (FS) endings respond only to tonic stretch. Muscle spindles are very complex organs that are responsible for controlling the coordination of our muscular behavior. The feedback, which they keep supplying continually, assures a constant adjustment of muscular contraction.

GOLGI TENDON ORGAN   In contrast to the muscle spindle, the *Golgi tendon organ,* when stretched, sends signals to the central nervous system and causes the muscle to relax rather than contract. It consists of a mass of nerve endings, which are enclosed within a connective tissue capsule and embedded in a muscle tendon (Figure 3–7). It is situated close to the junction of the tendon with the fleshy part of the muscle in such a way that it has an end-to-end relationship with the muscle fibers. As the muscle shortens in contraction, the tension in the tendon increases and the Golgi tendon organs are stretched and activated. They are much less sensitive to stretch than spindles and require a stronger stretch to be activated. When the stress is greater than the Golgi tendon organ stretch threshold, the reflex contraction due to spindle stimulation is overridden and the muscle relaxes. The Golgi tendon organ provides instantaneous information of the degree of tension on each small segment of muscle. It is therefore a protective mechanism and, when the tension is extreme, its inhibitory effect can be great enough to effect a whole muscle relaxation.

Joint and Skin Proprioceptors

Two important receptors located in the joints or skin are the *pacinian corpuscles* and the *Ruffini endings.* Pacinian corpuscles are found beneath the skin, concentrated in regions around the joint capsules and tendon sheaths. They are large end-organs consisting of a tip of nerve fiber surrounded by many concentric layers of capsule. They are activated by pressure which compresses and distorts the capsule, but only for a very brief period of time. Consequently they are important for detecting rapid changes in pressure but useless for constant pressure awareness. In running, the information provided by the pacinian corpuscles allows the nervous system to predict where the feet will be at any time so that appropriate adjustments in limb position can be anticipated and effected as needed (Guyton, 1976). *Ruffini endings* are also activated by mechanical deformation but, in contrast to the pacinian corpuscles, are important for signaling continuous states of pressure. They adapt slowly at first but then transmit a steady signal thereafter. Ruffini endings are located in the deep layers of the skin and are scattered throughout the collagenous fibers of the joint capsules. They are stimulated strongly by sudden joint movements and are thus important in sensing joint position and changes in joint angle of as little as two degrees. Each joint receptor monitors a specific section of the total range of motion of the joint. By knowing which receptor is stimulated, the brain can tell how far the joint is bent. The sensing of the complete movement by the central nervous system is the result of the integration of the stimuli received from the individual receptors.

Although *cutaneous* receptors are fundamentally exteroceptors, the ones that receive stimuli from touch, pressure, and pain serve as proprioceptors when they show sensitivity to texture, hardness-softness, and shape, and when they participate in the pain or flexion withdrawal reflex and the extensor thrust reflex.

Labyrinthine and Neck Proprioceptors

These proprioceptors detect sensations concerned with determination of body position and changes in position as they relate to equilibrium. The labyrinths detect orientation and movements only in the head, whereas the neck proprioceptors inform the nervous system of the orientation of the head to the body.

The labyrinths of the inner ear consist of the cochlea, the three semicircular canals, and the utricle and saccule. The cochlea is concerned with hearing but the rest of the labyrinth is concerned with the sense of balance, or equilibrium. Each of the canals contains a membranous tube, and the bony spaces for the macule of the utricle and the saccule contain membranous sacs correspondingly named. The entire membranous labyrinth, filled with fluid, consists of hair cells that are sensitive to the movement of the fluid as the head moves, and these are intimately related to branches of the eighth cranial nerve. Thus, movement of the head is translated into nerve impulses that reach the brain.

The hair cells located in the macule and the saccule have, in addition, an overlying gelatinous substance in which otoliths (small carbonate of lime crystals) are embedded. The otoliths accentuate the effects of gravity on the hair cells, and thus are able to detect changes in position that upset static equilibrium. They are also sensitive to linear acceleration by the head.

The semicircular canals are each in a different plane at right angles to each other. When the head turns, the canals move with it, but at first the fluid in them tends to remain stationary owing to inertia. When the head stops, the canals do also but again, because of inertia, the fluid does not stop moving immediately. This process enables the canals to detect any changes in angular velocity of the head. The anatomical arrangement of the entire labyrinth is such that some part of it is especially sensitive to any position or direction of movement of the head with respect to gravity.

The most important proprioceptive information needed for the maintenance of equilibrium is that provided by the joint receptors of the neck, since they are sensitive to the angle between the body and the head. When the head is bent in one direction, the impulses from the neck prevent the labyrinthine proprioceptors from producing a feeling of imbalance. They do this by sending signals exactly opposite to those transmitted by the labyrinth. If the entire body's orientation with respect to gravity is altered, however, the neck receptors do *not* counteract the labyrinthine receptors, and change in equilibrium is sensed.

Reflex Movement

Reflexes are integrated at various levels of the nervous system. A reflex movement is a specific pattern of response that occurs without volition and without the need of direction from the cerebrum. The anatomical basis for a reflex act is the reflex arc (Figure 3–9). This consists of an afferent neuron that comes from a receptor organ, enters the spinal cord, and there makes a synaptic connection either directly with the dendrites and the cell body of an efferent neuron, or indirectly through one or more connector neurons. The axon of the efferent neuron extends from the cord to the muscle where its distal branches terminate in muscle fibers. (It will be recalled that the axon of the efferent neuron together with all of the muscle fibers that it serves constitute a motor unit.) The point of contact between an axon and a muscle fiber is known as a myoneural junction, and also as a motor end-plate. The number of reflex arcs and the number of motor units involved depend both upon the nature of the reflex and upon the extent of muscular activity needed. Automatic reflex motions accompany all normal voluntary motion. Indeed, very few muscles in most movement patterns are under conscious control.

Exteroceptive Reflexes

Although there is some overlap, as could be inferred from the discussion of receptors, there are two main classes of reflexes related to skeletal movements, namely, exteroceptive and proprioceptive. Many of the exteroceptor reflexes exhibited by animals and man are familiar to us. A horse will twitch its skin when flies alight on it; a dog will scratch when its skin is irritated by a flea, or perhaps tickled by a man. A human being jumps when a sudden loud noise is heard. A person also blinks when a foreign body strikes the eyeball, or even threatens to strike it. Three exteroceptive reflexes which may be of special interest are the extensor thrust and flexor and crossed extensor reflexes.

Extensor Thrust Reflex

Pressure against the sole of the foot stimulates the pacinian corpuscles in the subcutaneous tissue and elicits the reflex contraction of the extensor muscles of the lower extremity. When the weight is supported by the feet the pressure of the floor is sufficient to bring about this reaction. As the weight is shifted to the balls of the foot in preparation for a jump, or to the palms of the hand in preparation for a handspring, the pressure results in the extensor thrust reflex facilitating the contractions of the

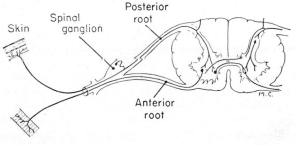

Figure 3–9 Reflex arc mechanism.

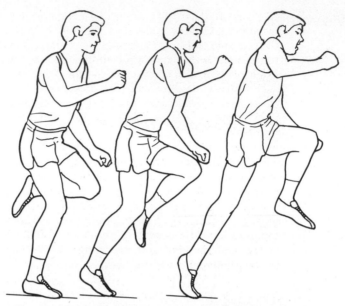

Figure 3–10   Extensor thrust reflex. As the weight is transferred to the ball of the foot in preparation for the hurdle, the concentrated pressure on the ball of the foot may enable the extensor thrust reflex to facilitate the push-off from the ground.

extensor muscles of the legs and arms, respectively, thus assisting the push-off from the floor (Deutsch, 1977; Gowitzke and Milner, 1980) (Figure 3–10). Some authorities classify this reflex as a proprioceptor rather than an exteroceptor reflex (Gellhorn, 1973) (see page 61).

Flexor Reflex

The flexor reflex most frequently operates in response to pain, and is a device for self-protection. Because of the flexor reflex we quickly withdraw a part of the body the instant it is hurt. If a finger is pricked by a pin or if it inadvertently touches a hot pan, we do not have to decide to remove our hand from the source of pain; we jerk it back even before we realize what has happened to it. Furthermore, all the necessary muscles for withdrawing it are innervated promptly, not just those in the immediate vicinity of the injury. Although we are all too aware of the pain, this awareness plays no part in the reflex action of withdrawal. The value of the awareness is rather in teaching us to avoid repetition of the act that caused the pain. This reflex is also called the withdrawal reflex.

Crossed Extensor Reflex

This reflex functions cooperatively with the flexor reflex in response to pain in a weight-bearing limb. For instance, when an animal injures its paw, the flexor reflex causes it to withdraw the paw. Simultaneously, owing to the crossed extensor reflex, the extensor muscles of the opposite limb contract to support the additional weight thrust upon it. Similarly, if a man who is barefoot happens to step on a tack with his right foot he quickly shifts his weight to his left foot and withdraws his right foot from the floor. As the flexors of his right limb contract to enable him to lift his foot, the extensors of his left limb contract more strongly to support the weight of his entire body.

Guyton (1974) also cites the example of a non-weight-bearing limb in man responding in like manner. For example, if a pain stimulus is applied to one hand, at the same moment that the hand is withdrawn, the opposite arm will extend as though to push the body away. Most authorities, however, appear to look upon the crossed extensor reflex as a mechanism for providing support for the body when one foot has been lifted.

Proprioceptive Reflexes

Earlier in this chapter receptors were classified as exteroceptors and interoceptors, the latter being subdivided into visceral receptors and proprioceptors. Proprioceptive reflexes are generally described as those reflexes that occur in response to stimulation of receptors located in the skeletal muscles, tendons, joints, and labyrinths of the inner ear. According to this interpretation the proprioceptive reflexes are those interoceptors related to motions and positions of the body. The stretch or myotatic reflex is always included among these. Some classifications also include the extensor thrust, the labyrinth and neck, and the tendon organ reflex.

Stretch Reflex

Many texts use the term *myotatic reflex* synonymously with *stretch reflex*; this would appear to be logical, since the word comes from the Greek words for muscle *(mys)* and stretching *(tasis)* (Gardner, 1975). Other authorities classify stretch reflexes as a special type of myotatic reflex. This should not disturb the student, however, for it is obvious that these classifications are man-made devices for facilitating study and research. It is not surprising for there to be discrepancies in such classifications and even in the interpretation of the same classification. This type of reflex is called the stretch reflex because stretch of the muscle excites the muscle spindle, causing in turn a reflex contraction of the muscle and relaxation of its antagonists. The muscle spindle picks up the stretch stimulus and transmits it by way of the afferent neuron to the spinal cord. There the central terminal branches of the sensory neuron synapse directly with the dendrites of the motor neuron, which innervates the same muscle fibers that were stretched. These fibers then contract. This is the simplest type of reflex arc and is commonly known as a monosynaptic arc. Gardner (1975) prefers the term "two-neuron reflex arc" and describes it as involving "one area of synaptic junction." This is more accurate, since an arc consisting of a single sensory neuron and a single motor neuron is not restricted to a single synapse. The important characteristic of this type of reflex arc is that it does not make use of connector neurons in the spinal cord. (Many authorities state that *all* stretch reflexes have this characteristic, but some state more cautiously that *most* of them do.)

Gardner (1969) classifies stretch reflexes as phasic and static (tonic) types. The phasic type is the kind described above, and includes familiar clinical tests, such as the knee jerk. Reflexes of this type are extremely rapid and the contraction is of brief duration. The word "jerk" gives an accurate picture. While it is true that the cause of the stimulus in this instance is exteroceptive in nature (a rubber-headed hammer or the edge of the hand) it is nevertheless classed as a proprioceptive reflex. If the stretch is sudden and sufficiently strong the stretched muscle contracts quickly and forcefully because of the response of the primary endings of the muscle spindles. The speed and extent of the preparatory movement (the stretch) affects the phasic and tonic response frequencies, which in turn affect the amount of involuntary contraction of the stretched muscle.

Movements that put muscles on a stretch in the backswing or preparatory phase can take advantage of the stretch reflex. If the desired outcome is a strong application of force the preparatory movement should be rapid to benefit from the *phasic* increase in spindle discharge and long to increase the *tonic* response. The backswing in forceful striking and throwing patterns, the crouch before a vertical jump, and the stretch before a tuck dive are all examples (Figure 3–11A). If, however, the desired outcome is accuracy, as in a badminton low serve or a golf putt, the backswing should be short and slow with a pause before the force application (Figure 3–11B). This approach allows the phasic frequencies of the primary endings to slow down to tonic level. (The spindle's phasic response occurs at a higher activity level than the spindle's tonic response.) (Deutsch, 1977; Gardner, 1969; Gowitzke and Milner, 1980).

In the static type of stretch reflex the muscle is stretched slowly. This causes primary and secondary endings of several spindles to be stimulated, and results in a more sustained muscular contraction. The importance of the static stretch is that it causes muscle contraction as long as a muscle is put on excessive stretch. When such a reflex is elicited by the stretch caused by the tendency of weight-bearing joints to flex, the response of the extensor muscles is commonly referred to as the *antigravity reflex*. This term is also used by some to include the response of lower extremity and trunk muscles to the involuntary forward-backward swaying that usually occurs when a person stands in one position for a long time.

Ralston and Libet, who have made extensive electromyographic studies of muscular action, apparently do not accept this concept of an antigravity reflex. In 1953 they stated that investigators did not find electrical activity accompanying stretch unless the stretch was of such speed that it invoked the jerk type of reflex. They also stated that the short bursts of activity that accompanied swaying were apparently not simple stretch reflexes, in spite of the fact that they were probably initiated by local stretch receptor impulses. As evidence of the latter conclusion they stated that the contraction of the tibialis anterior and the soleus, which had been observed in a ''standing at ease'' position, was initiated by a degree of angular motion at the ankle joint that they claimed was far less than that required to elicit a stretch reflex. They concluded that the hypothesis that stretch reflex discharge occurs automatically to help maintain a given postural attitude in normal man was not supported by the available evidence. In 1957 Ralston reaffirmed this conclusion. Clearly this matter needs further investigation.

There are instances when it would be desirable to minimize the effect of the stretch reflex, as in flexibility exercises. This can be done if the stretch is done slowly and is held, as in static stretching. A quick stretch or bounce will evoke the reflex contraction.

Tendon Reflex   When tension is produced by muscle fibers, the Golgi tendon organs, which are located at the musculoskeletal juncture, are stimulated and signals are sent to the spinal cord. The reflex effect is to inhibit impulses from the motor nerve to the muscle, thus causing the muscle to relax. When tension on the muscle is extreme, the Golgi tendon organs' inhibiting action results in sudden relaxation of the muscle. This effect is called the *lengthening reaction,* and undoubtedly serves as protection for muscles or tendons that could be torn or ruptured by the strong contractile force. Guyton (1976) has suggested that the tendon reflex serves as a feedback mechanism to control the tension in the muscle. If the tension in the muscle became too great, the inhibiting

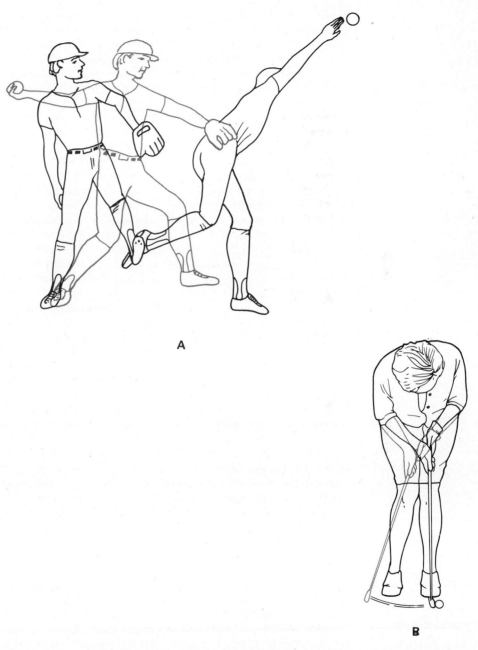

A

B

Figure 3–11 *A,* The phasic type of stretch reflex will facilitate force development if the backswing is long and rapid with little pause between the backswing and force phase as demonstrated in a forceful overarm throw. *B,* To take advantage of the tonic type of stretch reflex when accuracy is desired, the backswing should be short and slow, with a pause before the force phase. An example is the golf putt.

action of the receptors would cause relaxation. If the muscle tension became too little, the receptors would stop firing, and the muscle tension would be able to increase. The precise way in which this would happen is as yet unexplained.

The behavior of the tendon reflex in the performance of some skills by beginners is also a matter of interest. Gardner (1969) has speculated that the reason beginners do not follow through has to do with the fact that the tendon reflex causes relaxation of vigorously contracting muscle. It is suggested that until an increase in the Golgi tendon organ threshold develops with learning, beginners may need voluntary effort to counteract the inhibitory effect of the tendon organ reflex.

Labyrinth and Neck Reflexes

Newborn infants start out with very simple reflexes, which in the process of normal motor development are suppressed or modified. This phenomenon is especially evident in the labyrinth and neck reflexes. The tonic labyrinth reflexes emanate from utricle and semicircular canal receptors, which are sensitive to changes in position of the head with respect to gravity. Because of the primitive tonic labyrinth reflex present in the newborn child, a supine position of the head facilitates extension of the extremities, while a prone position inhibits extension and facilitates flexion. At a few months of age or more this primitive reflex is suppressed, and the labyrinth righting reflex is evident. In cooperation with other righting reflexes of the neck and eyes, it evokes muscular responses to restore the body to a normal upright position.

Righting reflexes can be demonstrated in adults. They respond to any body-tilting action by attempting to restore balance through facilitating limb actions, such as an arm or leg being thrust out. In spinning, the limbs facilitate restoration of the normal head position by actions that inhibit the rotation. The arm on the same side as the direction of the spin is thrust out during the spin, and the opposite arm is thrust out at the termination of the spin. This latter action is probably a response to the imbalance caused by the dizziness experienced at the conclusion of the spin.

Tonic neck reflexes are evident when the joint receptors in the neck are stimulated because of any movement in the neck. They are also present at birth and, even though they are masked by further development, they remain in adults. Like the tonic labyrinth reflex, they can also be demonstrated in adults. Actions due to tonic neck reflexes in the primitive infant form are predictable. If the head is flexed, flexion will occur in the upper extremities and extension in the lower ones. With head extension, the opposite occurs—extension in the upper extremities and flexion in the lower ones. Rotation of the head to the right is accompanied by extension and abduction of the limbs on the chin side, and flexion and adduction on the opposite side.

Tonic neck and tonic labyrinth reflexes become most apparent in adults in stressful situations. They are hard to distinguish from each other because movements of the head and neck occur together and labyrinth and neck receptors are stimulated simultaneously. In some instances they reinforce each other in their effect on joint actions of the extremities and in some instances they oppose each other. There are times when we should take advantage of them to facilitate actions, and other times when it would be beneficial to suppress them.

Gardner (1969) states that the neck reflexes are more effective in modifying upper extremity actions and the labyrinthine in modifying those of the lower extremities. There is no question that head position influences the actions of the arms. When a strong pulling action is required, flexion of the head will facilitate it. On the other hand, the neck reflex facilitation suggests that the head should be extended for strong pushing actions. For facilitating a one-armed pull, the head should be turned away in addition to being flexed and, in a one-armed push, the head should be turned toward the pushing arm. Other examples of reflex facilitation include extension of the head in a handstand to reinforce extension in the arms, flexion of the head to reinforce trunk, arms, and leg flexion in forward or backward rolls, and head rotation in archery to facilitate bow arm pushing on the chin side and bowstring arm pulling by the opposite side (Deutsch, 1977; Gowitzke and Milner, 1980).

Undoubtedly one of the difficulties in learning new motor skills is the failure to suppress reflex responses. In falling backward, our natural reaction is to extend the arms and throw the head forward. If a beginner did this in attempting a back dive, the entry into the water would be uncomfortable, to say the least. The labyrinth righting reflex must be suppressed consciously so that the head may be extended back and the body follow. Belly flops in front dives can also be attributed to the labyrinth righting reflex (Gardner, 1969).

Posture and Locomotor Mechanisms

Whether due to reflex action or to some other mechanism, it seems apparent that there are certain provisions in the human body for remaining more or less erect and for engaging in locomotion, and that these follow the general pattern of reflex behavior. The coordinated efforts of the body to resist the downward pull of gravity include the extensor thrust reflex, the static type of stretch reflex in response to gravitational pull, the muscular action evoked by forward-backward swaying, and the various mechanisms for preserving equilibrium, including visual orientation and labyrinthine reflexes.

In regard to locomotion, the action of the legs of a four-footed animal has been attributed to reflex action. Some classify this reflex as a division of the crossed extensor reflex (Ruch and Patton, 1979); others refer to it simply as a walking reflex (Guyton, 1974). Because research in this area has been done primarily on dogs and cats it has been suggested that this reflex exists only in quadrupeds. Nevertheless, it is logical to assume that it exists also in man inasmuch as the early forms of locomotion—creeping and crawling—resemble the locomotion of quadrupeds. Even after the erect position is assumed, the swing of the arms in opposition to the lower extremities reflects the earlier four-footed gait.

Volitional Movement

This topic involves such an extensive and complex body of knowledge that only the bare essentials and a few of the newer concepts can be touched upon here. The chief anatomical structures concerned with volitional movement, in addition to those mentioned earlier (skeletal muscle, basic nerve structures, motor units, and sensory receptors) are the cerebral cortex, the cerebellum, the brain stem, the corticospinal tracts, and the numerous motor pathways, both pyramidal and extrapyramidal.

The portion of the cerebral cortex in which impulses for the majority of volitional acts are thought to arise is the fold situated just in front of the transverse central fissure. Because of its location, this is known as the precentral gyrus, and because it was originally thought to consist entirely of motor cells, it is referred to as the motor

Figure 3–12 Integration of sensory signals from several different sources into a common thought by the common integrative area of the brain, showing also the primary and association areas for vision, for auditory sensations, and for somesthetic sensations. (From Guyton, A. C.: *Function of the human body.* 4th ed. Philadelphia: W. B. Saunders, 1974.)

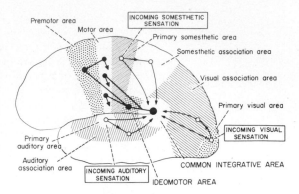

area of the cortex (Figure 3–12). In front of this area is another area having to do with movement. It is called the premotor area and is thought to be responsible for the more complex movement patterns (Gellhorn, 1973; Guyton, 1974).

Regarding the topography of the motor area, it used to be thought that this area was divided into distinct subareas, each of which was solely responsible for the contraction of particular muscles or groups of muscles. However, studies have revealed that there is considerable overlapping of motor unit territories (Gellhorn, 1973; Harrison, 1962). This appears to be a provision for the performance of complex movement patterns as well as for a variety of movement combinations.

The axons of the motor cells, called Betz's cells, descend through the brain stem and the spinal cord. Together these axons form the corticospinal tracts. They pass through the anterior portions of the medulla which constitute the pyramids, and it is here that most of the fibers cross to the opposite side. Because of their route through pyramids the fibers are known collectively as the pyramidal system and their cell bodies as pyramidal cells. The fibers from the premotor area and from other parts of the cortex do not pass through the medulla pyramids; hence they are referred to as the extrapyramidal system.

It was originally thought that the pyramidal system consisted exclusively of Betz cell axons. More recently, however, it has been discovered that the majority of pyramidal fibers actually come from cortical cells outside of the traditional motor area, and that the extrapyramidal system also includes many fibers from the motor area. Furthermore, the precentral gyrus is no longer thought to be exclusively a motor area, but rather a sensorimotor area because it is now known to receive some afferent impulses. There is experimental evidence to show that proprioceptive impulses have been received by the motor area after the sensory area in the postcentral gyrus had been removed (Gellhorn, 1973).

One of the most important of the concepts concerning volitional movement is that continued sensory stimulation is essential to motor unit function. There has been ample clinical evidence to show that when sensory innervation is impaired there is a noticeable impairment of volitional movement. It is realized now that for the successful and appropriate execution of volitional acts, sensory stimuli are as indispensable as motor stimuli. This is true throughout all stages of the movement (Gellhorn, 1973; Harrison, 1962). It is obvious from this that the stimulus-response concept, as formerly interpreted, is no longer adequate for explaining volitional acts (Harrison, 1962).

It has been discovered that the position of a limb is a factor in the intensity of response when a given muscle is made to contract by means of cortical stimulation.

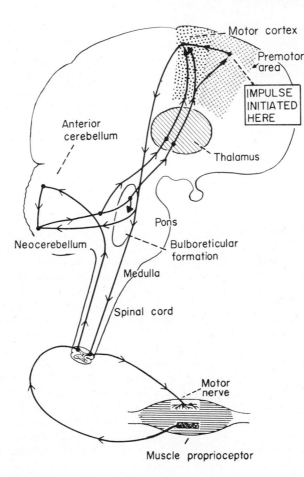

Figure 3–13 Feedback circuits of the cerebellum for damping motor movements. (From Guyton, A. C.: *Function of the human body.* 4th ed. Philadelphia: W. B. Saunders, 1974.)

For instance, in an electromyographic study of the triceps muscle, it was found that the response of the muscle to stimulation of the appropriate cortical area differed according to the size of the angle at the elbow joint. When the joint angle was acute, the response of the triceps to cortical stimulation was stronger than when the joint angle was obtuse. The significance of this experiment is the evidence it presents of the part played by the proprioceptors in relaying information about the position of the joint (Gellhorn, 1973; Harrison, 1962).

A concept that has received wide attention is known as the reafferent or servomechanism concept of overt behavior (Harrison, 1962). This mechanism is responsible for feeding back inhibitory impulses to motor neurons and thereby keeping the discharge frequency of the latter under control and safeguarding them against possible convulsive activity (Harrison, 1962; Loofbourrow, 1973).

Many of the structures and mechanisms that influence volitional movement belong to the extrapyramidal system. Among these is the cerebellum, which has the important task of controlling the timing and governing the intensity with which the muscles contract (Figure 3–13). There is also the reticular formation in the brain stem, a mechanism for exerting facilitatory and inhibitory influence on spinal centers, especially the centers for the antigravity muscles, and thus providing for finer coordinations (Loufbourrow, 1973). The thalamus in the brain stem is responsible for receiving sensory impulses and integrating them in coordinated patterns of movement, and the hypothalamus, which responds to emotional stimuli, is responsible for eliciting increased muscle power (Gellhorn, 1973). These are but a few of the ways in which the pyramidal and the extrapyramidal systems are seen to work together in volitional movement.

Kinesthesis

The conscious awareness of position of body parts and the amount and rate of joint movement is known as kinesthesis. Kinesthetic sensations originate primarily in the sensory receptors of the joint capsules and ligaments and include the Ruffini endings, pacinian corpuscles, and Golgi tendon organs. Signals from these receptors are transmitted rapidly to the cord and brain in beta type A nerve fibers so that the central nervous system is aware of the exact position of the body parts instantaneously. Without this rapid transmission and processing of information, accurately controlled movements could not proceed. Kinesthetic perception and memory are the basis of voluntary movement and motor learning. This perception and memory enables the performer to initiate a whole movement pattern or modify a part of it, such as the elimination or addition of a joint action, or a change in timing or speed of an action.

Reciprocal Innervation and Inhibition

One of the mechanisms that provides for economical and coordinated movement is the one known as reciprocal innervation and inhibition, first described by Sherrington. According to this concept, when motor neurons are transmitting impulses to muscles, causing them to contract, the motor neurons that supply their antagonists are simultaneously and reciprocally inhibited. The antagonistic muscles, therefore, remain relaxed and the movers, or agonists, contract without opposition. Reciprocal inhibition operates automatically in movements elicited by the stretch reflex and also in familiar volitional movements. In more complicated and in less familiar coordinations its operation depends upon the degree of skill developed by the performer.

Not all investigators are in agreement with respect to the operation of reciprocal innervation and inhibition in volitional movement. Some believe that muscles that are antagonistic to each other do contract concurrently under certain conditions, and they refer to this as cocontraction (see page 46). Others are of the opinion that simultaneous contraction of antagonistic muscles, when it does occur, is indicative of unskillful performance, and that skillful performance is characterized by the absence of antagonistic action (Basmajian, 1979; Gowitzke and Milner, 1980).

Laboratory Experiences

1. Engage a partner in Indian arm wrestling until one of you loses. Explain the *sudden* cessation of muscle tension in the loser which resulted in the end of the contest.

2. *a.* Practice throwing a badminton bird at a small target, such as a clipboard or notebook held by a partner 15–20 feet away from you. After several practice trials, close your eyes and throw at the target 10 times. After each throw your partner will tell you the result (too high, too low, too far left, and so forth, and the distance of 1, 2, 3, . . . , feet). Record the results after each throw.

    b. Change places with your partner, who will now have the same number of trials (10) with no practice and with eyes open. Record the results.

    c. Change places. With eyes open and no practice, take 10 trials to throw at the target. Record the results.

    d. Change places. Your partner should now throw 10 times with eyes closed and no practice trials. Report the results to your partner (as in *2a*) after each trial, recording the results.

    e. Compare the results in terms of success, order of sighted and unsighted throws, and effects of corrections. Discuss the involvement and influence of proprioceptors in this exercise.

3. Ask your partner to stand and face you with eyes closed. By moving body segments place your partner in some novel pose. Ask your partner, with eyes still closed, to describe the position exactly. After once again assuming the original standing position, ask your partner to reproduce the novel position. Explain the neuromuscular mechanisms that enable your partner to sense and reproduce the movement.

4. Record the distance of your best of three standing broad jumps. Repeat the jumps, but this time flex the head and neck vigorously as the legs are extended. After a few practice trials record the distance of the three jumps, which incorporate the reflex pattern. Compare your results with those of others in the class. What effect did the reflex pattern have? Explain.

5. Stand in a doorway with your arms at your side. Now press the backs of your hands strongly against the door jambs. Hold this position for at least 30 seconds. Step clear of the doorway and turn your head to the right. What happens to your arms? Explain.

6. Perform a headstand with the top of the head in contact with the supporting surface. Now repeat with the contact closer to the forehead so that the head is hyperextended. In terms of reflex facilitation, which position is better? Explain.

7. Look at the sequence of film tracings for the backward somersault depicted in Figure 5–6 in Appendix I. Which proprioceptive reflexes could be present in the position represented in Frame A? For each reflex named state the evidence which would suggest the presence of the reflex, the expected effect the reflex could have on the movement, and the verification of the effect as shown by the action in the next frames. Were there any expected reflex actions that apparently did not occur? Explain.

References

Basmajian, J. V. 1979. *Muscles alive.* 4th ed. Baltimore: Williams & Wilkins.

Deutsch, H. 1977. Inclusion of neuromuscular aspects of human motion in undergraduate kinesiology. In *Kinesiology: A national conference on teaching,* ed. C. J. Dillman and R. G. Sears, pp. 361–64. Urbana-Champaign: University of Illinois.

de Vries, H. A. 1974. *Physiology of exercise.* 2d ed. Dubuque, Iowa: William C. Brown.

Eldred, E. 1965. The dual sensory role of muscle spindles. *J. Am. Phys. Ther. Assoc.* 45:290–313.

Gardner, E. B. 1969. Proprioceptive reflexes and their participation in motor skills. *Quest,* monograph XII, 1:25

Gardner, E. 1975. *Fundamentals of neurology.* 6th ed. Philadelphia: W. B. Saunders.

Gellhorn, E. 1973. The physiology of the supraspinal mechanism. In *Science and medicine of exercise and sports,* 2d ed., ed. W. R. Johnson and E. Buskirk. New York: Harper & Row.

Gowitzke, B. A., and Milner, M. 1980. *Understanding the scientific bases of human movement.* 2d ed. Baltimore: Williams & Wilkins.

Guyton, A. C. 1974. *Function of the human body.* 4th ed. Philadelphia: W. B. Saunders.

Guyton, A. C. 1976. *Textbook of medical physiology.* 5th ed. Philadelphia: W. B. Saunders.

Harrison, V. F. 1962. Review of the neuromuscular bases for motor learning. *Res. Q. Am. Assoc. Health Phys. Educ.,* 33:59–69.

Huxley, H. E. 1958. The contraction of muscle. *Sci. Am.* (offprint).

Loofbourrow, G. N. 1973. Neuromuscular integration. In *Science and medicine of exercise and sports,* 2d ed., ed. W. R. Johnson and E. Buskirk. New York: Harper & Row.

Ralston, H. J. 1957. Recent advances in neuromuscular physiology. *Am. J. Phys. Med.* 36:94–120.

Ralston, H. J., and Libet, B. 1953. The question of tonus in skeletal muscle. *Am. J. Phys. Med.* 32:85–92.

Ruch, T. C., and Patton, H. D. 1979. *Physiology and biophysics.* 20th ed. Philadelphia: W. B. Saunders.

The Upper Extremity: The Shoulder Region

Objectives

At the conclusion of this chapter, the student should be able to:

1. Name, locate, and describe the structure and ligamentous reinforcements of the articulations of the shoulder region.
2. Name and demonstrate the movements possible in the joints of the shoulder region regardless of starting position.
3. Name and locate the muscles and muscle groups of the shoulder region, and name their primary actions as agonists, stabilizers, neutralizers, or antagonists.
4. Analyze the fundamental movements of the arm and trunk with respect to joint and muscle actions.
5. Describe the common athletic injuries of the shoulder region.

Introduction

Anatomical cooperation is beautifully illustrated in the movements of the arms on the trunk. The arm travels through a wide range of movements, and in each of these the scapula cooperates by placing the glenoid fossa in the most favorable position for the head of the humerus. When the arm is elevated sideward, for instance, the scapula rotates upward; when it is elevated forward, the scapula not only rotates upward but it tends to slide partially around the rib cage. Occasionally this movement is deliberately repressed, as in the arm placings and flingings of the old Swedish type of calisthenics, in stylized dance movements, and in some posture exercises, but in all natural movements, the scapula shares with the humerus in the movements of the arm on the trunk. In abduction, scapular and glenohumeral movements are continuous throughout the range of motion regardless of the resistance applied. After studying this relationship, Doody et al. (1970) concluded that:

> The movements of the scapula and humerus were continuous throughout the abduction, irrespective of the application of resistance, and without added stress, the scapular movement accounted for 58.62 degrees of the total movement, and the humerus for 112.52 degrees.
>
> What they called the "scapulohumeral rhythm" was found to vary among individuals, with some subjects experiencing a reverse rotation for the first 30 to 60 degrees of abduction.
>
> Although there was a relationship between the glenohumeral angle and the position of the arm, it could not be adequately described by a linear function.
>
> There was a continuous increase in the "mean relative amount of scapular movement" up to the position of maximum stress, which appeared to be between 90 and 140 degrees after which it fell off slightly.
>
> The scapulohumeral rhythm was affected by an increase in stress, it being noted that the scapula's major participation began earlier when stress was added and that its total contribution showed a slight decrease.

The upper extremity is suspended from the axial skeleton (head and trunk) by means of the shoulder girdle. The latter consists of the sternum and two clavicles in front, and two scapulae in back with their connecting joints, the sternoclavicular between the sternum and each clavicle and the acromioclavicular between the acromion process of each scapula and the corresponding clavicle. Since there is no union between the two scapulae in back, this is an incomplete girdle. The upper extremity's connection with the shoulder girdle is made through the glenohumeral joint, the joint between the head of the humerus and the glenoid fossa of the scapula, better known as the shoulder joint.

The sternoclavicular joint is an exceedingly small one, about the size of the joint between the great toe and the first metatarsal bone, yet it is the sole skeletal connection between the upper extremity and the trunk. This anatomical arrangement accounts for the extensive freedom of motion enjoyed by the upper extremity and is a vital factor n the superb cooperation that exists between the shoulder joint and the shoulder girdle. The upper arm has a remarkably wide range of motion owing largely to its ball and shallow socket construction. Its movements are further amplified by the cooperative actions of the shoulder girdle, as described above.

In order to understand and appreciate the great variety of movements of the arm on the trunk it is essential that one be thoroughly familiar with the structure and function of each joint involved and be able to distinguish between the contributions of each in any given movement.

The Shoulder Joint (Glenohumeral Articulation)

Structure

The shoulder joint is formed by the articulation of the spherical head of the humerus with the small, shallow, somewhat pear-shaped glenoid fossa of the scapula (Figure 4–1). It is a ball-and-socket joint. The structure of the joint and the looseness of the capsule (permitting between one and two inches of separation between the two bones) account for the remarkable mobility of the shoulder joint. Both the humeral head and

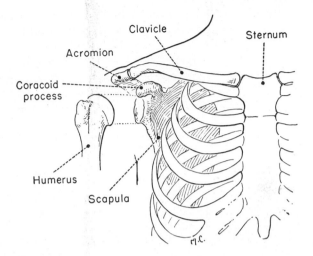

Figure 4–1 Anterior view of shoulder joint and shoulder girdle.

the glenoid fossa are covered with hyaline cartilage. The cartilage on the head is thicker at the center, while that which lines the cavity is thicker around the circumference. The glenoid fossa is further protected by a flat rim of white fibrocartilage, also thicker around the circumference. Called the glenoid labrum, this cartilage serves both to deepen the fossa and to cushion it against the impact of the humeral head in forceful movements (Figure 4–2).

The joint is completely enveloped in a loose sleevelike articular capsule which is attached proximally to the circumference of the glenoid cavity and distally to the anatomical neck of the humerus. The capsule is lined with synovial membrane which folds back over the glenoid labrum, covers all but the upper portion of the anatomical neck of the humerus, and extends through the intertubular groove in the form of a sheath for the tendon of the long head of the biceps. There are several bursae in the region of the shoulder joint. Among the larger are the one between the deltoid muscle and the capsule and the one on top of the acromion process.

Figure 4–2 Lateral view of right scapula showing glenoid cavity.

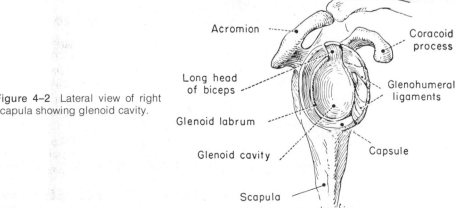

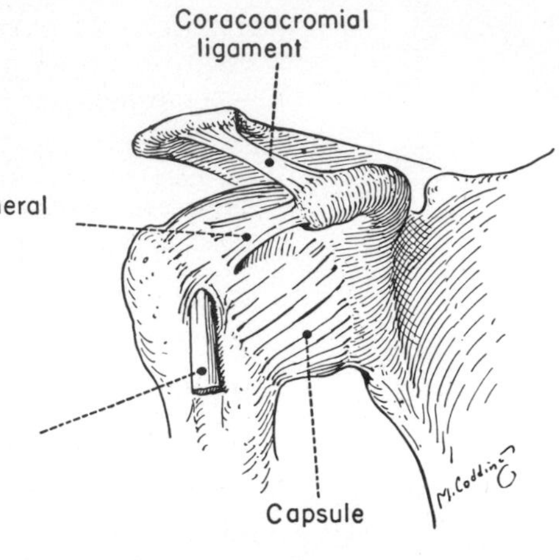

Figure 4–3 Anterior view of shoulder joint showing ligaments.

Ligamentous and Muscular Reinforcements

The shoulder joint is protected and stabilized by both ligaments and muscles. Inspection of the illustrations on these pages (supplemented by study of the table of muscular attachments in Appendix D) will help the reader to understand the relationships of the ligaments and muscles to the joints they reinforce.

The coracohumeral ligament, the three bands of the glenohumeral ligament, and the bridgelike coracoacromial ligament constitute the *ligamentous reinforcements* of the shoulder joint (Figure 4–3). *Muscular reinforcement* is provided above by the supraspinatus muscle and the long head of the biceps brachii, below by the long head of the triceps brachii, in front by the subscapularis muscle and the fibrous prolongations of both the pectoralis major and teres major muscles, and behind by the infraspinatus and teres minor muscles (see Figures 4–5 through 4–9).

Apparently these reinforcements do not prevent downward dislocation, however. Two electromyographic investigations have helped clarify the role of certain structures in stabilizing the shoulder joint and, in particular, preventing downward dislocation. In an extensive study of the shoulder region in 1944, Inman et al. noted the stabilizing function of the four muscles that constitute the "rotator cuff"—the supraspinatus, infraspinatus, teres minor, and subscapularis. In 1959 Basmajian and Bazant investigated the muscles whose fibers cross the shoulder joint vertically, as compared with those whose fibers cross it horizontally. To their surprise they discovered that it was the horizontal fibers and not the vertical that were active in preventing downward dislocation of the humerus. After doing a dissection of the shoulder joint, they agreed that the slope of the glenoid fossa was an important factor. Because of this slope, the head of the humerus was forced laterally as it was pulled downward, and it took the horizontally directed muscle fibers to check this lateral movement which, in turn, stopped the downward movement. They concluded that downward dislocation of the humerus was prevented primarily by three factors: (1) the slope of the glenoid fossa; (2) the tightening of the upper part of the capsule and of the coracohumeral ligament; and (3) the activity of the supraspinatus muscle and, to a lesser extent, of the posterior fibers of the deltoid (Basmajian, 1979).

Movements

The movements of the humerus, all of which take place at the glenohumeral articulation, are illustrated in Figure 4–4. The expected average ranges of these movements are summarized in Table 1–3. They are defined as follows:

FLEXION AND HYPERFLEXION A forward upward movement in a plane at right angles to the plane of the scapula. If the movement exceeds 180 degrees, it is hyperflexion.

EXTENSION Return movement from flexion.

HYPEREXTENSION A backward movement in a plane at right angles to the plane of the scapula.

ABDUCTION A sideward upward movement in a plane parallel with the plane of the scapula.*

ADDUCTION Return movement from abduction.

OUTWARD ROTATION A rotation of the humerus around its mechanical axis so that when the arm is in its normal resting position, the anteror aspect turns laterally.

INWARD ROTATION A rotation of the humerus around its mechanical axis so that when the arm is in its normal resting position, the anterior aspect turns medially. The full range of inward and outward rotation is best observed when the forearm is held in 90 degrees of flexion and the humerus is held in 90 degrees of abduction.

HORIZONTAL FLEXION A forward movement of the abducted humerus in a horizontal plane (i.e., from a plane parallel to the plane of the scapula to a plane at right angles to it).

HORIZONTAL EXTENSION A backward movement of the flexed humerus in a horizontal plane (i.e., from a plane at right angles to the plane of the scapula to a plane parallel to it).

CIRCUMDUCTION A combination of flexion, abduction, extension, hyperextension, and adduction performed sequentially in either direction so that the extended arm describes a cone and the fingertips a circle.

Muscles of the Shoulder Joint

Location

The muscles of the shoulder joint are listed according to their position in relation to the joint. This position is not always apparent, as a look at the illustrations will show. All muscles in this classification pass either from the trunk or the scapula to the arm.

Anterior
Pectoralis major
Coracobrachialis
Subscapularis
Biceps brachii

Posterior
Infraspinatus
Teres minor

Superior
Deltoid
Supraspinatus

Inferior
Latissimus dorsi
Teres major
Triceps brachii, long head

*Some authorities interpret abduction as the sideward movement of the arm away from the body, thus including the action of the shoulder girdle with that of the shoulder joint. When reading the literature, one should note which interpretation is intended.

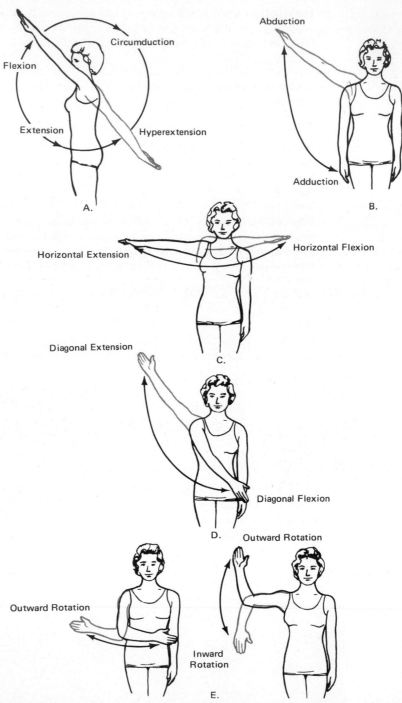

Figure 4–4 Movements of the humerus. *A,* Flexion, extension, hyperextension, circumduction. *B,* Abduction and adduction. *C,* Horizontal flexion and extension. *D,* Diagonal flexion and extension. *E,* Inward and outward rotation.

Characteristics and Functions

PECTORALIS MAJOR This large fan-shaped muscle of the chest (Figure 4–5) converges to a flat tendon, which, like that of the latissimus dorsi, twists on itself so that the lowest fibers become the uppermost at its point of attachment. The muscle is divided functionally into two parts, the clavicular and the sternal (or sternocostal). The clavicular portion lies close to the anteror deltoid muscle and acts with it in *flexion*, *horizontal flexion*, and *inward rotation* of the humerus. Participation in the latter movement, according to Scheving and Pauly, occurs only against resistance (Basmajian, 1979).

Ordinarily the line of pull of the clavicular portion of the pectoralis major lies below the axis of the shoulder joint. Steindler (1970) claims, however, that when the arm is raised sideward well above the horizontal, the line of pull of the upper clavicular fibers shifts above the center of the shoulder joint, and these fibers then cease to adduct and become abductors of the humerus (see Figure 2–4). The EMG study of Shevlin et al. (1969) supports this contention. They found that the clavicular fibers of the pectoralis major were significantly active in abduction at the level of 110 degrees. The sternocostal portion is generally antagonistic in its actions in the sagittal plane. It acts in downward and forward movements of the arm and in medial rotation when accompanied by adduction. The pectoralis major as a whole is most powerful for actions in the sagittal plane and is particularly important in all pushing, throwing, and punching activities. The clavicular portion may be palpated just below the medial two-thirds of the clavicle, the sternal portion just lateral to the sternum and below the clavicular part, and the muscle as a whole at the anterior border of the axilla.

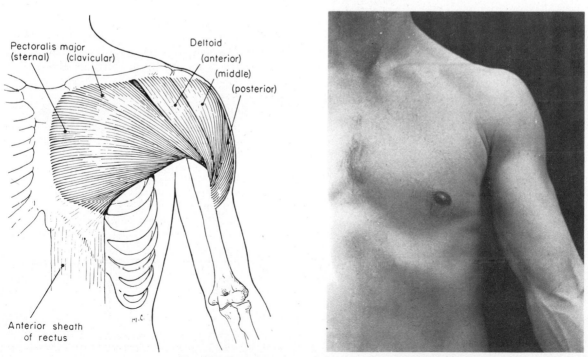

Figure 4–5   Anterior view of muscles of shoulder joint, superficial layer.

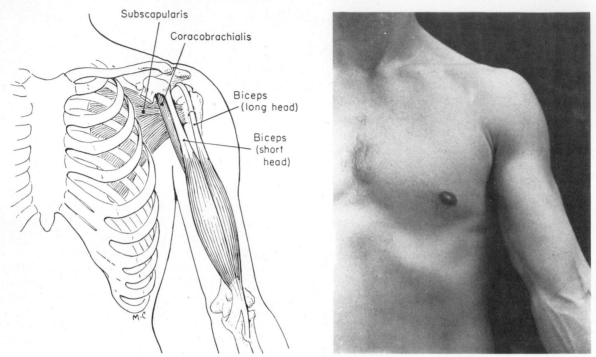

Figure 4–6   Anterior view of muscles of shoulder joint, deep layer.

CORACOBRACHIALIS   The muscle's line of pull passes in front of the shoulder joint (Figure 4–6), which suggests that it participates in *forward movements of the humerus.* Because the proximal attachment and line of pull of the coracobrachialis and the long head of the biceps are so similar it has been difficult to determine the specific actions of the coracobrachialis. However, Stevens et al. (1976) were successful in isolating and recording activity in the coracobrachialis, confirming that it serves as a main force in horizontal flexion movements. Their research also verified the belief that this muscle, the middle deltoid, and the long head of the triceps, acting like guy wires on a mast, serve to stabilize the shoulder joint. It may be palpated on the front of the upper arm between the anterior deltoid and the pectoralis major, but is a difficult muscle to identify. The method suggested by Brunnstrom (1972) is recommended.

SUBSCAPULARIS   As one of the *rotator cuff* muscles the subscapularis (Figures 4–6 and 4–7A) contributes significantly to stabilization of the glenohumeral joint, especially in the prevention of dislocation during forced lateral rotation of the abducted arm. It is also one of the depressors of the humeral head during abduction and flexion of the arm. Its chief action as a mover is inward rotation, which it performs most effectively when the arm is at the side or is elevated posteriorly. It has also shown significantly more electrical activity in horizontal extension than in horizontal flexion (Shevlin et al., 1969).

BICEPS BRACHII   Although essentially a muscle of the elbow joint, the biceps (Figure 4–6) crosses the shoulder joint and is active in some of the movements of the humerus. Both heads are always active in flexion and in abduction with resistance when the

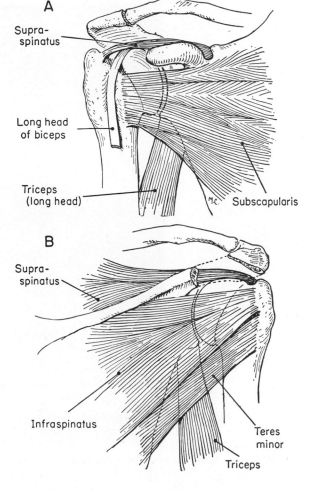

A

Supra-
spinatus

Long head
of biceps

Triceps
(long head)

Subscapularis

B

Supra-
spinatus

Infraspinatus

Teres
minor

Triceps

Figure 4-7 Muscular reinforcement of shoulder joint. *A*, Anterior view; *B*, posterior view.

elbow is straight. The muscle is also active in horizontal flexion and the short head sometimes participates in adduction against resistance and medial rotation.

DELTOID The complex structure of the deltoid (Figures 4–5 and 4–8), with the multipenniform arrangement of the bundles making up the middle portion, gives it a potential for great strength without undue bulk. The middle portion of the muscle is a *powerful abductor of the humerus*, its greatest activity occurring when the humerus is raised between 90 and 120 degrees, and it is capable of supporting the weight of the upper extremity for long periods while the hand is working at a height. The multipenniform arrangement of fibers compensates for the middle deltoid's rather poor angle of pull. The latter, however, serves the useful purpose of providing the muscle with a strong stabilizing component force. This is fortunate because in this position the shoulder joint depends more upon its muscles than upon its ligaments for holding the head of the humerus on the glenoid fossa. The middle portion has also been found to be active in horizontal extension.

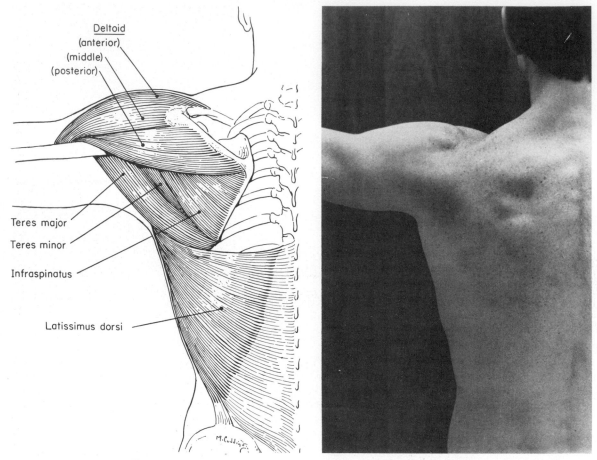

Figure 4–8   Posterior view of muscles of shoulder joint, superficial layer.

The anterior portion of the deltoid aids in *all forward movements* of the arm and in *inward rotation* of the humerus. It is also active in abduction. There is disagreement in the literature concerning the movements effected by the posterior deltoid but there seems to be sufficient evidence to conclude that, in addition to extension and lateral rotation, the lowest fibers, being situated below the axis of motion, assist in forceful adduction of the humerus from an overhead position. On the other hand, some of the upper fibers (those closest to the middle deltoid) probably act with the latter in contributing to abduction. In fact, Shevlin et al. (1969) stated that in their experiments the posterior deltoid elevated the humerus in the frontal plane (i.e., abduction) at all the levels tested (45, 90, and 110 degrees of elevation). Unfortunately they did not test above the 110-degree level; furthermore they used only one electrode for the posterior deltoid, placed "in the middle of its bulk."

SUPRASPINATUS   This muscle (Figures 4–7 and 4–9) acts together with the deltoid in abduction of the arm throughout the entire range. It also acts in flexion and horizontal extension. Action potentials reach their maximum when the arm is at 100

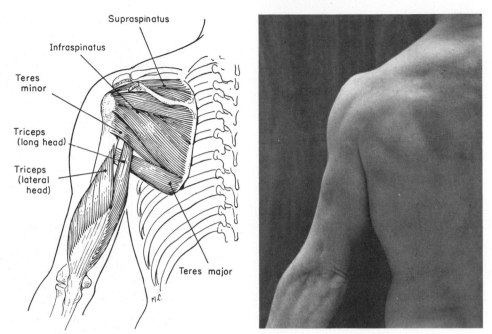

Figure 4–9 Posterior view of muscles of shoulder joint, deep layer.

degrees of flexion (Inman, 1962). As part of the rotator cuff it plays a significant part in the stability of the shoulder joint and is important in preventing downward dislocation (Basmajian, 1979). It may be palpated above the spine of the scapula, provided that the scapula is supported—e.g., when the armpit rests over the back of a chair.

INFRASPINATUS AND TERES MINOR In addition to their outward rotatory action these two muscles (Figures 4–7B, 4–8, and 4–9), which seem to act as one, have two additional noteworthy functions. Together with the subscapularis they depress the head of the humerus and thus prevent it from jamming against the acromion process during flexion and abduction of the arm. They are also part of the rotator cuff muscles (infraspinatus, teres minor, subscapularis, and supraspinatus) whose important function it is to aid materially in holding the head of the humerus in the glenoid fossa. Their important function in this capacity is to prevent dislocation of the shoulder joint, especially when the humerus is in the abducted position (Inman, 1962). They may be palpated on the posterior surface of the scapula, medial to and below the posterior deltoid muscle.

LATISSIMUS DORSI This is a broad sheet of muscle (Figure 4–8) that covers the lower and middle portions of the back. Coming mainly from the lower half of the thoracic spine and the entire lumbar spine, the fibers gradually converge as they pass upward and laterally toward the axilla. Here the fibers twist on themselves in such a way that the lowest fibers become the uppermost. They end in the narrow flat tendon of the distal attachment. The muscle has a favorable angle of pull for extension and adduction of the arm, particularly when the latter is raised between 30 and 90 degrees. Although EMG has confirmed the action of the latissimus dorsi in extension and adduction during static and dynamic, and resisted and unresisted movements, the same cannot be said for its action in medial rotation. Scheving and Pauly found it to be more important than the pectoralis major as an *inward rotator* of the humerus, but more recent investigators have rejected this view (Basmajian, 1979). The muscle may be palpated on the posterior border of the axilla just below the teres major.

TERES MAJOR   Structurally this muscle (Figures 4–8 and 4–9) appears to be in a favorable position to work with the latissimus dorsi in *downward* and *backward movements* of the humerus and also in *inward rotation*, but Basmajian (1979) detected no sign of activity in this muscle during these movements unless external resistance was applied. Against active resistance, activity was evident during rotation, adduction, and extension. No added resistance is needed, however, for the teres major to be active during hyperextension and adduction when the arm is behind the back.

TRICEPS BRACHII   Although primarily a muscle of the elbow joint, the triceps (Figures 4–7 and 4–9) is active in movements of the humerus because its long head crosses the shoulder joint. It assists in adduction, extension, and hyperextension of the humerus.

The Shoulder Girdle (Acromioclavicular and Sternoclavicular Articulations)

Structure of Acromioclavicular Articulation

The articulation between the acromion process of the scapula and the outer end of the clavicle (Figure 4–10) belongs to the diarthrodial classification. Within this group it is further classified as an irregular (arthrodial) joint. A small wedge-shaped disk may be found between the upper part of the joint surfaces, but this is frequently absent. The articular capsule is strengthened above by the acromioclavicular ligament, which passes from the upper part of the outer end of the clavicle to the upper surface of the acromion process, and behind by the aponeurosis of the trapezius and deltoid muscles. The clavicle is further stabilized by means of the coracoclavicular ligament (actually two ligaments, the conoid and the trapezoid), which, as the name suggests, binds the clavicle to the coracoid process.

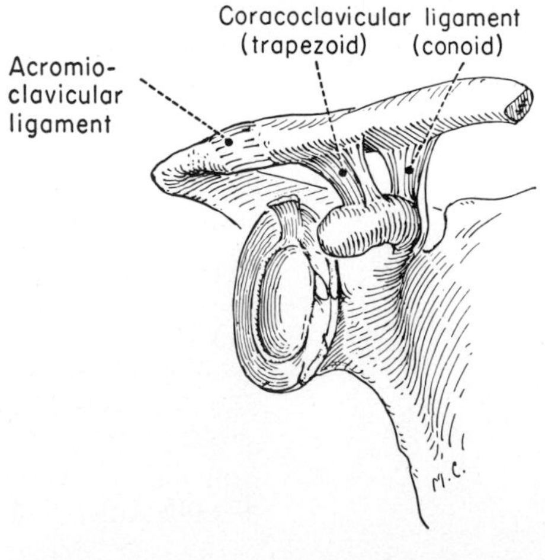

Figure 4–10 Anterior view of acromioclavicular articulation.

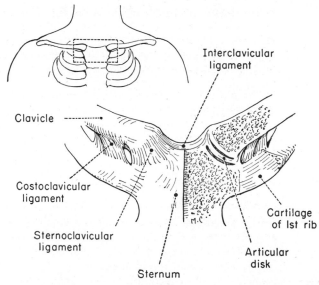

Figure 4–11   Anterior view of sternoclavicular articulation.

The conoid ligament passes from the base of the coracoid process to the conoid tubercle on the underside of the clavicle. The trapezoid ligament extends from the top of the coracoid process to the trapezoid ridge on the underside of the clavicle.

Structure of Sternoclavicular Articulation

The sternal end of the clavicle articulates with both the sternum and the cartilage of the first rib (Figure 4–11). It is classified as a double arthrodial joint because there are two joint cavities, one on either side of the articular disk. This round flat disk of white fibrocartilage is attached above to the upper and posterior border of the articular surface of the clavicle and below to the cartilage of the first rib near its junction with the sternum. The articular capsule is thin above and below but is thickened in front and behind by bands of fibers called the anterior and posterior sternoclavicular ligaments. The often overlooked importance of this capsule was demonstrated by Bearn (1967) in a series of experiments involving the loading of the lateral end of the clavicle both before and after cutting various structures. He presented convincing evidence that it is the capsule rather than the trapezius muscle that provides the chief support for the clavicle.

The movements of the clavicle at this joint are as follows: elevation and depression which occur approximately in the frontal plane about a sagittal-horizontal axis; horizontal forward-backward movements which occur in the horizontal plane about a vertical axis; and a limited degree of forward and backward rotation which occurs approximately in the sagittal plane about the bone's own longitudinal axis. (In forward rotation the top of the clavicle revolves forward-downward.)

The sternoclavicular articulation is of great importance in the movements of the shoulder girdle and of the arm as a whole. It permits limited motion of the clavicle in all three planes and, because of the bone's attachment to the scapula at its distal end, this articulation is partially responsible for the latter's movements. It is reinforced by four ligaments: the anterior sternoclavicular, a band of fibers blending with the anterior fibers of the articular capsule; the posterior sternoclavicular, which blends with the posterior fibers of the articular capsule; the interclavicular, consisting of a flat band which passes across the upper margin of the sternum and attaches to the sternal end of each clavicle; and the costoclavicular, a short strong band of fibers that connects the upper border of the first costal cartilage with the costal tuberosity on the underside of the clavicle.

Movements

It is customary to define the movements of the shoulder girdle (Figure 4–12) in terms of the movements of the scapulae. In doing this, there is some danger that the reader will visualize the movement as taking place solely in the joint between the scapula and the clavicle. It is well to emphasize the fact that every movement of the scapula involves motion in both joints, the acromioclavicular and the sternoclavicular.

The movements of the shoulder girdle expressed in terms of the composite movements of the scapula are as follows:

ELEVATION   An upward movement of the scapula (Figure 4–12A) with the vertebral border remaining approximately parallel to the spinal column. The elevation of the scapula is the direct result of elevation of the outer end of the clavicle, a movement that takes place at the sternoclavicular joint. This movement occurs to a slight extent during elevation of the humerus and to a greater extent in lifting the shoulders in a hunching gesture. The farther the clavicles depart from the horizontal position, the closer the scapulae move toward each other. The latter movement might well be called passive adduction since it is caused by the movement of the clavicles rather than by the adductor muscles of the scapulae.

DEPRESSION   The return from the position of elevation. There is no depression below the normal resting position.

ABDUCTION OR PROTRACTION   A lateral movement of the scapula away from the spinal column with the vertebral border remaining approximately parallel to it (Figure 4–12B). Pure abduction of the scapula is a hypothetical movement. Actually, because of two factors, the rounded contour of the thorax and the forward movement of the clavicle about a vertical axis at the sternoclavicular joint, a pure lateral movement of the scapula in the frontal plane is impossible. As the scapula abducts it turns slightly about its vertical axis in a movement known as a lateral tilt. This turning is characterized by a slight backward movement of the vertebral border and a corresponding forward movement of the axillary border. This movement causes the glenoid fossa to face slightly forward and the arms, if relaxed, to hang in a more forward position and in slight inward (medial) rotation.

ADDUCTION OR RETRACTION   A medial movement of the scapula toward the spinal column combined with a reduction of lateral tilt.

UPWARD TILT   A turning of the scapula on its frontal-horizontal axis so that the posterior surface faces slightly upward and the inferior angle protrudes from the back (Figure 4–12D). This is accompanied by a rotation of the clavicle about its mechanical axis so that the superior border turns slightly forward-downward and the inferior border backward-upward. It occurs only in conjunction with hyperextension of the humerus.

REDUCTION OF UPWARD TILT   The return movement from upward tilt.

UPWARD ROTATION   A rotation of the scapula in the frontal plane so that the glenoid fossa faces somewhat upward (Figure 4–12C). The movement occurs largely at the

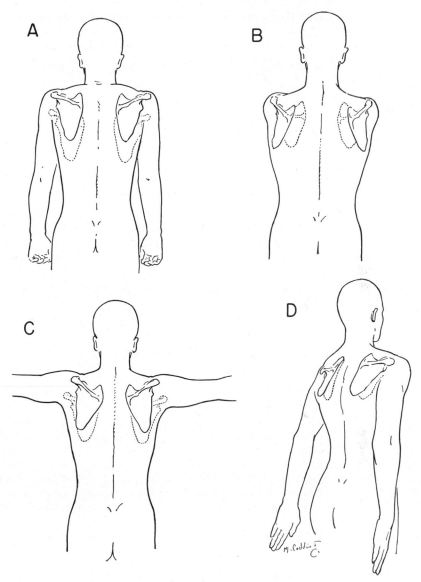

Figure 4–12 Movements of the shoulder girdle. *A*, Elevation. *B*, Abduction (combined with lateral tilt and upward rotation). *C*, Upward rotation. *D*, Upward tilt.

acromioclavicular joint but is accompanied by elevation of the outer end of the clavicle. Upward rotation is always associated with elevation of the humerus, either sideward or forward. It serves at least three useful purposes: (1) it puts the glenoid fossa in a favorable position for the upper extremity movement; (2) by positioning the small glenoid fossa beneath the larger head of the humerus it contributes significantly to the stability of the shoulder joint (Inman, 1962); and (3) by moving the origin of the deltoid medially at the same time that the latter muscle is elevating the humerus, the deltoid is prevented from shortening too much, thereby losing force too rapidly (Ralston, 1953).

DOWNWARD ROTATION   The return from the position of upward rotation. There may be slight downward rotation beyond the normal resting position so that the glenoid fossa faces slightly downward.

Muscles of the Shoulder Girdle

Location

The muscles of the shoulder girdle are classified as anterior or posterior muscles according to their location on the trunk.

Anterior	Posterior
Pectoralis minor	Levator scapulae
Serratus anterior	Rhomboids
Subclavius	Trapezius

Characteristics and Functions of Shoulder Girdle Muscles

PECTORALIS MINOR   This muscle (Figure 4–13) participates in several movements of the scapula—*downward rotation*, *upward tilt*, *depression*, and the combined movements of *abduction* and *lateral tilt*. In addition to its action on the scapula, an important function of the pectoralis minor is its lifting effect on the ribs, both in forced inspiration and in maintaining good chest posture. When the scapulae are stabilized by the adductors, contraction of the pectoralis minor *elevates* the third, fourth, and fifth ribs. Even without contracting it exerts a slight upward and outward pull on these ribs if the muscle is well developed. The pectoralis minor can therefore contribute either to good or to poor posture, depending upon whether its more effective pull is on the ribs or on the scapula. The key to its function as a muscle influencing good posture is stabilization of the scapulae by the adductors—i.e., the rhomboids and the middle trapezius. The pectoralis minor may be palpated midway between the clavicle and the nipple when the arm is elevated backward against resistance, provided the pectoralis major is relaxed, and also when the subject sits with the forearm resting on a table and pushes both downward and laterally simultaneously.

SERRATUS ANTERIOR   The upper portion causes *abduction* and *lateral tilt* of the scapula close to the ribs (Figures 4–13 and 4–16). The upper and lower portions of the serratus anterior and trapezius combine to form a force couple for upward rotation of the scapula. Activity of these muscles is especially evident during elevation of the arm, with the lower trapezius the more active of the two during abduction and the serratus anterior the more active during flexion. This muscle is important in reaching and pushing (Inman, 1962). A paralyzed serratus anterior prevents elevation of the arm above 100 degrees.

The muscle may be palpated on the anterior-lateral surface of the upper thorax, especially on a thin, muscular subject.

SUBCLAVIUS   The pull of this muscle (Figure 4–13), which is slightly *downward* and strongly toward the sternum, suggests that its chief function is to protect and stabilize the sternoclavicular articulation. It is also in a position to depress the scapula. It is not possible to palpate this muscle.

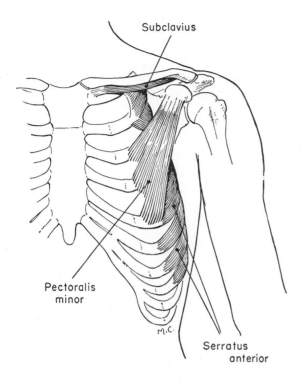

Figure 4–13   Anterior muscles of shoulder girdle.

LEVATOR SCAPULAE   This muscle is also listed with the muscles of the neck. Although one would expect the levator scapulae (Figure 4–14) to elevate and adduct the scapula, Bowen and Stone (1953) pointed out that it actually causes *elevation* and *downward rotation* when the trunk is in the erect position. Their explanation of this action is that the weight of the arm at the acromial end of the scapula pulls that end down at the same time that the levator is lifting the medial angle. Thus these two forces act as a force couple to rotate the scapula.

In more recent years Basmajian (1979) and Rasch and Burke (1978), who succeeded Bowen as authors of the textbook he originally wrote, appear to agree with Bowen in attributing the levator scapulae's movement of downward rotation to the weight of the arm and to the scapula's consequent need of postural support. Another author views this weight-supporting function as a cooperative action of the levator scapulae and the rhomboids lifting the medial border of the scapula, and of the upper trapezius lifting its lateral angle (Hollinshead, 1976). Still another claims that the levator together with the rhomboid minor tends to rotate the scapula downward in the early phase of contraction, preliminary to elevating it (Brunnstrom, 1972).

If the levator scapulae rotates the scapula downward only when the weight of the arm prevents it from adducting the scapula, it would be assumed that the trunk must be in the erect position for gravity to have this effect. In other positions, as in swimming, one would expect the levator to adduct as well as to elevate the scapula. It might be enlightening if an electromyographic study were to be made for the purpose of comparing the actions of the levator muscle when abduction of the humerus (and possible other movements) is performed from two different starting positions: erect standing or sitting, and prone lying.

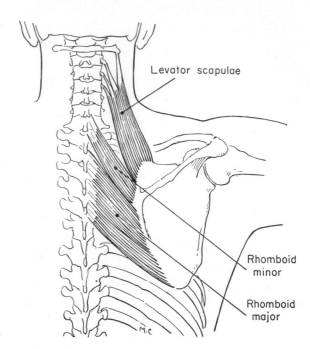

Figure 4–14 Posterior muscles of shoulder girdle, deep layer.

The muscle is a difficult one to palpate successfully. The reader is referred to Brunnstrom (1972) for one method of doing this.

RHOMBOIDS, MAJOR AND MINOR   Functionally, the rhomboids may be regarded as one muscle (Figure 4–14). They cause *downward rotation, adduction,* and *elevation* of the scapula. Their cooperative action with trapezius III (see below) is an important factor in the maintenance of good shoulder posture. When the tonus of these two muscles is deficient, the unbalanced pull of the pectoralis minor and the serratus anterior results in habitually abducted and tilted scapulae. This in turn results in the failure of the pectoralis minor and serratus anterior to hold the chest in good posture. Thus, one weak link in the chain of postural relationships leads to another. The rhomboids are also most active with the middle trapezius in stabilizing the scapula during abduction of the arm. During arm flexion there is little activity in these muscles until 150 degrees of flexion is reached, when it increases markedly (Inman et al., 1944).

These muscles are difficult to palpate, since they are completely covered by the trapezius. The technique suggested by Brunnstrom (1972) is recommended.

TRAPEZIUS   The trapezius (Figure 4–15) is a fascinating muscle to study. Because its location is directly under the skin it is easy to palpate. While some anatomists treat the muscle in three parts, it is more accurate to consider the four parts shown in Figure 4–15 separately. Parts I and II compose the upper trapezius, Part III the middle, and Part IV the lower. Its actions include the following:

Part I.   Elevation.

Part II.   Elevation; upward rotation; adduction.

Part III.   Adduction.

Part IV.   Upward rotation; depression; adduction.

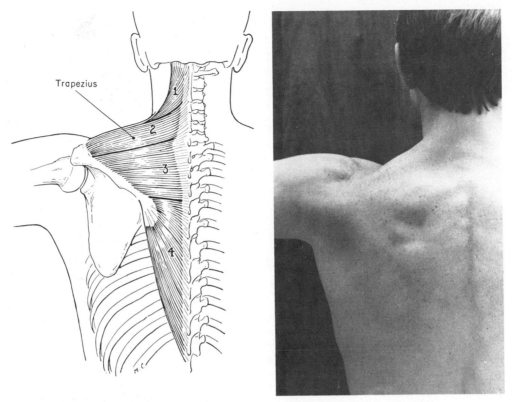

Figure 4–15   Trapezius.

In their 1952 study of the trapezius muscle, Wiedenbauer and Mortensen found that the trapezius showed definite activity during both elevation and retraction (adduction) of the scapula. In elevation the upper portion showed the greatest activity, and in retraction the middle and lower portions were most active. During abduction of the humerus and the accompanying upward rotation of the scapula the lower two-thirds of the trapezius was most active, and during flexion of the humerus the lower third was most active. The greatest activity of the muscle as a whole was seen in the upward rotation of the scapula accompanying abduction of the humerus (Basmajian, 1979).

The relation of the trapezius to the rhomboids and serratus is interesting. The rhomboids and Part III of the trapezius both adduct the scapulae, and have similar activity patterns during elevation of the arm. In these actions they are partners. Parts II and IV, however, rotate the scapulae upward; the rhomboids rotate them downward. In this respect, then, they are antagonists.

Trapezius III and the upper serratus are antagonistic, the former adducting and the latter abducting the scapulae, but Trapezius II and IV are partners with the lower serratus since they act on the scapula as a force couple to rotate the scapula upward, with Part II pulling up on the acromial end of the scapular spine and Part IV and the serratus pulling down on the medial end or root. (See the discussion of a force couple on pp. 353–354, and Figure 12–6.) This action facilitates elevation of the arm. The lower and middle parts of the trapezius are quite active during the entire range of abduction, but less so during the early stages of flexion when the scapula is being abducted. It is here that the serratus anterior, a scapular abductor as well as rotator, dominates.

Trapezius I and II have one important function that may be overlooked because there is little, if any, actual movement involved. This is support for the distal end of the clavicle and the acromion process of the scapula when a heavy weight is held by the hand with the arm down at the side. Anyone who has carried a heavy suitcase for a long distance has doubtless experienced tension and subsequent soreness in these parts of the muscle. When no weight is carried, however, the capsule of the sternoclavicular articulation provides all the support necessary for the fully depressed clavicle (Bearn, 1967).

These various combinations of function are an excellent illustration of the cooperative action of the muscles and of the astonishing versatility of the musculoskeletal mechanism.

Joint and Muscular Analysis of the Fundamental Movements of the Arm on the Trunk

As stated earlier, the movements of the arm on the trunk involve the cooperative action of the shoulder joint and the shoulder girdle, the latter including both the acromioclavicular and the sternoclavicular joints. In order to analyze correctly the great variety of movements of the upper extremity it is essential to understand this cooperative action of the three joints and their muscles.

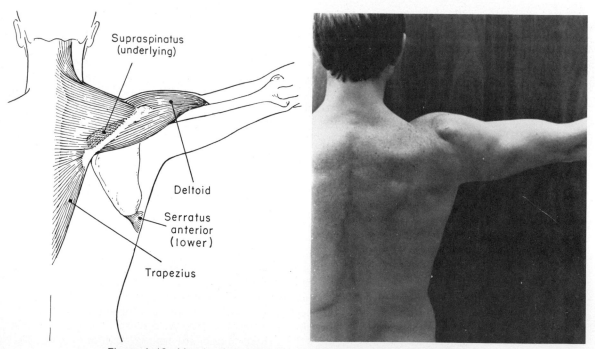

Figure 4–16 Muscles that contract to produce sideward elevation of the arm.

The fundamental movements of the arm on the trunk, together with the anatomical analysis of each, are presented below.

Sideward Elevation

This movement may occur from any distance up to the vertical (Figure 4–16).

SHOULDER JOINT   Abduction of the humerus by the deltoid and supraspinatus accompanied by slight depression of the humeral head due to the action of the subscapularis, infraspinatus, and teres minor. This is the least forceful of shoulder joint actions. True humeral abduction is the sideward elevation of the humerus in a plane parallel with the scapula. Hence, if the scapulae were slightly abducted and laterally tilted from poor posture, for instance, the abducted humeri would not be strictly in the frontal plane of the body but would be moving in an oblique plane, slightly anterior to the frontal plane.

Outward or lateral rotation by the infraspinatus and teres minor when palms are turned either out or up. Possible abduction by the biceps when the arm is in complete outward rotation.

SHOULDER GIRDLE   Upward rotation of the scapula by the serratus anterior and trapezius II and IV.

Sideward Depression

This movement may occur from any degree of sideward elevation, either against resistance or in any position that rules out the help of gravitational force (Figure 4–17).

SHOULDER JOINT   Adduction of the humerus by the latissimus dorsi, the teres major (against resistance), sternal portion of the pectoralis major, and probably the lowest fibers of the posterior deltoid. Reduction of outward rotation mainly by the subscapularis and the teres major.

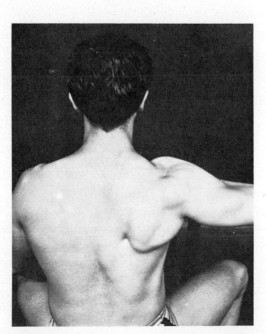

Figure 4–17   Sideward depression of the arm against resistance. The latissimus dorsi, teres major, and rhomboids are in strong contraction.

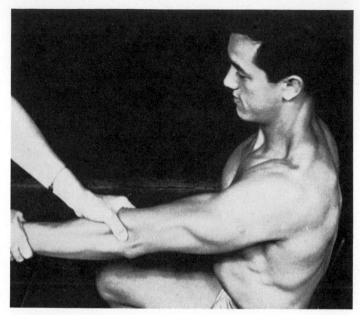

Figure 4–18 Forward elevation of the arm against resistance. The anterior and middle deltoid, upper trapezius, and serratus anterior are in strong contraction.

SHOULDER GIRDLE   Reduction of upward rotation by the rhomboids and pectoralis minor, with help from the levator scapulae.

Forward Elevation

This movement may occur up to the horizontal (Figure 4–18).

SHOULDER JOINT   Flexion of the humerus by the anterior deltoid and clavicular portion of the pectoralis major, with probably some participation of the coracobrachialis (against resistance) and biceps brachii.
   Slight outward rotation by the infraspinatus and teres minor.

SHOULDER GIRDLE   Upward rotation of the scapula by the serratus anterior and trapezius II and IV (slight).
   Abduction and lateral tilt of the scapula by the serratus anterior and pectoralis minor, unless intentionally inhibited.

Forward-Up-ward Elevation

This movement may occur from the horizontal to the vertical and beyond.

SHOULDER JOINT   Flexion of the humerus by the same muscles as above; hyperflexion if the humerus moves beyond the vertical.
   Continued outward rotation by the infraspinatus and teres minor if the palms turn to face each other when the arms reach the vertical.

SHOULDER GIRDLE   Upward rotation of the scapula by the serratus anterior and trapezius II and IV (increased).
   Slight to moderate elevation of the scapula by the levator scapulae, trapezius I and II, and rhomboids, unless effort is made to inhibit elevation. This action would be

evident in reaching activities like the high jump, long jump, or the pushing phase of the pole vault.

Reduction of abduction and lateral tilt mainly by virtue of the overhead position.

Forward-Down-ward Depression

This movement may occur from the overhead vertical to the starting position, either against resistance or in a position that rules out the help of gravitational force (Figure 4–19).

SHOULDER JOINT   Extension of the humerus by the sternal portion of the pectoralis major (diminishing as the movement progresses), teres major (against resistance), latissimus dorsi (especially during the lower 60 degrees of motion), and possibly the posterior deltoid and the long head of the triceps brachii. Extension is the most powerful of shoulder movements.

Reduction of outward rotation, probably by relaxation of outward rotator muscles but possibly aided by the subscapularis, teres major, latissimus dorsi, and pectoralis major.

SHOULDER GIRDLE   Reduction of elevation and upward rotation by relaxation of muscles. If the movement is performed against resistance, the pectoralis minor, trapezius IV, subclavius, and rhomboids would doubtless be active. In pulling movements like a chin-up, strong adduction of the middle trapezius and rhomboids and strong depression by the pectoralis minor and lower trapezius would also be evident.

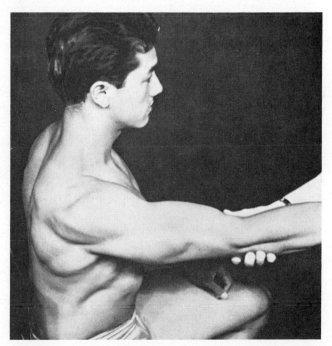

Figure 4–19 Forward-downward depression of the arm against resistance. The latissimus dorsi and teres major are in strong contraction.

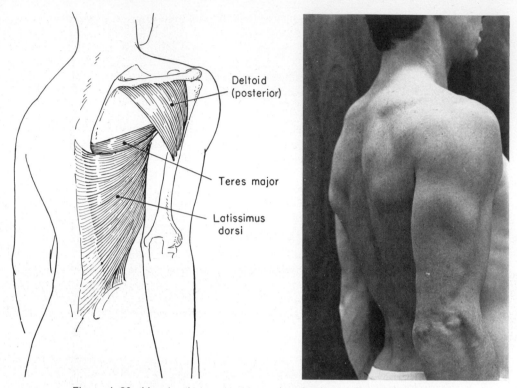

Figure 4–20   Muscles that contract to produce backward elevation of the arm.

Backward Elevation
(Figure 4–20)

SHOULDER JOINT   Hyperextension of the humerus by the posterior deltoid, latissimus dorsi, and teres major.

SHOULDER GIRDLE   Upward tilt of the scapula by the pectoralis minor.

Elevation if movement is carried to the extreme. Possibly the hyperextension of the humerus pushes the scapula into a position of slight elevation. If any scapular muscles are acting, they would probably be the levator scapulae, trapezius I and II, and rhomboids, with possibly the clavicular portion of the sternocleidomastoid (a neck muscle) helping.

Outward Rotation
(Figures 4–21 and 4–22)

SHOULDER JOINT   Outward rotation of the humerus by the infraspinatus and teres minor with the posterior deltoid acting only if the humerus is also being adducted and extended, as in a calisthenic or postural exercise.

SHOULDER GIRDLE   Adduction of the scapulae and reduction of any lateral tilt which may have been present by the rhomboids and trapezius III, with some involvement of trapezius II and IV.

Inward Rotation

SHOULDER JOINT   Inward rotation of the humerus by the subscapularis, teres major (against resistance), latissimus dorsi, anterior deltoid, and pectoralis major. If the upper extremity is in a position of outward rotation to start with, the coracobrachialis and short head of the biceps would be active in the first part of the movement.

SHOULDER GIRDLE   Abduction and lateral tilt by the serratus anterior and pectoralis

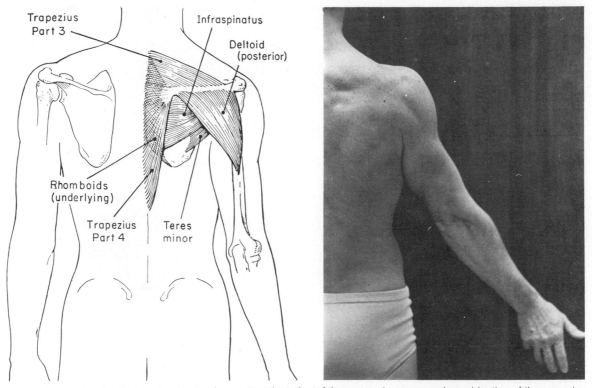

Figure 4–21   Muscles that contract to produce outward rotation of the arm and accompanying adduction of the scapula.

minor, with a tendency toward elevation by the levator scapulae, trapezius I and II, and rhomboids.

Horizontal Forward Swing from Side Horizontal Position

SHOULDER JOINT   Horizontal flexion of humerus by the pectoralis major, anterior deltoid, and coracobrachialis, with the short head of the biceps helping if the forearm is extended.

SHOULDER GIRDLE   Abduction and lateral tilt of scapula, unless deliberately inhibited. The movement is produced by the serratus anterior and pectoralis minor.

Horizontal Sideward Backward Swing from Forward Horizontal Position

SHOULDER JOINT   Horizontal extension of the humerus by the posterior deltoid, posterior portion of middle deltoid, infraspinatus, teres minor, and long head of the triceps.

SHOULDER GIRDLE   Adduction and reduction of lateral tilt of scapula by the rhomboids and trapezius III in particular, with II and IV also participating.

Shoulder Girdle Movements Not Involving the Arm

In addition to these coordinated movements of the arm on the trunk there are three movements of the shoulder girdle in which movements of the arm are passive because they are produced by the changes in position of the shoulder girdle from which they are suspended. These are (1) a lifting or hunching of the shoulders, (2) protraction of the shoulders, and (3) retraction of the shoulders.

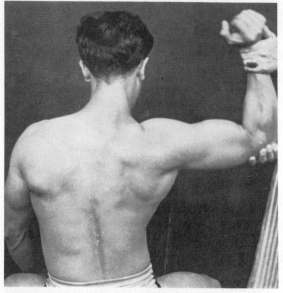 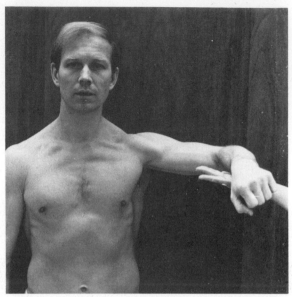

Figure 4–22 *A,* Outward rotation of the arm against resistance. The posterior deltoid, infraspinatus, and teres minor are in strong contraction. (The hyperextension and lateral flexion of the trunk are caused by the extreme effort. The latissimus is contracting because he is pushing his elbow down.) *B,* Inward rotation. The pectoralis major, anterior deltoid, teres major, and latissimus dorsi are in strong contraction.

SHOULDER LIFTING OR HUNCHING

Shoulder Girdle   Elevation by the levator scapulae, trapezius I and II, and rhomboids, with assistance by the sternocleidomastoid if the movement is performed against resistance. Reduction of the elevation is achieved by relaxing the muscles and letting the force of gravity have its way.

SHOULDER PROTRACTION

Shoulder Girdle   Forceful abduction and lateral tilt of scapula by the serratus anterior and pectoralis minor.

Shoulder Joint   Slight passive inward rotation.

Reduction of the movement is achieved by relaxation of the muscles but may be followed by slight retraction.

SHOULDER RETRACTION

Shoulder Girdle   Adduction and reduction of lateral tilt by the rhomboids, trapezius III, and possibly II and IV.

Diagonal Movements

Unless performing calisthenic or gymnastic exercises one rarely performs pure fundamental movements of the arm on the trunk. Most athletic and everyday movements are "in-between" or combination movements. In order to analyze these in terms of their muscular action, it is necessary to estimate the approximate proportions of the fundamental joint motions. For instance, the follow-through on a *tennis serve* might involve forward-downward depression of the arm (see shoulder joint and shoulder girdle analysis), or it might consist of forward-downward depression combined with a slight amount of "horizontal" forward swing. In other words, this could be described as a diagonal forward-downward and slightly inward movement of the arm, consist-

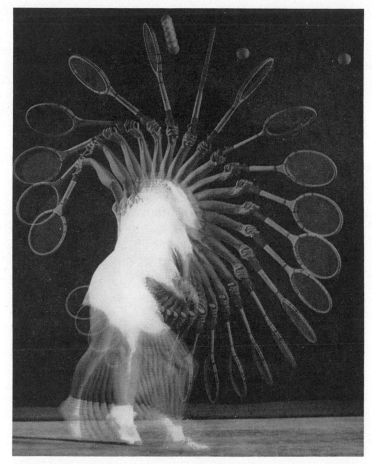

Figure 4–23   A tennis serve showing diagonal adduction of arm at shoulder joint during follow-through. (Courtesy of H. E. Edgerton.)

ing mainly of extension of the humerus combined with a slight degree of adduction. An appropriate term proposed by Logan and McKinney (1970) is "diagonal adduction" (Figure 4–23). After the server's racket is moved forward-upward to ball contact by inward rotation of the humerus at the shoulder and extension at the elbow, the arm movement is diagonally down and across the body in a combination of extension and adduction—i.e., diagonal adduction.

A true *forehand drive* might well consist of a pure horizontal forward swing from a side horizontal position (horizontal flexion of the humerus and abduction of the scapula), but the arm is more likely to start slightly above or below the horizontal and to move in a diagonal path.

An *underarm volleyball serve,* which is likely to have an upward as well as a forward component, would consist of a horizontal forward swing from the side horizontal position of the arm combined with a slight amount of forward-upward elevation. This would involve slight shoulder joint flexion accompanied by a combination of abduction, lateral tilt, and upward rotation of the shoulder girdle.

Common Athletic Injuries of the Shoulder Region

Acromioclavicu-lar Sprain

This occurs if the acromioclavicular joint is forced beyond its normal range of motion, such as from a downward blow against the outer end of the shoulder, causing the acromion to be driven downward away from the clavicle. It is also caused by a fall in which the person lands on an outstretched hand or flexed elbow when the arm is in a vertical position and at an angle of 45 to 90 degrees of flexion or abduction from the trunk. The damage consists of the tearing or severe stretching of the acromioclavicular ligaments.

Fracture of the Clavicle

A fracture of the clavicle in its middle third may result from the same type of injury that causes acromioclavicular sprains—namely, either a direct downward blow to the acromion process or, more commonly, landing on the hand from a fall with the arm rigidly outstretched. Such a fracture may be recognized or at least suspected if the injured person tends to support the arm with the good arm and carries the head tilted toward the injured side with his face turned to the opposite side. Teenagers and preteenagers are more likely to have a greenstick fracture from such injuries (Klafs and Arnheim, 1973).

Dislocation of the Shoulder

There are three types of these dislocations: forward or subcoracoid, downward or subglenoid, and posterior. The most common type among young athletes is the forward (subcoracoid) type, which is most likely to occur when the humerus is abducted and laterally rotated or when the pectoralis major is forcefully contracting. In this the head of the humerus, having slipped forward out of the glenoid fossa, comes to rest beneath the coracoid process (Figure 4–24A). The injured arm is usually held out from the side in a position of slight abduction and lateral rotation. The shoulder is well protected from downward dislocations because of the upward tilt of the glenoid fossa and the effectiveness of the supraspinatus, posterior deltoid, and the superior part of the capsule in tightening to hold the humeral head in the socket.

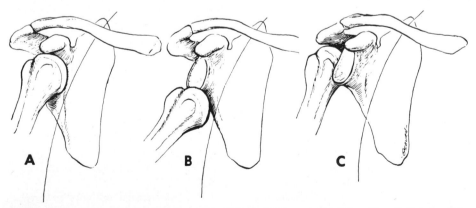

Figure 4–24   Dislocations of the shoulder. *A,* Typical subcoracoid dislocation. *B,* Subglenoid dislocation. *C,* Posterior dislocation. (From O'Donoghue, D. H.: *Treatment of injuries to athletes.* 3d ed. Philadelphia: W. B. Saunders, 1976.)

When these dislocations do occur, they are caused by a blow from the top of the shoulder and happen more easily when the arm is slightly abducted.

Chronic Disloca-tion of the Shoulder

This dislocation is usually forward and results either from a congenital abnormality or from repeated acute dislocations in an otherwise normal joint. With proper care following an acute dislocation there should be no recurrences. It is important to know which condition is the cause, since congenital abnormalities are likely to require surgery (O'Donoghue, 1976).

Laboratory Experiences

Joint Structure and Function

1. Facing your partner's back, hold your thumb against the inferior angle of one scapula and your index or middle finger against the root of the spine at the scapula. Try to follow the movements of the scapula as your partner performs all of the fundamental movements of the arm on the body.

2. Using a form like that in Appendix A, record the essential information regarding the glenohumeral, acromioclavicular, and sternoclavicular articulations. Study the movements of these joints both on the skeleton and on the living body.

3. In five different subjects measure the amount of abduction that occurs in the shoulder girdle (i.e., the separation of the scapulae) when the arms are raised to the forward horizontal position. How much can this vary in one individual? In measuring the distance between the scapulae, measure the horizontal distance between the midpoints of the vertebral borders.

4. Using a protractor-goniometer, measure the amount of upward rotation of the scapula which occurs when the arm is raised sideward-upward to the overhead position. To make this measurement, center the instrument over the medial angle of the scapula and adjust one of its arms in line with the normal resting position of the inferior angle and the other lin line with the inferior angle after maximum upward rotation of the scapula has taken place.

Muscular Action

Directions. Work in groups of three, with one person serving as the subject, the second as an assistant helping to support or steady the stationary part of the body and giving resistance to the moving part, and the third palpating the muscles and recording the results on the checklist found in Appendix E.

5. **SIDEWARD ELEVATION OF THE ARM.** Shoulder joint: abduction and possibly outward rotation; shoulder girdle; upward rotation.
Subject: In erect position, raise arm sideward to shoulder level, keeping elbow straight.
Assistant: Resist movement by exerting pressure downward on subject's elbow. See to it that subject does not elevate shoulder.
Observer: Palpate the three portions of the deltoid and tell which portions contract. Palpate the four parts of the trapezius. Which parts contract? Does the pectoralis major contract during any part of the movement?

6. **SIDEWARD DEPRESSION OF THE ARM** (Figure 4–17). Shoulder joint: adduction and possibly reduction of outward rotation; shoulder girdle: downward rotation.

Subject: In erect position with arm raised sideward to shoulder level, lower arm until 45 degrees from side.

Assistant: Place hand under subject's elbow and resist movement. (If no resistance is given, the muscle action will be the same as in elevation, except that the contraction will be eccentric instead of concentric.)

Observer: Palpate the latissimus dorsi, teres major, pectoralis major, and posterior deltoid. Do they each contract and, if so, during which part of the movement?

7. **FORWARD ELEVATION OF THE ARM** (Figure 4–18).   Shoulder joint: flexion; shoulder girdle: upward rotation and probably abduction.

Subject: In erect position, raise arm forward to shoulder level, keeping elbow straight.

Assistant: Resist movement by exerting pressure downward on the subject's elbow. See that subject does not elevate shoulder.

Observer: Palpate the anterior deltoid and the pectoralis major. Do both the sternal and clavicular portions of the latter muscle contract?

8. **FORWARD DEPRESSION OF THE ARM** (Figure 4–19).   Shoulder joint: extension; shoulder girdle: downward rotation and probably adduction.

Subject: In erect position with arm raised forward to shoulder level, lower it until 45 degrees from side.

Assistant: Resist movement at underside of elbow.

Observer: Palpate the latissimus dorsi and the pectoralis major. Do they contract with equal force throughout the movement?

9. **BACKWARD ELEVATION OF THE ARM** (Figure 4–20).   Shoulder joint: hyperextension; shoulder girdle: upward tilt.

Subject: Either in erect position or lying face down, raise arm backward, keeping elbow straight.

Assistant: Place hand over subject's elbow and resist movement.

Observer: Palpate the posterior deltoid, latissimus dorsi, and teres major.

10. **HORIZONTAL SIDEWARD-BACKWARD SWING OF THE ARM** (from forward horizontal position). Shoulder joint: horizontal extension and slight outward rotation; shoulder girdle: adduction and reduction of lateral tilt.

a. *Subject:* In erect position with arms raised forward to shoulder level, palms down, swing arms sideward in horizontal plane as far as possible.

Assistant: Stand facing subject between the arms and resist movement by grasping the outstretched elbows.

Observer: Palpate the posterior deltoid and latissimus dorsi. What other muscles can be palpated?

b. *Subject:* Lying face down on narrow plinth or on table close to edge with arm hanging straight down, raise arm sideward as far above the horizontal as possible.

Assistant: Resistance may be given at elbow, but is not necessary, since gravity furnishes sufficient resistance.

Observer: Same as in *a*.

11. **HORIZONTAL SIDEWARD-FORWARD SWING OF THE ARM** (from side horizontal position).   Shoulder joint: horizontal flexion and slight inward rotation; shoulder girdle: abduction and lateral tilt.

a. *Subject:* In erect position with arm raised sideward to shoulder level, palm down, swing arm forward in horizontal plane.

Assistant: Stand behind subject's arm and resist movement by holding elbow.

Observer: Palpate pectoralis major and anterior deltoid.

b. *Subject:* Lie on back on table with arm extended sideward, palm up. Raise arm to vertical position, keeping elbow straight.
Assistant: Resistance may be given at elbow, but is not necessary, since gravity furnishes sufficient resistance.
Observer: Same as in *a*.

12. **OUTWARD ROTATION OF ARM.**   Shoulder joint: outward rotation; shoulder girdle: possibly adduction and reduction of lateral tilt.
a. *Subject:* Lying face down on a table with upper arm at shoulder level, resting on table and forearm hanging down off edge of table. Keeping forearm at right angles to upper arm, raise hand and forearm forward-upward to limit of motion, without allowing upper arm to leave table.
Assistant: Steady upper arm and resist movement of forearm by holding wrist.
Observer: Palpate infraspinatus and teres minor.
b. *Subject:* Sitting erect with upper arm at side-horizontal position and elbow bent at right angles with forearm at forward horizontal position. Without moving upper arm raise forearm to vertical position (Figure 4–22).
Assistant: Support upper arm at elbow and give resistance to forearm at wrist.
Observer: Same as in *a*.

13. **INWARD ROTATION OF ARM.**   Shoulder joint: inward rotation; shoulder girdle: abduction and lateral tilt, and tendency toward elevation.
a. *Subject:* Same position as in 12*a*. Raise forearm backward-upward.
Assistant: Steady upper arm and resist movement of forearm by holding wrist.
Observer: Palpate teres major and latissimus dorsi.
b. *Subject:* Lie on back on table with upper arm at shoulder level resting on table and forearm raised to vertical position. Lower forearm forward-downward to the limit of motion.
Assistant: Steady upper arm and resist forearm motion by holding wrist.
Observer: Palpate anterior deltoid and clavicular portion of pectoralis major.

14. **ELEVATION OF SHOULDER**
Subject: In erect position, lift shoulder toward ear, keeping arm muscles relaxed.
Assistant: Resist movement by pressing down on shoulder.
Observer: Palpate trapezius I and II.

15. **DEPRESSION OF SHOULDER**
a. *Subject:* In erect position with shoulder raised and elbow flexed, push down with elbow, lowering shoulder to normal position.
Assistant: Resist movement by holding hand under elbow.
Observer: Palpate trapezius IV.
b. *Subject:* Take cross rest position between two chairs or parallel bars.
Observer: Palpate trapezius IV.

16. **ADDUCTION OF SHOULDER GIRDLE** (retraction)
Subject: In erect position with arms raised sideward, elbows flexed and fingers resting on shoulders, push elbows backward, keeping them at shoulder level.
Assistant: Stand facing subject and resist movement by pulling elbows forward.
Observer: Palpate middle and lower trapezius (Parts III and IV). (This movement is somewhat similar to the one in 10, but here the emphasis is on the shoulder girdle rather than on the arm.)

17. **ABDUCTION OF SHOULDER GIRDLE** (protraction)
Subject: In erect position with arms raised sideward, elbows flexed, and fingers resting on shoulders, pull elbows forward, attempting to touch them in front of chest.

Assistant: Stand behind subject and resist movement by pulling elbows back.
Observer: Palpate serratus anterior.

Action of the Muscles Other Than the Movers

18. STABILIZATION OF THE SCAPULA DURING FORCEFUL FORWARD DEPRESSION OF THE ARM
    Subject: In erect position with arm raised forward above shoulder level, lower arm against strong resistance.
    Assistant: Resist the arm movement by placing hand under the arm just above the subject's elbow.
    Observer: Palpate trapezius IV. Explain.

19. STABILIZATION OF SCAPULA DURING OUTWARD ROTATION OF HUMERUS
    Subject: Rotate the arm outward as it hangs at the side.
    Observer: Palpate the scapular adductors. Explain.

20. ROTATION OF ARM IN POSITION OF SIDE ELEVATION
    Subject: With one arm raised sideward to shoulder level, rotate it first outward, then inward.
    Observer: Palpate middle deltoid. Explain its action.

21. VIGOROUS ARM FLINGING SIDEWARD TO THE HORIZONTAL
    Subject: Fling arm vigorously to the side horizontal position.
    Observer: Palpate the adductors of the shoulder joint. Do they contract momentarily at the very end of the movement? Explain.

22. VIGOROUS ARM FLINGING DOWNWARD
    Subject: From an overhead position, fling arm vigorously forward-downward, stopping it at the body.
    Observer: Palpate the flexors of the shoulder joint. Do they contract momentarily at the end of the movement? Explain.

Applications

23. Work in groups of three with the members designated respectively as A, B, and C. Equipment for each group: a volleyball and an empty 12-ounce frozen juice can or other can of approximately same size.
    "A" stands at one end of playing area with left side toward the opposite end.
    "B" stands facing "A" about two arm lengths away and holds can vertically in right hand with arm extended forward and with volleyball balanced on open end of can.
    "A" adjusts distance and swings extended right arm horizontally backward with thumb side up and palm flat. "A" then swings arm vigorously forward and strikes ball forcefully with palm, attempting to project ball as far as possible.
    "C" observes "A's" action and writes answers to following questions without saying them aloud.
    a. What is the movement of "A's" humerus at the shoulder joint in the preparatory movement?
    b. Same for the striking movement?
    c. What is the position of "A's" humerus at the moment of impact?
    Repeat until each person has taken a turn at being A, B, and C. Report answers to the rest of group and discuss if not in agreement.

24. Work in partners with one observing while the other performs.
    Starting position: Hang from horizontal bar with palms facing body and with feet hanging clear or, if necessary, with toes just touching floor or bench.
    Movement: Chin self with steady pull and hold end position.
    Observer: Write joint analysis of *(a)* starting position of humerus at shoulder joint, and of scapulae; and *(b)* movement of each. Discuss with partner.

References

Basmajian, J. V. 1979. *Muscles alive.* 4th ed. Chapter 10. Baltimore: Williams & Wilkins.

Bearn, J. B. 1967. Direct observations on the function of the capsule of the sternoclavicular joint in clavicular support. *J. Anat.* 101:159–70.

Bowen, W. P., and Stone, H. A. 1953. *Applied anatomy and kinesiology.* 7th ed. Philadelphia: Lea & Febiger.

Brunnstrom, S. 1972. *Clinical kinesiology.* 3d ed. Philadelphia: F. A. Davis.

Conway, A. M. 1961. *Movements at the sternoclavicular and acromioclavicular joints. Phys. Ther. Rev.* 41:421–32.

Dempster, W. T. 1965. Mechanisms of shoulder movement. *Arch. Phys. Med. Rehabil.* 46:49–70.

Doody, S. G., Freedman, L., and Waterland, J. C. 1970. Shoulder movements during abduction in the scapular plane. *Arch. Phys. Med. Rehabil.* 51:595–604.

Hollinshead, W. H. 1976. *Functional anatomy of the limbs and back.* 4th ed. Philadelphia: W. B. Saunders.

Inman, V. T. 1962. The shoulder as a functional unit. *J. Bone Joint Surg.* 44A:977–78.

Inman, V. T., Saunders, J. B. deC. M., and Abbott, L. C. 1944. Observations on the function of the shoulder joint. *J. Bone Joint Surg.* 26:1–30.

Klafs, C. E., and Arnheim, D. D. 1973. *Modern principles of athletic training.* St. Louis: C. V. Mosby.

Logan, G. A., and McKinney, W. C. 1970. *Kinesiology.* Dubuque, Iowa: William C. Brown.

O'Donoghue, Don H. 1976. *Treatment of injuries to athletes.* 3d ed. Philadelphia: W. B. Saunders.

Ralston, H. J. 1953. Mechanics of voluntary muscle. *Am. J. Phys. Med.* 32:166–84.

Rasch, P. J., and Burke, R. K. 1978. *Kinesiology and applied anatomy.* 6th ed. Philadelphia: Lea & Febiger.

Shevlin, M. G., Lehmann, J. P., and Lucci, J. A. 1969. Electromyographic study of the function of some muscles crossing the glenohumeral joint. *Arch. Phys. Med. Rehabil.* 50:264–70.

Singleton, M. C. 1966. Functional anatomy of the shoulder. *J. Am. Phys. Ther. Assoc.* 46:1043–51.

Steindler, A. 1970. *Kinesiology of the human body.* Springfield, Ill.: Charles C Thomas.

Stevens, A. J., Rosselle, N. E., and Michels, A. A. 1976. Possibility of a selective activity in the coracobrachialis. In *Biomechanics V-A,* ed. P. V. Komi, pp. 267–71. Baltimore: University Park Press.

The Upper Extremity: The Elbow, Forearm, Wrist, and Hand

Objectives

At the conclusion of this chapter, the student should be able to:

1. Name, locate, and describe the structure and ligamentous reinforcements of the articulations of the elbow, forearm, wrist, and hand.
2. Name and demonstrate the movements possible in the joints of the elbow, forearm, wrist, and hand regardless of the starting position.
3. Name and locate the muscles and muscle groups of the elbow, forearm, wrist, and hand, and name their primary actions as agonists, stabilizers, neutralizers, or antagonists.
4. Analyze the fundamental movements of the forearm, hand, and fingers with respect to joint and muscle actions.
5. Describe the common athletic injuries of the forearm, elbow, wrist, and fingers.

In much the same way that the shoulder girdle's cooperation with the shoulder joint contributes to the wide range of motion available to the hand, the cooperative movements of the elbow, radioulnar, and wrist joints contribute to the versatility and precision of its movements. Although the hand is intrinsically skillful, its usefulness would be greatly impaired if anything interfered with the motions of the forearm or wrist. Injury to any one of the joints involved makes this painfully obvious to the sufferer.

The Elbow Joint

Structure

The elbow is far more complex than the simple hinge joint that it appears to be. The two bones of the forearm attach to the humerus in totally different ways. The humeroulnar joint is indeed a true hinge joint, but the humeroradial joint is far from it. It has been classified as an arthrodial or gliding type of joint, but it would be more accurately described as a restricted or atypical ball-and-socket joint. Inspection of the articulating surfaces as depicted in Figure 5–1 or of the skeleton itself will help to make this clear. The distal end of the humerus presents a spool-like process (trochlea) on the medial side and a spherical knob (capitulum) on the lateral side. The ulna articulates with the humerus by means of a semicircular structure that is cupped around the back and underside of the trochlea. The inner surface of this is known as the semilunar notch. It terminates below and in front in the small coronoid process, and above and in back in the broad olecranon process.

The radius articulates with the humerus by means of a slightly concave saucer-like disk, which is directly beneath the capitulum when the arm is hanging straight down. In spite of the joint's ball-and-socket structure the radius is unable to ab- or adduct because of the annular ligament that encircles the radial head and binds it to the radial notch of the ulna. Furthermore, because of this and other ligamentous connections with the ulna, the radius is unable to rotate independently (Figures 5–2 and 5–3). Hence, the only movements it is free to engage in at the elbow are flexion and extension. For this reason one is justified in classifying the elbow joint as a whole as a hinge joint.

The two articulations of the elbow joint, as well as the proximal radioulnar articulation, are completely enveloped in an extensive capsule. This is lined by synovial membrane, which extends into the proximal radioulnar articulation, covers the olecranon, coronoid, and radial fossae, and lines the annular ligament. The capsule is strengthened by four ligaments, the *anterior, posterior, radial collateral,* and *ulnar collateral.* The last named is the strongest. It is a thick triangular band, attached above by its apex to the medial epicondyle of the humerus and below by its base to the medial margins of the coronoid and olecranon processes of the ulna and the intervening ridge.

Movements

FLEXION From the anatomical position this is a forward-upward movement of the forearm in the sagittal plane (Figure 5–4A).

EXTENSION Return movement from flexion. A few individuals are able to hyperextend the elbow joint. This is probably because of a short olecranon process, rather than loose ligaments (Figure 5–4A).

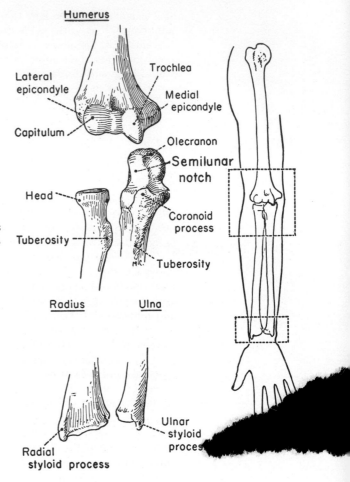

Figure 5–1 The bony structures of the elbow and radioulnar joints, anterior view.

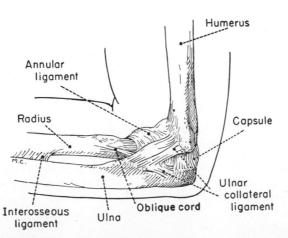

Figure 5–2 Medial aspect of elbow joint showing ligaments.

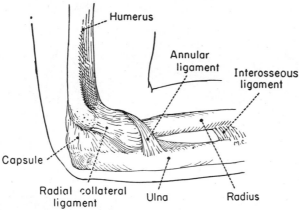

Figure 5–3 Lateral aspect of elbow joint showing ligaments.

The Radioulnar Joints

Structure of Proximal Radioulnar Joint

The disk-shaped head of the radius fits against the radial notch of the ulna and is encircled by the annular ligament (Figures 5–1, 5–2, and 5–3). The notch and annular ligament between them form a complete ring within which the radial head rotates. Inasmuch as the superior surface of the radial head articulates with the capitulum of the humerus, rotation must occur here too, although, strictly speaking, this is not part of the radioulnar joint. The three joints in this region, the humeroulnar, humeroradial, and proximal radioulnar, all share a common capsule.

Structure of Distal Radioulnar Joint

At the distal end of the forearm the radius articulates with the head of the ulna by means of a small notch (Figure 5–1). A triangular fibrocartilaginous disk lies between the head of the ulna and the proximal row of wrist bones (Figure 5–12) and serves to reinforce the joint, as well as to separate it from the wrist. The joint is also strengthened by the *volar radioulnar* and *dorsal radioulnar* ligaments. Both the proximal and distal radioulnar joints are classified as pivot joints.

Movements

PRONATION   This is a rotation of the forearm around its longitudinal axis in such a way that the palm turns medially. It corresponds to medial or inward rotation of the humerus.

SUPINATION   This is a rotation of the forearm around its longitudinal axis in such a way that the palm turns laterally. It corresponds to lateral or outward rotation of the humerus.

   Note: When the elbow is in an extended position, pronation of the forearm tends to accompany inward rotation of the upper arm, and supination tends to accompany outward rotation. In the anatomical position of the arm the humerus is rotated outward and the forearm is supinated. The full range of pronation and supination is best seen when the elbow is maintained at a 90-degree angle (Figure 5–4). When the upper arms are at the sides of the body and the forearms are extended forward in the horizontal position, the mid or neutral position relative to pronation and supination is with the thumbs up and the palms facing each other. An excellent way to study what happens to the two forearm bones in these movements is suggested in Exercise 4 of the Laboratory Experiences.

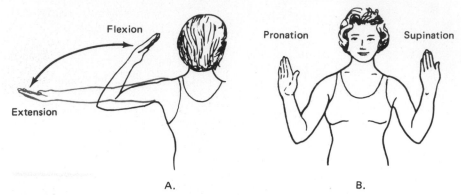

Figure 5–4   Movements of the elbow and radioulnar joints. *A*, Flexion and extension. *B*, Right radioulnar joints pronated; left radioulnar joints supinated.

Muscles of the Elbow and Radioulnar Joints

Location   The muscles of the elbow and radioulnar joints are listed below according to their positions relative to the joints involved:

Anterior (elbow region)	Posterior
Biceps brachii	Triceps brachii
Brachialis	Anconeus
Brachioradialis	Supinator
Pronator teres	
Anterior (wrist region)	
Pronator quadratus	

Characteristics and Functions of Individual Muscles

BICEPS BRACHII   This is primarily a muscle of the elbow and radioulnar joints (Figure 5–5) but, as noted in the last chapter, it also acts at the shoulder joint. Unless prevented from doing so (by the action of neutralizers or by fixation of the hand when the subject is hanging from a bar), it simultaneously *flexes* and *supinates* the forearm. The integrated EMG of the biceps is greater in the supinated than in the completely pronated position. Studies by Basmajian (1979) and others have shown that the biceps is active during flexion of the supine forearm under all conditions of static and dynamic contraction but, in most instances in which the forearm is pronated, the biceps shows little activity unless an external resistance is applied (Figure 5–6). External resistance is also necessary for the biceps to be active in supination of the extended arm. It may be palpated on the anterior surface of the upper arm when the forearm is flexed, especially in the supinated position.

BRACHIALIS   This muscle's (Figure 5–7) sole function is *flexion* of the elbow joint, and it is said to be the unexcelled flexor under all conditions (Basmajian, 1979). It is partially covered by the biceps but can be palpated just lateral to this muscle if the contraction is sufficiently strong, and especially if the forearm is maintained in the pronated position as it is being flexed (Figure 5–6). It is a spurt muscle.

BRACHIORADIALIS   In addition to its role as a contributor to elbow *flexion* (more active in a semiprone than a supine position), it has been suggested that this muscle

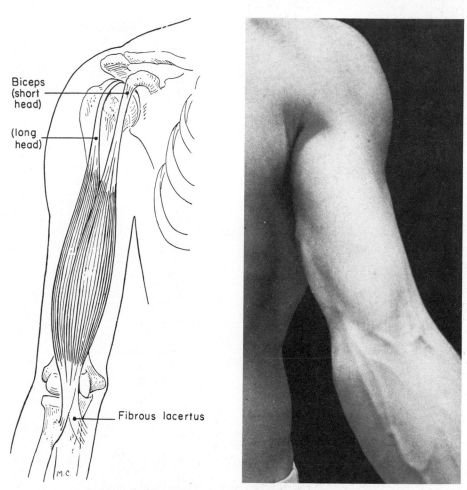

Figure 5–5   Biceps muscle of the arm.

(Figure 5–8) may tend to "derotate" the forearm as it flexes it, but this has not been confirmed by electromyographic research. It has been found, however, that the brachioradialis neither supinates nor pronates the fully extended forearm unless the movement is strongly resisted (Basmajian, 1979; De Sousa et al., 1961). It has also been noted that this muscle is most active in quick movements and is, therefore, a shunt muscle (Basmajian, 1979). It may be palpated on the anteroradial aspect of the upper half of the forearm.

PRONATOR TERES   This is primarily a pronator of the forearm (Figure 5–9), but it assists in flexing against resistance. The angle of the elbow joint does not influence the pronation activity of this muscle (Basmajian, 1979). It is difficult to palpate.

PRONATOR QUADRATUS   This muscle's (Figure 5–9) sole action is *pronation* of the forearm. EMG experiments have shown that the electrical activity of the pronator quadratus is definitely greater than that of the pronator teres, irrespective of the speed of the movement or the degree of elbow flexion. It is too deep to palpate successfully.

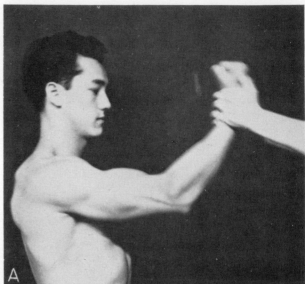

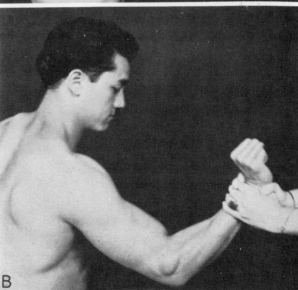

Figure 5–6 Flexion of the forearm. *A,* In a position of supination. *B,* In a position of pronation. The biceps brachii is less active when the forearm is pronated than when it is supinated.

TRICEPS BRACHII Virtually three muscles in one (Figures 5–10 and 5–11), the triceps covers the entire posterior surface of the upper arm. Its long head is the only one of the three to cross the shoulder joint. It is a powerful *extensor of the elbow joint* with two factors in its favor, a large physiological cross section (p. 309) and a favorable angle of pull (p. 310). Furthermore, it is a spurt muscle. In a comparison of the three heads it was noted that the medial head appeared to be the principal extensor of the elbow joint, usually accompanied by the lateral head. All three heads

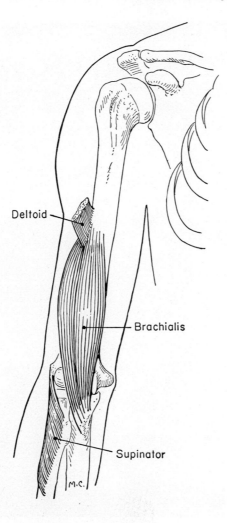

Deltoid

Brachialis

Supinator

M.C.

Figure 5–7   Deep muscles on front of right arm.

participate when there is resistance (Basmajian, 1979). The muscle is an easy one to see as well as to palpate.

ANCONEUS   This muscle *extends* (Figure 5–11) the forearm. In an EMG study of elbow joint muscles made in 1967, Pauly et al. found that this muscle initiates extension of the elbow, helps to maintain the extended position, and appears to stabilize the joint during other movements of the upper extremity. It was also noted that the muscle was moderately active during pronation and supination of the forearm (Basmajian, 1979; Provins and Salter, 1955). The muscle may be palpated on the back of the elbow at the lateral margin of the olecranon process.

SUPINATOR   Although assisted by others, this muscle (Figures 5–7 and 5–10) is the primary one for *supination* under all conditions. Palpation with any degree of success is extremely difficult.

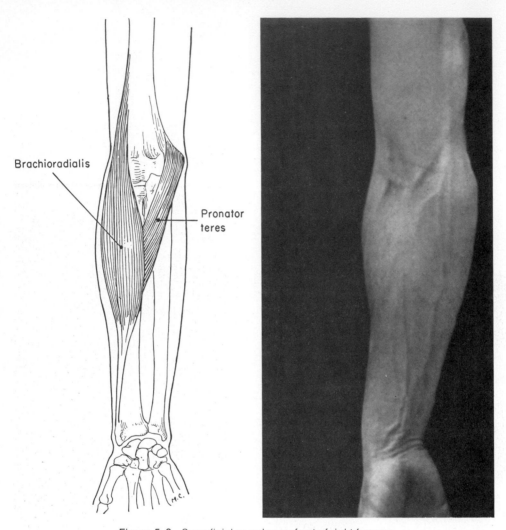

Figure 5–8   Superficial muscles on front of right forearm.

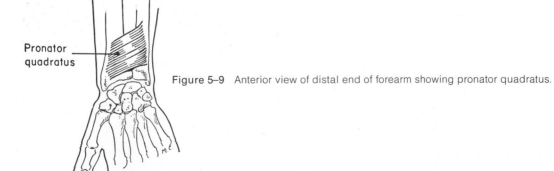

Figure 5–9   Anterior view of distal end of forearm showing pronator quadratus.

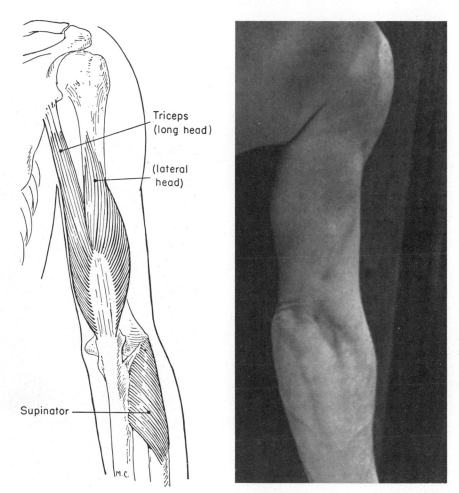

Figure 5–10   Triceps and supinator.

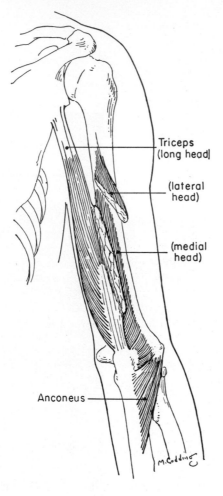

Figure 5–11   Triceps and anconeus.

Muscular Analysis of the Fundamental Movements of the Forearm

FLEXION   There are three important flexors of the forearm: the brachialis, brachiora-dialis, and biceps—the three Bs. Their relative participation in and contribution to flexion of the forearm has been the subject of much study. Since elbow flexion may be performed with the forearm pronated, semipronated, or supinated, with or without resistance, slowly or rapidly, with or against gravity, there have been many variables to study. Investigators agree that the brachialis serves as a flexor under all conditions, and there is general agreement that the biceps is more active in flexion when the arm is supinated than when it is pronated. Beyond that, opinions differ. These differences are quite evident if the results of the three research reports that follow are compared.

In their 1957 study of the biceps, brachialis, and brachioradialis, Basmajian and Latif noted that (1) the biceps flexed the supinated forearm and assisted in flexing the semiprone forearm when the movement was resisted; (2) the brachialis flexed the forearm under all conditions, it being the "work horse" of the elbow joint; and (3) the brachioradialis was a rapid flexor of the forearm in all positions, and was also moderately active in slow flexion of the prone or semiprone forearm. It was also found that the pronator teres contributes to flexion only when resistance is offered to the movement, and it was concluded that the three muscles act together with maximum electrical activity when the forearm is in the "semiprone" position; i.e., midposition, flexing against resistance (Basmajian, 1979).

As a result of a study of the relation of forearm position to the strength of elbow flexion, Larson (1969) concluded that during maximal isometric contractions (1) the biceps is most active electrically when the forearm is supinated and least active when it is pronated, (2) the brachioradialis is most active electrically when the forearm is either in the midposition or in supination and least active when the forearm is pronated, (3) the pronator teres, as a flexor, does not seem to be significantly affected by the position of the forearm, and (4) the isometric force exerted by the elbow flexors during maximal voluntary contractions is greatest when the forearm is supinated or in midposition and least when the forearm is pronated.

In a more recent study, Bouisset et al. (1975) recorded the activity of the three muscles simultaneously using surface and wire electrodes. It was established that during flexion performed in the horizontal plane, with the forearm in a semipronated position, there was a linear relationship between the integrated EMG and the work performed by each muscle, regardless of load and velocity. In addition high correlations between EMGs of the biceps and the brachialis and the biceps and the brachioradialis were obtained, leading to the conclusion that the work performed by each muscle appears to be a constant fraction of the total external mechanical work performed, regardless of the velocity and the resistance. Bouisset called this constant relation between the excitation level of the three muscles the *flexor equivalent*. These findings suggest that the brachialis, after all, should not be considered to be the *main* elbow flexor.

EXTENSION   When not produced by the force of gravity, extension of the elbow joint is effected by the triceps and anconeus.

PRONATION   Movement of the forearm at the two radioulnar joints. Produced by the combined action of the pronator teres and pronator quadratus.

SUPINATION   Movement of the forearm at the two radioulnar joints. Produced by the supinator and biceps brachii.

The Wrist and Hand

The hand and wrist owe their mobility to their generous supply of joints (Figure 5–12). The most proximal of these is the radiocarpal or wrist joint. Just beyond this are the two rows of carpal bones, each row consisting of four bones. The carpal joints include the articulations within each of these rows, as well as the articulations between the two rows. The carpometacarpal joints (Figure 5–13A) are located at the base of the hand. Closely associated with them are the intermetacarpal joints, those points of contact between the bases of the metacarpal bones of the four fingers. The fingers unite with the hand at the metacarpophalangeal joints. Within the fingers

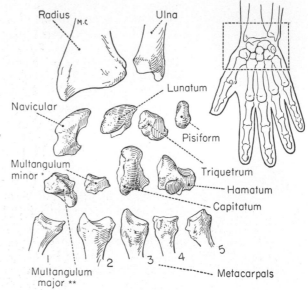

Figure 5–12 Bones of the wrist, anterior view.

*Also called Trapezoid.
**Also called Trapezium.

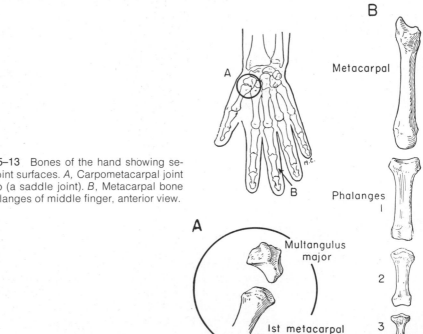

Figure 5–13 Bones of the hand showing selected joint surfaces. *A,* Carpometacarpal joint of thumb (a saddle joint). *B,* Metacarpal bone and phalanges of middle finger, anterior view.

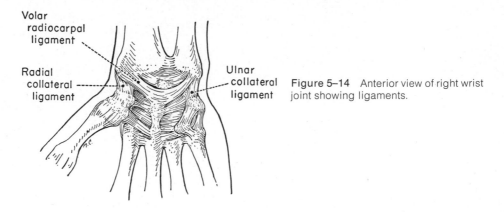

Volar
radiocarpal
ligament

Radial
collateral
ligament

Ulnar
collateral
ligament

Figure 5–14   Anterior view of right wrist joint showing ligaments.

themselves there are two sets of interphalangeal joints, the first between the proximal and middle rows of phalanges and the second between the middle and distal rows. The thumb differs from the four fingers in having a more freely movable metacarpal bone and in having only two phalanges instead of three. The metacarpal bone of the thumb is so similar to a phalanx that it might well be described as a cross between a phalanx and a metacarpal (Figure 5–13B).

Structure of the Wrist (Radiocarpal) Joint

The wrist joint is an ovoid (condyloid) joint formed by the union of the slightly concave, oval-shaped surface of the proximal row of carpal bones (i.e., the navicular, lunate, and triquetral bones, but not the pisiform). The distal radioulnar joint is in close proximity to the wrist joint and shares with it the articular disk that lies between the head of the ulna and the triquetral bone of the wrist. However, it is not a part of the wrist joint, for each joint has its own capsule. The capsule of the wrist consists of four ligaments that merge to form a continuous cover for the joint. These are the volar radiocarpal, dorsal radiocarpal, ulnar collateral, and radial collateral (Figures 5–14 and 5–15).

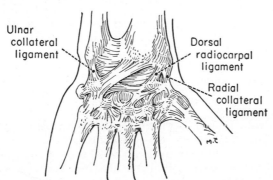

Ulnar
collateral
ligament

Dorsal
radiocarpal
ligament

Radial
collateral
ligament

Figure 5–15   Posterior view of right wrist joint showing ligaments.

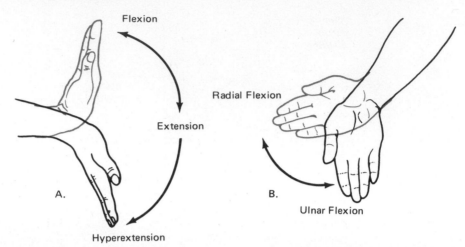

Figure 5–16   Movements of the hand at the wrist joint. *A*, Ulnar and radial flexion; *B*, Flexion, extension, and hyperextension.

Movements of the Hand at the Wrist Joint

FLEXION   From the anatomical position (Figure 5–16) this is a forward-upward movement in the sagittal plane, whereby the palmar surface of the hand approaches the anterior surface of the forearm.

EXTENSION   Return movement from flexion.

HYPEREXTENSION   A movement in which the dorsal surface of the hand approaches the posterior surface of the forearm—the exact opposite of flexion.

RADIAL FLEXION (ABDUCTION)   From the anatomical position this is a sideward movement in the frontal plane, whereby the hand moves away from the body with the thumb side leading (Figure 5–16B). The movement corresponds to abduction of the humerus.

ULNAR FLEXION (ADDUCTION)   From the anatomical position this is a sideward movement in the frontal plane, whereby the hand moves toward the body with the little finger side leading. The movement corresponds to adduction of the humerus.

CIRCUMDUCTION   A movement of the hand at the wrist whereby the finger tips describe a circle, and the hand as a whole describes a cone. It consists of flexion, radial flexion, hyperextension, and ulnar flexion occurring in sequence in either this or the reverse order. If there appears to be rotation when one performs this movement it is taking place in the radioulnar joints, not the wrist joint.

Structure and Movements of the Midcarpal and Intercarpal Joints

These are the joints within the wrist itself. The articulation between the four carpal bones in the proximal row with the four in the distal row is known as the midcarpal articulation.* The joints between the adjacent bones within either row are known as the intercarpal joints of the proximal and distal rows, respectively.* These joints are all diarthrodial in structure. Within this classification they belong to the nonaxial

*Anatomists differ in regard to these definitions. See both Gray's and Morris's anatomy textbooks (Goss, 1973; Schaffer, 1967).

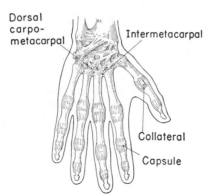

Dorsal
carpo-
metacarpal

Intermetacarpal

Collateral

Capsule

Figure 5–17 Posterior view of ligaments of right hand.

group and thus permit only a slight gliding motion between the bones. These slight movements, however, add up to a modified hinge type of movement for the midcarpal joint as a whole.

A further characteristic of the carpal region is that the bones are shaped and arranged in such a way that the anterior surface is slightly concave from side to side. This provides a protected passageway for the tendons, nerves, and blood vessels supplying the hand. Among the many carpal ligaments, the radiate is the strongest. Its fibers radiate from the capitate to the navicular, lunate, and triquetral bones on the anterior surface of the wrist.

Structure of the Carpometacarpal and Inter-metacarpal Joints (Figures 5–12, 5–17, and 5–18)

Although it has been customary to credit the carpometacarpal joint of the thumb with being the only saddle joint, the authors of this text agree with Fick who is quoted by Morris as describing the carpometacarpal joints of all the fingers as modified saddle joints, the joint of the little finger more nearly approaching a true saddle joint than any other except that of the thumb (Schaffer, 1967). The latter is a prime example of a saddle joint (Figure 5–13A). It is enclosed in an articular capsule that is stronger in back than in front. The capsule is thick but loose and serves to restrict motion rather than to prevent it. There are no additional ligaments.

The carpometacarpal joints of the four fingers are not only encased in capsules but are also protected by the dorsal, volar, and interosseous carpometacarpal ligaments (Figures 5–17 and 5–18). Closely associated with these joints are the intermetacarpal articulations, the joints between the bases of the metacarpal bones of the four

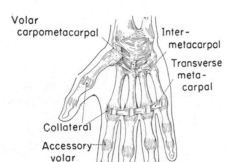

Volar
carpometacarpal

Inter-
metacarpal

Transverse
meta-
carpal

Collateral

Accessory
volar

Figure 5–18 Anterior view of ligaments of right hand.

fingers. These are irregular joints. They share the capsules of the carpometacarpal joints and are further reinforced by the dorsal, volar, and interosseous basal ligaments and also by the transverse metacarpal ligament, a narrow fibrous band that connects the heads of the four outer metacarpal bones.

Movements of the Carpometacarpal Joint of the Thumb

The names of the movements of the thumb may seem illogical until they are viewed in the context of the resting thumb position—i.e., turned on its axis so that it faces in a plane perpendicular to the other fingers.

ABDUCTION (Figure 5–19A)   A forward movement of the thumb at right angles to the palm.

ADDUCTION   Return movement from abduction.

HYPERADDUCTION (Figure 5–19B)   A backward movement of the thumb at right angles to the hand.

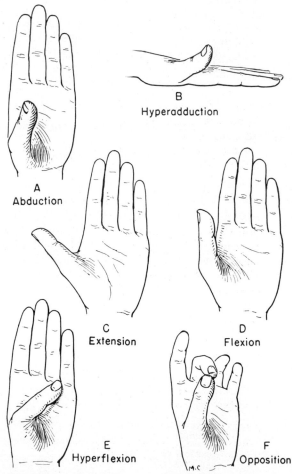

Figure 5–19   Movements of the thumb at the carpometacarpal joint.

EXTENSION (Figure 5–19C)   A lateral movement of the thumb away from the index finger.

FLEXION (Figure 5–19D)   Return movement from extension.

HYPERFLEXION (Figure 5–19E)   A medialward movement of the thumb from a position of slight abduction. The thumb slides across the front of the palm.

CIRCUMDUCTION   A movement in which the thumb as a whole describes a cone and the tip of the thumb describes a circle. It consists of all the movements described above, performed in sequence in either direction.

OPPOSITION (Figure 5–19F)   This movement, which makes it possible to touch the tip of the thumb to the tip of any of the four fingers, is essentially a combination of abduction and hyperflexion and, according to some investigators, slight inward rotation. Others claim that what appears to be inward rotation of the metacarpal is actually a slight medial movement of the greater multangular bone with which the metacarpal articulates. The movements of the metacarpal are accompanied by flexion of the two phalanges, especially the distal. The apparent rotatory movement is explained in part by the oblique axis of motion about which abduction and adduction of the thumb take place, and in part by the movement of the greater multangular bone that accompanies flexion of the thumb. The total movement of the thumb in opposition might well be described as a movement of partial circumduction.

Movements of the Carpometacarpal and Intermetacarpal Joints of the Fingers

Largely because of the short ligaments in this region, especially in the case of the second, third, and fourth digits, the motion in both the carpometacarpal and intermetacarpal joints is almost nonexistent, being limited to slight gliding. The fifth carpometacarpal joint is slightly more mobile and permits a limited motion of the fifth metacarpal bone, resembling in small degree the motion of the thumb.

Structure of the Metacarpophalangeal Joints
(Figures 5–13, 5–17, and 5–18)

The joint at the base of each of the four fingers, uniting the proximal phalanx with the corresponding metacarpal bone, is an ovoid (condyloid) joint. The oval, convex head of the metacarpal fits into the shallow oval fossa at the base of the phalanx. The fossa is deepened slightly by the fibrocartilaginous volar accessory ligament. The joint is encased in a capsule and is protected on each side by strong collateral ligaments.

The metacarpophalangeal joint of the thumb has flatter joint surfaces than do the corresponding joints of the four fingers and has more of the characteristics of a hinge joint. In addition to the articular capsule, it is protected by a collateral ligament on each side and by a dorsal ligament.

Movements of the Metacarpophalangeal Joints of the Four Fingers
(Figure 5–20)

FLEXION   The anterior surface of the finger approaches the palmar surface of the hand.

EXTENSION   Return movement from flexion. Most individuals are able to achieve slight hyperextension in these joints.

ABDUCTION   For the fourth, fifth, and index fingers this is a lateral movement away from the middle finger. This movement is limited and cannot be performed when the fingers are fully flexed.

ADDUCTION   Return movement from abduction.
Note: In ab- and adduction of the fingers a different point of reference is used than

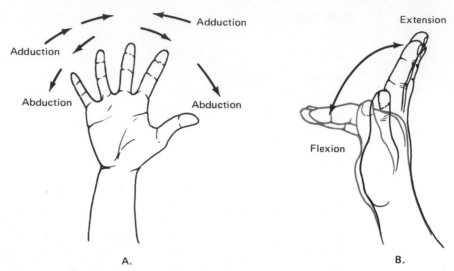

Figure 5–20   Movements of the metacarpophalangeal joints. *A*, Abduction and adduction. *B*, Flexion and extension.

in ab- and adduction of the hand as a whole. The center line of the hand—that is, the line passing through the middle finger when the latter is in its normal, extended position—is the reference line for the second, fourth, and fifth digits. Comparable movements of the middle finger are called radial and ulnar flexion.

These lateral finger movements are actually movements of the proximal phalanx with the action occurring at the metacarpophalangeal joint, but the entire finger moves as a unit since there is no lateral action possible at the interphalangeal joints.

CIRCUMDUCTION   The combination of flexion, abduction, extension, and adduction performed in sequence in either direction.

Movements of the Metacarpophalangeal Joints of the Thumb

FLEXION   The volar surface of the thumb approaches that of the thenar eminence (base of thumb).

EXTENSION   Return movement from flexion. Individuals vary greatly in their ability to hyperextend the thumb at this joint.

The Interphalangeal Joints

These are the joints between the adjacent phalanges of any of the five digits. They are all hinge joints; hence, their only movements are flexion and extension. These correspond to flexion and extension of the first phalanx at the metacarpophalangeal joints. Hyperextension is slight, if present at all. Each joint is enclosed within an articular capsule which is strengthened in front by an accessory volar ligament and on each side by a strong collateral ligament.

Muscles of the Wrist and Hand

Location

The muscles of the wrist, fingers, and thumb are classified according to their location on the forearm or the hand and within each group are listed alphabetically (Table 5–1). Of the 19 muscles of the fingers and thumb, 10 are located entirely within the hand and are called intrinsic muscles. Those located outside of the hand on the forearm but with tendon attachments on the thumb or fingers are extrinsic muscles.

Characteristics and Functions of Muscles

WRIST MUSCLES (Figures 5–21, 5–22, and 5–23A)   As one would expect from their location, the *flexor carpi radialis* and *flexor carpi ulnaris* are important flexors of the wrist. The palmaris longus, however, is a weak contributor to wrist flexion and may even be absent in some individuals. The flexor carpi radialis is also active in radial flexion (abduction) and the flexor carpi ulnaris in ulnar flexion. The tendons of these muscles may be readily palpated on the anterior surface of the wrist (Figure 5–21). The palmaris longus tendon, if present, is clearly visible if the hand is flexed against a slight resistance. The ulnaris tendon is best identified by its relation to the pisiform

TABLE 5–1 WRIST AND HAND MUSCLES

MUSCLES OF THE WRIST

Anterior	Posterior
Flexor carpi radialis	Extensor carpi radialis brevis
Flexor carpi ulnaris	Extensor carpi radialis longus
Palmaris longus	Extensor carpi ulnaris

MUSCLES OF THE FINGERS AND THUMB

On the Forearm (Extrinsic Muscles)	In the Hand (Intrinsic Muscles)
Fingers*	Fingers
Extensor digiti minimi	Abductor digiti minimi
Extensor digitorum	Flexor digiti minimi brevis
Extensor indicis	Interossei dorsales manus
Flexor digitorum profundus	Interossei palmaris
Flexor digitorum superficialis	Lumbricales manus
	Opponens digiti minimi
Thumb	Thumb
Abductor pollicis longus	Abductor pollicis brevis
Extensor pollicis brevis	Adductor pollicis
Extensor pollicis longus	Flexor pollicis brevis
Flexor pollicis longus	Opponens pollicis

*It is important to have an exact knowledge of the distal attachments of these muscles in order to understand their actions.

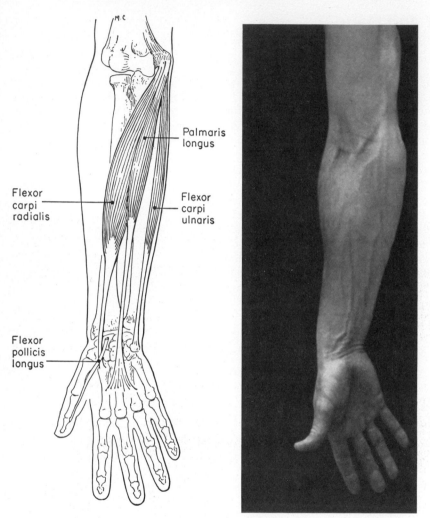

Figure 5–21   Superficial muscles on front of right forearm.

bone. It should not be confused with the tendon lying close on the ulnar side of the palmaris tendon. This is a tendon of the flexor digitorum superficialis, probably the one for the fourth finger (Figure 5–24A).

Both *radial extensor* muscles of the wrist are active in extension and radial flexion (abduction), with the *extensor carpi radialis brevis* more active in extension than the *extensor carpi radialis longus*. The *extensor carpi ulnaris* works cooperatively with the extensor carpi radialis muscles in wrist extension and participates in ulnar flexion (adduction).

The *three wrist extensor muscles* may be palpated on the dorsal surface of the forearm when the forearm and hand are resting palm down on a table, the *carpi radialis longus* on the radial side at elbow level and slightly below, the *brevis* slightly below the longus, and the *carpi ulnaris* on the ulnar margin of the dorsal surface

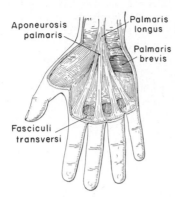

Figure 5–22 Palmar aponeurosis and palmaris muscles of right palm.

about midway between the elbow and wrist. The tendon of the carpi radialis longus may be palpated on the dorsal surface of the wrist in line with the index finger.

The *flexor carpi radialis* and *extensor carpi radialis longus*, together with the *abductor pollicis longus* of the thumb, team up to produce *radial flexion (abduction)* of the wrist, and the *extensor* and *flexor carpi ulnaris* muscles team up similarly to produce *ulnar flexion (adduction)*.

MUSCLES OF THE FINGERS AND THUMB (Figures 5–22 through 5–29) In most instances the names of the muscles of the finger and thumb indicate their chief function. These muscles will therefore not be discussed individually. Some of these muscles,

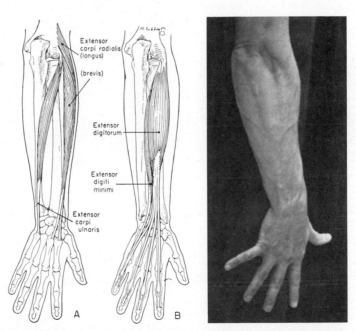

Figure 5–23 Muscles on back of right forearm. *A,* Extensor carpi radialis longus and brevis and extensor carpi ulnaris. *B,* Extensor digitorum and extensor digiti minimi.

however, have important additional roles, and these should be identified. In addition to being an extensor of the interphalangeal joints, the *extensor digitorum* is an important wrist extensor. Similarly, the flexor digitorum *superficialis* is active in wrist flexion as well as in flexion at the proximal phalangeal joints. The *abductor pollicis longus* both abducts and flexes the metacarpophalangeal joint of the thumb, and the *abductor pollicis brevis*, together with the *opponens pollicis*, is active in extension and abduction of the thumb. Both the *flexor and extensor pollicis longus* are active in adduction and opposition of the thumb, and the *adductor pollicis* participates in opposition and flexion.

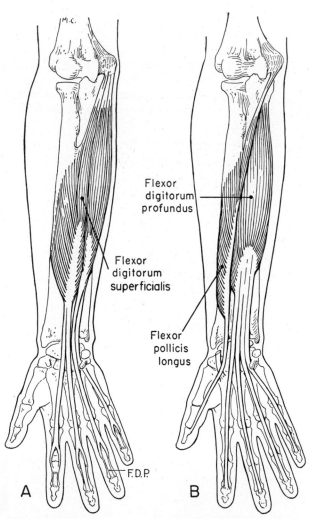

Figure 5–24   Deep muscles on front of right forearm. *A,* Flexor digitorum superficialis. *B,* Flexor digitorum profundus and flexor pollicis longus.

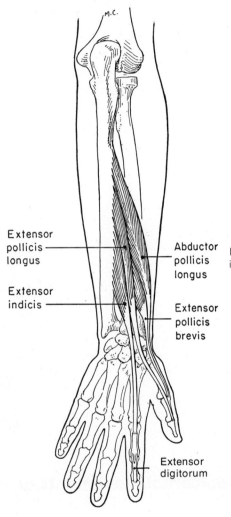

Extensor
pollicis
longus

Abductor
pollicis
longus

Extensor
indicis

Extensor
pollicis
brevis

Extensor
digitorum

Figure 5–25 Posterior muscles of the thumb and
index finger.

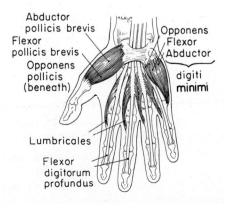

Abductor
pollicis brevis
Flexor
pollicis brevis
Opponens
pollicis
(beneath)

Opponens
Flexor
Abductor

digiti
minimi

Lumbricales

Flexor
digitorum
profundus

Figure 5–26 Anterior view of muscles of right
hand.

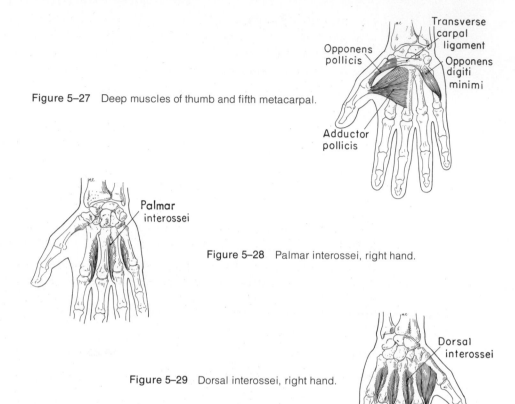

Figure 5–27   Deep muscles of thumb and fifth metacarpal.

Figure 5–28   Palmar interossei, right hand.

Figure 5–29   Dorsal interossei, right hand.

Muscular Analysis of the Fundamental Movements of the Wrist, Fingers, and Thumb

The Wrist

These are movements of the hand as a unit. They occur chiefly at the radiocarpal joint but involve the midcarpal and intercarpal joints when flexion or hyperextension is carried to the limit of motion.

FLEXION   Performed by the flexors carpi radialis, carpi ulnaris, digitorum superficialis, with possible help from the palmaris longus, flexor pollicis longus, and flexor digitorum profundus.

EXTENSION AND HYPEREXTENSION   Performed synchronously by the extensors carpi radialis longus, carpi radialis brevis, carpi ulnaris, and extensor digitorum, with possible help from the pollicis longus and extensors indicis and digiti minimi.

RADIAL FLEXION (ABDUCTION)   Performed by the extensors carpi radialis longus and brevis and flexor carpi radialis, with possible help from the abductor pollicis longus and the extensors pollicis longus and brevis.

ULNAR FLEXION (ADDUCTION)   Performed by the extensor carpi ulnaris and the flexor carpi ulnaris.

The Fingers

For a better understanding of all the actions of the finger and thumb muscles, they should be studied both on the skeleton (using an elastic band to represent muscles) and on another person. Particular attention should be paid to the relation of each muscle to every joint it crosses, to the muscle's line of pull, and to the leverage involved.

As an aid to recognizing the secondary actions of the muscles, a record of the joints crossed by all the finger and thumb muscles is summarized below.

FOREARM MUSCLES OF THE FINGERS   All five of these muscles cross four sets of joints: wrist, carpometacarpal, metacarpophalangeal, and proximal interphalangeal. The extensor digitorum and extensor digiti minimi also cross both the elbow and the distal interphalangeal joint, making a total of six joints crossed. The flexor digitorum superficialis crosses the elbow but not the distal interphalangeal, and both the extensor indicis and flexor digitorum profundus cross the distal interphalangeal joint but not the elbow.

INTRINSIC MUSCLES OF THE FINGERS   Of these six muscles, only the abductor digiti minimi and flexor digiti minimi brevis cross both the carpometacarpal and the metacarpophalangeal joints. The two interossei muscles, dorsales and palmares, and the lumbricales cross only the metacarpophalangeal joint, and the opponens digiti minimi, like the opponens pollicis, crosses only the carpometacarpal joint. The two work together in the cupping action of the palm as well as independently in other opposition movements.

FOREARM MUSCLES OF THE THUMB   All four of these muscles cross both the wrist and carpometacarpal joints, and all but the abductor pollicis longus also cross the metacarpophalangeal joint. The extensor and flexor pollicis longus muscles cross the interphalangeal joint as well. The thumb, of course, has no second interphalangeal joint.

INTRINSIC MUSCLES OF THE THUMB   All four of these muscles cross the carpometa-carpal joint and all but the opponens pollicis cross the metacarpophalangeal joint.

The muscular action of the fingers is given in terms of the movement of each phalanx. Movement of the proximal phalanx takes place at the metacarpophalangeal joint, of the middle phalanx at the proximal interphalangeal joint, and of the distal phalanx at the distal interphalangeal joint. For convenience in referring to individual fingers, numbers are assigned as follows: 2 for the index finger, 3 for the middle finger, 4 for the ring finger, and 5 for the little finger.

FLEXION

Proximal Phalanx   Flexed by the lumbricales manus (all fingers), interossei palmaris (palmar interossei) (2,4,5), interossei dorsales manus (2,3,4), flexor digiti minimi brevis (5), and opponens digiti minimi (5), with possible help from the flexors digitorum superficialis and profundus.

Middle Phalanx   Flexed by the flexor digitorum superficialis, which acts on all four fingers and at the same time contributes to flexion of the metacarpal bones.

Distal Phalanx   Flexed by the flexor digitorum profundus, which also acts on all four fingers and at the same time contributes to flexion of the proximal and middle phalanges.

EXTENSION

Proximal Phalanx   Extended by the extensor digitorum (all fingers), extensor indicis (2), and extensor digiti minimi (5). The extensor digitorum is also able to help extend the middle and distal phalanges.

Middle and Distal Phalanges   Extended by the lumbricales manus (all fingers) and interossei dorsales manus (dorsal interossei) (2,3,4). The abductor digiti minimi (5) and the extensor digitorum (all fingers) are also able to help extend the middle and distal phalanges at the same time that they are extending the proximal phalanx.

Note: When all the fingers flex or extend the antagonists relax in reciprocal innervation. However, if a single finger moves, the antagonists will contract in an attempt to keep the other fingers still.

ABDUCTION AND ADDUCTION   Abduction is brought about by the interossei dorsales manus (2,4) and abductor digiti minimi (5), and adduction by the interossei palmaris (2,4,5).

Radial and ulnar flexion of the middle finger is performed by the interossei dorsales manus (3).

OPPOSITION   The fifth digit, or little finger, being at the outer margin of the hand, has greater freedom of movement than do the other fingers. Through the action of the opponens digiti minimi the metacarpal bone of this finger can engage in a slight degree of opposition at the carpi metacarpal joint. Together with the thumb, it participates in this movement when the hand is "cupped," as when scooping up water, and also when the tip of the little finger is brought forcibly against the tip of the thumb.

The Thumb

The muscular action of the thumb is given in terms of the movements of the metacarpal bone and the two phalanges, proximal and distal.

The Thumb Metacarpal

FLEXION   The metacarpal is flexed and hyperflexed after being slightly abducted by the flexor pollicis brevis and the adductor pollicis. The flexor pollicis longus also participates and becomes more dominant when the action is full flexion (Basmajian, 1979).

EXTENSION   Performed chiefly by the abductor pollicis longus, with help from the opponens pollicis, the abductor pollicis brevis, and the extensors pollicis longus and brevis.

ABDUCTION   Four muscles are responsible for this movement, two from the forearm, the abductor pollicis longus and the extensor pollicis brevis, and two from the thenar eminence, the abductor pollicis brevis and the opponens pollicis. Under some conditions these may be helped by the flexor pollicis brevis.

ADDUCTION   This is performed mainly by the adductor pollicis, with some help from the flexor pollicis brevis and, in certain positions, from the extensor pollicis longus.

OPPOSITION   This is performed mainly by the opponens, but with appreciable help from the flexor pollicis brevis. As opposition is not a single, well defined movement but varies according to the finger that is being opposed and to the exact position of that finger, the muscles controlling the thumb must adapt to the demands of the situation. This includes the action of the phalanges as well as that of the metacarpal.

The Thumb Phalanges

FLEXION   The flexor pollicis longus flexes both of the phalanges. Additional flexors of the proximal phalanx include the flexor pollicis brevis and the adductor pollicis, with help from the abductor pollicis brevis when necessary.

EXTENSION   The extensor pollicis longus extends both of the phalanges. This is joined by the brevis in the extension of the proximal phalanx.

The plane in which flexion and extension of the thumb phalanges takes place is determined by the position of the metacarpal bone of the thumb.

Cooperative Actions of Wrist and Digits

Length of Long Finger Muscles Relative to Range of Motion in Wrist and Fingers

An interesting characteristic of the long finger muscles is that they do not have sufficient length to permit the full range of motion in the joints of the fingers and wrist at the same time. For instance, one cannot achieve complete flexion of the fingers and wrist simultaneously because the extensor digitorum will not elongate enough to permit it. If maximum *finger* flexion is maintained, the wrist is able to flex only slightly. And, similarly, if maximum *wrist* flexion is maintained, it will be impossible to achieve a real grip with the fingers. They flex incompletely and without appreciable force. Or, if one first makes a tight fist and then determines to flex the wrist completely, the individual will soon discover that the fingers loosen their grip and tend to open up in spite of efforts to prevent it. This is not caused by contraction of the finger extensors, but by their inability to elongate sufficiently.

The same type of reaction occurs if one attempts to achieve maximum extension of the fingers when the wrist is fully hyperextended. This involuntary movement due to the tension of opposing muscles is known as the tendon or pulley action of multijoint muscles. Because of this arrangement of the muscles, the strongest finger flexion can be obtained when the wrist is held rigid in either a straight or slightly hyperextended position and the strongest finger extension when the wrist is rigid in either a straight or slightly flexed position. The most powerful wrist action—either flexion or hyperextension—can take place only when the fingers are relaxed. In other words, strong finger action requires a rigid wrist; strong wrist action requires relaxed fingers. This aspect of wrist and finger action has been discussed exceptionally well by Wright (1962).

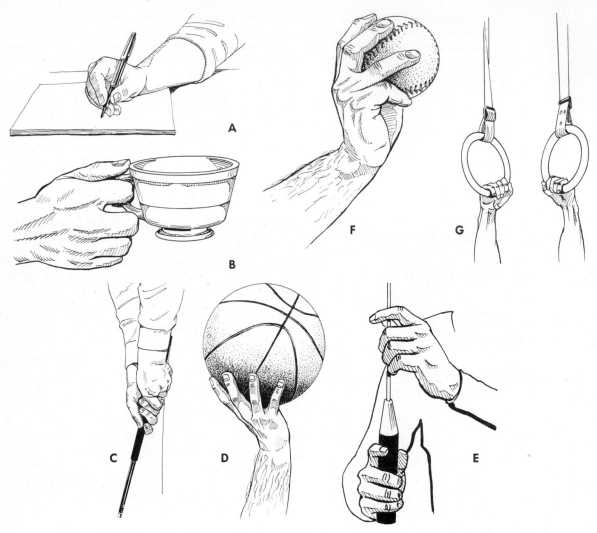

Figure 5–30   Examples of grasps. The muscular involvement depends on the nature of the grasp.

Examples of Using the Hands for Grasping

In sports and gymnastics there is probably less concern with the fine, precision movements of the fingers and thumb than with the grosser movements such as the grasping of balls, striking implements, and suspension apparatus. In general, grasping activities involve flexion of the fingers (usually all three joints), opposition of the thumb metacarpal, and flexion of the phalanges. The degrees of these movements, together with the degree of abduction that may be present in the fingers, depend upon the shape and size of the object being grasped, as well as on the purpose of the movement (Figure 5–30). The muscular involvement also depends upon the nature of the grasp. There is a complex interplay between the extrinsic and intrinsic muscular involvement, which varies with the force and spread of the grasp. Generally speaking the extrinsic rather than the intrinsic muscles appear to be the major force for compression actions, power gripping, and the gross movements associated with precision gripping. The intrinsic muscles are of greater significance in the refinements of precision movements and the rotation actions which are part of these movements. The wrist extensors are also active during grasping motions, since they stabilize the wrist against the flexion tendencies of those finger flexors which cross the front of the wrist joint (Basmajian, 1979).

Whether pitching, throwing for distance, or tossing a ball straight upward, the movements of the forearm and hand are of prime importance. The greater the force desired for moving the ball, the greater the contribution of the upper arm, but as this discussion applies only to the forearm and hand the upper arm is not considered here. Ignoring the finer movements, the essential action of the forearm in both overhand pitching and in throwing for distance is extension; of the wrist, "flexion" from the hyperextended to the extended position (with an abrupt check of the motion when the wrist is straight); and of the fingers, extension.

In a vertical toss, starting with the forearm forward at a slight downward slant— i.e., with the elbow at a slightly obtuse angle—the movements are elbow flexion followed by finger extension and wrist flexion from the hyperextended position. The active muscles are mainly the elbow flexors, the wrist flexors in static contraction, and the finger extensors. The reader may find it of interest to analyze the joint and muscle actions in other kinds of throws.

Common Athletic Injuries of the Forearm, Elbow, Wrist, and Fingers

Fractures of the Forearm

These are common among children and teenagers and are usually caused either by a direct blow or by falling on a rigidly outstretched arm. It is more usual for both the radius and ulna to break than for either one to break alone, and in the younger age group the fracture of either or both bones is likely to be of the greenstick type.

It is important to immobilize the elbow joint in the treatment of a fractured radius, even though the fracture is close to the wrist. This is because in pronation and supination, as the radial head rotates against both the capitulum of the humerus and the radial notch of the ulna, the broad distal end swings halfway around the ulna. The need for immobilizing the elbow joint in the event of a radial fracture should be apparent to anyone who is conversant with kinesiology.

Elbow Dislocation

The majority of these dislocations consist of the backward displacement of the ulna and radius in relation to the humerus. The most common cause is catching oneself from a fall by taking the weight on the outstretched hand with the elbow in rigid extension or hyperextension. This can be a very serious injury, since it is likely to involve blood vessels and nerves.

Elbow Fracture-Dislocation

Elbow dislocations are frequently accompanied by fractures, the most common being a fracture of the medial epicondyle, especially in the middle to late adolescent age group in those whose epicondylar epiphyses have not yet closed.

Sprained or Strained Wrist

This type of wrist injury is very common and, like so many of the other upper extremity injuries, is caused by catching oneself from a fall by thrusting the arm downward and taking the weight on the palm with the hand hyperextended at the wrist and the elbow rigidly extended. Although the injury is usually called a sprain, it is more likely to be a strain, since the site of the trouble tends to be at the tendon attachments rather than at the attachments of the anterior ligaments (Klafs and Arnheim, 1973; O'Donoghue, 1976). It may also involve the fracture of a carpal bone.

Injuries Caused by a Blow from a Ball Against the Tip of a Finger

These are the result of extending the fingers toward the oncoming ball when preparing to catch it. In a true baseball finger the ball forces the distal phalanx into flexion so sharply that the extensor digitorum tendon pulls off the bit of bone from the base of the phalanx to which it is attached (O'Donoghue, 1976). This type of injury is known as an avulsion fracture. Less severe injuries from the same cause may result in damage to an interphalangeal cartilage.

Tennis Elbow

Epicondylitis, or "tennis elbow," affects the lower end of the humerus on the lateral side. It is a chronic inflammation of the attachment of the extensor carpi radialis brevis and extensor digitorum to the lateral epicondyle. The condylar attachment of the radial collateral ligament may also be involved. It is believed that the inflammation occurs because of the mechanical construction of the elbow itself. The leverage is such that with each stroke the extensor attachments are subjected to repetitive pressures and strains. Any combination of inflexible and weak forearm musculature and rigid racket may result in chronic tennis elbow. When the condition occurs on the medial end it is called "golfer's elbow." The symptoms are the same for both maladies—painful to touch, with increased aggravation when the elbow is twisted (Nirschl, 1974).

Laboratory Experiences

Elbow and Forearm: Joint Structure and Function

1. Using a form like the one in Appendix A, record the essential information regarding the two articulations of the elbow joint and, likewise, the two radioulnar articulations. Study the movements of these joints both on the skeleton and on the living body.

2. Using a protractor-goniometer, measure the range of motion on five subjects for the following movements: flexion, pronation, and supination of the forearm.

3. Repeat Exercise 24 from Chapter 4, this time writing the joint analysis of *(a)* the starting position of the forearm at the elbow and radioulnar joints, and *(b)* the movement from the starting position to the final pull-up position. Discuss with partner.

4. Assume a handshaking grasp with a skeleton with the elbow flexed and the forearm approximately horizontal. Slowly pronate your forearm and note the movement of the skeleton's forearm. Observe carefully each end of the radius and ulna and describe what happens. Now supinate your forearm as far as possible and carefully observe the radioulnar movements of the skeleton. Note the way the edge of the radial head rotates against the notch of the ulna and the way the superior surface of the radial head revolves against the capitulum of the humerus. At the distal end note the way the broad articular process of the radius swings around the head of the ulna and the radial shaft crosses over that of the ulna. Note that the ulna itself does not rotate, although it may appear to do so when the elbow is fixed in extension and pronation of the forearm occurs in conjunction with inward rotation of the humerus.

Elbow and Forearm: Muscular Action

Record the results on a chart similar to the one in Appendix E.

5. **FLEXION**

    Subject: Sit with the entire arm resting on a table. Flex the forearm *(a)* with palm up (forearm supinated), *(b)* with thumb up (forearm in neutral position), and *(c)* with palm down (forearm pronated).

    Assistant: Resist the movement by holding the wrist. Steady the upper arm if necessary.

    Observer: Palpate as many of the forearm flexors as possible. Do you notice any difference in the muscular action in *a, b,* and *c*?

6. **EXTENSION**

    a. *Subject:* Lie face down on a table with one arm raised to shoulder level, with the upper arm resting on the table, the forearm hanging down. Extend the forearm without moving the upper arm.

    Assistant: Steady the upper arm and resist the forearm at the wrist.

    Observer: Palpate the triceps and anconeus.

    b. *Subject:* On hands and knees, bend and extend the elbows in a push-up exercise.

    Observer: Palpate the triceps and anconeus.

7. **SUPINATION**

    Subject: Assume a handshaking position with the assistant and turn your forearm outward.

    Assistant: Assume the same position with the subject and resist the movement.

    Observer: Palpate and identify the muscles which contract.

8. **PRONATION**

    Subject: Assume a handshaking position with the assistant and turn the forearm inward.

    Assistant: Assume the same position with the subject and resist the movement.

    Observer: Palpate and identify the muscles which contract. What is their function? Can you palpate the principal movers?

Action of Muscles Other Than Movers

9. **SUPINATION WITHOUT FLEXION**

    Subject: Sit with the arm supported, elbow in a slightly flexed position and relaxed. Supinate the forearm without increasing or decreasing flexion at the elbow.

    Observer: Palpate the triceps. Explain.

10. **VIGOROUS FLEXION OF FOREARM**

    Subject: Flex forearm vigorously, then check the movement suddenly before completing the full range of motion.

    Observer: Palpate the triceps. Does it contract during any part of the movement? Explain.

11. Perform a movement in which the supinator acts as a neutralizer.

Elbow and Forearm: Applications

12. Working with a partner execute a knee push-up, i.e., a push-up from the front lying position, onto the knees instead of the toes, until the elbows are fully extended. Keep the body straight from the knees to the top of the head. Return to the starting position slowly and in good form.

    a. Analyze the joint and muscular action of the elbows in the push-up.

    b. Do the same for the return movement.

    c. What force is responsible for the movement in *a*? In *b*?

    d. What is the chief difference in the type of muscular action used in the push-up and in the let-down (return movement)? (See last paragraph on page 342.)

13. In reading the section on Common Injuries it may have been noted that several injuries to the forearm, elbow, and wrist are caused by taking the weight on the outstretched hand with the elbow rigidly extended when catching oneself from a fall. The following exercise is designed

to accustom one to the practice of giving at the elbow and other upper extremity joints at the moment the hand strikes the ground. If practiced frequently this technique should become a habit.

Kneel on a gymnasium mat with the knees slightly separated, hips in extension, and body erect. Shift your weight to the side until you lose your balance and fall to a side-sitting position with your arm outstretched and your hand reaching to catch your weight. At the moment of contact let your elbow give (i.e., flex) and, if the force is sufficient, roll onto your shoulder and back with knees drawn up. Practice this many times, both to right and left. Experiment with variations.

Wrist and Hand: Joint Structure and Function

14. Using a form like the one in Appendix A, record the essential information regarding the radiocarpal, carpometacarpal, metacarpophalangeal, and interphalangeal articulations. Study the movements both on the skeleton and on the living body. Pay particular attention to the carpometacarpal joint of the thumb.

15. With a protractor-goniometer measure the amount of hyperextension possible at the wrist (*a*) with the fingers flexed, (*b*) with fingers extended. Likewise measure the amount of flexion possible at the wrist (*a*) with the fingers flexed, (*b*) with the fingers extended. Explain.

Wrist and Hand: Muscular Action

(See checklists in Appendix E.) If possible, get someone who plays the piano to serve as a subject.

16. **FLEXION AT WRIST**
Subject: Sit with forearm resting on a table with palm up. Flex hand at wrist.
Assistant: Resist movement by holding palm.
Observer: Palpate, identify, and explain the action of as many muscles as possible.

17. **EXTENSION AND HYPEREXTENSION AT WRIST**
Subject: Sit with forearm resting on a table with palm up. Flex hand at wrist.
Assistant: Resist movement by holding palm.
Observer: Palpate, identify, and explain the action of as many muscles as possible.

18. **RADIAL FLEXION AT WRIST**
Subject: Sit with forearm resting on a table, ulnar side (little finger side of hand) down. Keeping thumb against hand, raise hand from table without moving forearm.
Assistant: May give slight resistance to hand.
Observer: Palpate and identify the muscles responsible for radial flexion.

19. **ULNAR FLEXION AT WRIST**
Subject: Lie face down or bend forward in such a way that radial side of hand (thumb side) is on supporting surface, with forearm supported and wrist neither flexed nor hyperextended. Keeping little finger against hand, raise hand without moving forearm.
Assistant: May give slight resistance to hand.
Observer: Palpate and identify the muscles responsible for ulnar flexion.

20. **FINGER FLEXION**
Subject: Sit with forearm resting on a table with palm up. Flex fingers without flexing wrist.
Assistant: Resist movement by hooking own fingers over those of subject.
Observer: Palpate, identify, and explain the action of as many muscles as possible.

21. **FINGER EXTENSION**
Subject: Sit with forearm resting on a table with palm down, fingers curled over edge of table. Extend fingers.
Assistant: Resist movement by holding hand over subject's fingers.
Observer: Palpate, identify, and explain the action of as many muscles as possible.

22. ABDUCTION OF THUMB

Subject: Place the hand on a table with the palm up and the thumb slightly separated from the index finger. Abduct the thumb at the carpometacarpal joint by raising it vertically upward.

Assistant: Give slight resistance to the thumb at the proximal phalanx.

Observer: Palpate the abductor pollicis brevis in the thenar eminence.

23. HYPERFLEXION OF THUMB IN POSITION OF SLIGHT ABDUCTION

Subject: Place the hand on a table with the palm up and the thumb slightly raised from the table. Hyperflex the thumb at the carpometacarpal joint.

Assistant: Give slight resistance to the proximal phalanx of the thumb.

Observer: Palpate the flexor pollicis brevis in the thenar eminence.

24. EXTENSION OF THUMB

Subject: Rest the fully extended hand on its ulnar border with the thumb uppermost. Extend the thumb as far as possible.

Observer: Identify the tendons of the abductor pollicis longus, extensor pollicis longus, and extensor pollicis brevis.

25. OPPOSITION OF THUMB

Subject: Press the thumb hard against the tip of the middle finger.

Observer: Palpate and identify the opponens pollicis and adductor pollicis.

Action of Muscles Other Than Movers

26. Perform a movement in which the extensor carpi ulnaris and extensor carpi radialis longus and brevis act as neutralizers to prevent flexion at the wrist.

27. Perform a movement in which the extensor carpi ulnaris and flexor carpi ulnaris act as mutual neutralizers.

Hands: Application

28. In Figure 5–30 inspect the various styles of grasping sport objects and analyze a few of these. First identify the joint position of the wrist, fingers, and thumb, and then determine the chief muscular involvement.

References

Basmajian, J. V. 1979. *Muscles alive.* 4th ed. Baltimore: Williams & Wilkins.

Beevor, C. 1951. *The Croonian lectures on muscular movements.* Reprint ed. New York: Macmillan.

Bouisset, S., Lestienne, F., and Maton, B. 1975. Relative work of main agonists in elbow flexion. In *Biomechanics V-A,* ed. P. V. Koni, pp. 272–79. Baltimore: University Park Press.

DeSousa, O. M., DeMoraes, J. L., and Viera, F. L. de M. 1961. Electromyographic study of the brachioradialis muscle. *Anat. Rec.* 139:125–31.

Goss, C. M., ed. 1973. *Gray's anatomy of the human body.* 29th ed. Philadelphia: Lea & Febiger.

Klafs, C. E., and Arnheim, D. D. 1973. *Modern principles of athletic training.* St. Louis: C. V. Mosby.

Larson, R. F. 1969. Forearm positioning on maximal elbow-flexor force. *J. Am. Phys. Ther. Assoc.* 49:748–59.

Nirschl, R. P. 1974. The etiology and treatment of tennis elbow. *J. Sports Med.* 2:308–23.

O'Donoghue, D. H. 1976. *Treatment of injuries to athletes.* 3d ed. Philadelphia: W. B. Saunders.

Pauly, J. E., Rushing, J. L., and Scheving, L. E. 1967. An electromyographic study of some muscles rossing the elbow joint. *Anat. Rec.* 159:47–53.

Piscopo, J. 1974. Assessment of forearm positions upon upper arm and shoulder girdle strength performance. In *Kinesiology IV,* pp. 53–57. Washington, D.C.: American Association of Health, Physical Education and Recreation.

Provins, K. A., and Salter, N. 1955. Maximum torque exerted above the elbow joint. *J. Appl. Physiol.* 7:393–98.

Schaffer, J. P., ed. 1967. *Morris' human anatomy.* 11th ed. New York: Hafner Publishing.

Steindler, A. 1970. *Kinesiology of the human body.* Springfield, Ill.: Charles C Thomas.

Wright, W. G. 1962. *Muscle function.* New York: Hafner Publishing.

The Lower Extremity: The Hip Region

Objectives

At the conclusion of this chapter, the student should be able to:

1. Name, locate, and describe the structure and ligamentous reinforcements of the articulations of the hip and pelvic girdle.
2. Name and demonstrate the movements possible in the hip joint and pelvic girdle, regardless of starting position.
3. Name and locate the muscles and muscle groups of the hip and pelvis, and name their primary actions as agonists, stabilizers, neutralizers, or antagonists.
4. Analyze the fundamental movements of the thigh and pelvis with respect to joint and muscle actions.
5. Describe the common athletic injuries of the thigh, hip, and pelvis.

The Relationship Between the Hip Joint and the Pelvic Girdle

The relationship between the hip joint and the pelvic girdle is somewhat similar to that between the shoulder joint and shoulder girdle. Just as the scapula tilts or rotates to put the glenoid fossa in a favorable position for the movements of the humerus, so the pelvic girdle tilts and rotates to put the acetabulum in a favorable position for the movements of the femur. There are these differences, however. Whereas the left and right sides of the shoulder girdle can move independently, the pelvic girdle can move only as a unit. Furthermore, whereas the movements of the shoulder girdle take place in its own joints (sternoclavicular and acromioclavicular), the pelvic girdle is dependent for its movements upon the lumbosacral and other lumbar joints, and the hip joints. Hence, an analysis of the movements of the pelvic girdle must always be stated in terms of spinal and hip action.

The Hip Joint

Structure

The hip joint (Figure 6–1), a typical ball-and-socket joint, is formed by the articulation of the spherical head of the femur with the deep cup-shaped acetabulum. The latter, formed by the junction of the three pelvic bones (ilium, ischium, and pubis), is also described as horseshoe-shaped since there is a gap (the acetabular notch) at the lower part of the "cup." The entire acetabulum is lined with hyaline cartilage. This is thicker above than below, and the center is filled in with a mass of fatty tissue covered by synovial membrane. A flat rim of fibrocartilage, known as the *glenoid labrum,* is attached by its circumference to the margin of the acetabulum (Figure 6–2). It covers the hyaline cartilage and, since it is considerably thicker at the circumference than at the center, it adds to the depth of the acetabulum. Furthermore, being thicker above and behind, it serves to cushion the top and back of the acetabulum against the impact of the femoral head in forceful movements. The head also is completely covered with hyaline cartilage, except for a small pit near the center called the fovea capitis. The cartilage is thicker above and tapers to a thin edge at the perimeter.

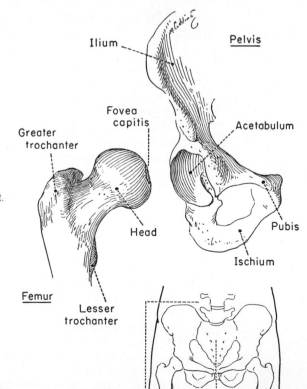

Figure 6–1   Bones of the hip joint.

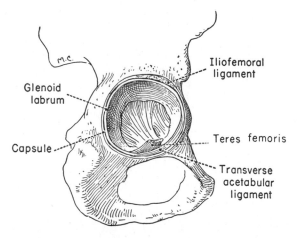

Figure 6–2 Acetabulum of right hip joint.

Ligamentous Reinforcements

The *transverse acetabular* ligament is a strong, flat band of fibers continuous with the glenoid, which bridges the acetabular notch and thus completes the acetabular ring.

The *teres femoris* is a flat, narrow triangular band attached by its apex to the fovea capitis near the center of the femoral head, and by its base to the margins of the acetabular ligament (Figure 6–3). Its function is to "tie" the head of the femur to the lower part of the acetabulum and thus provide the joint with reinforcement from within.

Outer reinforcement is provided by the three ligaments of the femoral neck, one for each of the pelvic bones that unite to form the acetabulum (Figures 6–4 and 6–5). The *iliofemoral* ligament, called the Y ligament because of its supposed resemblance to an inverted Y, is an extraordinarily strong band of fibers situated at the front of the capsule and intimately blended with it. Because of its position it serves to check extension and both outward (lateral) and inward (medial) rotation. The *pubofemoral* ligament consists of a narrow band of fibers at the medial anterior and lower portion of the capsule. It prevents excessive abduction and helps to check extension and outward rotation. The *ischiofemoral* ligament is a strong triangular ligament at the back of the capsule. It limits inward rotation and adduction in the flexed position.

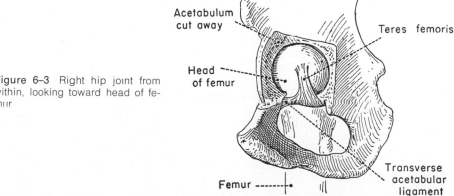

Figure 6–3 Right hip joint from within, looking toward head of femur

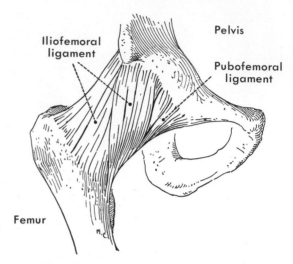

Figure 6–4 Anterior view of right hip joint.

Movements of the Femur at the Hip Joint

The movements of the femur (Figure 6–6) are similar to those of the humerus, but are not quite so free as the latter because of the deeper socket. In studying the movements of the femur the student should first be aware of the position of the femur in the fundamental standing position. If viewed from the front, it is seen that the shaft of the femur is not vertical but that it slants somewhat medialward. This serves to place the center of the knee joint more nearly under the center of motion of the hip joint. Hence, the mechanical axis of the femur—a line connecting the center of the femoral head with the center of the knee joint—is almost vertical (Figure 1–2). The degree of slant of the femoral shaft is related both to the size of the angle between the neck and shaft and the width of the pelvis.

As seen from the side, the shaft of the femur bows forward. These characteristics of the femur—the obtuse neck-shaft angle and the forward bowing of the shaft—are, as Steindler (1970) has explained, provisions for resisting the strains and stresses sustained in walking, running, and jumping, and for assuring the proper transmission of weight through the femur to the knee joint.

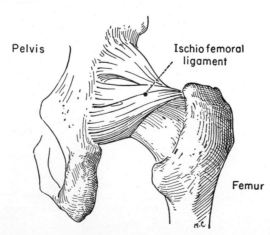

Figure 6–5 Posterior view of right hip joint.

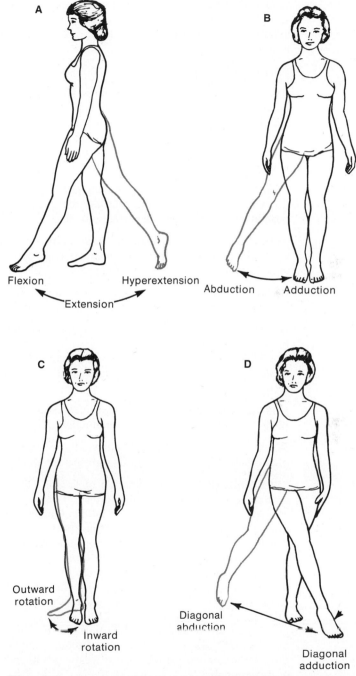

Figure 6–6 Movements of the hip joint. *A,* Flexion, extension, and hyper-extension. *B,* Abduction and adduction. *C,* Inward and outward rotation. *D,* Diagonal abduction and adduction.

FLEXION   A forward movement of the femur in the sagittal plane. If the knee is straight, the movement is restricted by the tension of the hamstring muscles. In extreme flexion the pelvis tilts backward to supplement the movement at the hip joint.

EXTENSION   Return movement from flexion.

HYPEREXTENSION   A backward movement of the femur in the sagittal plane. This movement is extremely limited. Except in dancers and acrobats, it is possible only when the femur is rotated outward and is probably completely absent in many individuals. The restricting factor is the iliofemoral ligament at the front of the joint. The advantage of this restriction of movement is that it provides a stable joint for weight-bearing without the need for strong muscular contraction.

ABDUCTION   A sideward movement of the femur in the frontal plane so that the thigh moves away from the midline of the body. A greater range of movement is possible when the femur is rotated outward.

ADDUCTION   Return movement from abduction. Hyperadduction is possible only when the other leg is moved out of the way. In extreme hyperadduction the teres femoris becomes taut.

OUTWARD ROTATION   A rotation of the femur around its longitudinal axis so that the knee is turned outward.

INWARD ROTATION   A rotation of the femur around its longitudinal axis so that the knee is turned inward.

The range of inward and outward rotation is affected by the degree of femoral torsion (twisting of the femur on its long axis so that one end is inwardly rotated with respect to the other).

HORIZONTAL FLEXION   A forward movement of the abducted thigh in a horizontal plane, probably accompanied by reduction of outward rotation.

HORIZONTAL ABDUCTION   A sideward movement of the flexed thigh in a horizontal plane, probably accompanied by outward rotation.

CIRCUMDUCTION   A combination of flexion, abduction, extension, and adduction performed sequentially in either direction.

An interesting study on the relation of femoral torsion to in-toeing and out-toeing during walking was reported by Crane (1959). He noted that the out-toeing group was capable of 60 to 80 degrees of lateral rotation but less than 20 degrees of medial rotation. The in-toeing group, on the other hand, was capable of only 10 to 20 degrees of lateral rotation and 60 to 80 degrees of medial rotation. X-rays showed abnormal femoral torsion in both of these groups. Although the cause could not be determined, Crane suggested that it might be traced either to fetal positions or, as was thought by Fitzhugh, to sleeping positions during infancy.

In comparing a group of "normal" children, aged 6 months to 9 years, with data on "normal" adults, he found that femoral torsion was three or four times greater during the first year of life than it was in adulthood and that the decrease in torsion occurred gradually.

A striking contrast was seen in a comparison of two young boys who had opposite patterns of sitting. Boy A, aged 7, habitually assumed a kneeling-sitting position with the knees close and the feet widely separated and everted like a letter W. Boy B, aged 5, habitually assumed the familiar position known as "tailor sitting" or "Indian sitting." Their rotation and torsion measurements were as follows:

	Lat. rot.	Med. rot.	Femoral torsion (anteversion)
Boy A	5–10°	75°	R 50; L 53°
Boy B	80°	10°	Less than 10°

Muscles of the Hip Joint

Location

The muscles acting at the hip joint are listed below according to their position in relation to the joint. They include several muscles which act with equal or greater effectiveness at the knee joint. These are known as the two-joint muscles of the lower extremity. Only their action at the hip joint is considered in this section.

Anterior
    Iliopsoas
    Pectineus
    Rectus femoris
    Sartorius
    Tensor fasciae latae

Posterior
    Biceps femoris ⎫
    Semimembranosus ⎬ "Hamstrings"
    Semitendinosus ⎭
    Gluteus maximus
    Six deep outward rotators

Medial
    Adductor brevis
    Adductor longus
    Adductor magnus
    Gracilis

Lateral
    Gluteus medius
    Gluteus minimus

Characteristics and Functions of Hip Joint Muscles

ILIOPSOAS (Figure 6–7; also listed with the spinal muscles)   Since the *psoas major* and *iliacus* muscles share a common distal attachment and act as one muscle at the hip joint, the usual practice of treating them as one muscle is followed here. The muscle is a *strong hip flexor*. Depending upon the circumstances it will either *flex the thigh on the trunk* or will *flex the trunk as a unit on the thighs* from a supine lying position, or in any position when the movement is performed against resistance. While some believe it helps to stabilize the hip joint in the standing position, others disagree. Results of EMG studies support either view (Basmajian, 1979; LaBan et al., 1965).

Considerable disagreement has arisen concerning additional functions. There has been some evidence of both outward and inward rotation but it would be well to follow Basmajian's (1979) advice concerning this and abandon the controversy, since there is insufficient evidence to support either side and the amount of activity during the rotation is minimal at best.

In regard to abduction and adduction, Steindler (1970) assumed that from its position the iliopsoas would *adduct* the femur but that such movement would be negligible. Both Basmajian and Close found in their EMG investigations that the iliopsoas was definitely active in *abduction*, especially as the limit of the range of motion was approached (Basmajian, 1979). It may be of interest to the reader to look at

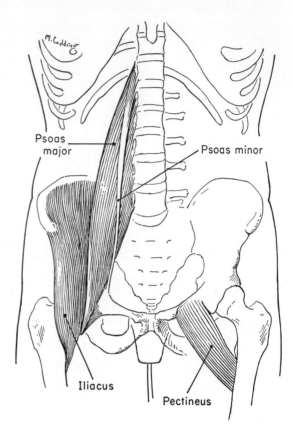

Figure 6–7 Anterior view of pelvic region showing psoas major and minor, iliacus and pectineus.

Figure 1–2, which depicts the mechanical axis of the femur, and visualize the lines of pull of the iliopsoas. It will be noted that the only fibers that appear to be in a position to abduct are the outermost fibers of the iliacus, which originate from the vicinity of the anterior superior iliac spine. As the limb is abducted, however, more fibers are in a position to contribute to the force for the abduction.

The muscle is extremely difficult to palpate. It is impossible to palpate the iliacus, but the *psoas major* may possibly be palpated on slender subjects who are able to keep the abdominal muscles relaxed during the testing. Two techniques are suggested:

1. The subject lies on the side, rolled toward the face, and flexes the thigh against slight resistance without contracting the abdominal muscles. The psoas may be palpated in the groin.
2. The subject lies on the back with the lower back arched as much as possible. From this position one thigh is flexed without contracting the abdominal muscles. An assistant should support the underside of the pelvis and try to keep it from moving. The psoas may be palpated through the abdomen.

PECTINEUS This muscle (Figure 6–7) is a short, thick, quadrilateral muscle situated lateral and superior to the adductor longus and more or less parallel to it. It *flexes the thigh* and possibly *assists in adduction* when the hip is in a flexed state. Whether it also contributes to outward rotation is debatable. As a flexor it has a good angle of pull

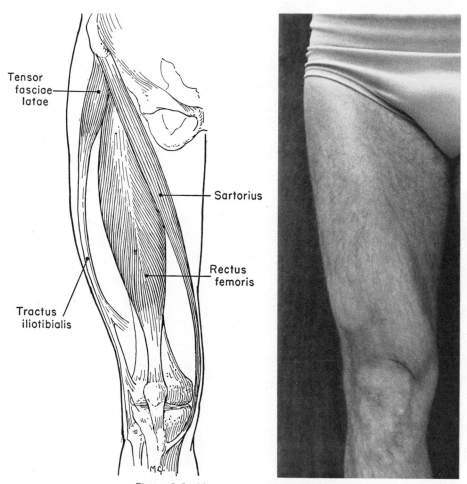

Tensor
fasciae
latae

Sartorius

Rectus
femoris

Tractus
iliotibialis

Figure 6–8   Muscles on front of right thigh.

that together with its internal structure accounts for its ability to overcome considerable resistance. It may be palpated at the front of the pubis, just lateral to the adductor longus, but it is difficult to distinguish from the latter muscle.

RECTUS FEMORIS (Figure 6–8; also listed with the knee muscles)   This muscle *flexes the thigh* and is also active during abduction and lateral rotation. It is a large bipenniform muscle, located superficially on the front of the thigh. It acts on the knee joint as well as the hip and is therefore a two-joint muscle. It shows maximum activity in single joint movements or in the countercurrent actions of hip flexion and knee extension. There is no activity when the hip flexion is concurrent with knee flexion. According to Wright (1962), the rectus femoris serves as an anterior ligament of the hip in addition to being a flexor. It may be palpated as well as seen on the anterior surface of the thigh.

SARTORIUS (Figure 6–8; also listed with the knee muscles)   This is also a two-joint muscle. Its action on the thigh is *flexion.* It also shows activity in abduction when

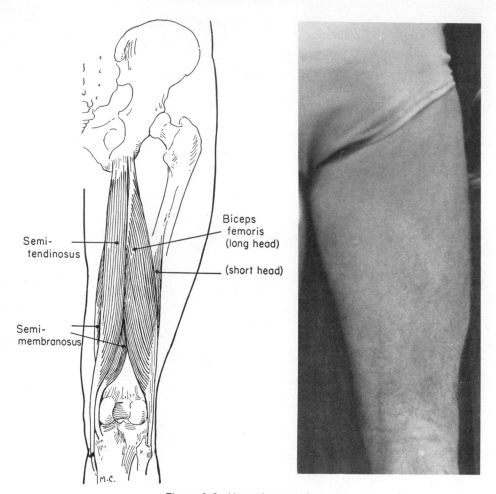

Figure 6-9   Hamstring muscles.

external resistance is offered, and in outward rotation while sitting (Stubbs et al., 1975). It is a long, slender, ribbonlike muscle directed obliquely downward and medialward across the front of the thigh. It is the most superficial of the anterior thigh muscles and may be readily seen and palpated on slender subjects. On others, it may be palpated at the anterior superior iliac spine. Its name is derived from its alleged function of enabling one to sit with the legs "tailor" fashion.

TENSOR FASCIAE LATAE   This muscle (Figures 6–8 and 6–11) *flexes* and *abducts the femur* and *tenses the fascia lata.* Apparently it also rotates the femur inward but its contribution appears to be minimal (Basmajian, 1979; Wheatley and Jahnke, 1951). It is a small muscle located close in front of and slightly lateral to the hip joint, and may be palpated about 2 inches anterior to the greater trochanter. Because its pull on the fascia lata is transmitted by means of the iliotibial tract down to the lateral condyle of the tibia, it helps to extend the leg at the knee. Together with the gluteus maximus,

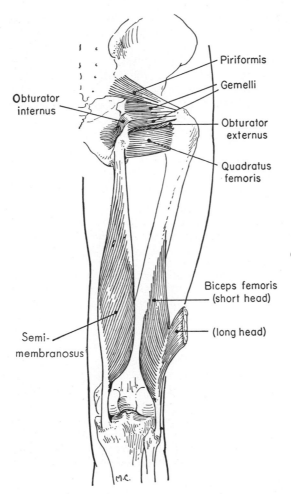

Obturator
internus

Piriformis

Gemelli

Obturator
externus

Quadratus
femoris

Biceps femoris
(short head)

(long head)

Semi-
membranosus

Figure 6–10   Deep posterior muscles of right thigh.

which also unites with the fascia lata, it helps to stabilize the knee joint in weight-bearing positions. When the lower extremities are fixed, both of these muscles help to steady the pelvis and trunk on the thighs.

THE HAMSTRINGS (Figures 6–9 and 6–10; also listed with the knee muscles)   The three hamstring muscles, *biceps femoris*, *semimembranosus*, and *semitendinosus*, are situated on the back of the thigh, extending from the tuberosity of the ischium down just below the knee joint, with the biceps femoris on the lateral aspect of the posterior surface and the two "semi" muscles on the medial aspect.

The biceps femoris is the lateral hamstring muscle. Only its long head crosses the hip joint; the short head, therefore, has no part in hip joint movements. The tendon may be palpated on the lateral aspect of the posterior surface of the knee.

Together the semimembranosus and semitendinosus constitute the medial component of the hamstring group. The *semimembranosus* lies anterior to the *semiten-*

dinosus and has a shorter, deeper tendon that is extremely difficult to palpate. The *semitendinosus* tendon may easily be palpated on the medial aspect of the posterior surface of the knee when the leg is flexed against resistance from the prone lying position. It should not be confused with the gracilis tendon, which lies slightly anterior to it. All three muscles *extend the femur* or, if the thighs are bearing weight as in either the standing or long sitting position, they will extend the forward flexed trunk as a unit—i.e., from the hips. (Spinal action must not be confused with hip action, or vice versa.) The effectiveness of the medial hamstrings as extensors of the hip is related to knee joint action. Fujiwara and Basmajian demonstrated that they show maximum activity during hip extension when the knee is either stabilized or flexed simultaneously (Basmajian, 1979). They were inactive, however, during simultaneous hip and knee extension.

Basmajian (1979) reports that some investigators found that all three hamstrings, in addition to extending the hip, help to stabilize it, except in erect standing. Also, they adduct the femur from the abducted position when the movement is resisted and help to rotate the extended femur, the long head of the biceps femoris rotating it laterally and the inner hamstrings rotating it medially.

GLUTEUS MAXIMUS (Figures 6–11, 6–12, and 6–13)   This is the largest and most superficial of the three buttock muscles. It is a potentially *powerful hip extensor*. It also *rotates the femur outward* when the latter is extended. The *lower portion assists in adduction* from an abducted position if the movement is resisted. The *upper portion abducts* against strong resistance (MacConaill and Basmajian, 1969). One can understand these seemingly contradictory functions more readily after studying the relation of the muscle to the hip joint's center of motion as seen from behind. Figure 6–13 shows that roughly one-third of the muscle lies above the center of motion and two-thirds below it. This puts the uppermost fibers in a position for abducting the thigh and the lower fibers in a position for adducting the thigh, whereas the fibers lying directly behind the femoral head are not in position for doing either. The entire muscle may easily be palpated on the posterior surface of the buttock.

The gluteus maximus has been the subject of much EMG study. Contrary to what one might think because of its size and prominence, the gluteus maximus has been shown to be active during the motions named above only when moderate to heavy resistance to the movement exists. And, even though it displays bursts of activity during brief periods of normal and fast walking, its participation is not essential. Duchenne (1959) has demonstrated that ordinary walking is not affected by complete paralysis of the gluteus maximus.

The activity of the gluteus maximus in stair climbing has been confirmed in studies conducted by the Prosthetic Devices Research Project in Berkeley (1953) and by Merrifield (1961). It has also been found to be active in walking up an inclined plane, in extending the femur against resistance, in abducting the femur, especially against resistance and when rotated outward, and in adducting the femur against resistance when in an abducted position (Merrifield, 1961). Surprisingly, Houtz and Fischer, the only investigators who have reported on its role in bicycling, stated that it was unimportant in this activity (Basmajian, 1979). In a later more extensive study of gluteus maximus function, the same investigators had some additional surprising results. After testing their subjects in the performance of several exercises commonly prescribed for strengthening the gluteus maximus, they found that the movements which elicited the greatest electrical activity were as follows: hyperextension movements of the thigh performed against resistance from the erect standing position,

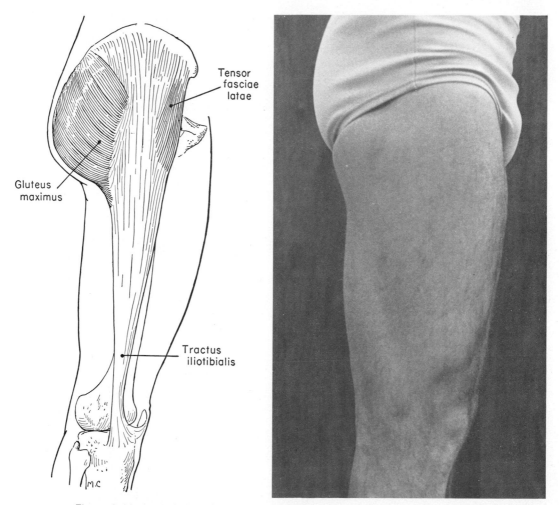

Figure 6–11   Lateral view of gluteus maximus, tensor fasciae latae, and iliotibial tract.

muscle setting, and vigorous hyperextension of the trunk from an erect position. Furthermore, they found that lifting a 25-pound weight from both a squat position and from a straight leg, trunk bend position elicited relatively minor electrical activity (Fischer and Houtz, 1968).

If an individual stands erect with feet parallel, voluntary contraction of the gluteus maximus, achieved by "pinching the buttocks together," produces two interesting postural effects. The pull on the femur causes a slight outward rotation at the hip joint, but since friction between the soles of the feet and the floor prevents the feet from turning laterally, the rotatory force is transmitted from the femur to the talus and thence to the other tarsal bones, resulting in supination of the foot and a lifting of the medial aspect of the longitudinal arch. At the same time the pull at the muscle's proximal attachment decreases the lumbar lordosis. This setting or tensing of the gluteus maximus is frequently advocated as a corrective postural exercise.

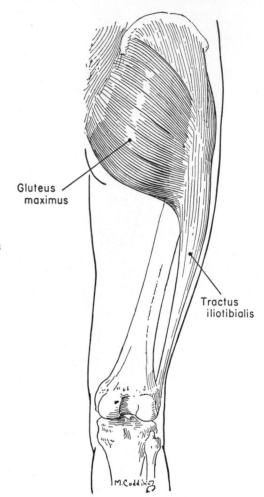

Figure 6–12 Posterior view of gluteus maximus and iliotibial tract.

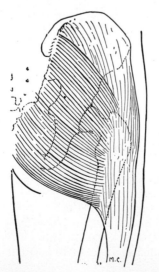

Figure 6–13 Diagram showing relation of gluteus maximus to hip joint.

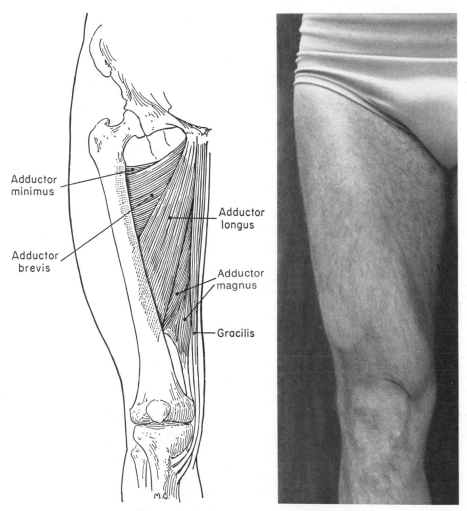

Figure 6–14   Adductor muscles of right thigh.

THE SIX DEEP OUTWARD ROTATORS   These six muscles (obturator externus and internus, gemellus superior and inferior, quadratus femoris, and piriformis) (Figure 6–10) form a compact group behind the hip joint. Their fibers run horizontally for the most part. The piriformis, the most superior of the group, is slightly above the joint and the quadratus femoris, the most inferior, is slightly below it. Some of the muscles have a secondary function such as ab- or adduction, but neither of these functions compares in importance with that of *outward rotation*. They are favorably situated for helping to hold the femoral head in the acetabulum.

ADDUCTOR BREVIS   This muscle (Figure 6–14) lies just above the adductor longus and consists of fibers that are almost horizontal when the thigh is in its normal resting or standing position. From this position it both *adducts* and *aids in flexing the femur*, but if the hip is flexed to a marked degree it combines extension with adduction, against resistance. It is also active in inward rotation.

ADDUCTOR LONGUS   This muscle (Figure 6–14) *adducts* and *flexes the femur.* Steindler (1970) has pointed out that, while it ordinarily helps to flex the thigh, when the flexion exceeds about 70 degrees it becomes an extensor as a result of a shift in the relationship between the muscle's line of pull and the joint's center of motion. In an EMG study made in 1966, de Sousa and Vitti found that this muscle was always active during free adduction and inward rotation (Basmajian, 1979). The muscle may be palpated just below its proximal attachment at the medial aspect of the groin.

ADDUCTOR MAGNUS   This muscle (Figure 6–14) *extends the thigh as well as adducting it,* and the condyloid or *lowest portion also assists in inward rotation.* De Sousa and Vitti have noted that this muscle was not active during free adduction and extension unless the movement was performed against resistance (Basmajian, 1979). Like the other adductors, it was found to be active in inward rotation. The adductor magnus may be palpated on the medial aspect of the middle half of the thigh. The uppermost portion of the muscle—i.e., the portion that comes from the pubis—is sometimes treated as a separate muscle called *adductor minimus.*

GRACILIS (Figure 6–14; also listed with the knee muscles)   This muscle *adducts* and *flexes the femur.* As the name indicates, it is a slender muscle. Being an adductor, it is sometimes called the adductor gracilis and, like the hamstrings, sartorius, and rectus femoris, it is a muscle of the knee as well as the hip joint. EMG studies have shown that it participates in hip flexion only when the knee is extended and that it is most active during the first part of flexion; it also helps to rotate the femur medially (inward) (Steindler, 1970).

GLUTEUS MEDIUS   This muscle (Figure 6–15A) is essentially an *abductor of the femur.* The *anterior fibers also rotate the thigh inward.* The muscle may be palpated about 2 or 3 inches above the greater trochanter.

The muscle is an important one in walking and in standing in good posture. When the weight is shifted onto one foot, tension of the gluteus medius and other abductors is an important factor in stabilization of the hip. Lack of such stabilization results in an exaggerated sideward thrust of the supporting hip and a drop of the pelvis on the opposite side (Trendelenburg sign). Paralysis of this muscle causes a typical limping gait known as the gluteus medius gait. When the weight is borne on the affected side, the trunk tilts strongly to that side and the opposite hip is thrust into prominence.

Figure 6–15 Gluteus medius and minimus.

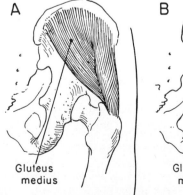

Gluteus medius

Gluteus minimus

GLUTEUS MINIMUS   This muscle (Figure 6–15B) *rotates inward and abducts*. It is smaller than the gluteus medius and is situated beneath it. Whereas the medius is primarily an abductor and secondarily an inward rotator, the minimus is primarily an inward rotator and secondarily an adductor. The muscles appear to work cooperatively, each one assisting in the other's primary function.

Muscular Analysis of the Fundamental Movements of the Thigh

FLEXION   This movement is performed chiefly by the tensor fasciae latae, pectineus (both of these especially during the first half of range), iliopsoas, rectus femoris, and sartorius. The gracilis and adductors longus and brevis assist in flexion in selected positions.

EXTENSION   The three hamstring muscles are the chief hip extensors. The gluteus maximus extends only against resistance. The three adductors also extend against resistance and when the thigh is flexed beyond a 45-degree angle.

ABDUCTION   The chief abductors are the gluteus medius and minimus, the former being the more effective of the two. The sartorius and rectus femoris are active against resistance; the uppermost fibers of the gluteus maximus abduct against resistance during the early part of the movement, and the tensor fasciae latae abducts the thigh when it is extended.

ADDUCTION   The adductor longus is the primary adductor. Other important adductors are the adductors magnus and brevis and the gracilis. The pectineus adducts the flexed thigh, and the lower third of the gluteus maximus assists in the movement when it is performed against resistance. The hamstrings adduct the abducted thigh against resistance.

OUTWARD ROTATION   This movement is performed by the six deep outward rotators, biceps femoris, and gluteus maximus.

INWARD ROTATION   The chief inward rotators are the gluteus medius and minimus, the latter being the more effective of the two. They are assisted by the semimembranosus, semitendinosus, gracilis, and adductor longus. The lower fibers of the adductor magnus rotate the thigh inward when it is extended. Some say that the tensor fasciae latae also helps, but this is debatable.

HORIZONTAL FLEXION   Probably performed by the adductors longus and brevis, gracilis, iliopsoas, pectineus, rectus femoris, sartorius and tensor fasciae latae, and accompanied by the relaxation of the outward rotators.*

HORIZONTAL ABDUCTION   Probably performed by the gluteus medius, minimus and upper maximus, and the six deep outward rotators.*

*So far as the authors know these movements have not yet been analyzed electromyographically.

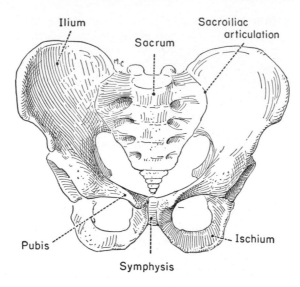

Figure 6–16   Anterior view of pelvis.

The Pelvic Girdle

Structure

The pelvis (Figure 6–16) is a rigid bony basin, which serves as a massive connecting link between the trunk and the lower extremities. Each pelvic bone (os innominatum) is made up of three bones—the ilium, ischium, and pubis. These bones become fused into a single bone by about the time of puberty. The two hip bones together form the pelvic girdle. This bony girdle or basin is firmly attached to the sacrum at the sacroiliac articulation, an articulation that is difficult to classify. It presents some of the characteristics of a diarthrodial joint, an articular cavity being present for part of the articulation. It is unlike other diarthrodial joints in one important respect, however. No movement can be voluntarily effected at the sacroiliac joint. Any movement which does occur is involuntary. Just how much motion can take place at the sacroiliac joint is debatable. Some anatomists say that a slight "giving" may occur there as a shock absorption device; others claim that no motion occurs at the joint normally, except in women during pregnancy and parturition, when the ligaments relax in order to permit a slight spreading of the bones.

The sacrum is firmly bound to the two iliac bones by means of the anterior, posterior, and interosseous sacroiliac ligaments (Figures 6–17 and 6–18). It is further reinforced by the iliolumbar, sacrotuberous, and sacrospinous ligaments and by the lower portion of the erector spinae muscle. Because of this firm attachment, the sacrum might well be considered a part of the pelvic girdle. From the point of view of function it is more truly a part of the pelvis than of the spine.

Movements of the Pelvis

Changes in the position of the pelvis are brought about by virtue of the motions of the lumbar spine and the hip joints. Movements in these joints permit the pelvis to tilt forward, backward, and sideward, and to rotate horizontally.

INCREASED INCLINATION (FORWARD TILT) (Figure 6–19C)   A rotation of the pelvis in the sagittal plane about a frontal-horizontal axis in such a manner that the symphysis pubis turns downward and the posterior surface of the sacrum turns upward.

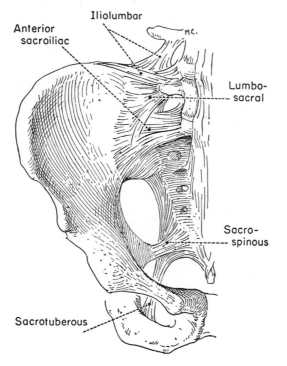

Figure 6–17   Anterior view of sacro-iliac articulation showing ligaments.

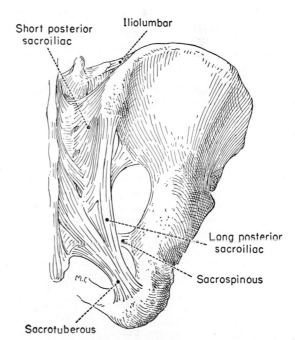

Figure 6–18   Posterior view of sacroili-ac articulation showing ligaments.

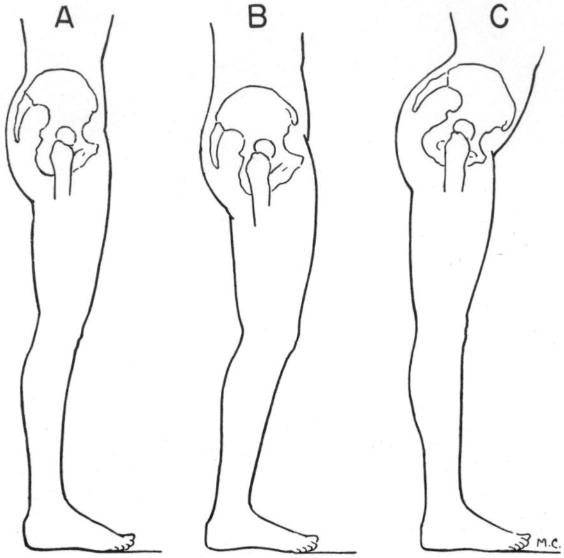

Figure 6–19 Anteroposterior inclinations of the pelvis. *A*, Mid-position. *B*, Decreased inclination (backward tilt). *C*, Increased inclination (forward tilt).

DECREASED INCLINATION (BACKWARD TILT) (Figure 6–19B)   A rotation of the pelvis in the sagittal plane about a frontal-horizontal axis in such a manner that the symphysis pubis moves forward-upward and the posterior surface of the sacrum turns somewhat downward.

LATERAL TILT (Figure 6–20A)   A rotation of the pelvis in the frontal plane about a sagittal-horizontal axis in such a manner that one iliac crest is lowered and the other is raised. The tilt is named in terms of the side which moves downward. Thus, in a lateral tilt of the pelvis to the left, the left iliac crest is lowered and the right is raised.

ROTATION (LATERAL TWIST) (Figure 6–20B)   A rotation of the pelvis in the horizontal plane about a vertical axis. The movement is named in terms of the direction toward which the front of the pelvis turns.

Muscles of the Pelvis

All the muscles that attach to the pelvic bones or to the sacrum serve either to initiate or to control pelvic movements. As one would expect, these are all muscles either of the hip joint or of the lumbar spine, including the lumbosacral junction. The precise combination of movements at these joints depends upon whether the pelvic movement is primary or whether it is secondary, supplementing either the spinal movements or those of the hip joint.

Muscles providing the force for primary movements of the pelvis when one is standing with both feet facing forward could be as follows:

INCREASED TILT   Hip flexors and lumbosacral spinal extensors.

DECREASED TILT   Hip extensors and lumbosacral spinal flexors.

LATERAL TILT TO THE RIGHT   Left lateral lumbosacral flexors, right hip abductors, and left hip adductors.

ROTATION TO RIGHT   Left lumbosacral rotators, left hip outward rotators, and right hip inward rotators.

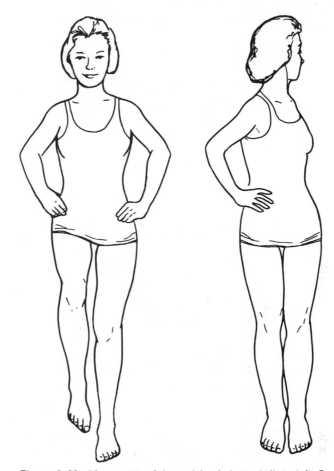

Figure 6–20   Movements of the pelvis. *A*, Lateral tilt to left. *B*, Rotation (lateral twist) to left.

The Relationship of the Pelvis to the Trunk and Lower Extremities

Architecturally, the pelvis is strategically located. Linking the trunk with the lower extremities, it must cooperate with the motion of each yet at the same time contribute to the stability of the total structure. When the body is in the erect standing position, the pelvis receives the weight of the head, trunk, and upper extremities, divides it equally, and transmits it to the two lower extremities. Whenever an individual stands on only one foot, the pelvis automatically adapts itself to this position and transmits the entire weight of the upper part of the body to one of the lower extremities. It requires a fine adjustment to do this in such a way that the balance of the total structure is preserved.

Since the pelvis depends upon the joints of the lower spine and those of the hips for its movements, it is not surprising that its motion is sometimes associated with the motion of the trunk or spine, and sometimes with that of the thighs. In such cases the movement of the pelvis may be said to be *secondary* to that of the spine, or of the thighs, as the case may be. In fact, most of its motion belongs in one or the other category. Occasionally, however, the movement seems to be initiated in the pelvis itself, with the spine and thighs cooperating with it. In such an event, the movement of the pelvis might be considered *primary,* and that of the spine and hips secondary. One sees this type of movement when the individual "tucks the hips under" as one would have to do to change from C to B, or even C to A, in Figure 6–19.

It is not always easy to judge the habitual tilt of the pelvis from the contour of the body. Prominent buttocks, heavy layers of fat, or an unusually convex sacrum can easily mislead the observer. Figure 6–21 shows a sketch based on an x-ray that illustrates a type of build in which the contour of the lower back and pelvic region does not correspond to the bony structure. In this illustration the tilt, as judged by the position of the sacrum, is greater than it appears to be from the contour of the lower back. This observation is of importance to those who tend to place emphasis on the position of the pelvis in giving posture instruction.

The joint analyses of the primary and secondary movements of the pelvis are given below.

Primary Movements of Pelvis

JOINT ANALYSIS OF THE PRIMARY MOVEMENTS OF THE PELVIS AS PERFORMED FROM THE FUNDAMENTAL STANDING POSITION

Pelvis	Spinal Joints	Hip Joints
Forward tilt	Hyperextension	Slight flexion
Backward tilt	Slight flexion	Complete extension
Lateral tilt to left	Slight lateral flexion to right	R: Slight adduction L: Slight abduction
Rotation to left (without turning the head or moving the feet)	Rotation right	R: Slight outward rotation L: Slight inward rotation

Secondary Movements of Pelvis

JOINT ANALYSIS OF MOVEMENTS OF THE PELVIS SECONDARY TO THOSE OF THE SPINE

Spine	Pelvis
Flexion	Backward tilt
Hyperextension	Forward tilt
Lateral flexion to left	Lateral tilt to left
Rotation to left	Rotation to left

MOVEMENTS OF THE PELVIS SECONDARY TO THOSE OF THE LOWER EXTREMITY   The pelvis moves with the lower extremity for the purpose of supplementing the latter's range of motion for three types of lower extremity movements: (1) movements of both limbs acting in unison, as when swinging them forward or backward in suspension; (2) movements of both limbs acting in opposition, as when walking, running, or doing a flutter kick in swimming; and (3) movements of one limb, as when kicking or

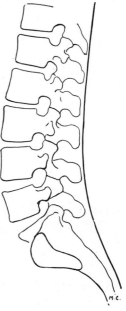

Figure 6–21 Lumbar and lumbosacral regions of the spine showing discrepancy in the lower lumbar curve as seen in the vertebral bodies and as seen in the contour of the back. (The sketch is based on an x-ray.)

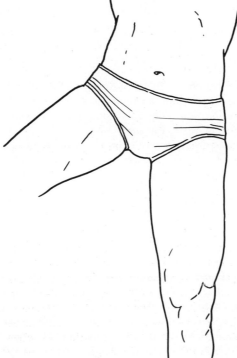

Figure 6–22 Lateral tilt of pelvis secondary to abduction of thigh at hip.

when raising one leg to the side. In double leg swinging the pelvis tilts backward (decreased inclination) when the thigh is flexed at the hip joint and forward (increased inclination) when the thigh is raised backward in apparent hyperextension. In opposition movements, when one leg is placed forward and the other backward, the pelvis rotates in the horizontal plane about a vertical axis. This pelvis orientation places the forward flexed leg in slight outward rotation and the extended rear leg in slight inward rotation at the hip joint. When one thigh is moved sideward in wide abduction, the pelvis tilts laterally, lifting on the side of the abducted leg and lowering on the side of the vertical support leg. Slight abduction of the support leg at the hip joint occurs as a necessary adjustment of the tilted pelvis (Figure 6–22). In each of these positions the pelvis positions itself so as to favor the movement of the thighs.

Common Athletic Injuries of the Thigh, Hip Joint, and Pelvis

Contusion of the Thigh Muscles

The muscles of the thigh are in a particularly vulnerable position in contact sports, especially in football. It is fortunate for the femur that it is so well protected in front by the heavy quadriceps muscles. It is likewise fortunate for the rectus femoris that the vasti muscles lie between it and the bone and thus cushion the former against the blows it frequently receives. In spite of such cushioning, however, and in spite of the external protection usually worn by the player, the quadriceps muscles do suffer contusions, the vasti lateralis and intermedius in particular but the rectus femoris also on occasion. The symptoms of thigh contusions tend to be delayed and more diffused than those of contusions occurring in less fleshy areas. Nevertheless, they can be severe, causing disability, especially when the injured muscle is put on a stretch such as when the knee is flexed beyond 90 degrees (O'Donoghue, 1976).

Myositis Ossificans

This is a condition in which calcification develops following repeated traumas of the muscle. It is likely to occur when the symptoms of muscle injury are so mild that the player insists on continuing to play. The front of the thigh and the brachialis muscle of the upper arm appear to be the most vulnerable area so affected. O'Donoghue, (1976) suggests that the frequency of this condition is caused in large part by poor treatment such as overvigorous massage, manipulation under anesthesia, overstrenuous exercise, and too early return to participation in the sport in which a severe muscle injury has occurred. In other words, myositis ossificans can often be prevented if muscle contusions are given proper treatment.

Strains of the Hamstring Muscle Group

There is high incidence of hamstring strains among athletes. These tend to occur in running more than in any other activity, especially when a muscular imbalance occurs through fatigue or other condition. A disturbance of the player's coordination often results. A frequent site of the strain is the distal attachment of the biceps femoris on the fibular head. This is close to the attachment of the collateral fibular ligament and it is often difficult to differentiate between strain of the bicipital tendon and sprain of the fibular ligament. At a slightly higher—i.e., more proximal—site at the junction of the tendon with the fleshy part of the muscle, it may be difficult to differentiate between a muscle strain and a contusion or hematoma (O'Donoghue,

1976). A correct diagnosis is essential in order that the appropriate treatment may be selected. It is therefore important that the diagnosis be made by a physician. A common strain in the pelvic area is one that occurs where the semitendinosus and the long head of the biceps femoris attach to the lower and medial impression on the tuberosity of the ischium. This is usually caused by a forceful movement of the lower extremity involving flexion of the thigh with the knees held in extension. In severe strains there may also be an avulsion fracture, especially if the ossification of the epiphysis is not yet complete.

Hip Conditions

Although this section is headed "Common Athletic Injuries of the Thigh, Hip Joint, and Pelvis," no hip conditions are discussed here. This is because of the relatively low incidence of hip joint injuries in athletics. The structure of the joint accounts for the rarity of dislocations, and fractures of the hip joint region are fortunately not a serious threat to athletes. The dangerous age when hip fractures are a real threat is old age when the bones have lost their toughness and have become brittle.

Contusion of Buttocks Area

This is common and not usually of serious consequence. If, however, the tuberosity of the ischium receives a direct blow, the contusion may be accompanied by a fracture.

Contusion and Strain of Iliac Crest (Hip Pointer)

This is likely to occur from a blow in football or other contact sport, especially if the crest is not adequately protected. The injury may consist of a simple contusion, or it may involve a strain of the muscles that attach to the crest or even a muscular avulsion, a condition in which the muscle pulls away from the crest, taking some bone with it. If the latter occurs and the injury is not properly diagnosed and therefore not adequately treated, there is likely to be a recurrence (Klafs and Arnheim, 1973; O'Donoghue, 1976).

Contusion of Sacrum and Coccyx

Contusion of the sacrum is a common injury in contact sports and can be very painful but is not usually serious, provided it is only a contusion and the bone is not cracked or fractured. It can be prevented or minimized by the wearing of adequate protection. Contusion of the coccyx may also result from a direct blow or from a fall in which the subject lands heavily in a sitting position.

Laboratory Experiences

Joint Structure and Function

1. Using a form like the one in Appendix A, record the essential information regarding the hip joint. Study the movements both on the skeleton and on the living body.

2. Using a protractor type of goniometer, measure the range of motion in the following joint movements on five different subjects:
   a. Hip flexion, with straight knee.
   b. Hip flexion, with flexed knee.
   c. Total abduction of both thighs.

3. From an erect standing position with the feet together take a fairly long step forward with the right foot, stopping with weight mostly over the right foot and with the left foot still in place but with the heel raised and the ball of the foot bearing just enough weight to maintain balance. Analyze the joint action that has taken place at each hip joint.

4. Analyze the joint action of each hip joint in each phase of riding a bicycle.

Muscular Action   (See Appendix E for muscle checklist.) Identify as many muscles as possible in the following experiments.

5. HIP FLEXION
   a. *Subject:* Sit on table with legs hanging over edge. Raise thigh.
      Assistant: Resist movement slightly by pressing down on knee.
      Observer: Palpate pectineus, tensor fasciae latae, sartorius, rectus femoris, and adductor longus. Does the gracilis contract?
   b. *Subject:* Lie on one side, rolled toward face. Flex thigh of top leg, allowing knee to flex passively.
      Assistant: Resist movement by pushing against knee.
      Observer: Palpate iliopsoas.

6. HIP EXTENSION
   a. *Subject:* Stand facing table with trunk bent forward until it rests on table. Grasp sides of table. Raise one leg, keeping the knee straight.
      Assistant: Resist movement by pushing down on thigh close to knee. Second time, give resistance at heel.
      Observer: Palpate gluteus maximus, adductor magnus, and hamstrings.
   b. *Subject:* Lie face down on table and raise one leg with knee straight.
      Assistant: Resist movement by pushing down on knee.
      Observer: Palpate same muscles as in *a.*

7. HIP ABDUCTION
   Subject: Lie on one side and raise top leg.
   Assistant: Resist movement by pushing down on knee.
   Observer: Palpate gluteus maximus, gluteus medius, and tensor fasciae latae.

8. HIP ADDUCTION
   Subject: Lie on one side with top leg raised; then lower it.
   Assistant: Resist movement by pressing up against knee.
   Note: Unless resistance is applied, the action will be performed by means of the eccentric contraction of the abductors.
   Observer: Palpate three adductors and name them.

9. OUTWARD ROTATION OF THIGH
   Subject: Stand on one foot with the other knee bent at right angles so that the lower leg extends horizontally backward. Rotate the free thigh outward by swinging the foot medially.
   Assistant: Steady subject's knee and resist movement of leg at ankle.
   Observer: Palpate gluteus maximus.

10. INWARD ROTATION OF THIGH
   Subject: Stand on one foot with other knee bent at right angles so that the lower leg extends horizontally backward. Rotate the free thigh inward by swinging the foot laterally.
   Assistant: Steady subject's knee and resist movement of leg at ankle.
   Observer: Palpate gluteus medius, tensor fasciae latae, and lower adductor magnus.

11. DECREASE OF PELVIC INCLINATION
   Subject: Lie on back with knees drawn up and feet resting on floor. Tilt pelvis in such a manner that lumbar spine becomes flatter.
   Assistant: Kneeling at subject's head and facing subject's feet, place thumbs on the anterior superior iliac spines and fingers under the lower back. Resist movement by pushing iliac spines toward subject's feet.

Observer: Palpate rectus abdominis and gluteus maximus. Palpate the hamstrings. Do they contract?

12. **INCREASE OF PELVIC INCLINATION**

Subject: In erect standing position, stiffen the knees and push the buttocks as far back as possible.

Observer: Palpate tensor fasciae latae, sartorius, pectineus, and iliocostalis. Does the adductor longus or gracilis contract?

13. **LATERAL TILT OF PELVIS**

Subject: Stand on one foot on stool with other leg hanging free. Pull free hip up as far as possible.

Assistant: Give slight resistance by holding ankle down.

Observer: Palpate oblique abdominals, iliocostalis, adductor magnus, adductor longus, and gracilis on side of free leg.

References

Advisory Committee on Artificial Limbs, National Research Council. 1953. *The pattern of muscular activity in the lower extremity during walking.* Berkeley, Cal.: Prosthetic Devices Research Project, Institute of Engineering Research, University of California, Series II.

Basmajian, J. V. 1979. *Muscles alive.* 4th ed. Baltimore: Williams & Wilkins.

Crane, L. 1959. Femoral torsion and its relation to toeing-in and toeing-out. *J. Bone Joint Surg.* 41A:421–28.

Duchenne, G. B. 1959. *Physiology of motion,* ed. and trans. E. B. Kaplan. Philadelphia: W. B. Saunders.

Fischer, F. J., and Houtz, S. J. 1968. Evaluation of the function of the gluteus maximus muscle. *Am. J. Phys. Med.* 47:182–91.

Inman, V. T. 1947. Functional aspects of the abductor muscles of the hip. *J. Bone Joint Surg.* 29A:607–19.

Klafs, C. E., and Arnheim, D. D. 1973. *Modern principles of athletic training.* St. Louis: C. V. Mosby.

LaBan, M. M., Raptou, A. D., and Johnson, E. W. 1965. Electromyographic study of function of iliopsoas muscle. *Arch. Phys. Med. Rehab.* 46:676–79.

MacConaill, M. A., and Basmajian, J. V. 1969. *Muscles and movements.* Baltimore: Williams & Wilkins.

Merrifield, H. H. 1961. An electromyographic study of the gluteus maximus, the vastus lateralis and the tensor fasciae latae. *Diss. Abstr.* 21:1833.

O'Donoghue, D. H. 1976. *Treatment of injuries to athletes.* 3d ed. Philadelphia: W. B. Saunders.

Steindler, A. 1970. *Kinesiology of the human body.* Springfield, Ill.: Charles C Thomas.

Stubbs, N. B., Capen, E. K., and Wilson, G. L. 1975. An electromyographic investigation of the sartorius and tensor fascia latae muscles. *Res. Q. Am. Assoc. Health Phys. Educ.* 46:358.

Wheatley, M. D., and Jahnke, W. D. 1951. Electromyographic study of the superficial thigh and hip muscles in normal individuals. *Arch. Phys. Ther.* 31:508–22.

Wright, W. G. 1962. *Muscle function.* New York: Hafner Publishing.

The Lower Extremity: The Knee, Ankle, and Foot

Objectives

At the conclusion of this chapter, the student should be able to:

1. Name, locate, and describe the structure and ligamentous reinforcements of the articulations of the knee, ankle, and foot.
2. Name and demonstrate the movements possible in the joints of the knee, ankle, and foot, regardless of starting position.
3. Name and locate the muscles and muscle groups of the knee, ankle, and foot, and name their primary actions as agonists, stabilizers, neutralizers, or antagonists.
4. Analyze the fundamental movements of the lower leg and foot with respect to joint and muscle actions.
5. Describe the common athletic injuries of the leg, knee, and ankle.

The Knee Joint

The knee joint is a masterpiece of anatomical engineering. Placed midway in each supporting column of the body, it is subject to severe stresses and strains in its combined functions of weight-bearing and locomotion. As Steindler (1970) has pointed out, it meets the requirements made of it with remarkable efficiency. To take care of the weight-bearing stresses it has massive condyles; to facilitate locomotion it has a

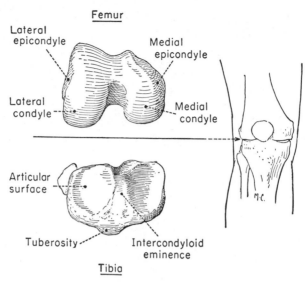

Figure 7–1 Articulating surfaces of knee joint.

wide range of motion; to resist the lateral stresses due to the tremendous lever effect of the long femur and tibia, it is reinforced at the sides by strong ligaments; to combat the downward pull of gravity and to meet the demands of such violent locomotor activities as running and jumping, it is provided with powerful musculature. It would be difficult, indeed, to find a mechanism better adapted for meeting the combined requirements of stability and mobility than the knee joint.

In this connection, however, mention should be made of two forms of malalignment at the knee joint, one of which is common. These are the conditions popularly known as "knock-knees" and "bowlegs." In knock-knees (genu valgum) the knees are closer to the midline of the body than is normal. In the standing position the knees are closer together than the feet, so that when the feet are placed side by side, the knees are either pressed together or are slightly overlapping with one behind the other. Mechanically, the condition means that the weight-bearing line of the lower extremity passes lateral to the center of the knee joint. This puts the medial ligament (tibial collateral) under increased tension and subjects the lateral meniscus to increased pressure and friction. Such a joint is an unstable one. Not only is it more prone to injury than a well aligned joint, but in all weight-bearing positions postural strains are constantly present. The condition of bowlegs (genu varum) is just the reverse of knock-knees, with the additional complication of the long bones themselves being curved laterally.

Structure

Although the knee is classified as a hinge joint, its bony structure resembles two ovoid or condyloid joints lying side by side, yet not quite parallel (Figure 7-1). The lateral flexion permitted in a single ovoid joint is not possible in the knee joint because of the presence of the second condyle. The two rockerlike condyles of the femur rest on the two slightly concave areas on the top of the tibia's broad head. These articular surfaces of the tibia are separated by a roughened area, called the intercondyloid eminence, which terminates both anteriorly and posteriorly in a slight hollow but

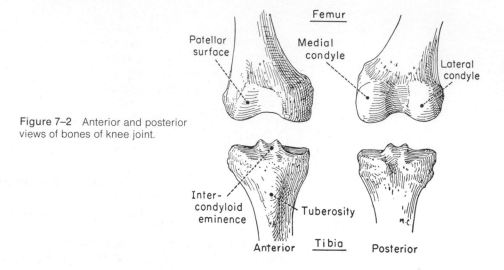

Figure 7–2 Anterior and posterior views of bones of knee joint.

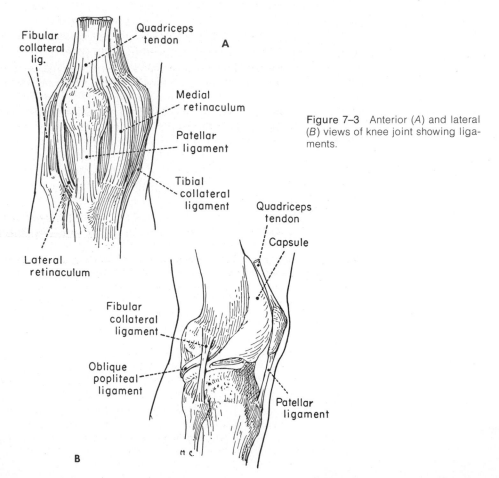

Figure 7–3 Anterior (*A*) and lateral (*B*) views of knee joint showing ligaments.

rises at the center to form two small tubercles not unlike miniature twin mountain peaks (Figure 7–2). The medial articular surface is oval; the lateral is smaller and more nearly round. Each is overlaid by a somewhat crescent-shaped fibrocartilage, known as a semilunar cartilage or meniscus.

The lower end of the femur terminates in the two rockerlike condyles already mentioned. The lateral condyle is broader and more prominent than the medial. The medial condyle projects downward farther than the lateral. This, however, is evident only when a disarticulated femur is held vertically. In its normal position in the body the femur slants inward from above downward. This slant is known as the obliquity of the femoral shaft. Observation of the mounted skeleton will show that the downward projection of the medial condyle compensates for the obliquity of the femoral shaft.

Another interesting feature of the condyles is that they are not quite parallel. While the lateral condyle lies in the sagittal plane, the medial condyle slants slightly medially from front to back. This is an important factor in the movements of the knee.

Anteriorly, the two condyles are continuous with the smooth, slightly concave surface of the patellar facet for the articulation of the patella. The patella, or knee cap, is a large sesamoid bone located slightly above and in front of the knee joint. It is held in place by the quadriceps tendon above, by the patellar ligament below, and by the intervening fibers that form a pocket for the patella (Figure 7–3).

The articular cavity is enclosed within a loose membranous capsule that lies under the patella and folds around each condyle but excludes the intercondyloid tubercles and cruciate ligaments. It is supplemented by expansions from the fascia lata, iliotibial tract, and various tendons. The oblique popliteal ligament covers the posterior surface of the joint completely, shielding the cruciate ligaments and other structures not enclosed within the capsule (Figure 7–4).

The synovial membrane of the knee joint is the most extensive of any in the body. It folds in and around the joint in a manner far too complicated to attempt to describe here. There are numerous bursae in the vicinity of the knee joint, among the largest and most important being the prepatellar, infrapatellar, and suprapatellar bursae.

The Semilunar Cartilages

These cartilages (Figure 7–5), or menisci as they are called, are somewhat circular rims of fibrocartilage, situated on the articular surfaces of the head of the tibia. They

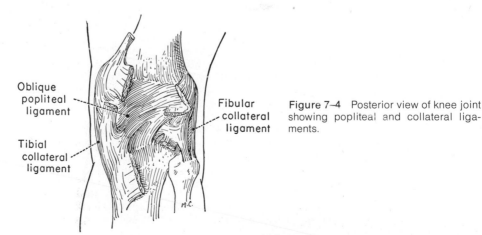

Oblique popliteal ligament

Tibial collateral ligament

Fibular collateral ligament

Figure 7–4   Posterior view of knee joint showing popliteal and collateral ligaments.

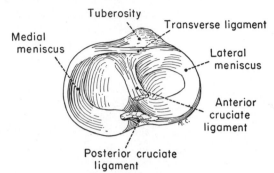

Figure 7–5 The menisci (semilunar cartilages) of the knee joint.

are relatively thick at their peripheral borders, but taper to a thin edge at their inner circumferences. Thus they deepen the articular facets of the tibia and, at the same time, serve in a shock-absorbing capacity. The inner edges are free, but the peripheral borders are attached loosely to the rim of the head of the tibia by fibers from the inner surface of the capsule.

The lateral semilunar cartilage forms an incomplete circle, conforming closely to the nearly round articular facet. Its anterior and posterior horns, which almost meet at the center of the joint, are attached to the intercondyloid eminence.

The medial cartilage is shaped like a large letter C, broader toward the rear than in front. Its anterior horn tapers off to a thin strand attached to the anterior intercondyloid fossa. It is not as freely movable as the lateral cartilage because of its secure anchorage to the tibial collateral ligament at the medial side of the knee. Largely because of this point of attachment, the medial cartilage is more frequently injured than the lateral.

Ligaments of the Knee*

PATELLAR LIGAMENT (Figure 7–3)   This is a strong, flat ligament connecting the lower margin of the patella with the tuberosity of the tibia. Passing over the front of the patella, the superficial fibers are continuations of the central fibers of the quadriceps femoris tendon.

COLLATERAL TIBIAL LIGAMENT (Figures 7–3A, 7–4, and 7–6)   This is a broad, flat, membranous band on the medial side of the joint. It is attached above to the medial epicondyle of the femur below the adductor tubercle, and below to the medial condyle of the tibia. It is firmly attached to the medial meniscus. This fact should be noted because of its significance in knee injuries. It serves to check extension and to prevent motion laterally.

COLLATERAL FIBULAR LIGAMENT (Figures 7–3, 7–4, and 7–6)   This is a strong, rounded cord, attached above to the back of the lateral epicondyle of the femur and below to the lateral surface of the head of the fibula. It serves to check extension and to prevent motion medially.

OBLIQUE POPLITEAL LIGAMENT (Figures 7–3B and 7–4)   This is a broad, flat ligament, covering the back of the knee joint. It is attached above to the upper margin of the intercondyloid fossa and posterior surface of the femur and below to the posterior margin of the head of the tibia. Medially, it blends with the tendon of the semimembranosus muscle and laterally with the lateral head of the gastrocnemius.

---

*Detailed descriptions of individual ligaments are included here because of their importance to a good understanding of the complex injuries experienced by this joint.

THE CRUCIATE LIGAMENTS (Figure 7–6)   These are two strong, cordlike ligaments situated within the knee joint, although not enclosed within the joint capsule. They are called cruciate from the fact that they cross each other, and are further designated anterior and posterior, according to their attachments to the tibia. They serve to check certain movements at the knee joint. They limit extension and prevent rotation in the extended position. They also check the forward and backward sliding of the femur on the tibia, thus safeguarding the anteroposterior stability of the knee.

Anterior Cruciate Ligament (Figure 7–6)   This passes upward and backward from the anterior intercondyloid fossa of the tibia to the back part of the medial surface of the lateral condyle of the femur.

Posterior Cruciate Ligament (Figure 7–6)   This is a shorter and stronger ligament than the anterior. It passes upward and forward from the posterior intercondyloid fossa of the tibia to the lateral and front part of the medial condyle of the femur.

TRANSVERSE LIGAMENT (Figure 7–5)   This is a short, slender, cordlike ligament, connecting the anterior convex margin of the lateral meniscus to the anterior end of the medial meniscus.

THE ILIOTIBIAL TRACT (Figures 6–11 and 6–12)   The iliotibial tract is said to act like a tense ligament that connects the iliac crest with the lateral femoral condyle and the lateral tubercle of the tibia. At the knee joint the tract serves as a stabilizing ligament between the lateral condyle of the femur and the tibia. The attachment to the femoral condyle is then a fixed point and the distal end moves forward in knee extension and backward in knee flexion (Kaplan, 1958).

Movements

The movements that occur at the knee joint are primarily flexion and extension. A slight amount of rotation can take place when the knee is in the flexed position and the foot is not supporting the weight (Figure 7–7).

FLEXION AND EXTENSION   The movements of flexion and extension at the knee are not as simple as are those of a true hinge joint. This can be demonstrated in the classroom by holding a disarticulated femur and tibia together in a position of extension and then, holding the tibia stationary, flexing the femur on the tibia as

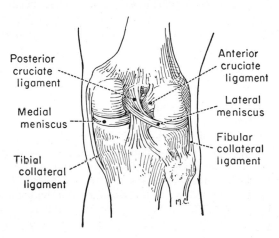

Posterior cruciate ligament

Medial meniscus

Tibial collateral ligament

Anterior cruciate ligament

Lateral meniscus

Fibular collateral ligament

Figure 7–6   Posterior view of knee joint showing cruciate ligaments.

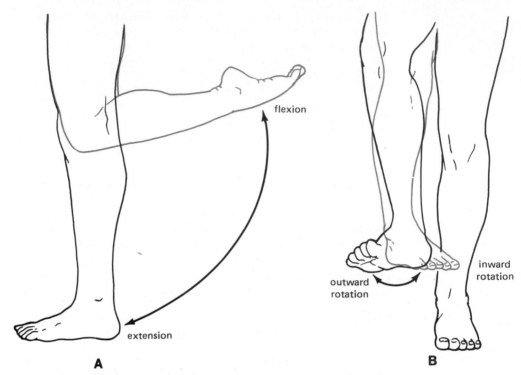

Figure 7–7 Movements of the knee joint. *A*, Flexion and extension. *B*, Inward and outward rotation (in flexed, non-weight-bearing position).

though the individual were assuming a squat or sitting position. If no other adjustment is made, the femoral condyles will roll back completely off the top of the tibia. What prevents this in real life is the fact that as the condyles roll backward they simultaneously glide forward and thus remain in contact with the menisci throughout each phase of the movement. Conversely, when the femur extends on the tibia, the forward roll of the femoral condyles is accompanied by a backward glide.

Because the femoral condyles are not quite parallel and differ in size, a slight degree of rotation occurs during the initial phase of flexion and the final phase of extension. This can be readily seen on the living subject if he stands with the knees slightly flexed and then extends them completely. The patellae are seen to turn slightly medialward, indicating slight inward rotation of the thighs. Because of the inequality of the two condyles, the medial condyle continues to roll forward after the lateral condyle has ceased its movement. The inward rotation of the femur that accompanies the completion of extension is commonly known as "locking" the knees. In persons who tend to hyperextend their knees habitually the rotation is more pronounced.

When the leg is flexed or extended in a non-weight-bearing position, the tibia rotates on the femur, instead of vice versa. The final phase of extension is accompanied by slight outward rotation of the tibia. At the beginning of flexion the tibia rotates inward until the midposition is attained (Schaeffer, 1953).

The rotation that occurs in the final stage of extension and the initial phase of flexion is an inherent part of these movements and should not be confused with the voluntary rotation that can be performed when the leg is not bearing weight and the knee is in a flexed position.

INWARD AND OUTWARD ROTATION IN THE FLEXED POSITION In spite of the fact that the knee joint is classified as a hinge joint, its condylar structure accommodates movement other than just flexion and extension under certain conditions. When the leg has been flexed at the knee, the collateral ligaments become slack and it is possible to rotate the leg on the thigh through a total range of about 50 degrees. This can occur, however, only when the leg is not bearing the body weight. It is impossible, for instance, to rotate either the leg or the thigh in this manner when the body is in a stooping position. A good way to demonstrate rotation of the tibia is to sit on a chair with the heel resting lightly on the floor. In this position, with the knee and thigh held motionless, the foot should be turned first in and then out. The action will be that of inward and outward rotation of the tibia. The movement taking place within the foot itself should be discounted. Taut collateral ligaments prevent rotation when the leg is extended at the knee, either in a weight-bearing or non-weight-bearing position (Klein, 1962). Inward or outward movements of the foot in the extended position are due to rotation at the hip joint.

Muscles of the Knee Joint

Location

The muscles acting on the knee joint are classified as anterior or posterior according to the relation of their distal tendons to the transverse axis of the joint.

Anterior	Posterior
Quadriceps femoris group	Hamstring group
Rectus femoris	Biceps femoris
Vastus intermedius	Semimembranosus
Vastus lateralis	Semitendinosus
Vastus medialis	Sartorius
	Gracilis
	Popliteus
	Gastrocnemius

Characteristics and Functions of Individual Muscles

QUADRICEPS FEMORIS GROUP This group (Figures 7–3, 7–8, and 7–9) consists of the rectus femoris and the vasti: vastus intermedius, vastus lateralis, and vastus medialis. Of these, only the rectus femoris, the most superficial of the four, crosses the hip joint. The vastus intermedius lies posterior to the rectus and is completely covered by it. The distal portions of the four muscles unite to form a single broad, flat tendon that attaches to the base of the patella, the base being the upper border. In some texts this is given as the distal attachment of the quadriceps group, with no further explanation. If this ended the matter, one would wonder how muscles that did not cross the knee joint could extend it. Obviously, the patellar ligament connecting the patella with the tuberosity of the tibia is a vital part of the quadriceps femoris. Actually, the patella is a sesamoid bone encased within the quadriceps tendon, with the patellar ligament being but a continuation of this and the tibial tuberosity the true distal point of attachment. All four muscles extend the leg at the knee joint.

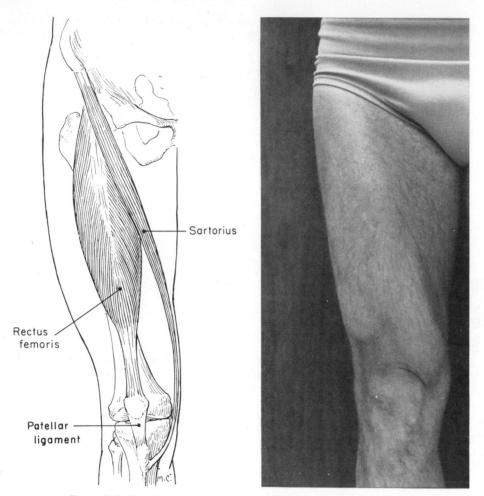

Sartorius

Rectus
femoris

Patellar
ligament

Figure 7–8   Front of thigh showing rectus femoris and sartorius muscles.

The vastus lateralis and vastus medialis, with their fibers converging toward the patella, together with the vastus intermedius and rectus femoris, with their longitudinal approach, serve to steady the knee joint in weight-bearing positions and to maintain a balanced tension on the patella. There is very little activity from these muscles, however, in relaxed standing. Because the three vasti are one-joint muscles they are *powerful knee extensors*, regardless of the position of the hip joint. Their greatest activity is during the last part of knee extension. The vastus medialis is the most active of the three throughout the greatest range of knee extension. Its lower portion is also important in preventing lateral dislocation of the patella. When the knee is fully extended, static contraction of the quadriceps serves to pull up or "set" the patella, a mild exercise used in rehabilitation of the injured knee. These muscles are not active in ordinary standing (Basmajian, 1979).

Pocock concluded from his EMG investigation of the quadriceps muscles that

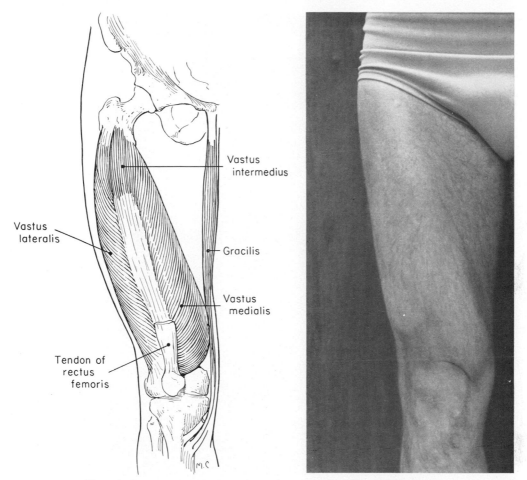

Figure 7–9   Front of thigh showing the three vasti muscles and the gracilis.

they function as a unit and do not have any particular timing pattern, as had been previously suggested (Basmajian, 1979).

The two-joint *rectus femoris* (also listed with the hip muscles) is of bipenniform structure with all except the lowest fibers slanting obliquely downward and sideward from the central tendon and the lowest fibers being approximately vertical (Figure 7–8). The upper three-quarters of the muscle consists of muscle fibers with the last quarter, down to the base of the patella, being the muscle's distal tendon. The entire muscle contracts regardless of whether it is producing movement at the hip joint or knee joint. The muscle may be palpated on the central-anterior surface of the thigh.

The majority of the *vastus lateralis* fibers slant downward and medialward to the tendon. The muscle may be palpated on the anterolateral aspect of the thigh, lateral to the rectus femoris.

Most of the fibers of the *vastus medialis* slant downward and lateralward to the tendon, with the lowest ones almost horizontal in direction. If the lateralis and medialis were looked upon as one muscle it would be considered to be of bipenniform

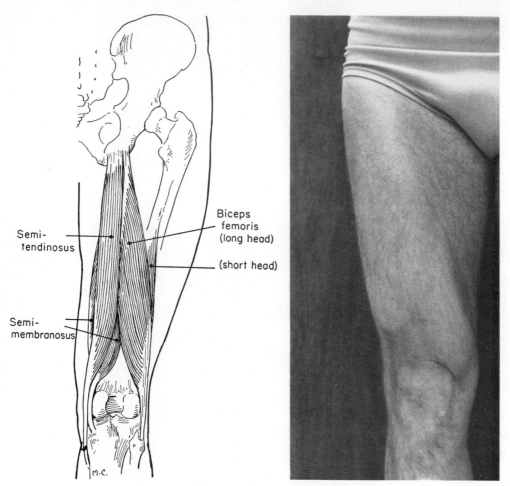

Figure 7–10   Hamstring muscles.

construction, with the fibers slanting in direct opposition to those of the rectus femoris. The fleshy part of both the medialis and lateralis extends down almost to the level of the base of the patella. The vastus medialis may be palpated on the anterome-dial aspect of the lower third of the thigh, medial to the rectus femoris.

HAMSTRING GROUP   (Also listed with the hip muscles.) The hamstrings (Figures 7–10 and 7–11), so named from their large, cordlike tendons behind the knee joint, consist of the biceps femoris, semimembranosus, and semitendinosus muscles. Although the *biceps femoris* constitutes the lateral hamstring, its long head lies approximately along the midline of the posterior aspect of the thigh, as far down as the popliteal space. The long head comes from the tuberosity of the ischium and the short head originates from the linea aspera on the posterior surface of the thigh. The two join at the distal tendon close to the lateral condyle of the femur, not far above the tendon's attachment to the head of the fibula. It is an important *flexor of the knee.*

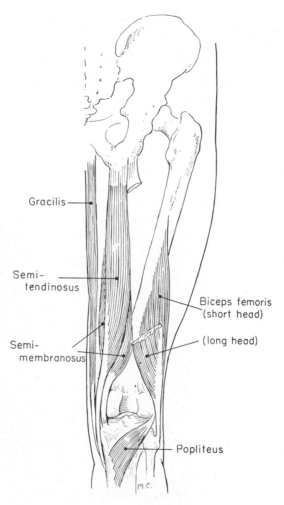

Figure 7–11 Posterior muscles of thigh and knee.

When the knee is flexed and not bearing weight, *the biceps can rotate the lower leg outward*. Its tendon may be palpated behind the knee on its lateral aspect. The long head is fusiform in construction; the short head is penniform.

The *semimembranosus* and *semitendinosus* constitute the medial hamstrings. The former lies deeper than the latter and attaches higher on the tibia. The semitendinosus is attached to the medial surface of the tibia below the head, just below the attachment of the gracilis and behind that of the sartorius. Like the biceps femoris, they *flex the knee joint*. The semitendinosus may be palpated on the medial aspect of the posterior surface of the knee. The tendon of the semimembranosus is almost impossible to palpate successfully as it is shorter than its partner and is partially covered by the latter, as well as by the gracilis tendon.

Although the hamstrings act at both the knees and the hips, their primary function is *knee flexion*. Wright (1962) called attention to the usefulness of the hamstrings in preventing hyperextension at the knee, and in unlocking the knee (i.e., reducing hyperextension) when one is returning from a position in which the line of gravity falls in front of the knee joints (e.g., inclining the trunk forward without bending the knees). Nearly everyone is familiar with the limiting effect of the hamstrings. The difficulty experienced by many in touching the toes with the fingers without bending the knees, and in sitting erect on the floor with the legs extended straight forward, is due to the fact that the hamstrings are frequently not long enough to permit such extreme stretching at the hips and knees simultaneously.

SARTORIUS   (Also listed with the hip muscles.) This is a long, slender, ribbonlike muscle (Figure 7–8), superficially located and directed obliquely downward and medialward across the front of the thigh. On its way to its distal attachment it curves around behind the bulge of the medial condyles in such a way that its line of pull is posterior to the axis of the knee joint. Thus, in spite of the fact that at least two-thirds of the muscle, including both its proximal and distal attachments, lies on the anterior aspect of the lower extremity, its action at the knee joint is generally *flexion,* not extension. With some subjects, however, more activity has been evident during extension than in flexion, a situation attributed to variations in insertion that could result in an anterior line of pull (Basmajian, 1979). It also assists in *inward rotation of the tibia when the knee is flexed.* Its line of pull is determined by the direction of its distal tendon between the latter's point of contact with the medial condyle of the tibia and its attachment to the upper anteromedial surface of the tibial shaft, almost as far forward as the anterior crest. It may be palpated at the anterior superior iliac spine, as well as along its entire length, where it is clearly visible on a thin, well-muscled subject.

GRACILIS   (Also listed with the hip muscles.) This is a long, slender muscle (Figures 7–9 and 7–11) situated on the medial aspect of the thigh. Its action at the knee joint is *flexion.* It also is slightly active in *inward rotation of the tibia when the knee is in a flexed position and the foot is not bearing weight.* It may be palpated on the medial aspect of the posterior surface of the knee, anterior to the semitendinosus tendon but close to it.

POPLITEUS   This muscle (Figure 7–11) *rotates the tibia inward* and *helps to flex the knee.* In structure and function it resembles the pronator teres muscle of the elbow. In a subject who is standing, it "unlocks" the knee joint preliminary to flexion. It also helps to protect and stabilize the knee joint from forward dislocation of the femur when a squatting position is assumed and maintained. During walking, it is active throughout most of the weight-bearing phase (Basmajian, 1979).

GASTROCNEMIUS   (Also listed with the ankle muscles.) This large calf muscle (Figure 7–23), although primarily a muscle of the ankle joint, has an important function at the knee joint. It is in a position to help *flex the knee* and does so when the leg is not bearing weight. However, according to Wright (1962), its most important function at the knee is serving as a *posterior ligament* to protect the joint in movements involving violent extension, as in running and jumping.

Hollinshead (1976) makes the interesting observation that, when the foot is fixed in weight-bearing, *the gastrocnemius can help to maintain knee extension.* It does this when the hip and knee are in strong extension and when plantar flexion of the ankle is inhibited. Under these circumstances the gastrocnemius is able to pull back and down on the femoral condyles, thus contributing to knee extension. Its activity in "relaxed standing at ease" was found in three-fourths of subjects tested barefooted. The wearing of high heels increased the frequency of subjects whose muscles were active. The muscle is easy to palpate, including both the muscle belly in the calf and the tendon behind the ankle.

Muscular Analysis of the Fundamental Movements of the Leg at the Knee Joint

FLEXION   The knee joint has five important flexors, namely the three hamstring muscles (biceps femoris, semimembranosus, and semitendinosus), the sartorius, and the gracilis; the latter is especially important during the early part of flexion, provided that the hip is not flexing simultaneously. Two additional muscles that help with flexion are the popliteus and gastrocnemius.

It should be remembered that when the weight is borne by the feet and the knees are allowed to flex, as in stooping, the knee flexors are not responsible for the movement. The flexion is produced by the force of gravity and is controlled by the extensor muscles that are contracting eccentrically—that is, in lengthening contraction.

The three adductors have also been shown to be active in most children during flexion and extension of the knee with or without external resistance. They were also active under the same conditions in most adults during knee flexion, but activity of these muscles during extension occurred only when resistance was applied (Basmajian, 1979).

EXTENSION   This action is performed by the four muscles that make up the quadriceps femoris group: the rectus femoris, vastus intermedius, vastus lateralis, and vastus medialis.

Muscles sometimes act in surprising ways. A good example of this is the action of the gastrocnemius at the knee when the weight is on the foot. When the weight is not on the foot, the gastrocnemius is an assistant flexor of the knee. Its primary function is extension (plantar flexion) of the ankle joint. When the foot is bearing weight, flexion of the knee cannot take place unless the ankle is dorsiflexing at the same time. If this dorsiflexion is prevented, the weight-bearing knee is unable to flex. Under these circumstances the gastrocnemius contracts in what might be called the reverse direction—that is, it acts on its proximal attachments and pulls backward and downward on the femoral condyles, and with the foot fixed this contributes to knee extension. It is because of such reversals as this that it is not desirable for a student to memorize muscular actions. The circumstances under which the movement is performed are of vital importance.

OUTWARD ROTATION OF THE TIBIA   This action is performed by the biceps femoris. It can occur only when the knee is flexed in a non-weight-bearing situation.

INWARD ROTATION OF THE TIBIA   This action is performed chiefly by the semimembranosus, semitendinosus, and popliteus, with possible help from the gracilis and sartorius. As with outward rotation, it can occur only when the knee is flexed and the foot is not bearing weight.

The Ankle and the Foot

The foot has two functions of great importance—support and propulsion. In studying the structure of the foot, these functions should be kept constantly in mind, for only by seeing the foot in terms of the combined static and dynamic demands made upon it can one fully appreciate its intricate mechanism.

The foot is united with the leg at the ankle joint. Within the foot itself are the seven tarsal bones. Two of the joints in this region are of sufficient importance to the kinesiologist to merit special attention. These are the subtalar and midtarsal joints, the latter including the talonavicular and calcaneocuboid articulations. The movements within the foot occur mainly at these two joints.

The structure of the ankle, tarsal joints, and toes will be described separately, but the muscles of these three regions will be discussed together as many of them act on more than one joint.

Structure of the Ankle

The ankle (Figures 7–12, 7–13, and 7–14) is a hinge joint. It is formed by the articulation of the talus (astragalus) with the malleoli of the tibia and the fibula. The latter bones, bound together by the transverse tibiofibular ligament, the anterior and posterior ligaments of the lateral malleolus, and the interossei, constitute a mortise into which the upper, rounded portion of the talus fits. The joint is surrounded by a thin, membranous capsule that is thicker on the medial side of the joint. In the back it is a thin mesh of membranous tissue and is not continuous, as are most capsules. It is reinforced by several strong ligaments.

Ligamentous Re-inforcement

The medial side of the ankle joint is protected by five strong ligamentous bands (Figures 7–13 and 7–14), four of them connecting the medial malleolus of the tibia with posterior tarsal bones; calcaneus, talus, and navicular. The fifth band (plantar calcaneonavicular) provides a horizontal connection between the navicular bone and the sustentaculum tali projection on the medial aspect of the calcaneus.

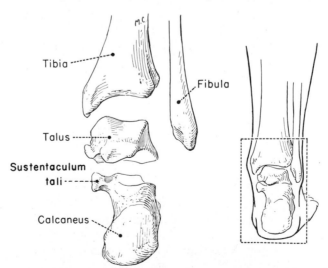

Figure 7–12   Bones of ankle and subtalar joints, posterior view.

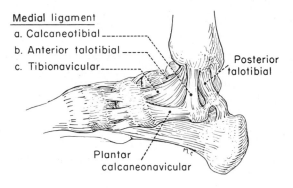

Medial ligament
a. Calcaneotibial
b. Anterior talotibial
c. Tibionavicular

Posterior
talotibial

Plantar
calcaneonavicular

Figure 7–13 Medial ligaments of ankle joint.

The lateral side of the ankle is reinforced by three ligaments which connect, respectively, the lateral malleolus with the upper lateral aspect of the calcaneus and with anterior and posterior portions of the talus. Inspection of Figures 7–13 and 7–14 gives one the impression that the lateral side of the ankle is less protected than the medial. If this is true, it might be a factor in the high incidence of ankle sprains.

Structure of the Foot

The foot (Figures 7–15 and 7–16) as a whole is usually described as an elastic arched structure, the keystone of the arch being the talus. This bone has several marks of distinction. Aside from being the connecting link between the foot and the leg, it is distinguished by having no muscles attached to it and by receiving and transmitting the weight of the entire body (with the exception of the foot itself), a function that requires great strength and firm support.

The foot has two arches, a longitudinal and a transverse. The longitudinal arch extends from the heel to the heads of the five metatarsals. It is sometimes described as being made up of an inner and an outer component. The outer component includes the calcaneus, cuboid, and fourth and fifth metatarsals (Figure 7–16A). The inner component consists of the calcaneus, talus, navicular, three cuneiforms, and the three medial metatarsals (Figure 7–16B). The outer component has a nearly flat contour and lacks mobility; hence, it is better adapted to the function of support, whereas the inner component with its greater flexibility and its curving arch is adapted to the function of shock absorption, so important in all forms of locomotion. Contrary to popular

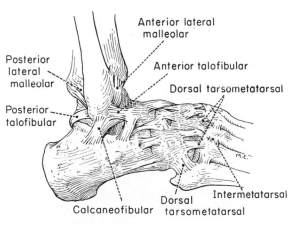

Anterior lateral
malleolar

Posterior
lateral
malleolar

Anterior talofibular

Dorsal tarsometatarsal

Posterior
talofibular

Figure 7–14 Lateral ligaments of ankle joint.

Calcaneofibular

Dorsal
tarsometatarsal

Intermetatarsal

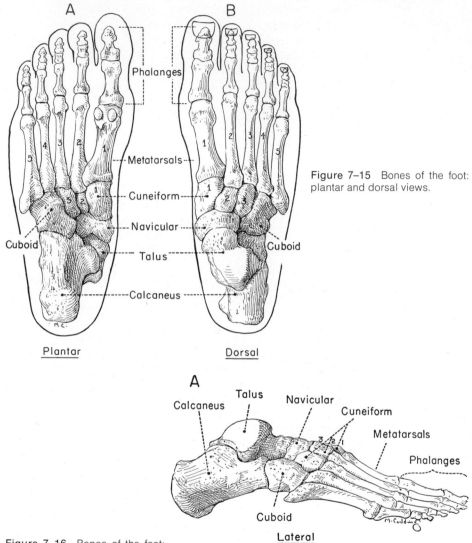

Figure 7–15 Bones of the foot: plantar and dorsal views.

Figure 7–16 Bones of the foot: lateral and medial views.

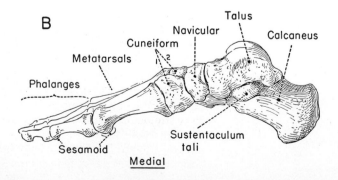

opinion, the height of the longitudinal arch is not indicative of the strength of the arch. Thus, a low arch is not necessarily a weak one, *provided it is not associated with a pronated (i.e., abducted and everted) foot.*

The transverse arch is the side-to-side concavity on the underside of the foot formed by the anterior tarsal bones and the metatarsals. The anterior boundary of this arch under the metatarsal heads is known as the metatarsal arch. There is some disagreement as to whether this should be called an arch, since it flattens completely when bearing weight. The metatarsal arch exists, therefore, only in non-weight-bearing situations.

The toes, especially the large and powerful "big toes," are largely responsible for propulsion. They provide the push-off at the end of the step. Their use in locomotion is directly proportional to the vigor and speed of the walk or run.

The strength and elasticity of the foot are due in large measure to the ligaments that bind the bones together and to the muscles that work to preserve the balance of the foot. Thus, both ligaments and muscles share the responsibility for maintaining the integrity of the feet. In a study of the flexibility and stability and other characteristics of the feet of 100 young women, Lawrence (1955) noted that there was no significant relationship between flexibility and stability, and that the size and weight of the body had very little effect upon the measurements of foot size, flexibility, stability, or degree of out-toeing. Lawrence also observed that long, narrow feet tended to be more flexible, but less stable, than feet of other proportions.

SUBTALAR JOINT This is the joint (Figure 7–17) between the underside of the talus and the upper and anterior aspects of the calcaneus or heel bone. It is reinforced by four small talocalcaneal ligaments. A fifth ligament, the *plantar calcaneonavicular,* is probably the most important of all. It is a broad, thick ligament that connects the sustentaculum tali projection of the calcaneus with the underside of the navicular bone. It passes under the talus and aids in supporting it. It is actually part of the subtalar joint, since it contains a fibrocartilaginous facet which is lined with synovial membrane. This is commonly called the *spring ligament* because of the yellow elastic fibers that give it its elasticity. The importance of this ligament can be readily seen when one remembers that the talus receives the weight of the entire body. The shock-absorbing function of this elastic support is obvious. It is probably equally obvious that excessive prolonged pressure on this ligament through improper use of the feet will cause it to stretch permanently and thus result in a lowered arch.

Unfortunately, Figure 7–17B gives a somewhat misleading picture of this ligament. Although it looks like a cord-shaped ligament on the medial aspect of the ankle, the part that shows in the picture is actually just the medial border of a broad ligament that extends beneath the head of the talus like a taut hammock.

MIDTARSAL JOINT (TRANSVERSE TARSAL; CHOPART'S) The midtarsal joint consists of two articulations, the lateral one being the calcaneocuboid joint and the medial one the talonavicular. On looking down on these from above, the continuous line of articulation—the talonavicular and calcaneocuboid—is seen to form a somewhat shallow letter S (Figures 7–15B and 7–18). The talonavicular joint is a modified ball-and-socket joint and permits somewhat restricted movements about three axes. The calcaneocuboid joint is nonaxial and permits only slight gliding motions. These seem to be supplementary or secondary to the freer motions of the talonavicular joint. There are several ligaments that reinforce these joints but the ones that give the most support are the *long and short plantar (calcaneocuboid) ligaments.* These are both wide, thick ligaments of great strength.

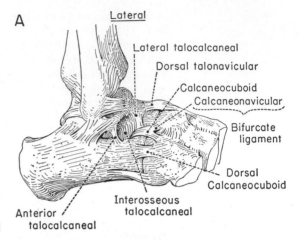

A   Lateral

Lateral talocalcaneal
Dorsal talonavicular
Calcaneocuboid
Calcaneonavicular
Bifurcate ligament
Dorsal Calcaneocuboid
Interosseous talocalcaneal
Anterior talocalcaneal

Figure 7–17 Ligaments of tarsal joints.

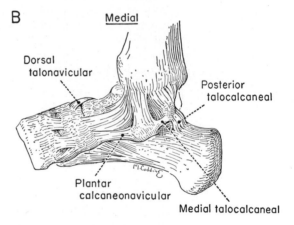

B   Medial

Dorsal talonavicular
Posterior talocalcaneal
Plantar calcaneonavicular
Medial talocalcaneal

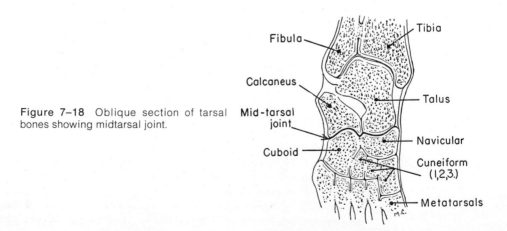

Fibula
Tibia
Calcaneus
Talus
Mid-tarsal joint
Navicular
Cuboid
Cuneiform (1,2,3.)
Metatarsals

Figure 7–18 Oblique section of tarsal bones showing midtarsal joint.

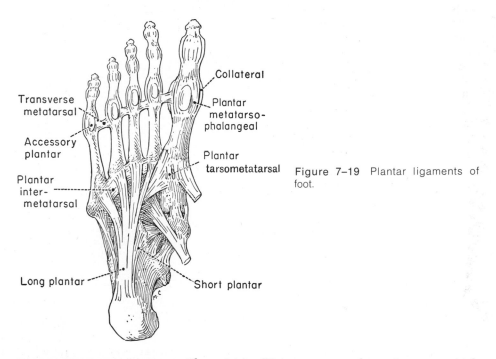

Figure 7–19 Plantar ligaments of foot.

TARSOMETATARSAL JOINTS   These joints (Figures 7–15 and 7–19) are nonaxial, with the possible exception of the great toe joint, which looks slightly like a saddle joint. The movements are of a gliding nature that resembles a restricted form of flexion, extension, abduction, and adduction.

INTERMETATARSAL JOINTS   These joints (Figures 7–14 and 7–19) include two sets of side-by-side articulations, those between the bases and those between the heads of the metatarsal bones. They are all nonaxial joints. The articulations between the heads of the metatarsal bones are an important part of the metatarsal arch. The total result of the movements occurring there is a spreading or flattening of the arch when the weight is on it and a return to its plantar concavity when the weight is taken off it.

METATARSOPHALANGEAL JOINTS   These joints (Figures 7–15 and 7–19) may best be described as a modified form of ovoid joint. The joint of the great toe differs from the others in that it is larger and has two sesamoid bones beneath it.

INTERPHALANGEAL JOINTS   As is true of the fingers, these are all hinge joints (Figures 7–15 and 7–19).

Movements of the Foot at the Ankle, Tarsal, and Toe Joints

ANKLE JOINT   The movements of the ankle joint occur about an axis that is usually described as frontal-horizontal but is actually slightly oblique, as evidenced by the slightly posterior position of the lateral malleolus relative to the medial. This is of minor significance but explains the tendency of the foot to turn out when it is fully elevated in dorsiflexion and to turn in when fully depressed in plantar flexion (Figure 7–20).

  Dorsiflexion (Flexion)   A forward-upward movement of the foot in the sagittal plane, so that the dorsal surface of the foot approaches the anterior surface of the leg.

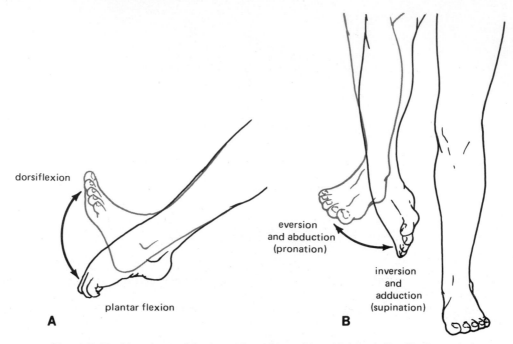

Figure 7–20   Movements of the foot at the ankle and tarsal joints. *A,* Dorsiflexion and plantar flexion. *B,* Supination and pronation (tarsal joint only).

Plantar Flexion (Extension)   A forward-downward movement of the foot in the sagittal plane, so that the dorsal surface of the foot moves away from the anterior surface of the leg.

TARSAL JOINTS   The movements that take place at the *midtarsal, subtalar,* and other *tarsal* joints occur together and are usually closely related to the ankle joint movements. Except for the talonavicular joint, which belongs to the ball-and-socket category, they are all nonaxial joints and therefore permit only slight gliding movements (Figure 7–20).

Dorsiflexion   Slight decrease in convexity of dorsal surface and in concavity of plantar surface of tarsal region. Accompanies dorsiflexion of ankle.

Plantar Flexion   Increase in convexity of dorsal surface and in concavity of plantar surface of tarsal region. Accompanies plantar flexion of ankle.

Inversion and Adduction (Supination)   A lifting of the medial border of the arch combined with a medial bending of the front of the foot.

Eversion and Abduction (Pronation)   A slight raising of the lateral border of the foot combined with a slight lateral bending of the front of the foot.

TARSOMETATARSAL AND INTERMETATARSAL JOINTS   Slight gliding motion. The first metatarsal bone has a slightly greater degree of motion at these joints than do the other metatarsals because of the absence of any ligament between its base and the base of the second metatarsal.

METATARSOPHALANGEAL JOINTS   Flexion, extension, and limited abduction and adduction.

INTERPHALANGEAL JOINTS   Flexion and extension; also hyperextension, especially of the great toe.

Muscles of the Ankle and Foot

Location

Eleven of the twenty-two muscles of the ankle and foot are intrinsic—i.e., they are located entirely within the foot. The other eleven are extrinsic; they have distal tendon attachments on the foot but are otherwise located outside of it (Table 7–1).

Characteristics and Functions of Individual Muscles

TIBIALIS ANTERIOR   This muscle (Figure 7–21A) lies along the full length of the anterior surface of the tibia from the lateral condyle down to the medial aspect of the tarsometatarsal region. Approximately one-half to two-thirds of the way down the leg it becomes tendinous. The tendon passes in front of the medial malleolus on its way to the first cuneiform. The muscle *dorsiflexes the ankle and foot,* and *supinates (inverts and adducts) the tarsal joints* when the foot is dorsiflexed (Kaplan, 1958). In an EMG study of the action of the leg muscles in movements of the free foot (the subject standing on the other foot), O'Connell (1958) found that the tibialis anterior initiates dorsiflexion. In other EMG studies it was found that one-half of the subjects in free standing had activity in the tibialis anterior that went away when the subjects leaned forward (Basmajian, 1979). The muscle may be palpated on the anterior surface of the leg just lateral to the tibia.

EXTENSOR DIGITORUM LONGUS   This muscle (Figures 7–21B and 7–22) *extends the four lesser toes.* It also *dorsiflexes both the ankle and the tarsal joints* and *helps to evert and abduct the latter.* It is a penniform muscle, situated lateral to the tibialis anterior muscle in the upper part of the leg and lateral to the extensor hallucis longus

TABLE 7–1 Ankle and Foot Muscles

EXTRINSIC MUSCLES	INTRINSIC MUSCLES
Anterior Aspect of Leg	Extensor digitorum brevis
Tibialis anterior	Flexor digitorum brevis
Extensor digitorum longus	Quadratus plantae
Extensor hallucis longus	Lumbricales
Peroneus tertius	Abductor hallucis
	Flexor hallucis brevis
Lateral Aspect of Leg	Adductor hallucis
Peroneus longus	Abductor digiti minimi
Peroneus brevis	Flexor digiti minimi brevis
	Dorsal interossei
Posterior Aspect of Leg	Plantar interossei
Gastrocnemius	
Soleus	
Tibialis posterior	
Flexor digitorum longus	
Flexor hallucis longus	

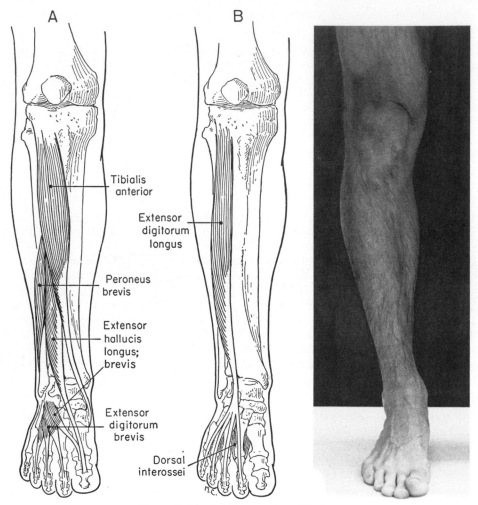

Figure 7–21   Anterior muscles of the leg.

in the lower part. Just in front of the ankle joint the tendon divides into four tendons, one for each of the lesser toes. The muscle may be palpated on the anterior surface of the ankle and the dorsal surface of the foot, lateral to the tendon of the extensor hallucis longus.

EXTENSOR HALLUCIS LONGUS   This muscle (Figure 7–21A) *extends and hyperextends the great toe.* It also *dorsiflexes the ankle and the tarsal joints.* Like the preceding muscle, it is penniform in structure. Its upper portion lies beneath the tibialis anterior and extensor digitorum longus, but about halfway down the leg the tendon emerges between these two muscles, thus becoming superficial. After it reaches the ankle the tendon slants medially across the dorsal surface of the foot to the top of the great toe. It may be palpated on the dorsal surface of the foot and great toe.

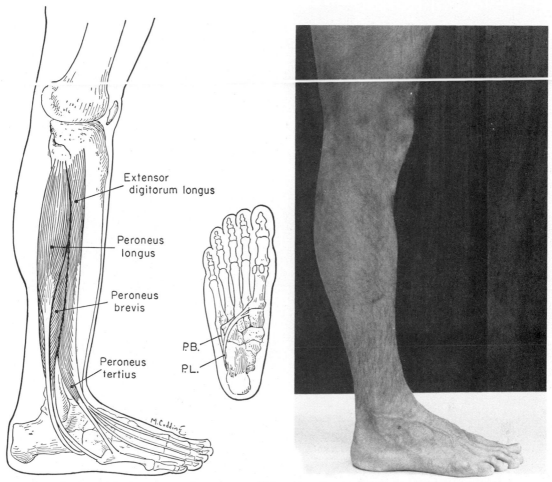

Figure 7–22 Lateral muscles of the leg. (P.B. = Peroneus brevis; P.L. = peroneus longus.)

PERONEUS TERTIUS   This muscle (Figure 7–22) *dorsiflexes and pronates (everts and abducts) the tarsal joints* and *dorsiflexes the ankle*. It is a small muscle that lies lateral to the extensor digitorum longus, sometimes described as the fifth tendon of the latter muscle. It may be palpated on the dorsal surface of the foot close to the base of the fifth metatarsal.

PERONEUS LONGUS   This muscle (Figure 7–22) *plantar flexes, everts, and abducts the tarsal joints,* and *plantar flexes the ankle*. It also is most active during the propulsive phase of walking. It is situated superficially on the lateral aspect of the leg with its distal tendon passing behind the lateral malleolus and proceeding forward and downward to the margin of the foot, where it passes behind the tuberosity of the fifth metatarsal. As this point it turns under the foot, passes through the peroneal

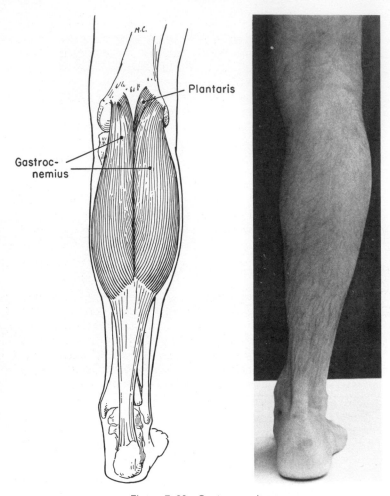

Figure 7–23   Gastrocnemius.

groove of the cuboid, and slants forward across the plantar surface of the foot to its attachment at the base of the first metatarsal and first cuneiform, not far from the attachment of the tibialis anterior. The muscle belly may be palpated on the lateral surface of the lower half of the leg and just above and behind the lateral malleolus.

PERONEUS BREVIS   This muscle (Figures 7–21A and 7–22) *plantar flexes and everts and abducts the tarsal joints* and *helps to plantar flex the ankle*. It is a penniform muscle, lying beneath the peroneus longus on the lower half of the lateral aspect of the leg. Its tendon passes behind the lateral malleolus immediately anterior to the tendon of longus and continues forward just above the longus tendon to its attachment on the tuberosity of the fifth metatarsal, below the attachment of the peroneus tertius. It may be palpated on the lateral margin of the foot, just posterior to the base of the fifth metatarsal.

GASTROCNEMIUS (Also listed with the knee muscles.) This is a powerful muscle (Figure 7–23) for *plantar flexing the foot at the ankle joint.* It is the most superficial muscle on the back of the leg and can be seen as two bulges in the upper part of the calf when it is well developed. Its two heads, together with the soleus, constitute the triceps surae. The lateral and medial portions of the muscle remain distinct from each other as far down as the middle of the back of the leg. Then they fuse to form the broad tendon of Achilles.

The most familiar function of this muscle is to *enable one to rise on the toes.* Many anatomists have thought that it acted only when the movement was resisted, but an EMG investigation by Sheffield et al. revealed that it was active in unresisted *plantar flexion* in subjects lying in the supine position (Basmajian, 1979). It has also been shown to be active in most individuals during normal relaxed standing. The muscle has a large angle of pull, approximately 90 degrees when the foot is in its fundamental position. Its internal structure and its leverage combine to make it an exceedingly powerful muscle. In a 1967 EMG study Herman and Bragin concluded that its most important role was plantar flexing in large contractions and in the rapid development of tension (Basmajian, 1979). It may be palpated in the calf of the leg and on the back of the ankle.

SOLEUS Like the gastrocnemius, this muscle (Figure 7–24) *plantar flexes the foot at the ankle joint.* It lies beneath the gastrocnemius, except along the lateral aspect of the lower half of the calf where a portion of it lies lateral to the upper part of the calcaneal tendon. Its fibers are inserted into the calcaneal tendon in a bipenniform manner. In an EMG study of the leg muscles, it was found that when the subjects balanced on one foot, the soleus was consistently more active than the gastrocnemius. In another study it was found that the soleus was most active in minimal contractions and when the foot was in a dorsiflexed position. This seems to imply that it was especially active in the reduction of dorsiflexion. Campbell et al., using five wire electrodes, have shown that the medial part of the soleus is a strong dynamic and static plantar flexor, whereas the lateral part is primarily a stabilizer (Basmajian, 1979). The muscle may be palpated slightly lateral to and below the lateral bulge of the gastrocnemius.

TIBIALIS POSTERIOR This muscle (Figure 7–25) *plantar flexes the tarsal joints and helps to plantar flex the ankle.* It participates in *supination (inversion and abduction)* when the foot is plantar flexed. It is the deepest of the muscles on the back of the leg. The main part of the muscle covers the intermuscular septum between the tibia and the fibula. In the lower front of the leg its tendon slants across the medial side of the ankle, passes behind the medial malleolus and above the sustentaculum tali, and then turns under the foot around the medial margin of the navicular bone to insert into its underside. The muscle is penniform in structure. Because of its direction of pull and its numerous attachments on the plantar surface of the tarsal bones, an important function of this muscle appears to be maintenance of the longitudinal arch.

FLEXOR DIGITORUM LONGUS This muscle (Figure 7–26) *flexes the four lesser toes, plantar flexes and helps to invert and adduct the tarsal joints, and helps to plantar flex the ankle.* It is situated on the medial side of the back of the leg behind the tibia. Penniform in structure, its distal tendon passes behind the medial malleolus between the tendons of the tibialis posterior and flexor hallucis longus. Beneath the tarsal bones it divides into four tendons that go to the distal phalanx of each of the four lesser toes.

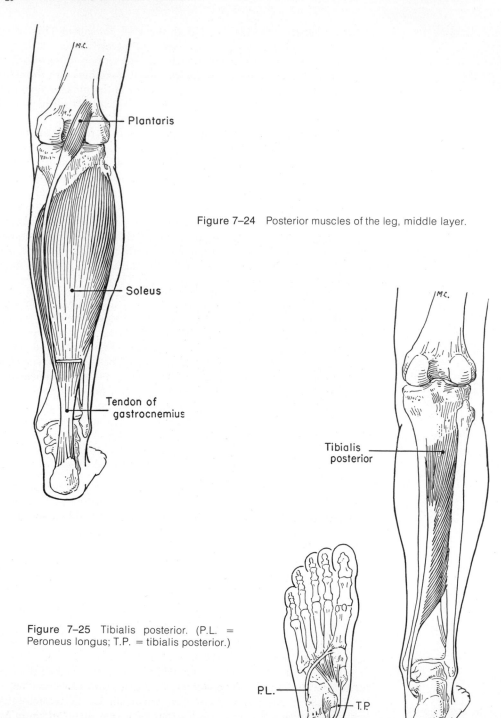

Figure 7–24   Posterior muscles of the leg, middle layer.

Figure 7–25 Tibialis posterior. (P.L. = Peroneus longus; T.P. = tibialis posterior.)

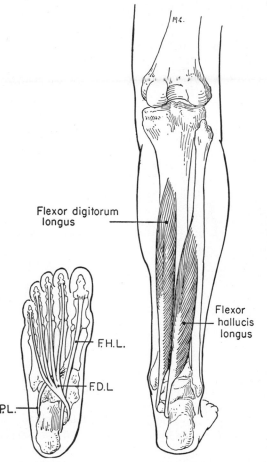

Flexor digitorum
longus

F.H.L.

F.D.L

P.L.

Figure 7–26 Flexor digitorum longus
and flexor hallucis longus; (F.H.L. =
flexor hallucis longus; F.D.L. = flexor
digitorum longus; P.L. = peroneus longus.)

Flexor
hallucis
longus

FLEXOR HALLUCIS LONGUS   This muscle (Figure 7–26) *flexes the great toe, plantar flexes and helps to invert and adduct the tarsal joints, and helps to plantar flex the ankle.* It is situated on the lateral side of the back of the leg, behind the fibula and the lateral portion of the tibia. The fibers unite with the distal tendon in a penniform manner. The tendon crosses behind the ankle to the medial side, passes behind and beneath the sustentaculum tali, the projection on the medial side of the calcaneus, and runs forward under the medial margin of the foot to the distal phalanx of the great toe. It is the most posterior of the three tendons that pass behind the medial malleolus. One of its important functions is to provide the push-off in walking, running, and jumping. It may be palpated on the medial border of the calcaneal tendon close to the calcaneus.

INTRINSIC MUSCLES OF THE FOOT   These muscles (Figures 7–27, 7–28, and 7–29) will be treated as a group rather than individually. There are eleven of these small muscles or muscle groups. All but one, the extensor digitorum brevis, are on the plantar surface and are usually described as being arranged in four layers. The dorsal

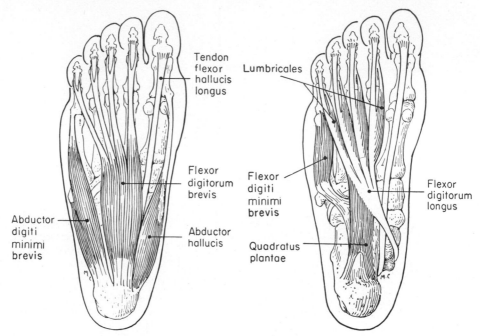

Figure 7–27 Plantar muscles of the foot, superficial layer.

Figure 7–28 Plantar muscles of the foot, middle layer.

interossei muscles, although included in the deepest layer, are situated between the metatarsal bones rather than on either surface (Figure 7–21B). The extensor digitorum brevis, which includes the hallucis, although the latter is sometimes described as a separate muscle, is situated on the dorsal surface of the foot (Figure 7–21A). With the exception of the *lumbricales* and the *quadratus plantae,* which help to flex the lesser toes, the names of these muscles indicate their functions. As one might expect, these intrinsic muscles are much more highly developed in primitive people than in people who habitually wear shoes.

Various research investigations have shown that the intrinsic muscles act as a functional unit, have a significant role in stabilization of the foot during propulsion, tend to show more activity in feet which are habitually pronated, do not show activity during relaxed standing in either normal or pronated feet and are not active in the normal *static* support of the longitudinal arches but do show definite activity in voluntary attempts to increase the height of the arches. They are also definitely active in the movement of rising on the toes.

PLANTAR FASCIA   On the plantar surface of the foot the muscles are covered by fascia (Figure 7–30), divided into medial, central, and lateral portions. The central portion, known as the plantar aponeurosis, is particularly strong and fibrous. It extends under the whole length of the foot, connecting the tuberosity of the calcaneus with the bases of the proximal phalanges of the five toes. This is an exceedingly strong band that serves as an effective binding rod for the longitudinal arch.

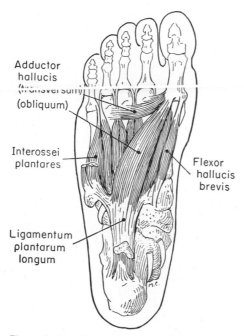

Adductor hallucis (transversum) (obliquum)

Interossei plantares

Flexor hallucis brevis

Ligamentum plantarum longum

Figure 7–29   Plantar muscles of the foot, deep layer.

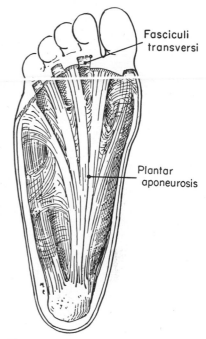

Fasciculi transversi

Plantar aponeurosis

Figure 7–30   Plantar fascia of the foot.

Muscular Analysis of the Fundamental Movements of the Ankle and Foot (Tarsal Joints and Toes)

The Ankle

DORSIFLEXION Performed by the tibialis anterior, peroneus tertius, extensor digitorum longus, and extensor hallucis longus.

PLANTAR FLEXION Performed by the gastrocnemius, soleus, and peroneus longus, with possible help from the tibialis posterior, peroneus brevis, flexor digitorum longus, and flexor hallucis longus.

The Tarsal Joints

DORSIFLEXION The same as for dorsiflexion of the ankle.

PLANTAR FLEXION Performed by the tibialis posterior, flexor digitorum longus, flexor hallucis longus, and peroneus longus and brevis.

SUPINATION (INVERSION AND ADDUCTION) (Figure 7–31B) Performed by the tibialis anterior (when the foot is dorsiflexed) and tibialis posterior (when the foot is plantar flexed), with possible help from the flexor digitorum longus and flexor hallucis longus (Basmajian, 1979; O'Connell, 1958).

PRONATION (EVERSION AND ABDUCTION) (Figure 7–31A) Performed by the peroneus longus, brevis, and tertius, with possible help from the extensor digitorum longus.

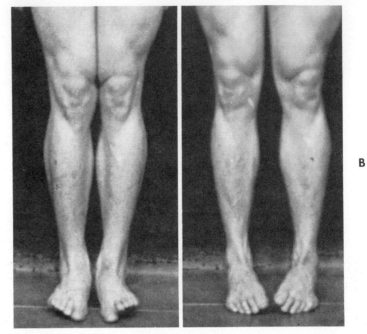

Figure 7–31 The feet and legs in weight-bearing position. *A*, In eversion and abduction. *B*, In inversion and adduction.

The Toes (Exclusive of the Intrinsic Muscles)

FLEXION   Performed by the flexor digitorum longus and flexor hallucis longus.

EXTENSION   Performed by the extensor digitorum longus and extensor hallucis longus.

Maintenance of the Arches

Many investigators have studied the structure of the arches and the role of muscles in maintaining them. Some have stated that the arch is supported by muscle contraction alone, while others have concluded that the arches are supported exclusively by passive structures, bones, and ligaments or the combination of muscular contraction and passive structures.

In 1963 Basmajian and Stecko investigated the activity of six muscles (tibialis anterior, tibialis posterior, peroneus longus, flexor hallucis longus, abductor hallucis, and flexor digitorum brevis) during static standing under various load conditions. Using twenty young men as subjects, they found that the subjects could support loads of 100 to 200 pounds, standing on one foot without any evidence of muscular action, and that with loads of 400 pounds some muscles became active but many still remained inactive. They concluded from these findings that the arches' first line of defense is ligamentous and that the muscles constitute a dynamic reserve, which is called into action reflexively when the load is excessive (Basmajian, 1979).

The electromyography of the static foot was also investigated by Gomez-Pellico and Llanos-Alcazar (1976). Five of the six muscles they investigated were the same as those selected by Basmajian and Stecko; the sixth was the abductor digiti minimi, rather than the flexor hallucis longus. Recordings were obtained on all six muscles for fifty subjects who stood first on both feet and then on one foot for five different slanting surfaces (horizontal, forward, backward, medial, and lateral). The results obtained led the authors to conclude that the activity of the studied muscles was almost nonexistent as an element of support of the plantar arch. In this regard their research agreed with the theory that the arch is supported by passive elements. On the other hand, they also determined that when the subject was resting on only one foot the muscular activity increased significantly. As mechanical stress on the arch increased there was a gradual increase in the participation of the active elements. They suggested that the muscles on the plantar arch are safety elements that operate progressively when the forces on the arch are higher than those that can be supported by the passive elements.

Common Athletic Injuries of the Leg, Knee, and Ankle

The Leg

Skin Bruises (Contusions)

These injuries are very common in sports because of the exposed position of the tibia and its lack of protection. A direct blow may cause an injury that varies in severity all the way from a simple bruise to a severe traumatic tibial periostitis, a condition in which the periosteum may be seriously damaged. Unlike the femur, the tibia has no anterior muscles to cushion it against sharp blows. It is important, therefore, to make every effort to protect the bone by the use of shin guards or other form of padding.

Shin Splints

This condition is usually associated with running or jogging, and produces symptoms of tenderness and pain on the medial surface of the tibia. The exact cause is unknown. The onset is gradual and the condition may be due to repeated tiny tears where the tibialis posterior attaches to the tibia or to tears or sprains in the interosseous membrane. Running on softer surfaces and support of the arches may be helpful in relieving the symptoms, but rest is essential for recovery. More precise treatment depends upon the diagnosis. Because there is considerable likelihood of a recurrence of the condition, it is important to supervise the player carefully when activity is resumed (Quigley, 1979).

Leg Fracture

The most common leg fracture experienced in athletics is that of the fibula, a fracture that tends to occur in the lower two-thirds of the leg. A fibular fracture is not usually of serious consequence, provided it is not accompanied by damage to the ankle joint, the condition of greatest concern being rupture of the tibiofibular ligament. A complicating condition that is likely to accompany this is displacement of the bones owing to the forceful pull of antagonistic muscles. If this results in instability of the ankle joint, the consequences can be extremely serious, causing a permanent disability (Klafs and Arnheim, 1973; O'Donoghue, 1976).

The Knee

Vulnerability of the Knee Joint

There can be no question as to the vulnerability of the knee. It is probably the most susceptible to injury of any of the joints in the body. Two factors appear to be responsible for this: its complicated structure and its position midway between the hip and the sole of the foot. Superficially, it looks like a hinge joint, but its action combines the movements of a hinge with the gliding of an irregular joint (p. 14). Furthermore, when it is flexed it is capable of a slight degree of medial and lateral rotation. Several writers have called attention to the strains and stresses to which the knee is subject, and have emphasized the need to be aware of these forces for knee function. Williams and Lissner (1963) have described methods for analyzing both tension and compression forces acting on the structures of the knee, and have suggested the application of these to exercise procedures.

Contusion

This condition occurs frequently among athletes and can be caused either by a fall or by a blow against the front or side of the knee. The problem presented by a contusion of the knee is that it often masks a more serious injury, the most likely being a tear of the medial collateral ligament at either its femoral or its tibial attachment, or severe damage to the lower part of the quadriceps tendon or to the patellar ligament and the attachment of the latter to the tuberosity of the tibia. O'Donoghue (1976) warns about the need for particular care in diagnosing the condition and recommends treating it, when in doubt, as though it were the more serious injury.

Collateral Ligament Sprain and the "Unhappy Triad"

This is doubtless one of the most, if not *the most*, frequently reported knee injury in the world of sports (Klafs and Arnheim, 1973). To understand the reason for this, a thorough knowledge of the structure of the joint is essential. Although classified as a hinge joint, it is by no means a typical one like the interphalangeal finger joints, for instance. In flexion and in the return from flexion, a certain amount of gliding occurs. When the knee is flexed it is capable of a slight amount of voluntary rotation. When it receives a blow from the side or when it is subjected to severe wrenching in the weight-bearing position, it can easily be forced beyond its normal range of rotatory motion. Furthermore, although abduction and adduction are not normal knee motions—that is, one cannot voluntarily perform them—the leg can be passively ab- or adducted by an outside force. A slight degree of this probably does no harm, but a severe lateral blow or violent wrenching is likely to tear the ligament on the opposite side.

The majority of knee sprains are caused by a blow from the lateral side toward the medial side or by a severe medialward twist (Klafs and Arnheim, 1973). This means that the leg has been violently adducted and medially rotated at the knee joint. O'Donoghue (1976) describes the classic athletic knee injury as follows: ". . . the foot is fixed to the ground, the thigh rotates inward and the leg outward, the knee is forced inward toward the opposite leg and the stress is primarily received on the ligaments on the inner side of the knee." If the force is great enough to be transmitted to the deep layer of this ligament, it is likely to affect the medial meniscus, which is attached to the ligament. In the severe triple injury known as the "unhappy triad," the two layers of the medial collateral ligament are torn near their attachment to the tibia, and both the medial meniscus and the anterior cruciate ligament are ruptured (Figure 7–32). The same type of injury can occur to the lateral side, but this is much less common. New light has been thrown on this problem by two investigations made during the early 1970s. Both were directed by C. A. Morehouse, and were undertaken because of the concern he and his coworkers felt regarding the high incidence of knee injuries in athletics, and because they were also disturbed by the lack of objective evidence to support the assumption of some authorities that ligaments are the first line of defense against knee injury and that a stretched ligament is inevitably a weaker one. They undertook to devise equipment for providing objective and reliable measurements of

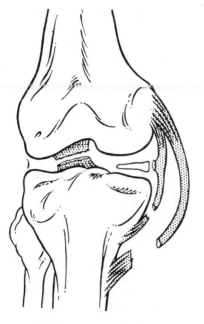

Figure 7–32 Triple injury to the knee involving sprain or, in more severe cases, rupture of medial collateral ligament and anterior cruciate ligament and damage to medial meniscus. (From O'Donoghue, D. H.: *Treatment of injuries to athletes*. 3d ed. Philadelphia: W. B. Saunders, 1976.)

knee stability as judged by the amount of abduction and adduction of which the knee was capable. Using this apparatus they investigated the effect of vigorous exercises, including squat jumps, on the lateral stability of knees, the possible relationship between knee stability and the occurrence of injuries to knee ligaments in college football, and the effectiveness of adhesive strapping in providing support to the knee joint prior to and following vigorous exercise.

To summarize their results briefly:

1. They developed an instrument with acceptable reliability but which they hoped to improve before using it for future studies.
2. The effects of football practice and scrimmage on knee stability yielded results that were inconclusive but tended to indicate a *decrease* in ab- and adduction.
3. Squat jumping was found *not* to increase ab- and adduction of the knee joint.
4. Adhesive strapping was found to provide support for a brief time but no support was apparent after 5 minutes of vigorous exercise.

When a number of cases of knee ligament injuries that occurred in football were analyzed, it was learned that this group had had less abduction rather than more. This suggested that the individual with more taut ligaments is more prone to injury (Morehouse, 1970).

In a follow-up study conducted by Goldfuss et al. (1973) a few years later for the purpose of investigating the effect of muscular tension on ab- and adduction of the leg at the knee joint, it was found that:

1. Unconscious muscular activity in the quadriceps and hamstring muscles had no effect on knee ab- and adduction measures.
2. Conscious contraction of the quadriceps and hamstring muscles was found to stabilize the knee joint against excessive ab- and adduction. The investigators felt

that this finding had important implications for the rehabilitation of injured knees, and that it indicated the need for maintaining the strength of these muscles during the recovery period of the injured joint.

Deep Knee Bending

Squatting, or deep knee bending, is a movement that is used in many ways, both in daily life activities and in sports and other physical education activities. It is used by the baseball catcher as his ready-to-catch position. It is also used as a starting position for running races, for executing various stunts, as an exercise for physical fitness or training, and for landing after jumping down from a height. In the home, on the street, and almost anywhere it is used for picking up objects from the floor or ground. Whether performed slowly or quickly, the basic muscular pattern is the same. In downward movement, the hip and knee joints are flexing and the ankle joints are dorsiflexing. The joint movements are *caused* by the force of gravity; they are *controlled* by the muscles that normally cause the opposite movements but that, for this purpose, are engaged in *eccentric contraction*. In the return movement—that is, the return to the erect standing position—the same muscles are working but this time in *concentric contraction*.

The demands placed on the muscles and ligaments of the knee joint during deep squats are severe, and there are some who denounce their use as taught in weight training and football conditioning. Such exercises, they believe, should be eliminated because they tend to weaken the ligaments and increase the instability of the joint (Morehouse, 1979). It is suggested that these factors be considered when contemplating the assignment of exercises involving repeated full squats or long-held squat positions, or stunts like the duck walk or the familiar Russian dance step.

The Ankle

Of all the injuries to which athletes are prone, those affecting the ankle joint have the highest incidence. One reason for this is thought to be the arrangement of the muscles. The long tendons cross the ankle in a way that makes for lack of bulkiness and for good leverage but contributes little to stabilization (Klafs and Arnheim, 1973). Consequently, this joint is unusually susceptible to strains, sprains, dislocations, and fractures.

Strains

A strain, it will be remembered, is a muscle injury. This includes the muscle tendon and the connective tissue by means of which the muscle is attached to the bone. Landing from jumping exposes the tendons of the ankle and foot muscles to the danger of strain. O'Donoghue (1976) points out the particular danger of broad jumping. As the jumper lands, the feet may be in severe dorsiflexion, and the impact of landing then forces them beyond their normal range of motion. This gives the Achilles tendon a sudden wrench that may cause tearing, either at the point of the tendon's attachment to the bone or at the junction between the tendon and the muscle belly.

The distal tendons of both the anterior and posterior tibial muscles are also subject to strain. The after-effects of each of these can be quite troublesome, since they are both inverters (supinators) of the foot, in addition to which the posterior tibial has the important function of helping to support the longitudinal arch.

Tenosynovitis   This is the term used for inflammation of the synovial membrane that surrounds a tendon, a condition that tends to follow strains. It occurs frequently at the ankle, but instead of resulting from a specific injury, it is caused most often by overuse of a tendon (O'Donoghue, 1976).

Sprains   A sprained ankle is all too familiar. It results from a sudden wrench or twist and is usually associated with forced inversion of the foot with the lateral ligaments being stretched or torn and sometimes ruptured or pulled off of the bone. The affected ligaments are any of those on the lateral aspect of the ankle—the calcaneofibular, anterior talofibular, and posterior talofibular. The interosseous talocalcaneal ligament, while not strictly an ankle ligament, may also be affected.

Fractures   Ankle fractures are usually caused by a sudden wrenching or twisting, the same factors that cause sprains but, whereas sprains are the result of excessive inversion of the foot, fractures result from excessive eversion. The majority of ankle fractures occur to the malleoli, especially the lateral malleolus. In the more serious fractures there is also likely to be some dislocation as the result of a separation between the tibia and fibula, with a consequent widening of the socket or mortise. Prompt and adequate treatment is all important if permanent damage is to be avoided. Emphasis is placed upon the importance of restoring the integrity of the mortise and maintaining the weight-bearing bones in proper relationship to one another (O'Donoghue, 1976).

Laboratory Experiences

Knee Joint: Joint Structure and Function

1. Using a form like that in Appendix A, record the essential information regarding the knee joint. Study the movements both on the skeleton and on the living body.

Muscular Action   (See Appendix E for muscle checklist.)

2. FLEXION AT KNEE
   Subject: Lie face down and flex leg at knee by raising foot.
   Assistant: Steady subject's thigh and resist movement by pushing down on ankle.
   Observer: Palpate biceps femoris, semitendinosus, gracilis, sartorius, and gastrocnemius.

3. EXTENSION AT KNEE
   a. *Subject:* Rise from a squat position.
      Observer: Palpate quadriceps femoris.
   b. *Subject:* Sit on table with legs hanging over edge. Extend leg.
      Assistant: Steady subject's thigh and resist movement by holding ankle down.
      Observer: Palpate quadriceps femoris.

4. OUTWARD ROTATION OF LEG WITH KNEE IN FLEXED POSITION
   Subject: Sit on table with legs hanging over edge. Turn foot laterally as far as possible without moving thigh.
   Assistant: Steady subject's thigh and give slight resistance by holding foot.
   Observer: Palpate biceps femoris.

5. INWARD ROTATION OF LEG WITH KNEE IN FLEXED POSITION
   Subject: Sit on table with legs hanging over edge. Turn foot medially as far as possible without moving thigh.

Assistant: Steady subject's thigh and give slight resistance by holding foot.
Observer: Palpate semitendinosus, gracilis, and sartorius.

Ankle and Foot: Joint Structure and Function

6. Using forms like the one in Appendix A, record the essential information regarding the ankle, subtalar, and midtarsal joints. Study the movements of these joints both on the skeleton and on the living body.

7. Using a protractor-goniometer, compare the total range of plantar and dorsiflexion of the ankle in a group of five or more subjects *(a)* with the knee straight, *(b)* with the knee flexed.

8. Make a similar comparison between two groups, one consisting of three to five varsity level swimmers and the other of the same number of recreational swimmers, or make a similar comparison between ballet and nonballet dancers.

Ankle and Foot: Muscular Action

(See Appendix E for muscle checklist.)

9. PLANTAR FLEXION
Subject: Perform each of the following actions: *a.* Stand and rise on the toes. *b.* Hold one foot off the floor and extend it vigorously.
Observer: Compare the muscular action of the leg in *a* and *b*.

10. DORSIFLEXION
Subject: Sit on a table with the legs straight and with the feet over the edge. Dorsiflex one foot as far as possible.
Assistant: Resist the movement by holding the foot.
Observer: Identify the tibialis anterior, peroneus tertius, extensor digitorum longus, and extensor hallucis longus.

11. PRONATION (EVERSION AND ABDUCTION)
Subject: In same starting position as in number 10, turn one foot laterally without extending it.
Assistant: Steady the leg at the ankle and resist the movement by holding one foot.
Observer: Identify the muscles that contract.

12. SUPINATION (INVERSION AND ADDUCTION)
Subject: In same position as above, turn one foot medially as far as possible.
Assistant: Steady the leg at the ankle and resist the movement by holding the foot.
Observer: Identify the muscles that contract.

References

Basmajian, J. V. 1979. *Muscles alive.* 4th ed. Baltimore: Williams & Wilkins.

Goldfuss, A. J., Morehouse, C. A., and LeVeau, B. F. 1973. Effect of muscular tension on knee stability. *Med. Sci. Sports* 5:267–71.

Gomez-Pellico, L., and Llanos-Alcazar, L. F. 1976. Electromyography of the static foot. In *Biomechanics V-A,* ed. P. V. Komi. pp. 289–94. Baltimore: University Park Press.

Hollinshead, W. H. 1976. *Functional anatomy of the limbs and back.* 4th ed. Philadelphia: W. B. Saunders.

Kaplan, E. B. 1958. The iliotibial tract. *J. Bone Joint Surg.* 40A:817–32.

Klafs, C. E., and Arnheim, D. D. 1973. *Modern principles of athletic training.* St. Louis: C. V. Mosby.

Klein, K. K. 1962. The knee and the ligaments. *J. Bone Joint Surg.,* 44A:1191–92.

Lawrence, S. 1955. A study of the flexibility and the stability of the feet of college women. Unpublished Master's thesis, Smith College.

Morehouse, C. A. 1970. Evaluation of knee abduction and adduction. The effects of selected exercise programs on knee stability and its relationship to knee injuries in college football. Washington, D.C.: Department of Health, Education, and Welfare. Final Project Report, Grant No. RD–2815M, Division of Research and Demonstration Grants, Social and Rehabilitation Service.

O'Connell, A. L. 1958. Electromyographic study of certain leg muscles during movement of the free foot and during standing. *Am. J. Phys. Med.* 37:289–301.

O'Donoghue, D. H. 1976. *Treatment of injuries to athletes.* 3d ed. Philadelphia: W. B. Saunders.

Quigley, T. B. 1979. Common musculoskeletal problems. In *Sports medicine and physiology,* ed. R. H. Strauss, pp. 217–18. Philadelphia: W. B. Saunders.

Schaeffer, J. P., ed. 1953. *Morris' human anatomy.* 11th ed. New York: McGraw Hill.

Steindler, A. 1970. *Kinesiology of the human body.* Springfield, Ill.: Charles C Thomas.

Williams, M., and Lissner, H. R. 1963. Biomechanical analysis of knee function. *J. Am. Phys. Ther. Assoc.* 43:93–99.

Wright, W. G. 1962. *Muscle function.* New York: Hafner Publishing.

The Spinal Column and Thorax

Objectives

At the conclusion of this chapter, the student should be able to:

1. Name, locate, and describe the structures and ligamentous reinforcements of the articulations of the spinal column and thorax.
2. Name and demonstrate the movements possible in joints of the spinal column and thorax, regardless of starting position.
3. Name and locate the muscles and muscle groups of the spinal column and thorax, and name their primary actions as agonists, stabilizers, neutralizers, or antagonists.
4. Analyze the fundamental movements of the spinal column and thorax with respect to joint and muscle actions.
5. Describe the common athletic injuries of the spinal column and thorax.

Structure and Articulations of the Spinal Column

If you were faced with the problem of devising a single mechanism that would simultaneously (1) give stability to a collapsible cylinder, (2) permit movement in all directions and yet always return to the fundamental starting position, (3) support

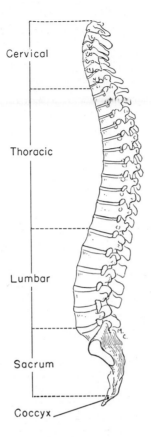

Cervical

Thoracic

Lumbar

Sacrum

Coccyx

Figure 8–1 Lateral view of the spinal column showing antero-posterior curves.

three structures of considerable weight (a globe, a yoke, and a cage), (4) provide attachment for numerous flexible bands and elastic cords, (5) transmit a gradually increasing weight to a rigid basinlike foundation, (6) act as a shock absorber for cushioning jolts and jars, and (7) encase and protect a cord of extreme delicacy, you would be staggered by the immensity of the task. Yet the spinal column fulfills all these requirements with amazing efficiency. It is at the same time an organ of stability and mobility, of support and protection, and of resistance and adaptation. It is an instrument of great precision, yet of robust structure. Its architecture and the manner in which it performs its many functions are worthy of careful study. From the kinesiological point of view, we are interested in the spine chiefly as a mechanism for maintaining erect posture and for permitting movement of the head, neck, and trunk.

In order to understand these functions of the spine, it is necessary to have a clear picture, first of the spinal column as a whole and second of the distinguishing characteristics of the different regions. The spinal column, consisting of seven cervical, twelve thoracic, and five lumbar vertebrae, the sacrum, and the coccyx, presents four curves as seen from the side. The cervical and lumbar curves are convex forward, the thoracic and sacrococcygeal curves convex to the rear (Figure 8–1). The thoracic and sacrococcygeal curves are called primary curves because they exist before birth. The cervical and lumbar curves develop during infancy and early childhood and hence are called secondary curves. From the first cervical to the fifth lumbar vertebra

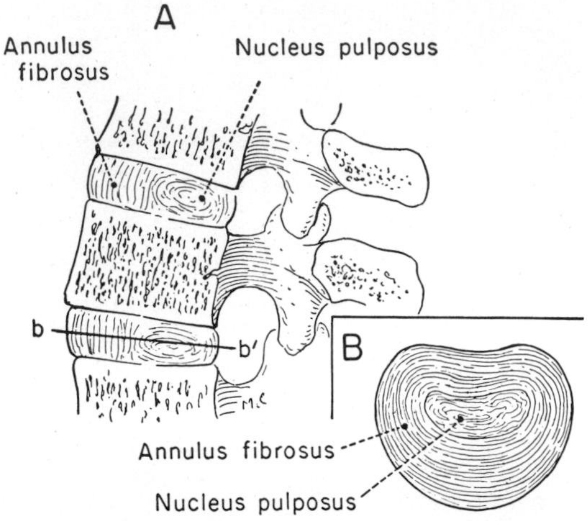

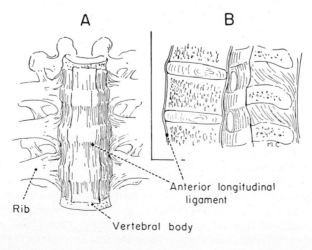

A

Annulus fibrosus   Nucleus pulposus

B

Annulus fibrosus
Nucleus pulposus

Figure 8–2   *A*, Sagittal section of lumbar vertebrae and intervertebral fibrocartilages. *B*, Transverse section of intervertebral fibrocartilage.

the vertebral bodies become increasingly larger, an important factor in the weight-bearing function of the spine.

There are two sets of interspinal articulations, those between the vertebral *bodies* and those between the vertebral *arches*. The latter are in pairs, with one on either side of each vertebra. The articulations of the first two vertebrae are atypical and will be described separately.

There is such a close relationship between the structure of the spinal column and the movements that take place in its different regions that the student will find it well worth the effort to acquire a thorough grasp of the structure, particularly of the joints, before proceeding to the movements. If possible, both a skeleton and a strung set of vertebrae should be referred to frequently while studying spinal structure.

Articulations of the Vertebral Bodies

These joints (Figure 8–2) are classified as synchondroses or cartilaginous joints. The bodies of the vertebrae are united by means of fibrocartilages, otherwise known as intervertebral disks. These correspond to the surfaces of the adjacent vertebral bodies, except in the cervical region where they are smaller from side to side. They adhere to

A   B

Rib

Anterior longitudinal ligament

Vertebral body

Figure 8–3   Anterior longitudinal ligament of the spine. *A*, Anterior view. *B*, Sagittal section of vertebrae showing lateral view of ligament.

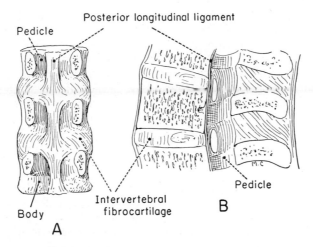

Pedicle

Posterior longitudinal ligament

Intervertebral fibrocartilage

Body

A

Pedicle

B

Figure 8-4 Posterior longitudinal ligament of spine. *A,* Frontal section of vertebrae showing posterior view of ligament. *B,* Sagittal section of vertebrae showing lateral view of ligament.

the hyaline cartilage both above and below, with no articular cavity in this type of joint. In thickness they are fairly uniform in the thoracic region but in the cervical and lumbar regions they are thicker in front than in back. Altogether, they constitute one-fourth of the length of the spinal column. Each disk consists of two parts, an outer fibrous rim and an inner pulpy nucleus known as the nucleus pulposus. This is a ball of firmly compressed elastic material, a little like the center of a golf ball. It constitutes a pivot of motion and permits compression in any direction, as well as torsion. The intervertebral disks are also important as shock absorbers.

Ligamentous Reinforcement

The joints of the spinal column are reinforced by several ligaments (Figures 8-3 and 8-4). The vertebral bodies are held together by two long ligaments, one in front and one in back. The *anterior longitudinal* ligament starts as a narrow band and widens as it descends from the occipital bone to the sacrum. The *posterior longitudinal* ligament, descending from the occipital bone to the coccyx, is relatively narrow throughout but has lateral expansions opposite each intervertebral fibrocartilage. Both ligaments are stronger in the thoracic region than in either the cervical or the lumbar region.

Figure 8-5 Sagittal section of vertebrae showing articulations of the vertebral arches.

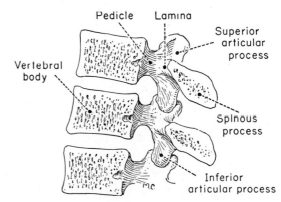

Pedicle   Lamina

Superior articular process

Vertebral body

Spinous process

Inferior articular process

Articulations of the Vertebral Arches

The articulations (Figure 8–5) between the facets of the vertebral arches are nonaxial diarthrodial joints. Each of these joints has an articular cavity and is enclosed within a capsule. A slight amount of gliding motion is permitted. The resultant movement of each vertebra is determined largely by the direction in which the articular facets face. The cervical spine appears to be somewhat of an exception, however. The facets in this region slant at about a 45-degree angle, lying halfway between the horizontal and the frontal planes (Figure 8–6A). Such a slant would seem to favor rotation and lateral flexion and to be unfavorable to flexion and hyperextension. Yet these latter movements occur as freely as does lateral flexion, whereas rotation from the second cervical vertebra down can be rated as only moderate. In the thoracic region they lie slightly more in the frontal and less in the horizontal plane than do the cervical articulations, and they have a slight inward and outward slant (Figure 8–6B). The upper facets face backward, slightly upward, and lateralward; the lower facets face forward, slightly downward, and medialward. They are adapted equally well to rotation and to lateral bending. In the lumbar region, except at the lumbosacral articulation, the articular facets lie more nearly in the sagittal plane (Figure 8–6C). The upper facets face inward and slightly backward; the lower facets face outward and slightly forward. Furthermore, the upper facets present slightly concave surfaces and the lower facets convex. By this arrangement of the facets, the lumbar vertebrae are virtually locked against rotation. The slight amount of rotation that does occur is made possible by the looseness of the capsules. At the lumbosacral articulation the facets lie somewhat more in the frontal plane than is true of the other lumbar joints.

The ligaments reinforcing these joints may be identified in Figure 8–7. The *ligamenta flava* and the *interspinous* and *supraspinous* ligaments are all thickest and strongest in the lumbar region. There remain two rather thin ligaments, the *intertransverse*, connecting the transverse processes of adjacent vertebrae, and the *ligamentum nuchae*, which is the continuation of the supraspinous ligament in the cervical region.

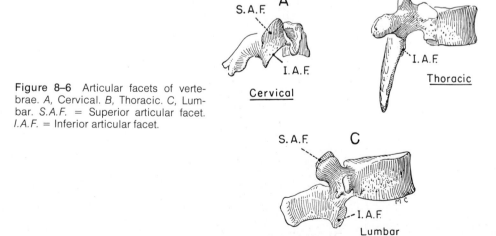

Figure 8–6   Articular facets of vertebrae. *A,* Cervical. *B,* Thoracic. *C,* Lumbar. *S.A.F.* = Superior articular facet. *I.A.F.* = Inferior articular facet.

A

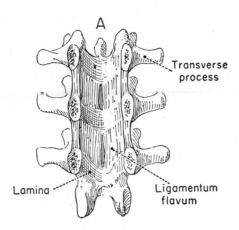

Transverse
process

Lamina

Ligamentum
flavum

B

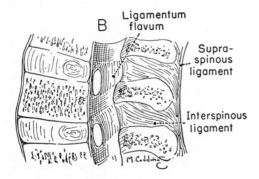

Ligamentum
flavum

Supra-
spinous
ligament

Interspinous
ligament

Figure 8–7 Ligaments of vertebral articulations. *A*, Frontal section of three lumbar vertebrae showing anterior view of vertebral arches and ligamenta flava. *B*, Sagittal view of lumbar vertebrae showing ligaments of vertebral arches. *C*, Side view of cervical spine showing ligamentum nuchae.

C

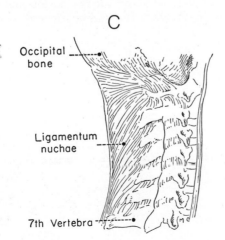

Occipital
bone

Ligamentum
nuchae

7th Vertebra

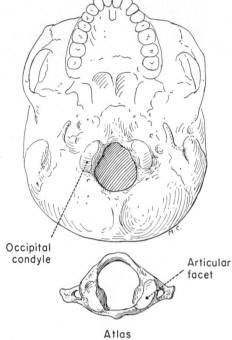

Figure 8–8 Bones forming atlanto-occipital articulation.

Atlanto-Occipital Articulation

This is the articulation (Figure 8–8) between the head and the neck. It consists of a pair of joints, one on each side. Each condyle of the occipital bone of the skull articulates with the corresponding superior articular fossa of the first vertebra, known as the atlas. Each articulation by itself belongs to the ovoid (condyloid) classification, but the movement that occurs in the two joints together is more like that of a hinge joint. The rigid relationship between the two joints results in a restriction of the lateral motion that would normally occur in an ovoid joint. The movements that take place at the atlanto-occipital articulation are chiefly flexion and extension, with a slight amount of lateral flexion (Figure 8–10A and B). There is no rotation.

Atlantoaxial Articulation

This is a perfect example of a pivot joint—a joint whose sole function is rotation (Figure 8–9). The toothlike peg (odontoid process or dens) that projects upward from the second cervical vertebra, otherwise known as the axis or epistropheus, fits into the ring formed by the inner surface of the anterior arch of atlas and the transverse

Figure 8–9 Atlantoaxial articulation. *A,* Posterior view. *B,* Superior view.

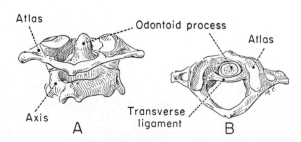

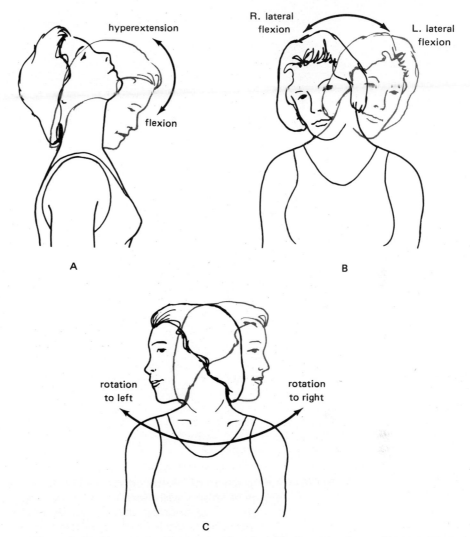

Figure 8–10 Movements of the head and neck. *A,* Flexion, extension, and hyperextension. *B,* Lateral flexion. *C,* Rotation.

ligament that bridges across the tips of the arch. Since no rotation occurs at the atlanto-occipital joint, rotation of atlas on axis will carry the head with it; thus the movement occurring at the atlantoaxial joint contributes to the movement of the head on the trunk (Figure 8–10C).

Atypical Spinal Contours

Wells (1947) investigated the spinal contours of 100 college women as recorded in routine anteroposterior posture photographs. These 100 photographs were selected from 1,200, 50 of them on the basis of a predominantly convex spine—that is, a spine in which the thoracic convexity involves a portion, possibly all, of the lumbar region—and 50 on the basis of a predominantly concave spine—that is, a spine in

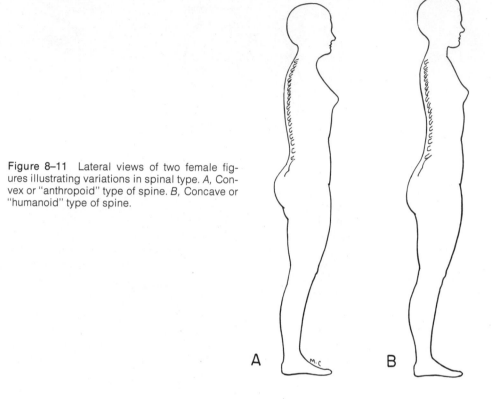

Figure 8–11 Lateral views of two female figures illustrating variations in spinal type. *A*, Convex or "anthropoid" type of spine. *B*, Concave or "humanoid" type of spine.

TABLE 8–1 Comparison of "Anthropoid" and "Humanoid" Types of Spines with Reference to the Depth and Length of the Anteroposterior Curves of the Thoracic and Lumbar Portions of the Spine*

ASPECT OF SPINE MEASURED	"ANTHROPOID" SPINE	"HUMANOID" SPINE
Total length of thoracic and lumbar portion of spine	3.54 cm	3.54 cm
Length of posterior convexity	2.79 cm (79%)	1.48 cm (42%)
Length of posterior concavity	0.75 cm (21%)	2.06 cm (58%)
Depth of posterior convexity	0.22 cm	0.08 cm
Depth of posterior concavity	0.06 cm	0.16 cm

* Mean values of measurements taken from the posture photographs of 100 college women, 50 representing the "anthropoid" type and 50 the "humanoid" type. (From Wells, 1947.)

which the lumbar concavity extends well up into the thoracic region. Because the convex spine is characteristic of the anthropoid apes, this group was called the "anthropoid spine" group, and because a lumbar curve is characteristic of the human spine, the second group was called the "humanoid spine" group (Figure 8–11). Measurements made on the photographs revealed that significant measurable differences existed between the two types of spine. The mean values of these measurements are presented in Table 8–1.

Movements of the Spine as a Whole

Individual Movements

The movements of the spinal column, which resemble those of a ball-and-socket joint, are described as follows.

FLEXION This is a forward-downward bending in the sagittal plane about a frontal-horizontal axis (Figure 8–12A). It involves a compression of the anterior parts of the intervertebral disks and a gliding motion of the articular processes. It occurs more freely in the cervical, upper thoracic, and lumbar regions. The cervical curve may be reduced to a straight line and the lumbar curve, in flexible individuals, may be reversed. The greatest anteroposterior motion in the lumbar spine usually occurs between the fifth lumbar vertebra and the sacrum.

EXTENSION AND HYPEREXTENSION Extension is the return movement from flexion (Figure 8–12B). Hyperextension is a backward-downward movement in the sagittal plane. It occurs most freely in the cervical and lumbar regions, and particularly at the lumbosacral junction. In the thoracic region hyperextension is limited by the overlapping of the spinous processes.

An interesting study of the flexibility of the spinal column of four individuals was made by Wiles (1935). Two of the subjects were normally active women; two were acrobatic dancers, one of them a child and the other a man. The photograph of Miss P. showed a spine of "normal" contours, that of Miss R. showed a long convexity or "anthropoid type" of spine, that of the child showed a marked lordosis, and that of the man showed a shallow but long concavity or "humanoid type" of spine. The range of motion in each spine, as measured on x-rays, is recorded in Table 8–2. The relationship between the type of spine and the degree and pattern of flexibility should be noted. The Wiles study, although it involved only four individuals, two of whom

TABLE 8–2 Anteroposterior Spinal Flexibility of Four Selected Cases*

SUBJECT	FLEXION	HYPEREXTENSION	TOTAL
Miss P.	64°	35°	99°
Miss R.	62°	19°	81°
Child	76°	39°	115°
Man	50°	71°	121°

* From Wiles, 1935.

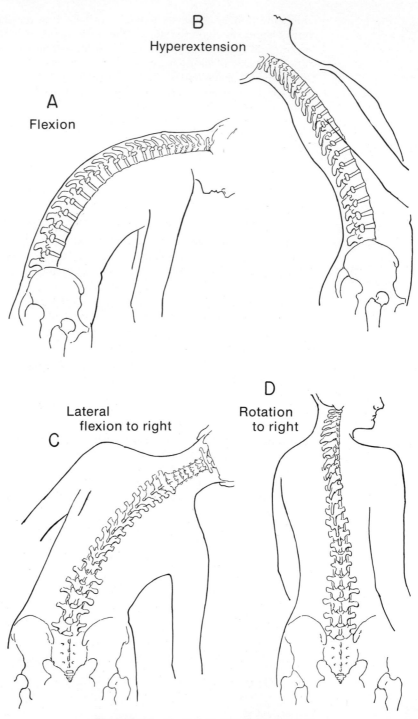

Figure 8–12   Movements of the spinal column.

were highly atypical from the point of view of agility, nevertheless suggests a relationship between structure and function. It is interesting to note that Miss R., whose spine seemed to be of the "anthropoid type," showed a marked limitation in hyperextension, whereas the adult male acrobat, who seemed to represent the extreme "humanoid type," showed extreme hyperextension but limited flexion. A study of the flexibility of a large sampling of these two spinal types might prove to be of value.

The significance of studies of the relationship between spinal contours and spinal flexibility lies in their implication for posture education and for recommendations regarding activity. Such studies are valuable to the degree that they give (1) a broad concept of the "normal," (2) an appreciation of the relatedness between structural type and physical skills, and (3) an awareness of the limitations characteristic of each type. Physical educators and therapists should realize that identical goals of posture, flexibility, and function cannot be laid down for all types of body build. Just what the specific abilities and limitations of each type are, and just what the goals for each type should be, are problems that are still open for investigation.

LATERAL FLEXION   This is a sideward bending in the frontal plane about a sagittal-horizontal axis (Figure 8–12C). It is freest in the cervical region and quite free in the lumbar region and at the thoracolumbar junction, but it is limited in the thoracic region by the presence of the ribs. Each rib (except the first, tenth, eleventh, and twelfth) articulates with two adjacent vertebrae and the intervening disk, and each rib (except the eleventh and twelfth) articulates with the transverse process of the lower of the two vertebrae (Figure 8–13). Thus it is seen that the ribs serve as splints, restricting lateral flexion of the thoracic spine to a marked degree. It is amazing that any motion can take place there at all.

For several reasons—the slant of the articular processes, the presence of the anteroposterior curves of the spine, and muscular and ligamentous tensions—lateral flexion is always accompanied by a certain amount of torsion. When lateral flexion is performed from the erect position, the maximum movement occurs in the lumbar region and at the thoracolumbar junction, with only slight involvement of the lower thoracic spine. (The cervical spine is excluded from this discussion.) The torsion occurs in the same part of the spine and consists in a turning of the vertebral bodies toward the side of the lateral flexion. Thus, if the spine bends to the right (forming a

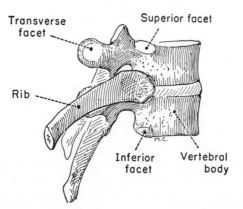

Transverse facet

Superior facet

Rib

Inferior facet

Vertebral body

Figure 8–13   Articulation of a rib with two adjacent vertebrae.

curve concave to the right), the vertebral bodies of the lumbar and lower thoracic vertebrae turn slightly to the right, with the spinous processes, therefore, turning to the left.

If the lateral flexion is performed from a position of hyperextension, and the hyperextension is maintained throughout the movement, the lateral flexion moves lower in the spine, occurring almost entirely below the eleventh thoracic vertebra. The torsion occurs in this same region and in the same manner that it does when the lateral flexion is performed from the erect position. The position of hyperextension seems to lock the thoracic spine against lateral movements.

If the lateral flexion is performed from a position of forward flexion, the movement occurs higher in the spine than ordinarily, the greatest deviation being at the level of the eighth thoracic vertebra. The torsion in this case reverses itself. Thus, in a side bend to the right, the vertebral bodies turn to the *left* and the spinous processes to the right. This reversal is not inconsistent. It is directly related to the anteroposterior curves of the spine. In the first two examples—that is, when the lateral flexion is performed either from the erect or from the hyperextended position—most of the movement takes place in the lower part of the spine, the part that is concave to the rear. The rotation that accompanies the side bend in these two cases is called concave-side rotation because the bodies turn in the direction of the concave or inner side of the laterally curved spine. When the side bend is performed from the flexed position, most of the movement takes place in the thoracic spine, the region that is convex to the rear. The rotation that accompanies the lateral flexion in this case is called convex-side rotation because the vertebral bodies turn in the direction of the convex or outer side of the laterally curved spine.

ROTATION   This is a rotatory movement of the spine in the horizontal plane about a vertical axis (Figure 8–12D). Spinal rotation is named by the way the front of the upper spine turns with reference to the lower part. Thus, a turning of the head and shoulders to the right constitutes rotation to the right. A turning of the legs and pelvis to the left, without turning the upper part of the body, also constitutes rotation of the spine to the right since the anatomical relationships are the same as in the former example. The movement of rotation is most free in the cervical region, with 90 per cent of the movement being attributed to the atlantoaxial joint. It is next most free in the thoracic region and at the thoracolumbar junction (Hollinshead, 1965). Owing to the interlocking of the articular processes, it is extremely limited in the lumbar region, there being only about 5 degrees of rotation to each side. In the cervical region there is no rotation between atlas and the skull, but free rotation at the pivot joint between atlas and axis. Whenever rotation occurs in the spine, it is accompanied by a slight amount of unavoidable lateral flexion to the same side.

When performed from the erect position, rotation of the spine (below the seventh cervical vertebra) occurs almost entirely in the thoracic region. When performed from the position of hyperextension, the movement shifts lower in the spine, occurring in the vicinity of the thoracolumbar junction. When performed from the flexed position, the rotation is higher than usual, occurring in the upper thoracic spine. Regardless of the position in which the rotation is performed—whether erect, flexed, or hyperextended—the slight lateral flexion which accompanies it is always to the same side as the rotation. Thus, if the spine rotates to the left, it flexes slightly to the left. This movement is very slight, however, and can scarcely be detected (Lovett, 1932).

CIRCUMDUCTION   This is a circular movement of the upper trunk on the lower, a combination of flexion, lateral flexion, and hyperextension, but not including rotation.

Summary of Spinal Movements

Flexion; extension; hyperextension
  Free in all three regions
  Cervical and thoracic curves may be reduced to straight lines
  Lumbar curve may be reversed in flexible subjects

Lateral flexion
  Free in cervical and lumbar regions
  Limited in thoracic region by rib attachments
  Accompanied by torsion

Rotation
  Freest at top, least free at bottom of spine
  Accompanied by slight lateral flexion

Circumduction
  Sequential combination of flexion, lateral flexion, and hyperextension

Regional Classification of Spinal Movements

Occipitoatlantal joint
  Flexion and extension
  Hyperextension
  Slight lateral flexion

Atlantoaxial joint
  Rotation

Remaining cervical joints
  Free flexion and extension
  Free hyperextension
  Free lateral flexion
  Free rotation

Thoracic region
  Moderate flexion
  Slight hyperextension
  Moderate lateral flexion
  Free rotation

Lumbar region
  Moderate to free flexion and extension
  Free hyperextension
  Free lateral flexion
  Slight rotation

Summary of Factors that Influence the Stability and Mobility of the Spinal Column

Before considering the muscular analysis of the spinal movements it would be advisable to review some of the special characteristics that contribute to the spine's stability and modify its mobility in one way or another.

PRESSURE AND TENSION STRESSES   The tendency of the compressed intervertebral disks to push the vertebrae apart, combined with the tendency of the ligaments to press them together, is an important factor in the stability of the spinal column.

ANTEROPOSTERIOR CURVES   The alternating anteroposterior curves of the spinal column influence the nature and the degree of movements that occur in the different regions. Individual variations from the so-called normal curves cause variations in the movement patterns. The anteroposterior curves are said to serve as a safeguard against the development of abnormal lateral curves (curvature of the spine, scoliosis).

RELATIVE THICKNESS AND SHAPE OF THE INTERVERTEBRAL DISKS   There is a direct relationship between the thickness of the disks and the degree of movement permitted, with greater freedom of motion where the disks are thick.

THICKNESS AND STRENGTH OF THE LIGAMENTS   These differ in the different regions and have a corresponding influence on the motions permitted in each region.

DIRECTION AND OBLIQUITY OF THE ARTICULAR FACETS   These are characteristic for each region and play an important part in determining the type of motion permitted in each.

SIZE AND OBLIQUITY OF THE SPINOUS PROCESSES   These overlap like shingles in the thoracic region, hence limiting hyperextension. In the lumbar region they are horizontal, and, although they are wide, they do not restrict motion.

ARTICULATIONS OF THE RIBS WITH THE VERTEBRAE   These limit lateral flexion in the thoracic region.

Muscles Operating the Spinal Column

Location

The muscles responsible for the movements of the spine, with the exception of two groups, have at least one attachment on the spinal column or the skull. The exceptions are the abdominal and the hyoid muscles. Both of these groups are superficially located on the front of the body. Nevertheless both groups, the abdominal muscles in particular, are effective movers or stabilizers of the spine. The muscles are listed below according to aspect and region.

Anterior Aspect
  Cervical Region
    Prevertebral muscles (longus capitis and colli, rectus capitis anterior, and lateralis)
    Hyoid muscles (suprahyoids and infrahyoids)
  Thoracic and Lumbar Regions
    Abdominal muscles
      Obliquus externus abdominis
      Obliquus internus abdominis
      Rectus abdominis
      Transversus abdominis

Posterior Aspect
  Cervical Region Only
    Splenius capitis and cervicis
    Suboccipitals (rectus capitis posterior major and minor, obliquus capitis superior and inferior)
  Cervical, Thoracic, and Lumbar Regions
    Erector spinae (iliocostalis, longissimus, and spinalis)
    Deep posterior spinal muscles (multifidi, rotatores, interspinales, intertransversarii, and levatores costarum)
    Semispinalis thoracis, cervicis, and capitis

Lateral Aspect
  Cervical Region
    Scalenus anterior, posterior, and medius (commonly called the three scalenes)
  Sternocleidomastoid
    Levator scapulae
  Lumbar Region
    Quadratus lumborum
    Psoas major

Characteristics and Functions of Individual Spinal Muscles

Anterior Aspect   **PREVERTEBRAL MUSCLES**   As Figure 8–14 shows, the longus colli and capitis extend vertically up the front of the vertebrae, the colli from the upper three thoracic to the first cervical (atlas) and the capitis from the lower cervical to the occipital bone. The rectus capitis muscles pass obliquely upward from the atlas to the skull, the anterior slanting medially and the lateralis laterally. With the exception of the longus colli, these muscles *flex the head and neck* when the left and right muscles act together. Acting separately, they *flex the head and neck laterally* or *rotate it to the opposite side*. The longus colli acts only on the neck and is active in resisted forward flexion, resisted lateral flexion, and rotation to the same side. It also stabilizes the neck during coughing, talking, and swallowing.

HYOID MUSCLES   Also called the strap muscles, these are small anterior muscles in the cervical region (Figure 8–15). There are four suprahyoids and four infrahyoids. Together they *flex the head and neck*. They are primarily muscles of some phase of swallowing, but they contract in cervical flexion whenever the movement is per-

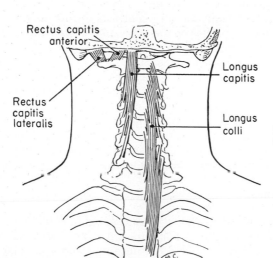

Rectus capitis anterior

Rectus capitis lateralis

Longus capitis

Longus colli

Figure 8–14   Prevertebral muscles of cervical spine (anterior view).

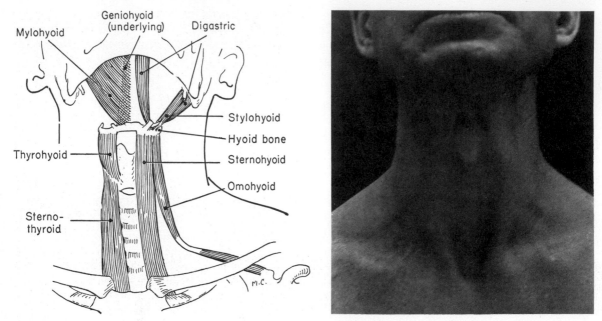

Figure 8–15 Hyoid muscles (Anterior view).

formed against resistance. By neutralizing one another's pull on the hyoid bone their action is transferred to the head and thence to the cervical spine. They may be palpated just below the jaw bone.

ABDOMINAL MUSCLES *Obliquus Externus Abdominis* The fibers of this muscle (Figure 8–16) run diagonally upward and outward from the lower part of the abdomen, the two muscles together forming an incomplete letter V, as seen from the front. When both sides contract they *flex the thoracic and lumbar spine* against gravity or other resistance. When only one side contracts in combination with other anterior, lateral, and posterior muscles on the same side, it *flexes the spine laterally*. When it combines with other spinal rotators, it *rotates the spine to the opposite side*—i.e., the right muscle rotates the spine to the left.

Investigators have found that the external obliques show the greatest activity in movements performed from the supine position—e.g., forward and lateral flexion of the spine, decrease of the pelvic tilt, forward flexion combined with rotation, and double knee circling (Partridge and Walters, 1959; Walters and Partridge, 1957). The external and internal obliques working together were found to show marked activity in two types of movement, namely straining and bearing down when the breath is held (Basmajian, 1979; Campbell, 1942) and forced exhalation (Basmajian, 1979; Campbell, 1942; Floyd and Silver, 1950). The external oblique may be palpated at the side of the abdomen.

Obliquus Internus Abdominis This muscle (Figure 8–17) lies beneath (i.e., deeper than) the external oblique. Its fibers fan out from the crest of the ilium, most of them passing diagonally forward and upward toward the rib cartilages and sternum, some horizontally forward toward the linea alba and some diagonally forward and

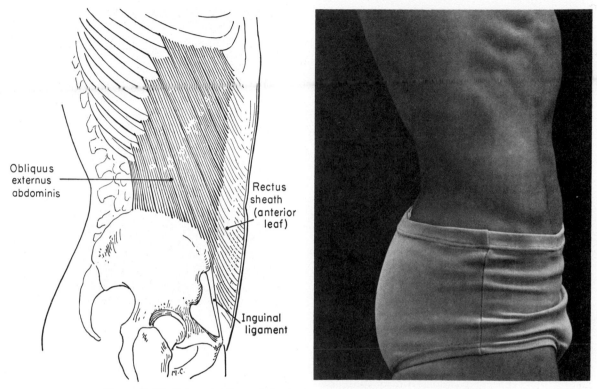

Figure 8–16   External oblique abdominal muscle (obliquus externus abdominis).

downward toward the crest of the pubis. Of the three abdominal muscles acting on the spine, this one is most active in rotation. EMG experiments have also shown it to have marked activity in the following movements: leaning backward, decreasing the pelvic tilt from the supine position, lifting the knees to the chest and lowering them from side to side, and lifting the knees over the head until the buttocks are raised from the supporting surface (Walters and Partridge, 1957). In summary, the internal oblique *flexes the lumbar and thoracic spine, flexes the spine laterally,* and *rotates the spine to the same side.* It may be palpated at the side of the abdomen, below the external oblique. It may also be palpated through the external oblique when the latter is relaxed, as in rotation.

Rectus Abdominis   This is the most superficial of the abdominal muscles (Figure 8–18). It is situated on the anterior surface of the abdomen on either side of the linea alba. It is a long, flat band of muscle fibers extending longitudinally between the pubis and the lower part of the chest. At three different levels transverse fibrous bands known as tendinous inscriptions cross the muscle fibers. The muscle is enclosed within a sheath formed by the aponeuroses of the other muscles making up the abdominal wall. EMG studies have shown the rectus to be strongly active in head raising from the supine position (Campbell, 1952; Floyd and Silver, 1950), and inclining the trunk backward from the erect position (Walters and Partridge, 1957; Partridge and Walters, 1959). The upper rectus was found to be more active in exercises involving the upper part of the body, such as spine flexion from the supine

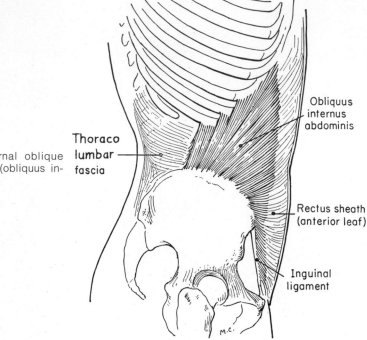

Figure 8–17 Internal oblique abdominal muscle (obliquus internus abdominis).

Thoraco lumbar fascia

Obliquus internus abdominis

Rectus sheath (anterior leaf)

Inguinal ligament

position (Walters and Partridge, 1957). In the latter movement it was also found to start contracting a moment before the lower rectus (Crowe et al., 1963). The lower rectus was found to be more active in movements involving a decrease of pelvic tilt—e.g., in the supine position bending the knees and lifting them toward the face until the fifth lumbar vertebra is raised approximately 5 inches above the supporting surface (Walters and Partridge, 1957). In brief, the rectus abdominis *flexes the lumbar and thoracic spine,* and *one side working alone helps to flex the spine laterally.* The muscle may be palpated on the front of the abdomen about 2 or 3 inches from the midline, from the pubis to the sternum.

Transversus Abdominis   This muscle (Figure 8–19) is made up of a broad sheet of fibers that run horizontally from the thoracolumbar fascia and cartilages of the lower ribs forward to the linea alba. Unlike the other abdominal muscles, it is *not* a mover of the spinal column; its pull is inward against the abdominal viscera and hence it is a strong muscle of *exhalation* and *expulsion.* It does, however, help to *stabilize the trunk* when acts requiring great effort are performed.

THE ABDOMINAL MUSCLES AS SPINAL FLEXORS   The rectus abdominis and the external and internal obliques work together to flex the lumbar and thoracic spine. They play a small part, however, in flexing the spine from an erect position. This movement is produced by the force of gravity and controlled by the extensors in eccentric contraction. Contraction of the rectus occurs only toward the end of the movement if the trunk is forced downward into full flexion against resistance (Flint, 1965). The only circumstance that would necessitate continued contraction of the abdominal muscles would be if the spine were being flexed against resistance, such as

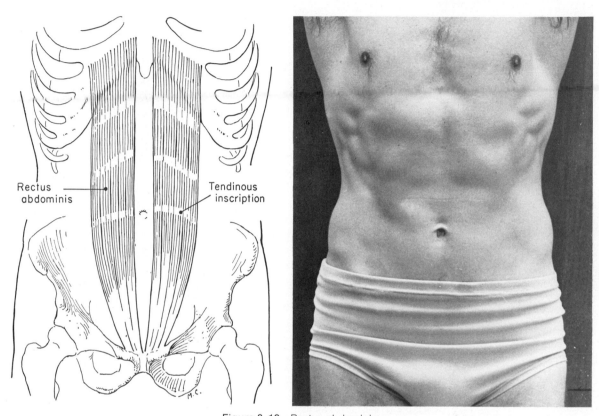

Figure 8–18   Rectus abdominis.

would occur if a person were lifting a weight by pulling down on a pulley rope and were supplementing arm strength by flexing the spine instead of by the more efficient method of bending the knees and using the body weight.

The abdominal muscles are markedly active when the spine is being flexed from a supine polition, especially at the beginning of this movement before the hips start to flex. Their activity is increased if a weight is held against the chest or on top of the head. (Obviously, the head and neck flexors are also working hard.) Once the hips start to flex, the abdominal muscles play a double role—namely, as movers in flexing the spine and as stabilizers of the pelvis against the pull of the hip flexors.

When a staight spine sit-up is performed, the abdominal muscles *do not act as movers* at all. In this exercise, the trunk as a whole is flexing at the hip joints on the lower extremities. As the hip flexors are attached to the movable pelvis, the latter needs to be stabilized against their pull, and this is done by means of the *static contraction* of the abdominal muscles. If the latter are not strong enough to prevent the tilting of the pelvis, the abdominal action then becomes involuntary eccentric or lengthening contraction. If the student is thoroughly familiar with the attachments of the abdominal muscles, he or she will know that they cannot be *movers* in this exercise since they *do not cross the hip joints*. A detailed analysis of the abdominal muscles in sit-ups and related exercises appears in Chapter 21.

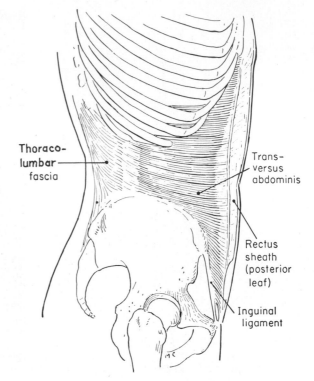

Figure 8-19 Transversus abdominis.

THE ABDOMINAL WALL   The abdominal wall consists of the four abdominal muscles. Together, these muscles form a strong anterior support for the abdominal viscera. They are subject to considerable stress from the pressure of the latter against their inner surface. The more stretched they become, as in the case of a protruding abdomen, the more heavily the organs rest upon the abdominal wall, subjecting it to direct gravitational stress. Thus a vicious circle is set in motion. The pressure against the lower abdominal wall stretches it still more, causing its protrusion to increase and subjecting it to ever-increasing gravitational stress. As is so often the case, correction of this postural fault is much more difficult than its prevention. A strong abdominal wall is greatly to be desired.

Posterior Aspect   **SPLENIUS CAPITIS AND CERVICIS**   These two muscles consist of bands of parallel fibers, slanting outward as they ascend from their centrally located lower attachments to their more laterally located upper attachments. The capitis is much broader than the cervicis. Figure 8–20 clearly shows the left cervicis and the right capitis muscles. The viewer should try to visualize both muscles on both sides. When the left and right sides contract together, they serve to *extend and hyperextend the head and neck*. They also help to *support the head* in erect posture. One side contracting alone can *flex the head and neck laterally* and also *rotate them to the same side*. The muscles may be palpated on the back of the neck just lateral to the trapezius and posterior to the sternocleidomastoid above the levator scapulae, especially if the head is extended against resistance in the prone position and the shoulders are kept relaxed. It is difficult to identify them, however.

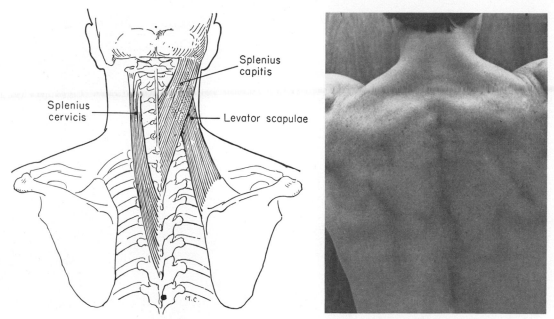

Figure 8–20 Posterior and lateral muscles of cervical spine.

SUBOCCIPITAL GROUP   This is a group of four short muscles (Figure 8–21) situated at the back of the lower skull (occipital bone) and upper two vertebrae (atlas and axis). It includes the obliquus capitis superior and inferior, and the rectus capitis posterior major and minor. Acting together on both sides, this group *extends and hyperextends the head*. When one side acts alone it *flexes the head laterally* or *rotates it to the same side*.

ERECTOR SPINAE   The muscle (Figure 8–22) commences as a large mass in the lumbosacral region but soon divides into three branches.

The *iliocostalis* branch consists of lumbar, thoracic, and cervical portions which are named *lumborum, thoracis,* and *cervicis,* respectively. It receives an additional tendon of origin from each rib throughout the thoracic region and gives off small slips to insert into the ribs in the thoracic region and into the transverse processes of the vertebrae in the cervical region.

The *longissimus* branch consists of three distinct portions which, in fact, appear to be three separate muscles (Figure 8–22). *Longissimus thoracis* is a broad band lying against the angles of the ribs, *longissimus cervicis* is narrower and lies slightly closer

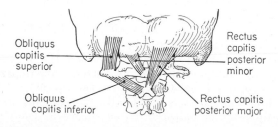

Figure 8–21 Suboccipital muscles (posterior view).

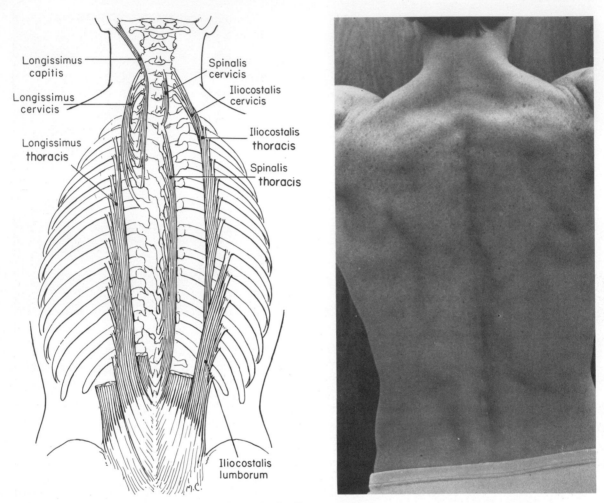

Figure 8-22   The erector spinae.

to the spine, connecting the transverse processes of the upper thoracic vertebrae with those of the lower cervical vertebrae, and *longissimus capitis* is a thin strand that lies against the vertebrae for its lower two-thirds and then slants outward and upward to the mastoid process of the temporal bone.

The *spinalis* branch lies against the vertebrae and is attached by separate slips to the spinous processes. It is of significance in the thoracic region only.

Electromyographic studies have shown that the erector spinae contributes little to the maintenance of erect posture unless a deliberate effort is made to extend the thoracic spine more completely or unless the weight is carried forward over the balls of the feet, in which case some static contraction of the muscle is required. In ordinary standing the level of activity is quite low (Basmajian, 1979).

In forward flexion from the standing position, the erector spinae undergoes eccentric contraction until the weight of the trunk is supported by the ligaments. When the trunk returns from this position the muscle contracts concentrically until the body is again erect and balanced (Basmajian, 1979). Pauly (1966) found that in almost all vigorous exercises performed from the standing position, the most active part of the erector spinae was the spinalis and the least active was the iliocostalis lumborum.

The muscle engages most forcefully in its functions of extension, hyperextension, and lateral flexion when these movements are performed against gravity or other resistance. Hyperextension from the prone lying position is considered the best exercise for strengthening the erector spinae (Pauly, 1966).

In brief, when the two sides of the muscle contract with equal force, the erector spinae *extends the head and spine* (assuming that all of its branches are contracting). When one side contracts alone, especially in conjunction with lateral and anterior muscles of the same side, it causes *lateral flexion*. And when one side alone contracts in a certain precise combination with lateral and anterior muscles—some on the same side, some on the opposite—it *rotates the head and spine to its own side*. The lumbar and lower thoracic portions of the muscle may be palpated in the two broad ridges on either side of the spine.

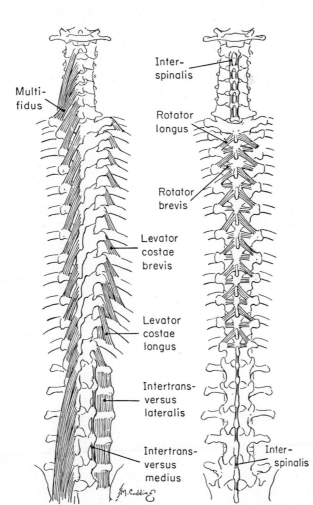

Figure 8–23 Deep posterior muscles of the spine.

DEEP POSTERIOR SPINAL MUSCLES   This group (Figure 8–23) includes the *multifidi*, *rotatores, interspinales, intertransversarii,* and *levatores costarum*. The latter is primarily a muscle of the thorax but is included here as a possible assistant in extension and lateral flexion. These muscles consist of small slips, in most cases inserting into the vertebrae immediately above their lower attachments. Some of the fibers run vertically, and some slant medially as they ascend. The former are best developed in the cervical and lumbar regions where their action is that of extension. The latter are best developed in the thoracic region where they either extend or rotate. It has been suggested that the muscles in this group are responsible for localized movements. It seems likely that they also help to stabilize the spine. In brief, acting symmetrically they *extend and hyperextend the spine* and acting asymmetrically they *rotate the spine to the opposite side* and *assist in lateral flexion.*

SEMISPINALIS THORACIS, CERVICIS, AND CAPITIS   These muscles (Figure 8–24) lie close to the vertebrae beneath the erector spinae. The thoracis and cervicis portions consist of small bundles of fibers that slant medially as they ascend to the spinous processes several vertebrae above. The lower portion of the semispinalis capitis—that is, the portion starting from the upper thoracic vertebrae—have a slight medial slant, but the bundles in the cervical region attaching to the occipital bone are vertical. Like

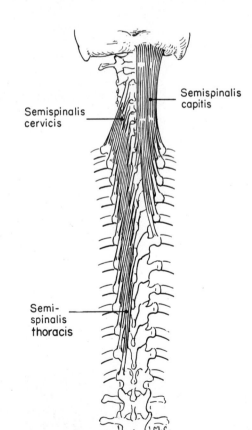

Figure 8–24   Semispinalis (posterior view).

Semispinalis cervicis

Semispinalis capitis

Semi-spinalis thoracis

the muscles in the preceding group they *extend and hyperextend the thoracic and cervical spine* when both sides contract together, and when only one side contracts they cause *lateral flexion and rotation to the opposite side.*

TRANSVERSOSPINALIS   This is not a different muscle from those already listed but represents a different organization of the deep muscles of the back. Some texts use this term for the three spinal muscles whose fibers slant medially as they ascend, namely the *semispinalis, multifidi,* and *rotatores* (Figures 8–23 and 8–24).

THORACOLUMBAR FASCIA   Although not a muscle, the thoracolumbar fascia (Figure 8–19) is described here because of its importance to the deep muscles of the spine and erector spinae. It binds these muscles together, holding them close to the skeletal structure and separating them from the more superficial muscles of the back. In the lumbar region it curves around the lateral margin of the erector spinae and folds in front of it to attach to the tips of the transverse processes of the vertebrae and to the intertransverse ligaments. Its lateral portion provides attachment for the transverse abdominis (Figure 8–19), and its posterior portion blends with the aponeurosis of the latissimus dorsi (Figure 4–20).

Lateral Aspect

SCALENUS ANTERIOR, POSTERIOR, AND MEDIUS   The three scalenes (Figure 8–25) run diagonally upward from the sides of the two upper ribs to the transverse processes of the cervical vertebrae. Acting together, they *flex the cervical spine* and, acting on one side at a time, they *flex the neck laterally.* They also serve to elevate the upper ribs in forced inspiration. They may be palpated on the side of the neck between the sternocleidomastoid and the upper trapezius but are difficult to identify.

STERNOCLEIDOMASTOID   This muscle (Figure 8–26) arises from two heads, one from the top of the sternum and the other from the top of the clavicle about 2 inches lateral to the first. They unite to attach to bones of the skull close below and behind the ear.

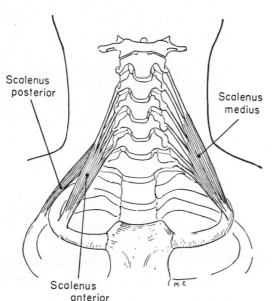

Scalenus
posterior

Scalenus
medius

Scalenus
anterior

Figure 8–25   The scalenes—anterior, posterior, and medius (anterior view).

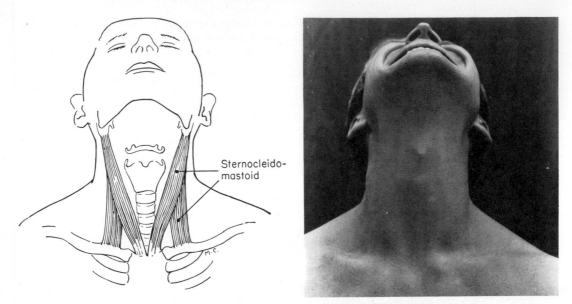

Figure 8–26   Sternocleidomastoid muscle.

Acting together, they *flex the head and neck.* Acting on one side at a time, they *flex the head and neck laterally;* they also *rotate them to the opposite side* (Figure 8–28A). They may be easily palpated, as well as seen, on the side of the neck from just under the ear to the front of the neck on either side of the sternoclavicular joint.

Campbell (1952) observed that both the sternocleidomastoid and the three scalenes show marked activity as soon as a person begins to raise the head from a supine position and Vitti et al., in a 1973 EMG study, confirmed the movements stated in the preceding paragraph (Basmajian, 1979).

LEVATOR SCAPULAE (Figure 8–20)   (Also listed with the muscles of the shoulder girdle.) When one scapula is fixed, the muscle on that side will help to *flex the cervical spine laterally.* If both muscles contract at the same time when both scapulae are fixed, they neutralize each other without effecting any movement. This action may possibly help to stabilize the neck, especially when the body is in the prone position, supported on "all fours."

QUADRATUS LUMBORUM   This flat muscle (Figure 8–27) is situated behind the abdominal cavity at the side of the lumbar spine. It extends from the crest of the ilium to the lowest rib and has slips branching medially to attach to the tips of the transverse processes of the upper four lumbar vertebrae. Acting bilaterally, it is credited with *stabilizing the pelvis and lumbar spine.* Acting unilaterally, it *flexes the lumbar spine to the same side.* In a 1972 EMG study, Waters and Morris found that together with other posterior spinal muscles, as well as with the abdominal muscles, it contracted regularly in each cycle of walking. According to the electromyogram reproduced in *Muscles Alive* (Basmajian, 1979), its action appears to coincide with the moment of heel contact. The muscle may be palpated on a thin, muscular subject just lateral to the erector spinae in the lumbar region.

PSOAS (Also listed with the muscles of the hip.) Like the quadratus lumborum, the psoas (Figure 6–7) is situated at the back of the abdominal cavity. Together, these two form the posterior abdominal wall. Although the psoas is primarily a muscle of the hip joint, its action on the lower spine and pelvis is of interest. Because the psoas major muscle at its proximal end attaches to the sides of the bodies and to the front and lower borders of the transverse processes of all the lumbar vertebrae, it has been thought to be a mover of the lumbar portion of the spinal column. A review of textbooks of kinesiology and of corrective exercises shows that there are conflicting statements concerning such movements. Some say that when its distal attachment is fixed, it *flexes* the lumbar spine; some say that it *hyperextends* it; others believe that sometimes it flexes and sometimes it hyperextends, according to the current relation of its line of pull to the lumbar joints. This relationship is thought to be affected by the position of the body, the anteroposterior postural curve of the lumbar spine, and its current status, whether in a position of flexion or hyperextension.

In the hope of resolving these apparent differences, the writings of four experimental clinicians, physicians, or physical therapists known for their wide experience in observing the muscular action of patients, and the statements of four researchers (or teams of researchers) based on their electromyographic experimentation were carefully examined. Unfortunately, this served only to uncover more conflicting statements (Brunnstrom, 1966; Crowe et al., 1963; Kendall and Kendall, 1943; Wright, 1962; Flint, 1965; Keagy et al., 1966; La Ban et al., 1965; Partridge and Walters, 1959).

What is the reader to conclude from this? Does it actually imply opposing points of view? On the contrary, there may be a number of logical explanations for the seeming disagreements. For instance, the writer may not have been explicit regarding techniques used or specific conditions at the time of examining or experimenting, the terminology used may be subject to misinterpretation, and variations in muscular action may have been caused by variations in anatomical structure or in habitual posture.

When there appear to be diverse opinions regarding muscular actions, it seems likely that the differences are not of great importance. Frequently, when there is lack of agreement regarding movement, one may safely assume that the true function of the muscular contraction, with reference to the joints in question, is more likely to be stabilization or balance than purposeful movement. This, in fact, has been suggested as a function of the psoas muscle by Keagy et al. (1966) and Nachemson (1969).

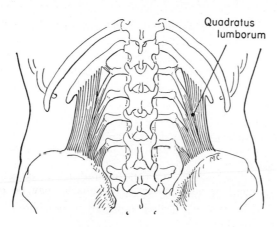

Figure 8–27   Quadratus lumborum (posterior view).

Brunnstrom (1966) has described this type of action with unusual clarity. She likens the muscles that are situated near the spinal column (erector spinae, psoas major, and so on) to guy ropes supporting an upright pole. When the pole starts to tip, the tension of the ropes on the opposite side increases. In like manner, if a person starts to lean backward, possibly to favor weak posterior muscles, the muscles on the front of the spine spring into action. Thus, it would appear that the most important role of the psoas is *stabilization or balancing of the spine* in response to other forces acting on the latter. In addition, unilateral contraction contributes to *lateral flexion* of the lumbar spine.

Muscular Analysis of the Fundamental Movements of the Head and Spine

In general, the muscles situated anterior to the spine flex it, those posterior to it extend it, and those lateral to it, when acting on one side only, either flex it laterally or rotate it, depending upon the requirements of the intended movement. *Because of the effect of gravity, however, the anterior muscles fulfill their function as flexors most successfully when the body is supine, the posterior muscles as extensors when the body is prone, and the lateral muscles as lateral flexors when the body is resting on the side.* These facts should be kept in mind when one is analyzing the muscular actions of the fundamental movements.

Cervical Spine and Atlanto-Occipital Joint

FLEXION   This is performed chiefly by the sternocleidomastoid, the three scalenes, and the prevertebral muscles. The supra- and infrahyoid muscles, whose chief function is to move the hyoid bone up or down in movements related to swallowing and vocalizing, give added force to cervical flexion when they contract together and movements of the mouth are prevented.

EXTENSION AND HYPEREXTENSION   Many muscles contribute to these movements: the splenius capitis and cervicis, the capitis and cervicis portions of the erector spinae, semispinalis, deep posterior spinal muscles, and the suboccipitalis. When the left and right sides of trapezius I contract together, they also help to extend the head and neck.

LATERAL FLEXION   This is performed by the simultaneous contraction of the extensors and flexors of the same side. Specifically, the chief lateral flexors include the capitis and cervicis portions of the splenius, erector spinae, semispinalis, three scalenes, and sternocleidomastoid. The suboccipitals, cervical portions of the deep posterior spinal muscles, and levator scapulae are in a position to aid in lateral flexion when they are needed.

ROTATION   The sternocleidomastoid and deep posterior spinal muscles rotate the head and neck to the opposite side and the splenius, erector spinae, and occipitals rotate them to the same side (Figure 8–28).

Thoracic and Lumbar Spine

FLEXION   This is performed by the three abdominal muscles: the rectus abdominis and external and internal obliques. As an aid to their effective action the pelvis must often be stabilized by the hip flexors, especially when the movement is performed from the supine position.

A

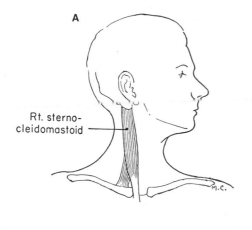

Rt. sterno-
cleidomastoid

M.C.

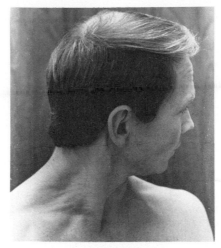

B

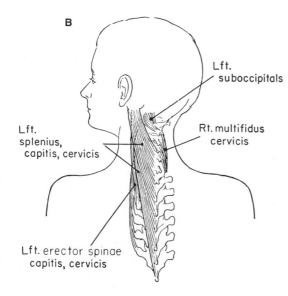

Lft.
suboccipitals

Lft.
splenius,
capitis, cervicis

Rt. multifidus
cervicis

Lft. erector spinae
capitis, cervicis

Figure 8–28 Muscles that contract
to rotate the head and neck to the
left.

EXTENSION AND HYPEREXTENSION   The thoracic and lumbar portions of the erector
spinae and the semispinalis thoracis are the chief extensors, but the deep posterior
spinal muscles also have a significant role. When hyperextension is performed from
the prone lying position, the erector spinae is particularly active.

LATERAL FLEXION   Many muscles are active in this movement—the erector spinae,
internal and external oblique abdominals, and quadratus lumborum in particular,
with the semispinalis thoracis, rectus abdominis, deep posterior spinal muscles,
psoas, and latissimus dorsi supplying additional force if needed. When the trunk is
flexed to the right from a side lying position on the left, the working muscles are those
on the right side of the trunk.

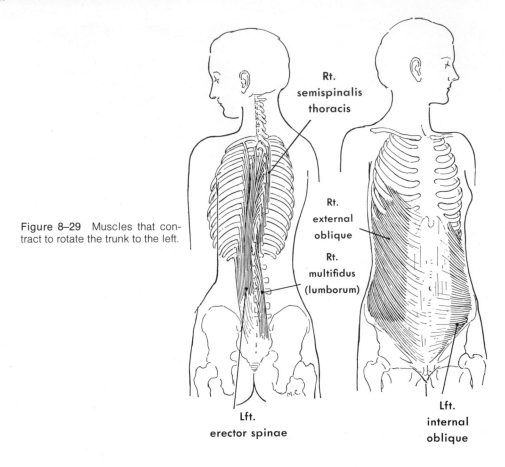

Figure 8–29   Muscles that contract to rotate the trunk to the left.

ROTATION   Rotation to the left (Figure 8–29) is effected by the left internal oblique abdominal muscle and the thoracic and lumbar portions of the left erector spinae, especially the iliocostalis thoracis branch, the right external oblique abdominal muscle, semispinalis thoracis, multifidus, and other deep posterior spinal muscles.

Structure and Articulations of the Thorax

The thorax is a bony-cartilaginous cage with an inverted V-shaped opening in front beneath the sternum (Figure 8–30). It is formed mainly by the ribs and their cartilages but also includes the sternum, which constitutes the anterior base of attachment for the ribs, and the thoracic portion of the spine, which provides the posterior base of attachment. The upper seven ribs whose cartilages articulate directly with the sternum are called true ribs and the remaining five, false ribs. This is a misleading term, the only difference being that the latter do not articulate with the sternum. In each case the cartilages of the eighth, ninth, and tenth ribs unite with the cartilage above; the eleventh and twelfth ribs, known as the "floating ribs," have no anterior attachment but end anteriorly in cartilaginous tips.

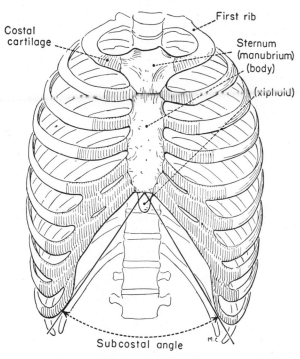

Figure 8–30 Anterior view of thorax.

The angle formed by the margins of the lower rib cartilages at the front of the chest is known as the subcostal angle. This is characteristically wider in individuals of stocky build than in those of slender build. The thorax is wider from side to side than it is from front to back and is slightly flattened in front. An infant or young child has a more "barrel-shaped" chest than does an adult—that is, a thorax whose antero-posterior diameter more nearly approaches its transverse diameter than is the case in an adult.

Before studying the articulations and the movements of the thorax, the student should review the ribs by observing them on a skeleton, noting especially their shape and the way in which they twist. If no skeleton is available, he or she should look carefully at pictures of the ribs, such as those shown in Figure 8–31.

All but the lowest two ribs articulate anteriorly with the sternum, either directly or indirectly, and all articulate posteriorly with the vertebrae. More specifically, with the exception of the first, tenth, eleventh, and twelfth ribs, the head of each rib articulates with two adjacent vertebrae, thus spanning the disk between (Figure 8–32). Each of the other ribs articulates with a single vertebra. Except in the case of the last two ribs, each rib has an additional vertebral articulation between the tubercle of the rib and the adjacent transverse process of the vertebra (Figure 8–33). All of these articulations are nonaxial, diarthrodial joints and permit only a slight gliding action.

There are four groups of sternocostal articulations: (1) the *sternocostal joints* between the costal cartilages and the sternum; (2) the joints between each rib and its cartilage, known as the *costochondral joints*; (3) the joints between one costal cartilage and another, called the *interchondral joints*; and (4) the two *intersternal joints*, one between the manubrium and body of the sternum, the other between the body and the xiphoid process (Figure 8–34).

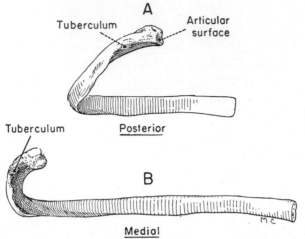

Figure 8–31 Rib. *A*, Posterior view. *B*, Medial view.

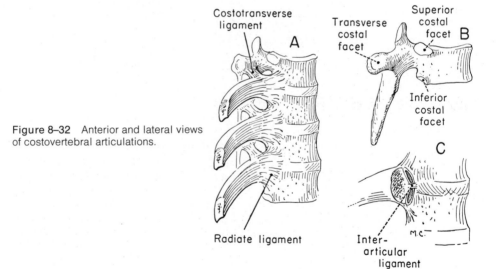

Figure 8–32 Anterior and lateral views of costovertebral articulations.

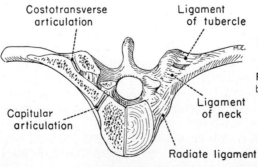

Figure 8–33 Superior view of costovertebral articulations.

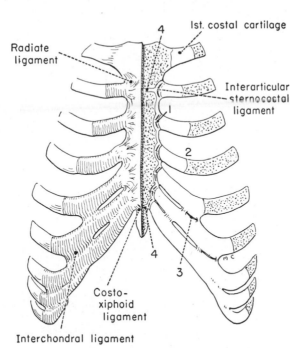

Radiate
ligament

4

Ist. costal cartilage

Interarticular
sternocostal
ligament

Figure 8–34 Sternocostal articulations. Key: *1*, Sternocostal; *2*, costochondral; *3*, interchondral; *4*, intersternal.

2

4

3

Costo-
xiphoid
ligament

Interchondral ligament

Movements of the Thorax

Because most of the ribs are attached both posteriorly and anteriorly, their movement is extremely limited. In the thoracic expansion associated with inhalation the anterior ends of the ribs are elevated in a flexion type of movement. This is accompanied by a slight eversion in which the lower margin of the central portion of the rib turns upward and lateralward, the inner surface being made to face somewhat downward. As the anterior ends of the upper ribs move upward they also push forward, carrying the sternum forward and upward with them. In the case of the lower ribs the anterior ends move laterally, thus "opening" the chest and widening the subcostal angle.

Although expansion of the thorax is ordinarily associated with inhalation for the purpose of providing the body with oxygen, there is another purpose. Whenever one exerts maximal muscular effort of short duration, a deep breath is taken and held while exerting the effort. This serves the purpose of stabilizing the ribs and sternum and thus provides firm anchorage for the upper extremity and trunk muscles that are used in forceful lifting, pushing, and pulling.

Enlargement of the Thorax in Inhalation

In inhalation the thorax is enlarged in three diameters: transverse, anteroposterior, and vertical.

INCREASE IN THE TRANSVERSE DIAMETER   This effect (Figure 8–35) results from the elevation and eversion of the lateral portion of the ribs. The shape and twist of the ribs together with their anterior and posterior attachments are responsible for what has so aptly been called their "bucket handle inspiratory movement." The elevation of the

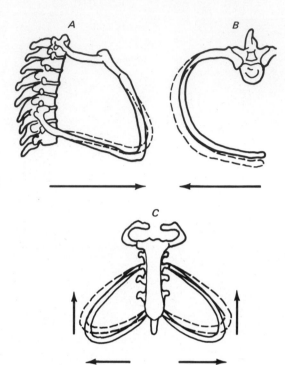

Figure 8–35 Expansion of thorax during inhalation. *A*, Lateral view. *B*, Superior view. *C*, Anterior view.

lower ribs is accompanied by a lateral movement of their anterior ends. This widening of the lower thorax increases the power of the diaphragm by putting it on a stretch.

INCREASE IN THE ANTEROPOSTERIOR DIAMETER   This effect (Figure 8–35) is produced by the elevation of the anterior ends of the obliquely placed ribs and of the body of the sternum, the latter being caused by the rib movement. The elevation of the anterior ends of the ribs causes the ribs to assume a more horizontal position and results in a straightening of the costal cartilages. The movements of the thorax in the anteroposterior and transverse diameters are inseparable. The expansion in both directions when the ribs are elevated is the inevitable result of their shape and of the oblique direction of their axes in motion.

INCREASE IN THE VERTICAL DIAMETER   This effect is brought about primarily by the depression of the central tendon of the diaphragm, but elevation of the upper two ribs makes a slight contribution. In forced inspiration the thoracic spine may extend to its limit, and this also contributes to a further increase in the vertical diameter.

Phases of Respiration

Basing his conclusions on his own findings as well as on those of several other investigators, Basmajian (1979) recognizes four phases of respiration. In brief, these are as follows:

PREINSPIRATION   This is a brief static phase that precedes the intake of air.

INSPIRATION   This phase is characterized by expansion of the thorax and the taking in of air.

PRE-EXPIRATION This is a brief static phase that follows inspiration and precedes expiration.

EXPIRATION This phase is characterized by an outflow of air accompanying a decrease in thoracic volume.

Muscles of Respiration

The muscles associated with respiration may be divided into two groups. The first group consists of the muscles of the thorax, and includes those muscles associated with the ribs whose primary function is respiration. The second group consists of those muscles of the spine and shoulder girdle whose functions in respiration, although important, are not their primary functions. Since only their activity in respiration is described here, the reader is directed to other sections of the text for additional information on the muscles included in this latter group.

Muscles with Primary Function of Respiration
  Diaphragm
  Intercostales, externi and interni
  Levatores costorum
  Serratus posterior inferior
  Serratus posterior superior
  Transversus thoracis

Muscles with Secondary Function of Respiration
  Abdominals
  Erector spinae
  Extensors of cervical and thoracic spine
  Pectoralis major and minor
  Quadratus lumborum
  Scalenes, anterior, posterior, and medius
  Sternocleidomastoid
  Trapezius I and II

Characteristics of Individual Muscles with Primary Function of Respiration

DIAPHRAGM This muscle (Figure 8–36) is a dome-shaped sheet that separates the thoracic and abdominal cavities from each other. Its contraction causes depression of its central tendon, and this increases the vertical dimension of the thorax. It also has a tendency to lift the lower ribs, but this appears to be resisted by the quadratus lumborum and iliocostalis lumborum. As the diaphragm moves downward it presses against the abdominal organs which, in turn, push forward against the relaxed abdominal wall. By increasing the intra-abdominal pressure it helps in defecation, vomiting, and other forms of expulsion. Although primarily a muscle of *inspiration*, a number of EMG studies have revealed the presence of electrical activity in the diaphragm during both the pre-expiratory and expiratory phases (Basmajian, 1979). It was suggested that this continuation of activity in the expiratory phase might be a braking action that serves the purpose of resisting or slowing down the elastic recoil of the lungs. This appears to imply that the contraction is eccentric or lengthening in nature, much like the action of the knee and hip extensors in resisting gravitational force in a slow, deep knee bend. The finding that the diaphragm did not show any activity in forced expiration would seem to bear this out. Two other findings were also

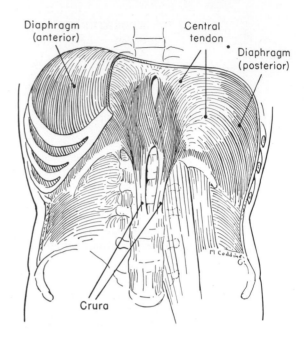

Figure 8–36   The diaphragm.

revealed by EMG studies—(1) that all portions of the diaphragm contract simultaneously, a positive indication that the muscle functions as a unit, and (2) that the
diaphragm is unquestionably the chief muscle of inspiration (Basmajian, 1979).

INTERCOSTALES, EXTERNI AND INTERNI   These muscles (Figure 8–37) are two layers
of similar sets of muscles, each set consisting of short parallel fibers that connect
adjacent ribs. The fibers of the outer set slant downward and forward from one rib to
the rib below, and those of the inner set slant in the reverse direction—that is,
downward and backward. An interesting point is that the slant of each set is similar to
the slant of the corresponding oblique abdominal muscle. Both sets extend posteriorly
as far as the angles of the ribs. In front, the external layer extends only as far forward
as the costal cartilages whereas the internal extends to the sternum. Hence the anterior
portion of the internal intercostals is not covered by the external layer.

These muscles have long been regarded as important respiratory muscles, second
only to the diaphragm, but for many years there has been a lack of agreement
concerning their specific functions. Some investigators have claimed that both sets
elevate the ribs, some that one set elevates and the other depresses, and some that both
the external intercostals and the anterior (uncovered) position of the internal layer
elevate, and the remainder of the internal depresses. Even electromyographic research
has not settled the question of functions. One reason may be that, as refinements are
made in techniques, investigators do not want to repeat the old methods, thus making
comparisons invalid. If several research teams could agree on using the same techniques under similar conditions, the findings of one or more studies might confirm
those of others.

In the past, it has been assumed that if a muscle is active during a certain phase of
breathing it is making a direct contribution to the movement characteristic of that

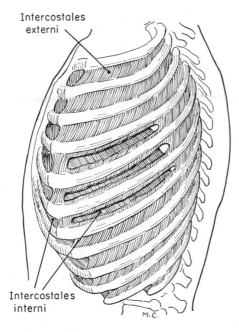

Intercostales externi

Intercostales interni

Figure 8–37   The intercostal muscles.

phase. For instance, if a muscle that attaches to the ribs, as do the intercostals, were to contract during the inspiratory phase, it would be assumed that it was helping to expand the thorax. Jones et al., however, have suggested a theory concerning the intercostals that deserves serious consideration. In a 1958 study their group noted that both sets of intercostals were constantly active during quiet breathing, but showed no rhythmic fluctuation as one would expect if they were causing the rhythmic movements of the thorax. They explained this observation by suggesting that the function of the intercostals was to supply the tension needed to keep the ribs at a constant distance from each other and to increase the intrathoracic pressure.

At the risk of putting too much emphasis on the findings from a single study, the results of Taylor's EMG investigation of the intercostal muscles, in which he used very fine needle electrodes, are briefly reported below (Basmajian, 1979).

External intercostals:
    A. No action at all in quiet breathing.
    B. Where two layers of muscles are present (i.e., both external and internal), the external acts in inspiration only. (In the light of the first notation it is assumed that this means in deep or forced inspiration.)

Internal intercostals:
    A. Where two layers of muscles are present, the internal acts during expiration only. This was noted in the lower lateral part of the thorax during quiet expiration.
    B. In the cartilaginous region in front where the internal is not covered by the external, electrical activity was noted during inspiration.

LEVATORES COSTARUM   These little muscles (Figure 8–38), slanting down and slightly outward from the tip of the transverse process of each vertebra to the rib below, with additional bands in the case of the seventh, eighth, ninth, and tenth vertebrae passing to the second rib below, are in a position to exert a lifting effect on the ribs, but have poor leverage for this as their attachments to the ribs are quite close to the costovertebral joints. In spite of this, it is assumed that they help to elevate the ribs during inspiration.

SERRATUS POSTERIOR INFERIOR   Like four chevrons, these broad bands (Figure 8–39) connect the lower borders of the lowest four ribs with the spinous processes and ligaments of lower vertebrae (lower two thoracic and upper two or three lumbar). They are assumed to *depress the four ribs and to stabilize them* against the pull of the diaphragm. They are too deep to palpate or to test electromyographically by present techniques.

SERRATUS POSTERIOR SUPERIOR   Like four steeply slanted, inverted chevrons, these bands (Figure 8–39) connect the upper borders of the second, third, fourth, and fifth ribs with the spinous processes and ligaments of the lower two or three cervical and the upper two thoracic vertebrae. They are assumed to help *elevate* the *four* ribs and in so doing to *expand the upper thorax*. Like the inferior, this muscle is too deep to palpate or to check by present EMG means.

TRANSVERSUS THORACIS   This muscle (Figure 8–40) connects the lower half of the inner surface of the sternum and adjoining costal cartilages with the lower borders

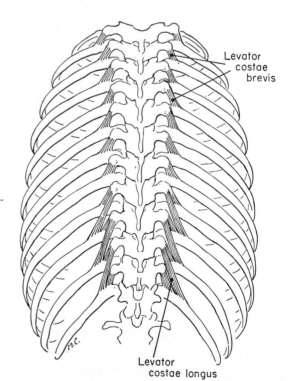

Figure 8–38   Levatores costarum (levator costae).

Levator costae brevis

Levator costae longus

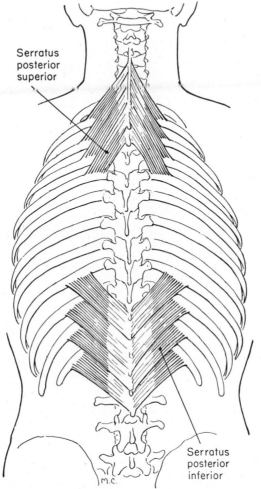

Figure 8–39   Serratus posterior superior and inferior.

and inner surfaces of the costal cartilages of the second, third, fourth, fifth, and sixth ribs. It consists of flat bands that radiate upward and outward from the inner surface of the sternum to the ribs, the lowest fibers being continuous with those of the transversus abdominis.

Characteristics of Individual Muscles with Secondary Function of Respiration

ABDOMINALS   The abdominals (Figures 8–16, 8–17, and 8–18) are considered to be the most important muscles for *expiration*, yet they do not become active until the expiration is forced. Normal quiet breathing is considered passive, and there is very little muscular activity during it. The *transversus abdominis* and the *two obliques* were found by Campbell (1952) to be the most important muscles of *forced expiration*. It was also noted that they do not initiate expiration but help to complete it. Although the rectus also contracts in expiration, it was found to be of little importance as

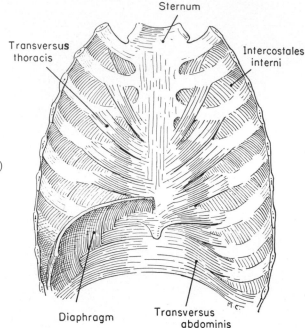

Sternum

Transversus
thoracis

Intercostales
interni

Figure 8–40 Posterior (inner)
view of anterior wall of thorax.

Diaphragm

Transversus
abdominis

compared to the other abdominals. Vigorous contraction of the abdominals is present in all expiratory actions such as coughing, sneezing, straining, or vomiting.

ERECTOR SPINAE   This extensive muscle (Figure 8–22) of the back serves to *stabilize the spine and pelvis* against the pull of the abdominal muscles. By resisting the tendency of the latter to flex the spine, it forces them to concentrate their activity on abdominal compression.

EXTENSORS OF CERVICAL AND THORACIC SPINE   These muscles (Figures 8–23 and 8–24) *stabilize the head and neck* against the pull of the scalenes and the sternocleidomastoid.

PECTORALIS MAJOR AND MINOR   A few investigators have reported activity of the pectoralis major (Figures 4–5 and 4–13) in deep inspiration but have not made it clear what function the muscle is performing. It seems reasonable to assume that when an individual holds the arms vertically upward or is suspended by the hands the *pectoralis major* would help to *elevate the sternum* and *upper six ribs*. The *pectoralis minor* is likewise in a position to *lift the third, fourth,* and *fifth ribs* when the thoracic spine is extended and the scapulae are stabilized.

QUADRATUS LUMBORUM   An EMG study conducted in 1965 by Boyd et al. confirms the assumption that this muscle (Figure 8–27) anchors the last rib against the pull of the diaphragm, which would otherwise tend to lift it and, in so doing, lose some of the force for depressing its central tendon (Basmajian, 1979).

SCALENES, ANTERIOR, POSTERIOR, AND MEDIUS   These three muscles (Figure 8–25) are assuming greater importance as respiratory muscles as the result of EMG research. They connect the transverse processes of the cervical vertebrae with the first two ribs.

They were formerly thought to be primarily lateral flexors of the neck and secondarily accessory or stabilizing muscles of respiration, their function being to anchor the first two ribs for the intercostals. Results of two investigations over ten years apart give strong evidence of *the scalenes' role as true respiratory muscles in quiet inspiration as well as in forced* (Basmajian, 1979). These muscles may be palpated on the side of the neck between the sternocleidomastoid and upper trapezius muscles.

STERNOCLEIDOMASTOID   As an accessory muscle of respiration, this muscle (Figure 8–26) showed marked electrical activity in *forced inspiration*. It helps to *elevate the sternum and clavicle.* In vigorous inspiration the head is usually held firmly erect and, instead of flexing the head and neck, the sternocleidomastoid has a slight lifting effect on the sternum and sternal end of each clavicle. It may be palpated on the side of the neck just below the ear and on the front of the neck at the junction of the clavicle and sternum.

TRAPEZIUS I AND II   In reviewing EMG studies of the trapezius, Basmajian (1979) was unable to find confirmation of Duchenne's inclusion of this muscle (Figure 4–15) as an accessory in respiration. It is included here as a possible stabilizer of the shoulder girdle against the downward pull of the pectoralis minor. As yet, there is no confirmation of this theory.

Muscular Analysis of Respiration

On the whole, EMG studies have tended to reinforce the muscular analysis of respiration as presented in older kinesiology texts, but there have been some unexpected revelations. The student who is interested in pursuing this subject is advised to read Basmajian's (1979) excellent summaries of EMG investigations before examining the original reports of individual studies.

Inspiration

The action of the diaphragm accounts for about one-third of the air exchanged in normal breathing. Action in the scalenes and the intercostals (especially the external) also occurs in quiet inspiration. With forced inspiration, these major muscles of inspiration, as well as the sternocleidomastoid, serratus posterior superior, levatores costorum, quadratus lumborum, erector spinae, and pectoralis major and minor, are active.

Expiration

Quiet expiration is generally considered to be a passive act. However, some activity has been recorded in the intercostals, serratus posterior muscles, diaphragm, and quadratus lumborum. The major muscles of forced expiration are the transversus abdominis and oblique abdominals. The erector spinae are active as stabilizers against the pull of the abdominals. Other participants include the transversus thoracic and intercostals.

Common Athletic Injuries of the Neck, Back, and Thorax

Neck Injuries

While these fortunately are not common among athletes, they are of prime concern. If there is the slightest suspicion of serious injury it is literally of vital importance that the individual not be moved *at all* until after having been examined by a physician, and then only under the physician's close supervision. *The danger of death or paralysis from the neck down cannot be overemphasized.*

Contusions of the Spine

These are undoubtedly much more common among athletes than among nonathletes. The muscles involved are usually those on either side of the spinous processes. Ordinarily the contusion is not serious but it may cause a hematoma. Another possible complication is painful stiffness, which may last for several days. Muscle spasm often occurs in the more severe contusions of the lower back.

Back Strains and Sprains

Strains (injuries to muscles) and sprains (injuries to ligaments) are both common in athletics, largely because there are so many muscles and ligaments in the region of the spine. In the early stages of these injuries it is often difficult to distinguish between them. The strain is usually the result of either a violent contraction or a movement which causes the muscles to overstretch (O'Donoghue, 1976). A sprain may be caused by the same kind of movements that cause a strain, but in the latter case the damage is a tearing of the ligaments.

An acute back *strain* that is not given proper treatment is likely to develop into a chronic strain and become a perpetual problem. This is usually more common in the lower back than in the upper. Prevention of back strain and sprain is of major concern in the planning of conditioning programs.

Fractures of Transverse Process of Lumbar Vertebra

These occur quite frequently in sports, either from a severe blow or from a violent muscular contraction. In either case, the damage to the muscle that attaches to the bone is of greater significance than the damage to the bone itself (O'Donoghue, 1976). This is understandable when one reviews the attachments of the back muscles, especially those of the semispinalis muscle and the deep posterior muscles of the spine.

Herniated Disk

O'Donoghue (1976) believes that the conditions that cause this, namely the compression of two adjacent vertebrae with such magnitude that the annulus fibrosus is ruptured, is rarely brought about by participation in sports. Repeated heavy lifting with the body in poor alignment is a more likely cause. If this has happened to an athlete, however, participation in athletics is unwise until the rupture can be repaired. Otherwise the nucleus pulposus is likely to protrude through the break in the disk and press on the spinal cord or a spinal nerve. The area most likely to be affected is the lumbar spine, especially between the fourth and fifth lumbar vertebrae. This condition can be very painful.

Rib Fractures

These are fairly common in contact sports like football and wrestling. The usual causes are either direct blows or forceful compressions. Sudden, violent, muscular contraction may also be a cause. In most fracture injuries two or more ribs are likely to be involved. A fracture should be suspected if breathing is accompanied by severe pain. A possible serious complication of rib fractures is damage to the soft tissues when the broken ends of the bone are pushed inward (Klafs and Arnheim, 1973; O'Donoghue, 1976).

Laboratory Experiences

Joint Structure

1. Study the bones of the spinal column and then fill out an outline like the one in Appendix A for each of the following joints, including the articulations of both the bodies and the arches.
   a. Atlanto-occipital.
   b. Atlantoaxial.
   c. A middle cervical joint.
   d. The joint between the seventh cervical and the first thoracic vertebra.
   e. A middle thoracic joint.
   f. The joint between the twelfth thoracic and the first lumbar vertebra.
   g. A middle lumbar joint.
   h. The lumbosacral joint.

Joint Action

2. Have a subject sit tailor fashion on a table and flex the spine as completely as possible. Observe the shape of the spine as seen from the side. Compare the three regions of the spine as to forward flexibility. Make a line drawing of the side view of the spine.

3. Have a subject sit astride a chair, facing its back, and hyperextend the spine as completely as possible. Observe and record the shape of the spine, as in 2.

4. Have a subject sit astride a bench and bend sideward as far as possible, first to one side and then to the other. Observe from the rear and draw a line representing the spine in maximum lateral flexion, both left and right.

5. Have a subject sit astride a bench with the hands at the neck, then rotate the trunk as far as possible, first to one side, then to the other. Observe and compare the regions of the spine as to rotating ability.

6. Observe flexion, hyperextension, lateral flexion, and rotation of the spine in several subjects, preferably subjects representing different body builds, and note individual differences.

7. Have a subject lie face down on a table with the legs and pelvis supported on the table, the trunk extending forward beyond the table, and the hands clasped behind the neck.
   a. Have the subject bend laterally. Compare the thoracic and lumbar regions. Note the torsion accompanying the lateral flexion.
   b. Have the subject flex the spine and then flex it laterally. Observe as in a.
   c. Have the subject hyperextend the spine (with someone helping to support the elbows) and then flex laterally. Observe as in a.
   d. Have the subject rotate the trunk to one side as far as possible. Compare the thoracic and lumbar regions. Is any lateral bending apparent in the spine?
   e. Have the subject flex the spine and then rotate it. Observe as in d.
   f. Have the subject hyperextend the spine and then rotate it. Observe as in d.

8. MOVEMENT OF THE THORAX IN RESPIRATION
   Subject: Breathe naturally for a while, then as deeply as possible.
   Observer: (a) Place the hands on the sides of the thorax and note the movement in the lateral diameter. (b) Place one hand on the ribs at the subcostal angle (just below the sternum) and the other hand against the back at the same level. Note the movement in the anteroposterior diameter. (c) Place the fingers on the sternum. Can you detect any movement in normal respiration? in deep respiration?

Muscular Action

The purpose of these exercises is not to test the strength of the muscles but to enable the observer to study the action of the muscles in simple movements of the body. The procedure, therefore, is quite different from that followed by the physical therapist in testing muscle strength. It is suggested that students work in groups of three: one acting as the subject, one as an assistant helping to support or steady the stationary part of the body and giving resistance to the moving part, and one palpating the muscles and recording the results. The checklists in Appendix E may be used for this purpose. They may also be used for the analysis of other movements.

9. FLEXION OF THE NECK
   a. *Subject:* Lie on the back and lift the head, bringing the chin toward the chest.
      Observer: Palpate and identify as many of the contracting muscles as possible.
   b. *Subject:* Lie on the back and lift the head, leading with the chin.
      Observer: Compare the action of the sternocleidomastoid in *b* with its action in *a*.

10. EXTENSION AND HYPEREXTENSION OF THE NECK
   a. *Subject:* Lie face down on a table with the head over the edge. Raise the head as far as possible, hyperextending both the head and the neck.
      Assistant: May resist the movement if stronger muscular action is desired.
      Observer: Palpate and identify as many of the contracting muscles as possible.
   b. *Subject:* Lie face down on a table with the head over the edge. Raise the head as far as possible with the chin tucked in.
      Assistant: Resist the retraction of the chin.
      Observer: Compare the muscular action in *b* with that in *a*.

11. LATERAL FLEXION OF THE HEAD AND NECK
   Subject: Lie on one side and raise the head toward the shoulder without turning the head or tensing the shoulder.
   Assistant: Give slight resistance at the temple.
   Observer: Palpate and identify as many muscles as possible.

12. ROTATION OF THE HEAD AND NECK
   Subject: Sit erect and turn the head to the left as far as possible.
   Assistant: Give fairly strong resistance to the side of the jaw.
   Observer: Palpate the sternocleidomastoids. Which one contracts?

13. FLEXION OF THE THORACIC AND LUMBAR SPINE
   Subject: Lie on the back with the arms folded across the chest. Raise the head, shoulders and upper back from the table, keeping the chin in. There is no need to come to a sitting position, since this is intended as a movement of spinal, not hip, flexion.
   Assistant: Hold the thighs down.
   Observer: Palpate the rectus abdominis and the external oblique abdominal muscle.

14. EXTENSION AND HYPEREXTENSION OF THE THORACIC AND LUMBAR SPINE
   Subject: Lie face down with the hands on the hips. Raise the head and trunk as far as possible.
   Assistant: Hold the feet down.
   Observer: Palpate the erector spinae and the gluteus maximus. What is the function of the latter muscle in this movement?

15. LATERAL FLEXION OF THE THORACIC AND LUMBAR SPINE
   Subject: Lie on one side with the under arm placed across the chest and the hand resting on the opposite shoulder, and with the hand of the top arm resting on the hip. Raise the trunk sideways.
   Assistant: Hold the legs down. If necessary, help the subject by pulling at the elbow.
   Observer: Palpate the rectus abdominis, external oblique abdominal muscle, erector spinae, and latissimus dorsi.

16. ROTATION OF THE THORACIC AND LUMBAR SPINE

Subject: Sit astride a bench with the hands placed behind the neck. Twist to one side as far as possible without leaving the bench.

Assistant: Resist the movement by grasping the subject's arms close to his shoulders and pushing (or pulling) in the opposite direction.

Observer: Palpate as many of the spinal and abdominal muscles as possible. Disregard the muscles of the scapula and arm.

17. MUSCULAR ACTION IN FORCED INHALATION

a. *Subject:* Inhale through a small rubber tube, pinching it slightly in order to furnish resistance.

Observer: Note the action of the sternocleidomastoid, cervical and thoracic extensors, and upper trapezius. Can any other muscular action be detected? If so, explain.

b. *Subject:* Run in place or around the room until short of breath. Hang from a horizontal bar.

Observer: Can you detect any action of the pectoralis major accompanying inhalation? (By stabilizing the arms, the hanging position causes the pectoralis major to act on the ribs.)

18. MUSCULAR ACTION IN VIGOROUS EXHALATION

Subject: Blow through a small rubber tube, pinching it slightly or holding a finger loosely over the end or blow into a spirometer, flarimeter, or toy balloon.

Observer: Note the action of the abdominal muscles and the erector spinae. Explain.

Action of the Muscles Other Than the Movers

19. SIT-UP

Subject: Lie on the back and come to a sitting position, keeping the spine as rigid as possible.

Assistant: Hold the feet down.

Observer: Palpate the abdominal muscles, erector spinae, and sternocleidomastoid. Explain the function of each.

20. DOUBLE LEG LOWERING

Subject: Lie on the back. Raise both legs, then slowly lower them half way.

Observer: Palpate the abdominal muscles and erector spinae. Explain the function of each.

21. TRUNK BENDING FORWARD

Subject: Stand with the feet slightly separated. Bend forward from the hips, keeping the back flat.

Observer: Palpate the erector spinae. Explain its function.

22. PUSH-UP

Subject: Assume a front-leaning-rest position on the hands and toes with the body straight. Let the elbows bend until the chest almost touches the floor, then push up again, keeping the body straight the entire time. Do not let it sag or hump.

Observer: Palpate the abdominal muscles. Explain their function.

References

Basmajian, J.V. 1979. *Muscles alive*. 4th ed. Baltimore: Williams & Wilkins.

Brunnstrom, S. 1966. *Clinical kinesiology*. 2d ed. Philadelphia: F. A. Davis.

Campbell, E. J. M. 1952. An electromyographic study of the role of the abdominal muscles in breathing. *J. Physiol*. 177:222–33.

Clarke, H. H., ed. 1976. Exercise and abdominal muscles. In *Physical fitness research digest.* Washington, D.C.: President's Council on Physical Fitness and Sport.

Crowe, P., O'Connell, A. L., and Gardner, E. B. 1963. An electromyographic study of the abdominal muscles and certain hip flexors during selected sit-ups. Report presented at National Convention of the American Association for Health, Physical Education, and Recreation.

Flint, M. M. 1965. An electromyographic comparison of the function of the iliacus and the rectus abdominis muscles. *J. Am. Phys. Ther. Assoc.* 45:248–52.

Floyd, W. F., and Silver, P. H. S. 1950. Electromyographic study of patterns of activity of the anterior abdominal wall muscles in man. *J. Anat.* 84:132–45.

Giordin, Y. 1973. EMG action potentials of rectus abdominis muscle during two types of exercise. In *Biomechanics III,* ed. S. Cerquiglini et al., pp. 301–08. Baltimore: University Park Press.

Hollinshead, W. H. 1965. Anatomy of the spine. *J. Bone Joint Surg.* 47A:209–15.

Jonsson, B. 1973. Electromyography of the erector spinae muscle. In *Biomechanics III,* ed. S. Cerquiglini et al., pp. 294–300. Baltimore: University Park Press.

Keagy, R. D., Brumlik, J. B., and Bergan, J. J. 1966. Direct electromyography of the psoas major muscle in man. *J. Bone Joint Surg.* 48A:1377–82.

Kendall, H. O., and Kendall, F. P. 1943. The role of abdominal exercises in a program of physical fitness. *J. Health Phys. Educ.*–14:480, 481, 504–06.

Klafs, C. E., and Arnheim, D. D. 1973. *Modern principles of athletic training.* St. Louis: C. V. Mosby.

LaBan, M. M., Raptou, A. D., and Johnson, E. W. 1965. Electromyographic study of function of iliopsoas muscle. *Arch. Phys. Med. Rehab.* 46:676–79.

LeVeau, B. 1974. Axes of joint rotation of the lumbar vertebrae during abdominal strengthening exercises. In *Biomechanics IV*, ed. R. C. Nelson and C. A. Morehouse, pp. 361–64. Baltimore: University Park Press.

Lipetz, S., and Gutin, B. 1970. An electromyographic study of four abdominal exercises. *Med. Sci. Sports.* 2:35–38.

Lovett, R. W. 1931. *Lateral curvature of the spine and round shoulders.* 5th ed. Philadelphia: P. Blakiston's Son, chapter 3.

Nachemson, A. *Quoted in* Jonsson, B. 1969. Morphology, innervation, and electromyographic study of the erector spinae. *Arch. Phys. Med. Rehab.* 50:638–41.

O'Donoghue, D. H. 1976. *Treatment of injuries to athletes.* 3d ed. Philadelphia: W. B. Saunders.

Partridge, M. J., and Walters, C. E. 1959. Participation of the abdominal muscles in various movements of the trunk in man. *Phys. Ther. Rev.* 39:791–800.

Pauly, J. E. 1966. An electromyographic analysis of certain movements and exercises. I. Some deep muscles of the back. *Anat. Rec.* 155:223–34.

Walters, C. E., and Partridge, M. J. 1957. Electromyographic study of the differential action of the abdominal muscles during exercise. *Am. J. Phys. Med.* 36:259–68.

Wells, K. F. 1947. An investigation of certain evolutionary tendencies in the female human structure. *Res. Q. Am. Assoc. Health, Phys. Educ. Rec.* 18:260–70.

Wiles, P. 1935. Movements of the lumbar vertebrae during flexion and extension. *Proc. R. Soc. Med.* 28:647–51.

Wright, W. G. 1962. *Muscle function.* New York: Hafner Publishing.

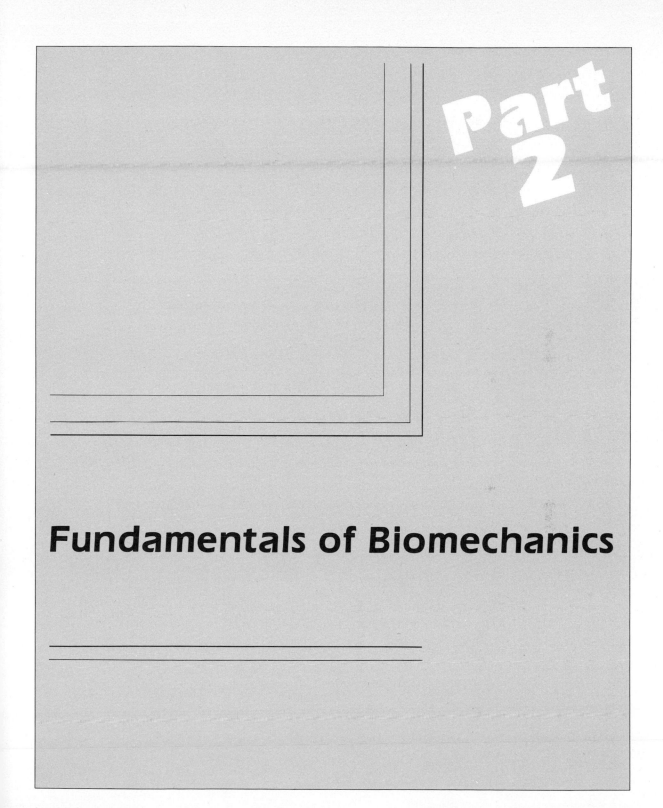

Part 2

Fundamentals of Biomechanics

Introduction to Part 2

As seen by the kinesiologist, the human body is a highly complex machine constructed of living tissue. As such it is subject to the laws and principles of mechanics as well as those of biology. The principles of mechanics are directly applicable both to the movements of the human body and to the implements it handles. Principles of balance and equilibrium, motion, and the application of forces apply equally to man in motion as they do to rockets and wheels, gears and missiles. A study of the fundamental principles of mechanics as they apply to movement skills will aid the teacher, therapist, and coach in the analysis of skills for the intelligent evaluation of technique and correction of error. Applications in research can lead to the determination of the relative merits of existing techniques as well as to the development of techniques yet unknown.

Interest in mechanical analysis and study as part of physical education was due in large measure to the influence of three pioneers. C. H. McCloy, University of Iowa, toured the country in the late 1930s and 1940s giving lectures with demonstrations showing specific ways in which performance could be improved by the application of appropriate mechanical principles. He was the first to develop a course in the mechanical analysis of motor skills. Pioneer efforts in cinematographic analysis by Ruth Glassow at the University of Wisconsin also contributed to interest in the application of the fundamental principles of mechanics and physics to sports skills among physical educators in the United States. During this same period Thomas Cureton, whose undergraduate degree was in electrical engineering, taught mechanics of sports and physical activities at Springfield College. His research and writing at this time concentrated on the applications of physics to physical education and on the principles of cinematographic analysis (Atwater, 1980). During the 1950s and early 1960s research on the mechanics of sports activities increased in scope and variety as others became involved and as methodology and equipment improved, but it was in the late 1960s and early 1970s that a lively interest in the mechanical analysis of humans in motion emerged. Graduate programs designed to prepare specialists in the mechanics of human motion appeared, and the results of vastly improved research methodology, technology, and instrumentation became apparent in a growing body of literature. There was a new area of study that many have named biomechanics of sport and others have called mechanical kinesiology.

In the branch of science called biomechanics, the principles and methods of mechanics are applied to the structure and function of biological systems (Atwater, 1980). Since biology is concerned with all living things, biomechanics is a very broad branch of science, and the biomechanics of sport is only one of the applied areas in which applications are made of the same common core of knowledge and fundamental research found in physics, mathematics, anatomy, and physiology. Other fields of applied biomechanics include industrial engineering and ergonomics, physical rehabilitation, medicine and biomedical physics, and aerospace science.

Of the fields of applied biomechanics the biomechanics of sport, dance, and physical education is the least advanced, but increased availability and use of advanced technology in the form of computers and electronic recording devices has resulted in research and study that formerly was almost prohibitive because of the agonizing amount of time it consumed. Additional impetus has also been supplied through the founding in 1973 of the International Society of Biomechanics (ISB) and, in 1977, the American Society of Biomechanics (ASB). The influence of these societies in stimulating study and disseminating knowledge through international meetings has done much to advance knowledge in this fascinating field of applied biomechanics, the biomechanics of sport, and physical education.

Part Two introduces the student to some elementary concepts necessary for understanding the biomechanics of sport and physical education. Chapter 9 presents mechanical concepts and terminology basic to the study of mechanics as an aspect of kinesiology. The need for understanding basic mathematical concepts for using appropriate formulas and understanding basic principles is also identified in this chapter. It is important to note here that the level of mathematics needed for this and subsequent chapters is relatively elementary and, with the aid of the examples given and the mathematics review in Appendix F, the average kinesiology student should have no difficulty. Under no circumstances, however, should the student become so involved with juggling numbers in this part that the sight of the forest is lost for the trees.

Part Two continues with a chapter on the fundamentals of motion description, with particular emphasis placed upon an understanding of projectiles and "free flight." Specific applications are made to sport and physical education activities. A similar approach is followed in subsequent chapters on the conditions of linear motion, the conditions of rotatory motion, and the center of gravity and stability. Each chapter concludes with a variety of problems and exercises designed to help the student understand the direct application of principles of mechanics to the execution of skills in sport and physical education.

References

Atwater, A. E. 1980. Kinesiology/biomechanics: Perspectives and trends. *Res. Q. Exercise Sport* 51:193–218.

Nelson, R. C. 1971. Biomechanics of sport: An overview. In *Selected Topics in Biomechanics,* ed. J. M. Cooper. Chicago: The Athletic Institute, pp. 31–7.

Wartenweiler, J. 1979. The manifold implications of biomechanics. In *Biomechanics IV,* ed. R. C. Nelson and C. A. Morehouse. Baltimore: University Park Press, pp. 11–14.

Terminology and Measurement in Biomechanics

Objectives

At the conclusion of this chapter, the student should be able to:

1. Define the terms mechanics and biomechanics, and differentiate between them.
2. Define the terms kinematics, kinetics, statics, and dynamics, and state how each relates to the structure of biomechanics study.
3. Convert the units of measurement employed in the study of biomechanics from the English system to the metric system, and vice versa.
4. Describe the nature of scalar and vector quantities, and identify such quantities as one or the other.
5. Demonstrate the use of the graphic method for the combination and resolution of two-dimensional vectors.
6. Demonstrate the use of the trigonometric method for the combination and resolution of two-dimensional vectors.

Introduction to Terminology

As it is presently constituted, kinesiology is an area of study concerned with the musculoskeletal analysis of human motion and the study of mechanical principles and laws as they relate to the study of human motion. Students of human motion capable of accurately analyzing the musculoskeletal actions occurring in the execution of a movement are well on their way toward knowing what is happening during that movement. Those who have taken the further step of acquiring a working knowledge of how human motion is governed by physical laws and principles have added an additional dimension of understanding how and why the motion occurs as it does. Together, all this information provides a scientific foundation upon which to make appropriate decisions concerning the most effective execution of any movement pattern. It is only through such study that definitive answers may be found concerning the "best" way for an individual to perform a skill and the reasons *why* the method selected is indeed the "best." The record-breaking "form" of one person may or may not be appropriate for another of different body build and size. In fact, although they break records, top performers' techniques may include actions which, if eliminated, would result in even greater performance. Unless subjected to scientific scrutiny, discrimination between the success factors and deterrent factors may be confused or not even identified.

Mechanics

Where *forces* and *motion* are concerned, the area of scientific study that provides accurate answers to what is happening, why it is happening, and to what extent it is happening is called *mechanics.* It is that branch of physics concerned with the effort that forces have on bodies and the motion produced by those forces. The study of mechanics is engaged in by those people whose occupations or professions require an understanding of force, matter, space, and time. Engineers, to a large extent, are involved with the application of mechanics. Navigation, astronomy, space, and communications experts all study mechanics. The same is true of individuals concerned with the study of human motion and the forces causing it. The laws and principles used to explain the motion of planets or the strength of buildings and bridges apply equally to humans. *All* motion, including motions of the human body and its parts, is the result of the application of forces and is subject to the laws and principles that govern force and motion.

Biomechanics

When the study of mechanics is limited to living structures, especially the human body, it is called *biomechanics.* Biomechanics is an interdisciplinary science based on many of the fundamental disciplines found in the physical and life sciences. Generally, biomechanics is considered to be that aspect of the science concerned with the basic laws governing the effect forces have upon the state of rest or motion of animals or humans, whereas the applied areas of biomechanics deal with solving practical problems. Anatomists, orthopedists, space engineers, industrial engineers, specialists in physical medicine, physical educators, dancers, and coaches all have an interest in biomechanics and in applying its principles to the improvement of human movement. Professional applications may differ, but the same basic laws of biomechanics provide a common foundation for all. In this context the part of biomechanics that applies to sport, dance, and physical education may be considered to be that part of kinesiology that involves the mechanics of human motion. Both terms, the biomechanics of sport and mechanical kinesiology, are currently in use as names for this applied area of study.

STATICS AND DYNAMICS   The study of biomechanics is divided into two areas, *statics* and *dynamics.* Statics covers situations in which all forces acting on a body are *balanced* and the body is in equilibrium. With a knowledge of the principles of statics one may have a better understanding of levers and a greater ability to solve problems such as locating the body's center of gravity or center of buoyancy. That branch of biomechanics dealing with bodies subject to *unbalanced* forces is called dynamics. Principles of dynamics explain circumstances in which an excess of force in one direction or a turning force causes an object to change speed or direction. Principles of work, energy, and accelerated motion are included in the study of dynamics.

KINEMATICS AND KINETICS   The terms *kinematics* and *kinetics* are also part of the vocabulary of the study of mechanics. Kinematics has been referred to as the geometry of motion. It describes the motion of bodies in terms of time, displacement, velocity, and acceleration. The motion occurring may be in a straight line (linear kinematics) or about a fixed point (angular kinematics). Kinematics is concerned only with the analytical and mathematical descriptions of all kinds of motion, and *not* with the forces that cause the motion. The branch of mechanics that considers the *forces* that produce or change motion is called kinetics. Admittedly the most complex of biomechanics studies, it is the area least developed in physical education and sport, and of most challenge to research today. Linear kinetics is concerned with the causes of linear motion, and angular kinetics deals with the forces that cause angular motion.

Quantities in Biomechanics

The Language of Science

In the study of human motion, as in the study of any science, careful measurement and the use of mathematics are essential for the classification of facts and the systematizing of knowledge. Mathematics is the language of science. It enables us to express relationships quantitatively rather than merely descriptively. It provides objective evidence of the superiority of one technique over another and thus forms the basis for developing effective measures for improving performance. Furthermore, it makes possible continuing advancement of knowledge through research. Had it not been for the use of mathematics, the contributions of great scientists like Archimedes, Galileo, and Newton would not have been possible.

In the biomechanical aspects of kinesiology, as in all mechanics, the depth of understanding of the principles and laws that apply to it is greatly increased through experimental and mathematical evidence. Hence, it is to the kinesiologist's advantage to become conversant with appropriate mathematical concepts and techniques. The mathematics needed for the quantitative treatment of the simple mechanics discussed in this text is not difficult. It consists of elementary algebra and right triangle trigonometry. A review of these essential mathematical concepts is presented in Appendix F.

Units of Measurement

The units of measurement employed in the study of biomechanics are expressed in terms of space, time, and mass. Presently there are two systems of measurement having units for these quantities, the English system and the metric system. Since both systems are currently used in research and literature, a comparison of equivalent values is helpful. Table 9–1 presents some common units used in biomechanics study and their English-metric equivalents.

LENGTH   In the metric or decimal system, all units differ in size by a multiple of ten. In ascending order, linear units are millimeters, centimeters, meters, and kilometers. In the English system the basic unit of length is the foot. Other possible units are inches, yards, and miles.

AREA OR VOLUME   In the metric system, square centimeters or square meters are used for area, and cubic centimeters, liters, or cubic meters are used for volume. In the English system, area units are square inches or feet, and cubic inches, cubic feet, quarts, or gallons denote volume.

MASS AND FORCE (WEIGHT)   *Mass* is the quantity of matter a body contains. The *weight* of a body depends upon its quantity of matter and the strength of the gravita-

**TABLE 9–1   Comparison of English and Metric
Systems of Measurement**

UNIT	METRIC SYSTEM	ENGLISH SYSTEM	EQUIVALENTS
Length	centimeter (cm) meter (m) = 100 cm kilometer (km) = 1000 m	inch (in) foot (ft) mile (mi) = 5280 ft	1 in = 2.54 cm 1 cm = 0.3937 in 1 ft = 0.305 m 1 m = 3.28 ft 1 mi = 1.609 km 1 km = 0.621 mi
Area	square meter (100 cm²)	square foot (144 in²)	1 in² = 6.45 cm² 1 cm² = 0.155 in²
Volume	cubic cm (cm³) liter (1000 cm³)	cubic in (in³) quart (57.75 in³)	1 qt = 0.946 liter 1 liter = 1.06 qt 1 in³ = 16.39 cm³ 1 cm³ = 0.06 in³
Mass	kilogram (kg)	slug (32 lb)	1 kg = 0.068 slug 1 slug = 14.6 kg
Force (weight)	newton (0.102 kg)	pound (lb)	1 lb = 0.454 kg 1 kg = 2.21 lb 1 N = 0.225 lb
Time	second	second	

tional attraction acting on it. The measure of gravitional *force* is called weight. The mass of an object will not change even if taken to the moon, but its weight will. The kilogram, equal to the mass of a liter of water, is the unit of mass in the metric system. The unit of force (weight) is the newton (N), and for most of the United States a mass of one kilogram weighs approximately 9.80 newtons. In the English system the pound is the basic unit of force (weight). The mass unit is the slug (from the English word for sluggish). A mass of one slug weighs approximately 32 pounds for the gravitational pull present at the latitude and longitude of most of the United States.

TIME   The basic unit of time for both systems of measurement is the second.

Scalar and Vector Quantities

The units of measure described in the previous section are quantities that possess size or amount. Units of length, volume, area, mass, and time are examples of such quantities. They are called *scalar* quantities or scalars. When one knows that a person has run 8 kilometers one has an indication of the *amount* of distance run. Distance is a measure of magnitude; it is a scalar. Similarly, the rate of running (speed) of 8 kilometers per hour, a temperature of 70 degrees, an area of 2 square miles, and a mass of 10 kilograms are all magnitude or scalar measures.

Quantities that are not completely described by a magnitude measure alone also exist. For a full description of these quantities, a knowledge of both magnitude and direction is needed. These quantities are called *vector* quantities. If two people on opposite sides of a door push with equal amounts of force, the door will not move. If, on the other hand, they both push on the same side of the door, thus changing the *direction* of one of the forces, the result will be very different. The nature of the movement of the door depends upon both the *amount* and *direction* of the force. Force, therefore, is a vector quantity. If the individual who ran 8 kilometers runs 8 more kilometers, the total distance run will be 16 kilometers. If, however, the runner goes 8 kilometers in one direction, reverses, and runs back to the starting point, the change in position or *displacement* is zero. The runner is zero kilometers from the starting point. Displacement, then, is also a vector quantity possessing both magnitude and direction. Numerous quantities in biomechanics are vector quantities. In addition to force, displacement, and velocity already mentioned, some other examples are momentum, acceleration, friction, work, and power. Vector quantities exist whenever *direction* and *amount* are inherent characteristics of the quantities.

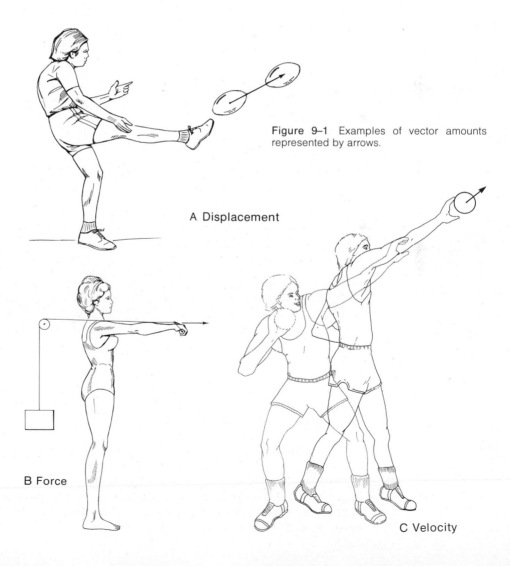

Figure 9–1 Examples of vector amounts represented by arrows.

A Displacement

B Force

C Velocity

Vector Analysis

Vector Representation

A vector is represented by an arrow whose length is proportional to the magnitude of the vector. The direction in which the arrow points indicates the direction of the vector quantity. Figure 9–1 shows examples of arrows indicating the vector quantities of force, displacement, and velocity.

Vector quantities are equal if magnitude and direction are the same for each vector. Although all the vectors below are of the same length (magnitude) only two are equal vector quantities. They are the two which also have the same direction (*d* and *f*).

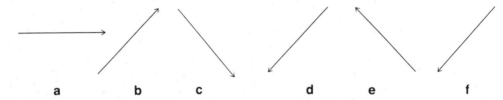

a   b   c   d   e   f

Combination of Vectors

Vectors may be combined by addition, subtraction, or multiplication. They are added by joining the head of one with the tail of the next while accounting for magnitude and direction. The combination results in a new vector called the *resultant*. The resultant vector is represented by the distance between the last head and the first tail. Figure 9–2 shows examples of vectors which have been combined by addition. Note that the head of the resultant, R, meets the *head* of the last component vector. These drawings also show that very different component vectors may produce the same resultant. The subtraction of vectors is done by changing the sign of one vector (multiply by −1) and then adding as before (Figure 9–3A). The multiplication of a vector by a number changes its magnitude only, not its direction (Figure 9–3B).

Resolution of Vectors

As just explained, the combination of two or more vectors results in a new vector. Conversely, any vector may be broken down or resolved into two component vectors acting at right angles to each other. The vector in Figure 9–1C represents the velocity with which the shot was put. Should one wish to know how much of that velocity was in a horizontal direction and how much in a vertical direction, the vector must be

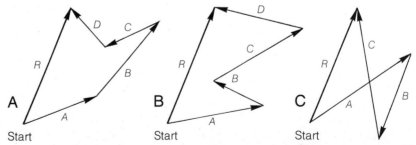

Figure 9–2 Vectors are added by joining the head of one with the tail of the next. The same resultant vector R, in examples A, B, and C, may be obtained from the combination of dissimilar components.

A. Subtraction

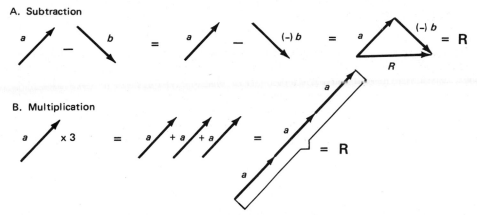

B. Multiplication

Figure 9–3   Vectors may be combined by subtraction or multiplication.

resolved into horizontal and vertical components. In Figure 9–4, A and B are the vertical and horizontal *components* of resultant R. The vector addition of these components once again would result in the resultant vector R. The arrows over A, B, and R indicate that they are vector quantities.

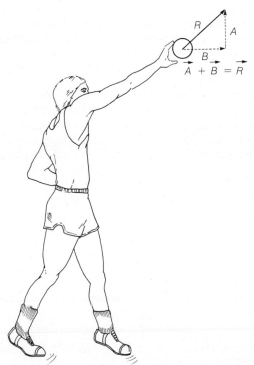

Figure 9–4   A resultant vector may be re-solved or broken down into two component vectors acting at right angles to each other. The velocity vector R has a horizontal component B and a vertical component A.

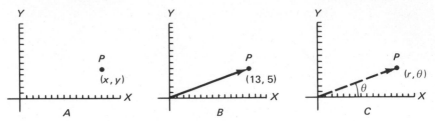

Figure 9–5   A point in space may be located in two dimensions using an x and y axis as a frame of reference. In A, point P is x units from the y axis and y units from the x axis. In B, point P is $13x$ units from the y axis and $5y$ units from the x axis. In C, point P is r units from the x, y intersection and θ degrees from the x axis.

Location of Vectors in Space

In describing motion it is helpful to have a frame of reference within which one can locate a position in space or change in position. It is possible to locate an object in three dimensions, but to simplify understanding, the description that follows is limited to motion in two dimensions—i.e., one plane.

The position of a point, P, can be located using either rectangular coordinates or polar coordinates. In the two-dimensional rectangular coordinate system, the plane is divided into four quadrants by two perpendicular intersecting lines. The horizontal line is the x axis and the vertical line is the y axis. Values along either axis are measured from the point of intersection of the two axes where x and y are both equal to zero $(0, 0)$. The location of point P is represented by two numbers, the first equal to the number of x units and the second to the number of y units away from the intersection or origin. In Figure 9–5, the rectangular coordinates for point p are (x, y) in A and $(13, 5)$ in B. In this latter example, point P is at the head of vector R and, since the location of the vector tail is at the origin, this vector's location in space is established. The tail is at $(0, 0)$, and the head is at $(13, 5)$.

Point P may also be described using polar coordinates. These consist of the distance (r) of point P from the origin and the angle (θ) that the line r makes with the x axis. The polar coordinates for point P in Figure 9–5C are (r, θ). If P is the vector head, r equals the vector's magnitude and θ is equal to its direction. In polar terms the vector's description is (r, θ).

In these coordinate systems degrees are customarily measured in a counter-clockwise direction. Also, by convention, x values to the right of the y axis are positive $(+)$ and those below are negative $(-)$. Y values above the x axis are positive and those below are negative. Point A in Figure 9–6 has (x, y) coordinates of $(4.3, 2.5)$ and (r, θ) coordinates of $(5, 30°)$. The (x, y) coordinates for point B are $(-1.5, -3)$ and the polar coordinates are $(3.4, 240°)$.

Graphic Resolution and Combination of Vectors

Within this frame of reference, quantities encountered in the study of biomechanics may be portrayed and handled graphically. Consider a broad jumper who takes off with a velocity of 31.6 ft/sec at an angle of 18 degrees. Since the takeoff velocity has both magnitude and direction, it is a vector quantity and may be *resolved* into its components. By selecting a linear unit of measurement to represent a unit of velocity, such as 0.25 inch to represent 4 feet per second of velocity, and by constructing a line of the appropriate length at an angle of 18 degrees to the x axis, one can determine the horizontal and vertical components of velocity for that jump. This is done by con-

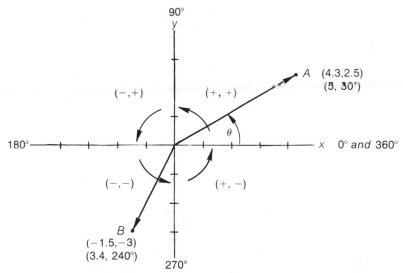

Figure 9–6 Coordinate quadrants. Values of x and y are positive in upper right quadrant and negative in lower left. X is negative in upper left and y is negative in lower right.

structing a right triangle in which the hypotenuse is the vector, representing the total velocity of the jump, the vertical side is the vertical velocity, and the horizontal side is the horizontal velocity (Figure 9–7). The horizontal and vertical velocity components are determined by carefully measuring the lengths of the respective sides of the triangle and converting those amounts to velocity values by using the conversion factor. In this illustration, the conversion factor selected was 0.25 in = 4 ft/sec. The values obtained from measuring the lengths of the sides and applying the conversion factor were 30 ft/sec, horizontal velocity component, and 10 ft/sec of vertical velocity.

The *combination* of vectors to determine the resultant vector may also be obtained graphically by the construction of a parallelogram, the sides of which are linear representations of the two vectors. The first step is to mark a point, P, on a piece of pa-

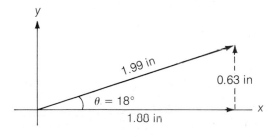

Given
Velocity of jump = 31.6 ft/sec
Angle of takeoff = 18°

Solution
Let 0.25 inch = 4 ft/sec

Then: velocity of jump = 1.99 in
Horizontal velocity x = 1.88 inches = 30 ft/sec and vertical velocity y = 0.63 in = 10 ft/sec

Figure 9–7 Graphic method of vector resolution. The horizontal and vertical velocity components of broad jump with initial velocity of 31.6 ft/sec at a direction of 18 degrees are determined by drawing vector components to scale.

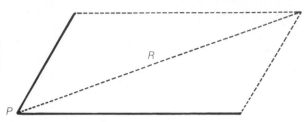

Figure 9–8   A "parallelogram of forces" used for determining the composite effect of two forces applied to the same point.

per. This represents the point at which the two vectors are applied. From this point two vector lines are drawn to scale, with the correct angle between them—that is, the same angle that actually exists between the two vectors. By using these two lines as two sides, a parallelogram is constructed with the addition of two more lines to form the other two sides (Figure 9–8). The diagonal is then drawn from the point of application, P, to the opposite corner. This diagonal represents both in magnitude and direction the composite effect of the two separate vectors. It is the resultant vector, R.

When one wishes to determine the resultant of *three* or more vectors acting at one point a similar procedure is followed. First, the resultant of two of the vectors is found. A second parallelogram is then constructed using the third vector as one side and the resultant of the first two vectors as the second side. The resultant vector of this second parallelogram is the resultant of all three vectors (Figure 9–9).

Another graphic method combines the vectors by adding them head to tail. Suppose Muscle J has a force of 1000 newtons and is pulling on bone E–F at an angle of 10 degrees, and Muscle K has a force of 800 newtons and is pulling at an angle of 40 degrees (Figure 9–10A). The composite effect of these two muscles may be described in terms of the amount of force and the direction or angle of pull of that composite force. Again a linear unit of measure is selected to represent a unit of force, and the vectors are placed in reference to the x, y axes so that the tail of the force vector for Muscle K is added to the head of the force vector for Muscle J (Figure 9–10B). The scale used in this example is 1 cm = 400 newtons. The resultant vector was drawn connecting the tail of J with the head of K. Its length represents the resultant force of the two muscles. The force in newtons was obtained by multiplying the vector length by the conversion factor, 1 cm = 400 N. The direction of the resultant force is indicated by the angle between the x axis and the resultant (measured with a protractor). Careful use of a protractor and ruler produced an r of 4.4 cm, which is equivalent to 1760 newtons pulling in a direction of 23.5 degrees. Like the parallelogram technique, this method is not limited to two vectors. Any number of vectors may be combined in this fashion.

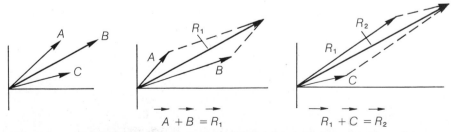

$$A + B = R_1 \qquad R_1 + C = R_2$$

Figure 9–9   Parallelogram method used for determining the composite effect of three or more forces applied to the same point, R_1 is resultant of combined forces A and B. R_2 is resultant of combined forces R_1 and C. Thus $\vec{A} + \vec{B} + \vec{C} = \vec{R_2}$.

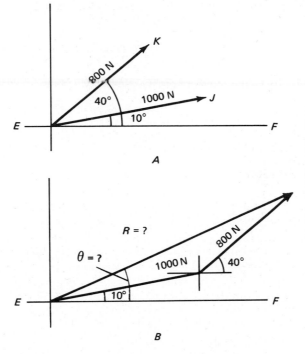

Figure 9–10 Combination of vectors using graphic method. Vector J is added to Vector K taking into account magnitude and direction. Resultant R is drawn by connecting tail of J to head of K. When measured with a ruler R equals 7 cm, which according to the scale is equivalent to 1750 N. The resultant angle θ, when measured with a protractor, is 23.5°.

Trigonometric Resolution and Combination of Vectors

Although the graphic method has value for portraying the situation, it does have serious drawbacks when it comes to calculating results. Accuracy is difficult to control in the drawing and measuring process, and the procedure is slow and unwieldy. A more accurate and efficient approach makes use of trigonometric relationships for both combining and resolving vectors.

Any vector may be resolved into horizontal and vertical components if the trigonometric relationships of a right triangle are employed. Let us use the previous example of the broad jumper whose velocity at takeoff was 31.6 ft/sec in the direction of 18 degrees with the horizontal (Figure 9–7). To find the horizontal velocity (V_x) and vertical velocity (V_y) at takeoff a right triangle is constructed. With the takeoff velocity (R) as the hypotenuse of the triangle, the vertical and horizontal components of velocity become the vertical and horizontal sides of the triangle (Figure 9–11). To obtain the values of V_x and V_y the sine and cosine functions are used as shown in Figure 9–11.* The horizontal velocity of the jump V_x turns out to be 30 ft/sec and the vertical velocity V_y is 10 ft/sec.

The combination of vectors is also possible with the use of right triangle trigonometric relationships.

If two vectors are applied at right angles to each other the solution should appear reasonably obvious since it is the reverse of the example just explained. If a baseball is thrown with a vertical velocity of 50 ft/sec and a horizontal velocity of 86.6 ft/sec the velocity of the throw and the angle of release may be determined as shown in Figure 9–12. The resultant velocity—i.e., the velocity of the throw—is 100 ft/sec and the angle of projection is 30 degrees.

*Refer to trigonometric table in Appendix G for values of trigonometric functions.

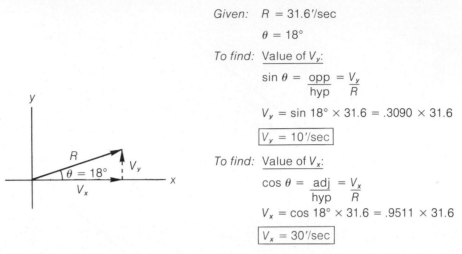

Given: $R = 31.6'/sec$

$\theta = 18°$

To find: Value of V_y:

$\sin\theta = \dfrac{opp}{hyp} = \dfrac{V_y}{R}$

$V_y = \sin 18° \times 31.6 = .3090 \times 31.6$

$\boxed{V_y = 10'/sec}$

To find: Value of V_x:

$\cos\theta = \dfrac{adj}{hyp} = \dfrac{V_x}{R}$

$V_x = \cos 18° \times 31.6 = .9511 \times 31.6$

$\boxed{V_x = 30'/sec}$

Figure 9–11   Resolution of a vector using the trigonometric method. Horizontal and vertical components are determined using cosine and sine functions.

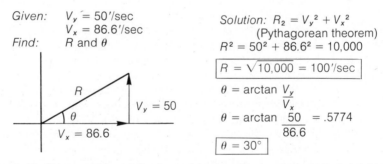

Given: $V_y = 50'/sec$
$V_x = 86.6'/sec$

Find: R and θ

Solution: $R_2 = V_y{}^2 + V_x{}^2$
(Pythagorean theorem)
$R^2 = 50^2 + 86.6^2 = 10,000$

$\boxed{R = \sqrt{10,000} = 100'/sec}$

$\theta = \arctan \dfrac{V_y}{V_x}$

$\theta = \arctan \dfrac{50}{86.6} = .5774$

$\boxed{\theta = 30°}$

Figure 9–12   Trigonometric solution to combination of two vectors applied at right angles.

If more than two vectors are involved or if they are not at right angles to each other as shown in previous examples, the resultant may be obtained by determining the x and y components for each individual vector and then summing these individual components to obtain the x and y components of the resultant. Once the x and y components are known, the magnitude and direction of R may be obtained. Let us consider the problem treated graphically in Figure 9–10, in which we were interested in determining the composite force of the two muscles and the resultant direction or angle of pull. To solve this problem trigonometrically, the horizontal and vertical components for each muscle must first be determined, as shown at the top of the opposite page:

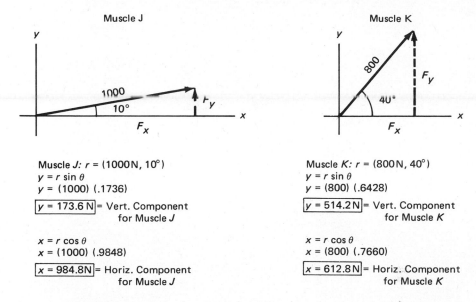

Muscle J: $r = (1000\,\text{N}, 10°)$
$y = r \sin \theta$
$y = (1000)\,(.1736)$
$\boxed{y = 173.6\,\text{N}}$ = Vert. Component
for Muscle J

$x = r \cos \theta$
$x = (1000)\,(.9848)$
$\boxed{x = 984.8\,\text{N}}$ = Horiz. Component
for Muscle J

Muscle K: $r = (800\,\text{N}, 40°)$
$y = r \sin \theta$
$y = (800)\,(.6428)$
$\boxed{y = 514.2\,\text{N}}$ = Vert. Component
for Muscle K

$x = r \cos \theta$
$x = (800)\,(.7660)$
$\boxed{x = 612.8\,\text{N}}$ = Horiz. Component
for Muscle K

Next, to obtain the y component of the resultant effect of the **two** muscles, the y values for Muscles J and K are summed: ($\Sigma y = 173.6 + 514.2$; $\Sigma y = 687.8$ N). Similarly, the x component for R is the sum of the x values for J and K: ($\Sigma x = 984.8 + 612.8$; $\Sigma x = 1597.6$ N).

As we have seen before, a knowledge of the horizontal (x) and vertical (y) components makes it possible to determine the resultant vector. A triangle is formed and the unknown parts are found. Figure 9–13 presents the solution once the x and y values for Muscles J and K have each been summed. The summed F_y and F_x values form the two sides of the triangle and the unknown resultant force is the hypotenuse. Using the tangent relationship between the two sides, the resultant angle of pull of the two muscles was calculated to be 23.3 degrees. With this additional information, the composite or resultant force of 1739 newtons was found using the $\sin \theta = \dfrac{\text{opp}}{\text{hyp}}$ relationship.

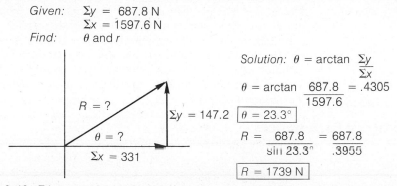

Given: $\Sigma y = 687.8$ N
$\Sigma x = 1597.6$ N
Find: θ and r

Solution: $\theta = \arctan \dfrac{\Sigma y}{\Sigma x}$
$\theta = \arctan \dfrac{687.8}{1597.6} = .4305$
$\boxed{\theta = 23.3°}$
$R = \dfrac{687.8}{\sin 23.3°} = \dfrac{687.8}{.3955}$
$\boxed{R = 1739\text{ N}}$

Figure 9–13   Trigonometric combination of summed vectors. The sum of all x components becomes the horizontal vector component; the sum of all y components becomes the vertical vector component. R and θ are determined by combining Σx and Σy.

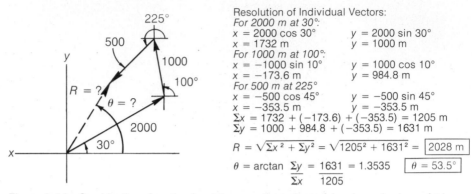

Resolution of Individual Vectors:
For 2000 m at 30°:
$x = 2000 \cos 30°$ $y = 2000 \sin 30°$
$x = 1732$ m $y = 1000$ m
For 1000 m at 100°:
$x = -1000 \sin 10°$ $y = 1000 \cos 10°$
$x = -173.6$ m $y = 984.8$ m
For 500 m at 225°
$x = -500 \cos 45°$ $y = -500 \sin 45°$
$x = -353.5$ m $y = -353.5$ m
$\Sigma x = 1732 + (-173.6) + (-353.5) = 1205$ m
$\Sigma y = 1000 + 984.8 + (-353.5) = 1631$ m

$R = \sqrt{\Sigma x^2 + \Sigma y^2} = \sqrt{1205^2 + 1631^2} = \boxed{2028 \text{ m}}$

$\theta = \arctan \dfrac{\Sigma y}{\Sigma x} = \dfrac{1631}{1205} = 1.3535 \quad \boxed{\theta = 53.5°}$

Figure 9–14   Combination of vectors involving negative values of x and y and values of θ larger than 90 degrees.

In the explanation of coordinate systems it was shown that values of x and y may be negative and that values of θ may exceed 90 degrees (Figure 9–6). An example of a problem with these additional factors is that of the hiker who plots the stated course and then must determine the resultant displacement at the completion of the course:

A hiker walks the following course: 2000 meters at 30 degrees, 1000 meters at 100 degrees, and 500 meters at 225 degrees. What is her resultant displacement? The solution is presented in Figure 9–14.

Value of Vector Analysis

The ability to handle variables of motion and force as vector or scalar quantities should improve one's understanding of motion and the forces causing it. The effect that a muscle's angle of pull has on the force available for moving a limb is better understood when it is subjected to vector analysis. Similar study of the direction and force of projectiles improves one's understanding of the effect of gravity, angle of release, and force of release upon the flight of a projectile. The effect of several muscles exerting their combined forces on a single bone is also clarified when treated quantitatively as the combination of vector quantities to obtain a *resultant*. Indeed, the effect that a change in any variable may produce becomes much more apparent. Without the use of a vector relationship, it would be difficult if not impossible to describe motion and forces in meaningful, quantative terms.

Laboratory Experiences

1. Express the following units in metric terms:
   a. a force of 25 pounds.
   b. a mass of 5 slugs.
   c. a distance of 11 inches.
   d. a velocity of 20 feet per second.
   e. a volume of 3 quarts.

2. Determine the distance between each set of points (scale: 1 unit = 10 cm).
   a. (2, 3); (5, 7).
   b. (1, 2); (3, 3).
   c. (1.5, 3.0); (6, 6).
   d. (0, 0); (6.2, 3.6).

3. Find the x and y component for each of the following vectors.
   a. 45 ft/sec at 25°.
   b. 85 lb at 135°.
   c. 118 kg at 310°.
   d. 25 m/sec² at 210°.

4. Express the following units in the English system:
   a. a mass of 40 kilograms.
   b. a force of 67 newtons.
   c. a distance of 36 kilometers.
   d. a volume of 7 liters.
   e. a linear acceleration of 5 meters/sec².

5. A basketball official runs 60 ft along the sideline in one direction, reverses, and runs 25 ft. What is the distance run? What is the displacement? Draw a vector diagram.

6. The muscular force of a muscle is 160 pounds and the muscle is pulling on the bone at an angle of 15 degrees. What are the vertical and horizontal components of this force?

7. At the moment of release, a baseball has a horizontal velocity component of 25 meters per second and a vertical velocity component of 14 meters per second. At what angle was it released, and what was its initial velocity in the direction of the throw in meters/sec? in feet/sec?

8. A child is being pulled in a sled by a person holding a rope that has an angle of 20 degrees with the horizontal. The total force being used to move the sled at a constant forward speed is 25 pounds. How much of the force is horizontal? vertical?

9. An orienteer runs the following course: 1000 meters at 45°, 1500 meters at 120°; 500 meters at 190°.
   a. Draw the course to scale accurately.
   b. Determine the resultant displacement graphically.
   c. Determine the resultant displacement trigonometrically.
   d. Explain any differences you have between your graphic and trigonometric results.
   e. Express the orienteer's position at the end of the course in terms of rectangular coordinates; polar coordinates.

10. A football lineman charges an opponent with a force of 175 pounds in the direction of 310 degrees. The opponent charges back with a force of 185 pounds in the direction of 90 degrees. What is the resultant force and in what direction will it act?

11. Referring to Figures 1–2 and 6–14, make a tracing of the femur and adductor longus muscle. Draw a straight line to represent the mechanical axis of the femur and another to represent the muscle's line of pull.
    a. Using a protractor, determine the angle of pull of the muscle (angle formed by muscle's line of pull and mechanical axis of bone).
    b. Assuming a total muscle force of 250 pounds, calculate the force components.

12. Muscle A has a force of 100 pounds and is pulling on a bone at an angle of 15 degrees. Muscle B has a force of 150 pounds and is pulling on the same bone at the same spot but at an angle of 30 degrees. Muscle C has a force of 75 pounds and is pulling at the same spot

with an angle of pull of 10 degrees. What is the composite effect of these muscles in terms of amount of force and direction?

13. Name as many vector and scalar quantities as you can think of which are part of the games of football, tennis, or golf.

References

Atwater, A. E. 1980. Kinesiology/biomechanics: Perspectives and trends. *Res. Q. Exercise Sport* 51:193–218.

Basford, L. 1966. *The science of movement.* London: Sampson Low Marston.

Cromer, A. H. 1977. *Physics for the life sciences*, 2d ed. New York: McGraw Hill.

Evans, F. G. 1971. Biomechanical implications of anatomy. In *Selected topics on biomechanics*, ed. J. M. Cooper. Chicago: Athletic Institute, pp. 3–30.

Hay, J. G. 1973. *The biomechanics of sports techniques.* Englewood Cliffs, N.J.: Prentice-Hall.

Kelley, D. L. 1971. *Kinesiology—fundamentals of motion description.* Englewood Cliffs, N.J.: Prentice-Hall.

Nelson, R. C. 1971. Biomechanics of sport: An overview. In *Selected topics on biomechanics,* ed. J. M. Cooper. Chicago: Athletic Institute, pp. 31–37.

Widule, C. J. 1974. *Analysis of human motion—experiences, experiments and problems.* Lafayette, Ind.: Balt Publishers.

The Description of Human Motion

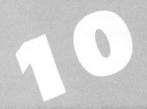

10

Objectives

At the conclusion of this chapter, the student should be able to:

1. Name the kinds of motion experienced by the human body, and describe the factors that cause and modify motion.

2. Name and use properly the terms that describe linear and rotatory motion— position, displacement, distance, speed, velocity, and acceleration.

3. Explain the interrelationships that exist among displacement, velocity, and acceleration, and use the knowledge of these interrelationships to describe and analyze human motion.

4. Describe the behavior of projectiles, and explain how angle, speed, and height of projection affect that behavior.

5. Describe the relationship between linear and rotatory movement, and explain the significance of this relationship to human motion.

Motion

If we are to understand the movements of the human musculoskeletal system and the implements put into motion by this system, we need first to turn our thoughts to the concepts of motion itself. What is motion? What determines the kind of motion that will result when an object or a part of the human body is made to move? How is motion described in mechanical terms? How do these generalities about motion apply to movements of the musculoskeletal system? Indeed, how does one know that motion is occurring?

Relative Motion

Motion is the act or process of changing place or position with respect to some reference object. Whether or not a body is at rest or in motion depends totally upon the reference. When walking down the street or riding a bicycle or serving a tennis ball, it seems obvious that movement is involved. Less obvious is the motion status of the sleeping passenger in a smoothly flying plane or of an automobile parked at a curb. If the earth is the reference point, all but the parked car are in motion relative to the earth, and even the parked car is in motion if the reference point is the sun. On the other hand, if the bicycle is the reference point, the person riding it is at rest relative to the bicycle, and the sleeping passenger is at rest with respect to anything in the plane. The *relative* motion of each is defined in relation to the specific reference object or point. It is possible, therefore, to be at rest and in motion at the same time relative to different reference points. The sleeping passenger is at rest relative to the plane and in motion relative to the earth. The relative motion of two bodies depends entirely upon their relative velocities through space. Two joggers running at 8 km/hr in the same direction are at rest with respect to each other. However, if one jogs at 8 km/hr and the other at 10 km/hr, the former would be considered to be at rest with respect to the latter but the latter would be in motion both with respect to the slower runner and to the earth.

Cause of Motion

It is difficult to think of motion without visualizing a specific object in the act of moving. If we did not actually see how it changed from a stationary condition to a moving one, we might wonder what caused it to be set in motion. Did someone pull on it, or push against it, or perhaps blow on it or even attract it with a magnet? What are these assumed causes of motion? Without exception, they are a form of force. *Force* is the instigator of movement. If we see an object in motion, we know that it is moving because a force has acted upon it. We know, too, that the force must have been sufficiently great to overcome the object's inertia, for unless a force is greater than the resistance offered by the object it cannot produce motion. We can push against a stone wall all day without moving it so much as 1 millimeter, but a bulldozer can knock the wall down at the first impact. The magnitude of the force *relative to the magnitude of the resistance* is the determining factor in causing an object to move.

Kinds of Motion

What are the ways in which an object may move? A hockey puck slides across the ice without turning. On the other hand, it may revolve as it slides. A figure skater spins in place. Arrows, balls, and jumpers move through the air in a pathway known as a parabola. The hand moves in an arc when the forearm turns at the elbow joint and the neighboring joints are held motionless. As we note the different ways in which objects move, we are impressed with the almost limitless variety in the patterns of movement. Objects move in straight paths and in curved paths, they roll, slide, and fall, they bounce, they swing back and forth like a pendulum, they rotate about a center, either partially or completely, and they frequently rotate at the same time that they move as a whole from one place to another. Although the variety of ways in which objects move appears to be almost limitless, careful consideration of these ways reveals the fact that there are, in actuality, only *two* major classifications of movement patterns. These are *translatory*, or *linear*, and *rotatory*, or *angular*. Either an object moves in its entirety from one place to another or it turns about a center of motion. Sometimes it does both simultaneously.

Figure 10–1   An example of rectilinear motion.

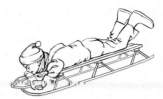

TRANSLATORY MOVEMENT   This kind of movement is termed translatory because the object is translated as a whole from one location to another. Translatory movement is commonly called linear motion, and is further classified as rectilinear or curvilinear. *Rectilinear motion* is the straight-line progression of an object as a whole with all its parts moving the same distance in the same direction at a uniform rate of speed. The child on the sled in Figure 10–1, a water skier pulled by a boat, or a bowling ball moving in a straight path are examples of rectilinear motion. *Curvilinear* motion refers to all curved translatory movement—that is, the object moves in a curved pathway. The paths of a ball or any other projectile in flight, the wrist during the force phase in bowling (Figure 10–2), or a skier in a sweeping turn are all examples of curvilinear motion. A special form of curvilinear motion, which on the surface does not appear to be translatory, is that called *circular* motion. This type of motion occurs when an object moves along the circumference of a circle—i.e., a curved path of constant radius. The logic for calling this type of motion linear relates to the fact that it occurs when an unbalanced force acts on a moving body to keep it in a circle. If that unbalanced force stops acting on the object and the object is free to move, it will move in a linear path tangent to the direction in which it is moving at the moment of

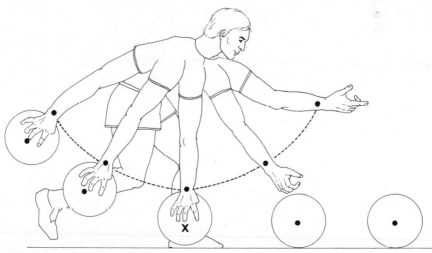

Figure 10–2   The wrist follows a curvilinear path during the delivery of a bowling ball. (Drawn from motion picture film tracing.)

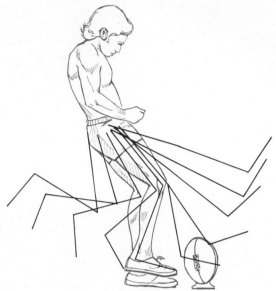

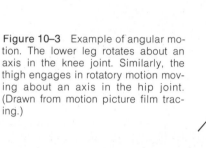

Figure 10–3 Example of angular motion. The lower leg rotates about an axis in the knee joint. Similarly, the thigh engages in rotatory motion moving about an axis in the hip joint. (Drawn from motion picture film tracing.)

release. The path of a ball held in the hand as the arm moves around in windmill fashion is an example of circular motion. If the ball is released during the motion, it will fly off at a tangent and continue in a straight line until gravity forces it into a curved path. Other examples of bodies in circular motion are the gondola on a moving Ferris wheel or the knot on the ring of a spinning lariat.

ROTATORY OR ANGULAR MOTION   This is the kind of motion that is typical of levers and of wheels and axles. Rotatory or angular motion occurs when any object acting as a radius moves in a circular path about a fixed point. The distance traveled may be a small arc or a complete circle. Most human body segment motions are angular movements in which the body part moves in an arc about a fixed point. The arm engages in rotatory motion when it moves in windmill fashion about a fixed point or axis in the shoulder. The head's motion in the act of indicating "no," the lower leg in kicking a ball, or the hand and forearm in turning a door knob are all examples of rotatory or angular motion. In each instance the moving body segment may be likened to the radius of a circle. The arm moving in windmill fashion and the lower leg and foot in kicking are the radii. In the "no" action of the head and in the door knob being turned by the forearm and hand, the radius is perpendicular to the long axis running vertically through the middle of the head and lengthwise through the middle of the forearm and hand, respectively (Figure 10–3). These movements are not to be confused with circular motion. Circular motion describes the motion of any *point* on the radius whereas angular motion is descriptive of the motion of the entire radius.

OTHER MOVEMENT PATTERNS   *Reciprocating* motion denotes repetitive movement. The use of the term is ordinarily limited to repetitive translatory movements, as illustrated by a bouncing ball or the repeated blows of a hammer, but technically it includes all kinds. The term *oscillation* refers specifically to repetitive movements in an arc. Familiar examples of this type of movement are seen in the pendulum, metronome, and tuning fork.

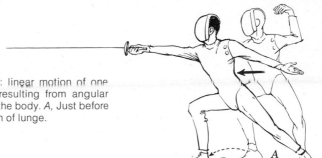

Figure 10–4   General motion: linear motion of one part of the body (the hand) resulting from angular motion of several segments of the body. *A,* Just before lunge (thrust). *B,* At completion of lunge.

Often, an object displays a combination of rotatory and translatory movement. This is sometimes referred to as *general motion.* The bicycle, automobile, and train move linearly as the result of the rotatory movements of their wheels, provided there is enough friction between the wheels and the supporting surface to keep the former from spinning in place. Likewise, people, as they walk or run down the street, experience translatory motion because of the angular movement of their body segments. The angular motions of several segments of the body are frequently coordinated in such a way that a single related segment will move linearly. This is true in throwing darts, in shot-putting, and in a lunge in fencing (Figure 10–4). Because of the angular motions of the forearm and upper arm, the hand travels linearly and thus is able to impart linear force to the dart and to the shot prior to their release, and to the foil.

Kinds of Motion Experienced by the Body

The human body experiences all kinds of motion. Because most of the joints are axial, the body segments must undergo primarily angular motion (Figure 10–5). A slight amount of translatory motion is seen in the gliding movements of the plane or irregular joints but these movements are negligible in themselves. They occur chiefly in the carpal and tarsal joint and in the joints of the vertebral arches in conjunction with angular movements in neighboring axial joints. The body as a whole experiences rectilinear movement when it is acted upon by the force of gravity, as in coasting (Figure 10–1), or in a free fall (Figure 10–7), and likewise when acted upon by an external force, as in water skiing (Figure 10–6). It experiences general motion in forward and backward rolls on the ground and in somersaults in the air, and rotatory motion in twirling on ice skates. It experiences curvilinear translatory motion in diving, broad jumping, high jumping, and hurdling, and it experiences reciprocating motion on the trampoline and when swinging back and forth on the rings, trapeze, or horizontal bar.

Factors That Determine the Kind of Motion

Thus far we have considered the cause of motion and the various kinds of motion based on movement patterns or paths. Now we must turn to another question. What determines the kind of motion that will result when an object is made to move? The best way for the student to discover the answer is to produce each kind of motion and then to analyze what was done to obtain the desired kind of motion.

In order to make an object move linearly, we discover that it must be free to move and that either we must apply force uniformly against one entire side of the object or we must apply it directly in line with the object's center of gravity. The object will

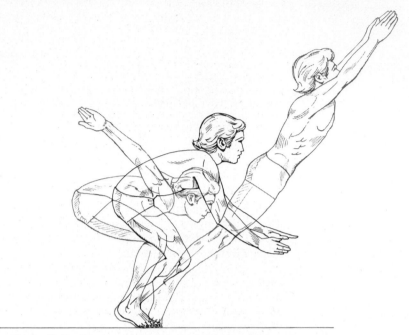

Figure 10–5   An example of movement of the body caused by the body's own muscular activity. Movements of individual body segments are primarily angular. (Drawn from motion picture film tracing.)

move in a straight line provided it does not meet an obstacle or resistance of some sort. If its edge hits against another object or encounters a rough spot, the moving object will turn about its point of contact with the interfering obstacle. If we attempt to push a tall cabinet across a supporting surface that provides excessive friction, such as a cement floor, the cabinet will tip, even though we place our hands exactly in line with the cabinet's center of gravity and push in a horizontal direction. In order to move it linearly it will be necessary to apply the push lower than the cabinet's center of gravity to compensate for the friction.

Figure 10–6   An example of movement of the body caused by an external force.

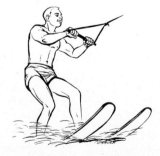

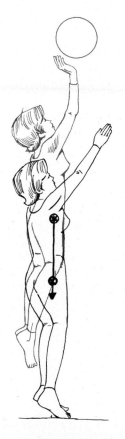

Figure 10–7 Landing from a vertical jump. An example of linear movement of the body caused by the force of gravity. (Drawn from motion picture film tracing.)

If one part of an object is "fixed," rotatory motion will occur when sufficient force is applied on any portion of the object that is free to move. A lever undergoes rotatory motion because, by definition, some portion of it remains in place. If it is desired to move an object in the manner of a lever it is necessary to provide a "fulcrum" and to apply force to the object at some point other than at the fulcrum. Thus, if rotatory motion of a freely movable object is desired, it is necessary to apply force to it "off center" or to provide an "off center" resistance that will interfere with the motion of part of the object.

Reciprocating motion is caused by a uniform repetition of opposing force applications, and the oscillation of a pendulum is produced by repeated applications of gravitational force to a suspended object that is free to move back and forth and that is in any position other than its resting position.

In summary, it may be said that the kind of motion that will be displayed by a moving object depends first of all upon the kind of motion permitted that particular kind of object. If it is a lever, it is permitted only angular motion, if it is a pendulum, oscillatory motion, and so on. If it is a freely movable object, it is permitted either translatory or rotatory motion, depending upon the circumstances. These circumstances include the point at which force is applied with reference to the object's center of gravity, the environmental pathways of movement available to the object, and the presence or absence of additional external factors that modify the motion.

Factors Modifying Motion

Motion is usually modified by a number of external factors, such as friction, air resistance, and water resistance. Whether these factors are a help or a hindrance depends upon the circumstances and the nature of the motion. The same factor may facilitate one form of motion, yet hinder another. For instance, friction is a great help to the runner because maximum effort may be exerted without danger of slipping, yet, on the other hand, friction hinders the rolling of a ball, as in field hockey, golf, and croquet. Again, wind or air resistance is indispensable to the sailboat's motion, but unless it is a tail wind it impedes the runner. Likewise, water resistance is essential for propulsion of the body by means of swimming strokes and of boats through the use of oars and paddles, yet at the same time it hinders the progress of both the swimmer and the boat, especially if these present a broad surface to the water. It is for this reason that swimmers keep the body level and that boats are streamlined. One of the major problems in sports is to learn how to take advantage of these factors when they contribute to the movement in question and, on the other hand, how to minimize them when they are detrimental to the movement. A more detailed discussion of forces influencing motion is presented in the chapter on the conditions of linear and rotatory motion.

There are also anatomical factors that modify the motion of the segments of the body. These include friction in the joints (minimized by synovial fluid), tension of antagonistic muscles, tension of ligaments and fasciae, anomalies of bone and joint structure, atmospheric pressure within the joint capsule, and the presence of interfering soft tissues. Except for the limitations due to fleshiness, these modifying factors are classified as internal resistance.

Kinematic Description of Motion

Motion has been defined as the act or process of changing place or position with respect to some reference point. Thus, in order to talk about motion, a starting point must be identified. Once this is done the resultant motion, regardless of whether it is translatory or rotatory, may be characterized according to the distance and direction away from the starting point, the speed of the movement, and any change in speed that may occur. This kind of motion study is called *kinematics*. Motion is described in terms of displacement, velocity, and acceleration with no consideration of or reference to the forces that cause or modify the motion. Linear kinematics is concerned with translatory motion and angular kinematics with rotatory motion.

Linear Kinematics

Distance and Displacement

The distance an object is removed from a reference point is called its *displacement*. Displacement does not indicate how far the object travels in going from point *A* to point *C*. It only indicates the final change of position. A person who walks north for 3 kilometers to point *B* and then east for 4 kilometers to point *C* has walked a *distance* of 7 kilometers, but the *displacement* with respect to the starting point is only 5 kilometers (Figure 10–8). Similarly, a basketball player who runs up and down the court several times has traveled a considerable distance, but the displacement with respect to one of the end lines may be zero. Or consider the poor golfer who, blinded

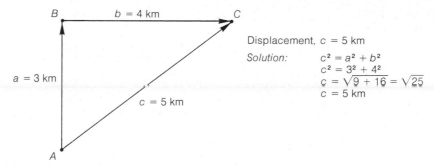

Figure 10–8 Displacement is the resultant distance an object is removed from its starting point.

by the late afternoon sun, hits the ball so erratically that the route to the green, 450 yards away, crosses and recrosses the fairway many times. Regardless of the zigzag path to the green and the many changes of direction needed to get there, the ball's displacement is the straight-line distance from the tee to the green.

Displacement is a vector quantity having both magnitude and direction. It is not enough to indicate only the amount of positional change. That alone would be distance, a scalar quantity. The direction of the vector must also be defined. When the golfer finally reaches the green, the displacement from the hole to green is 450 yards west. And the walker's displacement in Figure 10–8 is 5 km, in a northeast direction.

Speed and Velocity

Speed and velocity are two words that are frequently used to describe how fast an object is moving. These terms are often used interchangeably, but in fact there is a significant difference. Speed is related to distance and velocity to displacement. Speed tells how fast an object is moving—i.e., the distance an object will travel in a given time—but it tells nothing about the direction of movement.

$$\text{average speed} = \frac{\text{distance traveled}}{\text{time}} \quad \text{or} \quad = \frac{d}{t}$$

Examples of speed measurements are an auto traveling at 7 km/hr, the wind blowing at 60 mph, a ball thrown with a speed of 100 ft/sec, or a sprinter running at 10 m/sec.

Velocity, on the other hand, involves direction as well as speed. Speed is a scalar quantity, while velocity is a vector quantity. In most sports activities this difference is of no concern, but in others it is of extreme importance. The speed of a football player carrying the ball may be impressive but, if not directed toward the opponent's goal, it is not providing yardage for a first down. Although the speed may be great, the velocity in the desired direction may indeed be zero. Velocity is speed in a given direction. It is the amount of displacement per given unit of time. This is the same as saying that velocity is the rate of displacement, or

$$\text{average velocity} = \frac{\text{displacement}}{\text{time}}$$

In the diagrams in Figure 10–9, displacement values (s) are represented on the y axis and the time values (t) are on the x axis. If displacement values are plotted to correspond with their time values, the line formed by connecting these plotted values

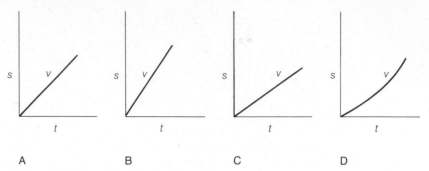

Figure 10–9 Examples of displacement–time graphs for uniform and nonuniform motion. The velocity in *A, B, C* is constant.

represents the rate of displacement or velocity (*v*). When the rate of displacement does not change—i.e., when the distance and direction traveled is the same for each equal time period—the velocity is constant and the velocity line on the diagram is a straight line. In Figures 10–9A, B, and C the velocity is constant, but in Figure 10–9D the curved line indicates that the rate of displacement changes, and therefore the velocity is not constant. When there is greater displacement per unit of time the velocity increases, as does the slope of the velocity line in the diagram. Figure 10–9B shows the fastest velocity and C the slowest. In D, the displacement starts at a slow rate and then increases. If A, B, C, and D represent runners on a straight track, A, B, and C would each be running at a constant but different velocity, with B's velocity the fastest and C's the slowest. Runner D starts out at a slow velocity but increases the rate of displacement until the resultant velocity is the fastest of all four.

Where velocity is constant, as in A, B, and C, the motion is said to be uniform. When the amount of displacement per unit of time varies, nonuniform motion occurs. Uniform motion is not a common characteristic of human motion, since most human movements are likely to have many variations in the rate of displacement. When the velocity of human motion is given, it is usually an average velocity that tells only the total displacement occurring in a stated period of time. Although a long distance runner who ran the Boston Marathon, a distance of 26 miles, 385 yards, in 2½ hours had an average velocity of 10.4 mph, it is doubtful that the velocity was uniformly 10.4 mph through the run. If one were to record the time at which the runner passed frequent and equally spaced distance points along the route, a displacement-time graph could be prepared to show the variations in the runner's speed at various points in the course of the race. This kind of information can be quite useful in helping a coach or participant to analyze the performance and strategy of the race, and to plan changes where needed. The narrower the distance intervals used, the greater is the possibility that critical variations in speed will become apparent. The use of cinematography permits a similar analysis of brief and fast events. The distance and time data necessary for graphing and analyzing the motion patterns are obtained indirectly from the film record.

In equation form, average velocity is

$$\bar{v} = \frac{s}{t}$$

The symbol $\bar{v}$ represents average velocity, s represents displacement, and t represents time. The average velocity of a tennis ball served 58 feet in 0.35 seconds is 58 divided by 0.35, or 165 ft/sec in the direction of the service court.

Acceleration

When velocity changes, its rate of change is called acceleration. A sprint runner has an initial velocity of 0 ft/sec. When the gun signals the beginning of a race, the sprinter's velocity begins to change by increasing. The rate of change in velocity is *acceleration*. Acceleration may be positive or negative. An increase is considered positive and a decrease such as slowing down at the end of the race is negative. Negative acceleration is also called deceleration. When velocity is plotted against time, as shown in Figure 10–10, the line formed by connecting the value of the velocity for the corresponding unit of time represents acceleration. In Figure 10–10A the velocity does not change. It remains constant and therefore there is no acceleration. In B the acceleration is positive and uniform. As t increases, v increases at a constant rate. In C acceleration is negative and uniform. As t increases, v decreases a constant amount per unit of time. In D acceleration is positive but nonuniform. Its rate of change is not constant. Again, taking the case of the runners on a straight track, the runner in A established a steady pace which, during the time represented on the graph, neither slowed down nor speeded up. The velocity remained constant, and there was no acceleration. The runner in B started at 0 velocity and increased the velocity at a constant rate such as might occur at the beginning of a race. The runner in C, at the end of a race, steadily decreased the velocity at a constant rate until it was 0, while in D the runner's acceleration (rate of velocity change) was initially slow but then proceeded to increase.

In equation form acceleration is expressed as

$$\bar{a} = \frac{v - u}{t}$$

where $\bar{a}$ represents average acceleration, v is the final velocity, u is the initial velocity, and t is time. A runner whose velocity changes from 2 ft/sec at the end of the first second of a race to 6 ft/sec at the end of the third second has accelerated 2 ft/sec for each of the 2-second time intervals measured. That is, the rate of change of velocity, $\bar{a}$, equals the difference between the final velocity (6 ft/sec) and the initial velocity (2 ft/sec) divided by the time interval (3 sec less 1 sec).

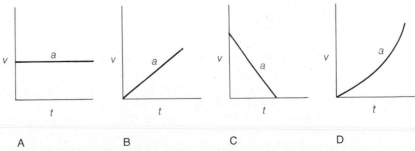

A   B   C   D

Figure 10–10 Examples of velocity–time graphs. *A,* Constant velocity; no acceleration. *B,* Uniform increasing acceleration. *C,* Uniform decreasing acceleration. *D,* Nonuniform increasing acceleration.

Since velocity is always displacement divided by time and acceleration is velocity divided by time, acceleration is really displacement divided by time divided by time, and the units for measurement must reflect this. The time unit must appear twice in acceleration units. The logic for this is apparent when the units of ft/sec are used for velocity in the equation for average acceleration:

$$\bar{a} = \dfrac{\dfrac{\text{final ft}}{\text{sec}} - \dfrac{\text{initial ft}}{\text{sec}}}{\text{sec}}$$

After the subtraction is completed this equation becomes $\bar{a} = \dfrac{\frac{ft}{sec}}{sec}$ or, as commonly written, ft/sec/sec or ft/sec². Thus, the average acceleration of the runner in the example is 2 ft/sec/sec, or 2 ft/sec².

One usually thinks of acceleration in terms of a change in the amount of distance covered in equal units of time. Acceleration also occurs when, although the speed remains constant, there is a change in *direction*. The example given for Figure 10–10A was that of a runner keeping a steady pace on a straight track with no acceleration. If the runner, still running at the same speed, shifts to a circular track, acceleration occurs because of the change in direction, and the velocity-time graph would look more like Figure 10–10B.

Uniformly Accelerated Motion

When the acceleration rate is constant, the velocity change is the same during equal time periods. Under these conditions motion is said to be *uniformly* accelerated. This type of acceleration does not occur with great frequency, since the change in velocity of bodies in motion is usually irregular and complicated. However, there is one common type of uniform acceleration that is important in sport and physical education, the acceleration of freely falling bodies.

Neglecting air resistance, objects allowed to fall freely will speed up or accelerate at a uniform rate owing to the acceleration of gravity. Conversely, objects projected upward will be retarded at a uniform rate that is also due to the acceleration of gravity. The value for the acceleration of gravity changes with different locations on the earth's surface, but for most of the United States this value can be considered to be 32 ft/sec² or 9.80 m/sec². Regardless of its size or density, a falling object will be acted on by gravity so that its velocity will increase 32 ft/sec each second it is in the air. A dropped ball starting out with a velocity of 0 ft/sec will have a velocity of 32 ft/sec at the end of 1 second, 64 ft/sec at the end of 2 seconds, 96 ft/sec at the end of 3 seconds, and so on. A second ball weighing twice as much will fall with exactly the same acceleration. It too will have a velocity of 96 ft/sec at the end of 3 seconds. Of course this example does not take into consideration the resistance or friction of air, which can be appreciable. The lighter the object the more it is affected. After an initial acceleration light objects such as feathers or snowflakes may stop accelerating entirely and fall at a constant rate. Consider, for instance, the difference between the behavior of a badminton shuttle and a golf ball when dropped from a height.

The denser and heavier the free-falling object, the less it is affected by air friction, especially if the distance of the fall is not too great. Even heavy objects, such as skydivers falling from great distances, eventually reach a downward speed large enough to create an opposing air resistance equal to the accelerating force of gravity. When this happens, the diver no longer speeds up but continues to fall at a steady speed. This speed is called *terminal* velocity and amounts to approximately 120 mph (176 ft/sec) for a falling skydiver. With the parachute open, the diver's velocity decreases to 12 mph steady velocity.

LAWS OF UNIFORMLY ACCELERATED MOTION   In spite of the reality of air resistance, much can be learned about the nature of free falling bodies and uniform acceleration through a knowledge of the *laws of uniformly accelerated motion*. Because the acceleration of gravity is constant, the distance traveled by a freely falling body, as well as its downward velocity, can be determined for any point in time by application of these laws. Expressed in equation form, they are

$$v = u + at \tag{1}$$

$$s = ut + \tfrac{1}{2}at^2 \tag{2}$$

$$v^2 = u^2 + 2as \tag{3}$$

Galileo's experiments with inclined planes enabled him to work out these equations. They apply to any type of linear motion in which acceleration is uniform. Their specific application to the effect of gravity on freely falling objects is presented in Table 10–1. If the initial velocity (u) is zero, as it is when an object is allowed to fall freely from a stationary position, the equations may be simplified:

$$v = at \tag{1}$$

$$s = \tfrac{1}{2}at \tag{2}$$

$$v^2 = 2as \tag{3}$$

The student may also discover that some authors, when applying these equations specifically to gravity, replace *a*, the symbol for acceleration, with the symbol g.

The time it takes for an object to rise to the highest point of its trajectory is equal to the time it takes to fall to its starting point. Similarly, the release speed and landing

TABLE 10–1 Effect of Gravity on a Freely Falling Object

	TIME	DISTANCE TRAVELED $s = ut + \tfrac{1}{2}at^2$	FINAL VELOCITY $v = u + at$	AVERAGE VELOCITY $\overline{v} = \dfrac{u + v}{2}$
English $a = 32$ ft/sec^2	1 sec	16 ft	32 ft/sec	16 ft/sec
	2 sec	64 ft	64 ft/sec	32 ft/sec
	3 sec	144 ft	96 ft/sec	48 ft/sec
	4 sec	256 ft	128 ft/sec	64 ft/sec
	5 sec	400 ft	160 ft/sec	80 ft/sec
Metric $a = 9.80$ m/sec^2	1 sec	4.9 m	9.8 m/sec	4.9 m/sec
	2 sec	19.6 m	19.6 m/sec	9.8 m/sec
	3 sec	44.1 m	29.4 m/sec	14.7 m/sec
	4 sec	78.4 m	39.2 m/sec	19.6 m/sec
	5 sec	122.5 m	49 m/sec	24.5 m/sec

speed are the same. Other than the fact that the directions are reversed, the upward flight is a mirror image of the downward flight. Proof that the release velocity and landing velocity are equal in amount but opposite in direction can be shown mathematically by substitution of values in the motion equations. Following vector conventions velocities upward are positive and those downward are negative. Thus the acceleration of gravity is treated as a negative value.

Example: Assuming that a ball is thrown upward so that it reaches a height of 5 meters before starting to fall, what is its initial velocity as it leaves the hand? What is its final velocity as it lands in the hand?

UPWARD THROW VELOCITY

Given: $v = 0$
$a = -9.80$
$s = 5$
Find: $u = ?$

DOWNWARD LANDING VELOCITY

Given: $u = 0$
$a = -9.80$
$s = 5$
Find: $v = ?$

Solution: Using Equation 3: $v^2 = u^2 + 2as$

$v^2 = u^2 + 2as$
$u^2 = v^2 - 2as$
$u^2 = 0 + (2 \times 9.8 \times 5)$
$u^2 = 98.0$
$u = \sqrt{98.0}$

$\boxed{u = 9.90 \text{ m/sec}}$

$v^2 = u^2 + 2as$

$v^2 = 0 - (2 \times 9.8 \times 5)$
$v^2 = -98.0$
$v = -\sqrt{98}$

$\boxed{v = -9.90 \text{ m/sec}}$

Projectiles

Vertical Projections

When a ball is allowed to fall freely its behavior is determined by gravity. When it is thrown straight up, its upward flight is governed by the *upward force of the throw and the downward force of gravity.* Objects projected upward are decelerated by the downward force of gravity at the same rate that those allowed to fall downward are accelerated (Figure 10–11). Consequently a ball thrown upward will have the same speed when it falls again into the hand as it did at the moment of leaving the hand.

When any object is thrown upward, it continues to slow down until it reaches a point at which the force of the velocity upward is neutralized by the downward force of gravity, and the resultant velocity is zero. This is the peak of the throw and the point at which, for a brief instant, the object seems suspended in air before it starts to drop. The greater the force of the upward projection, the longer it takes for the upward velocity to be reduced to zero by the force of gravity and the higher the ball will go. Referring to Table 10–1 it can be seen that a ball thrown upward with an initial velocity of 32 ft/sec will rise 16 feet and take 1 second to reach its high point, while a ball thrown upward with an initial velocity of 64 ft/sec will continue upward for 64 feet, reaching its peak in 2 seconds. It is important to reiterate that the time in the air, as well as the vertical distance, increases as the initial upward velocity becomes greater. Consequently, upward velocity should be emphasized in activities when it is desirable to allow as much time as possible in the air. Gymnasts and divers who wish

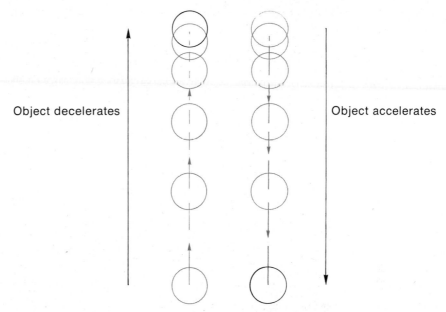

Object decelerates   Object accelerates

Figure 10–11   Objects projected upward are decelerated by the downward force of gravity at the same rate as those allowed to fall downward are accelerated. Both objects will cover the same distance in the same time. (Drawn from motion picture film tracing.)

to perform intricate stunt patterns in the air need as much time as possible, and therefore would benefit from the increased height that is a result of increased vertical velocity. It is also important to remember that the total time in the air is equal to twice the amount of time necessary to reach zero velocity at the high point of the projection.

Horizontal Projections

The flight path of a ball thrown horizontally is governed by the same two factors as that of a vertically projected ball—namely, the force of the throw and the downward force of gravity. A horizontally projected object starts out horizontally but immediately begins to follow a downward curved path because of the additional effect of gravity's force acting on it. The resultant displacement of the object is the sum of the horizontal displacement vector due to the force of the projection and the vertical displacement vector resulting from the force of gravity (Figure 10–12). Balls thrown horizontally from the same level but with different forces will have differing horizon-

Figure 10–12   Resultant displacement of a horizontally projected object.

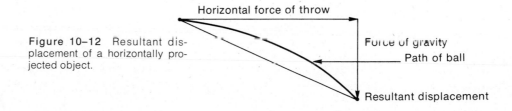

Horizontal force of throw

Force of gravity

Path of ball

Resultant displacement

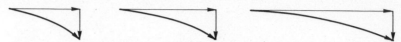

Figure 10–13 Flight path of balls with different horizontal velocities. Each ball is released at the same height as the other balls, and therefore each remains in the air for the same amount of time as the other balls before hitting the ground.

tal velocities and will travel different horizontal distances in a given time ($s = v/t$), but they all will travel the same vertical distance downward since the vertical drop depends entirely upon the time that gravity has to act on the object ($s = \frac{1}{2}at^2$), and the acceleration due to gravity does not change ($a = 32$ ft/sec^2). From this it can be seen that the horizontal force or velocity of a projected object is independent of the vertical force or velocity of the object (Figure 10–13).

The horizontal force influences *only* the horizontal distance that the object will cover while it remains in the air and not the vertical distance or the related amount of time that the object remains in the air. It follows, then, that an object projected horizontally from the same height and at the same time as one allowed to drop directly downward will land at the same level as the dropped object in the same amount of time. As with a vertically projected object, the time that a horizontally projected object remains in the air is totally dependent upon the amount of vertical distance between the landing point and the high point ($s = \frac{1}{2}at^2$).

The horizontal distance a projectile travels is governed by both the horizontal velocity of the object and the amount of time the object is able to remain in the air before it hits the ground. A ball thrown horizontally from a height of 3 m above the ground with a horizontal velocity of 25 m/sec will go 19.5 m horizontally before hitting the ground. A ball thrown with the same velocity but from a height of 2 m will hit the ground just 16 horizontal meters from its release point. Because of the increased height of release of the first ball, there was more *time* for its horizontal force to carry it horizontally before it hit the ground.

These values were determined as follows:

Example

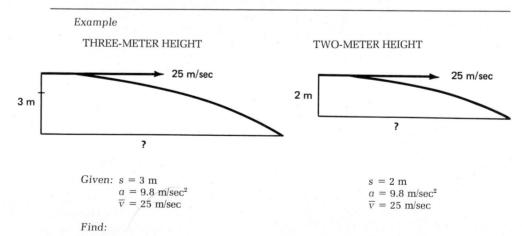

THREE-METER HEIGHT

25 m/sec

3 m

?

TWO-METER HEIGHT

25 m/sec

2 m

?

Given: $s = 3$ m
$a = 9.8$ m/sec^2
$\bar{v} = 25$ m/sec

$s = 2$ m
$a = 9.8$ m/sec^2
$\bar{v} = 25$ m/sec

Find:

1. The **time** object will be in the air before it drops to the ground. Use Equation 2, $s = \frac{1}{2}at^2$, and solve for t:

$$s = \tfrac{1}{2}at^2$$
$$t^2 = \frac{2s}{a}$$
$$t = \sqrt{\frac{6}{9.8}}$$

$$\boxed{t = .78 \text{ sec}}$$

$$s = \tfrac{1}{2}at^2$$
$$t^2 = \frac{2s}{a}$$
$$t = \sqrt{\frac{4}{9.8}}$$

$$\boxed{t = .64 \text{ sec}}$$

2. The **horizontal distance** the object will travel before it hits the ground. Use the velocity equation, $\bar{v} = s/t$, and solve for s:

$$\bar{v} = s/t$$
$$s = \bar{v}t$$
$$s = 25 \times 0.78$$

$$\boxed{s = 19.5 \text{ meters}}$$

$$\bar{v} = s/t$$
$$s = \bar{v}t$$
$$s = 25 \times 0.64$$

$$\boxed{s = 16 \text{ meters}}$$

Diagonal Projections

More often than not, objects put in flight will be sent in directions other than exactly vertical or horizontal. They will be projected at some angle with respect to the horizontal or vertical. If no other force acts on such an object except that which propels it into space, the object's inertia will cause it to continue to move at the same speed and in the same direction it had at the moment of release. Released at the angle shown in Figure 10–14, it would move toward point A. But the projectile does not do this. As with the horizontally projected object, this object begins dropping the instant it is projected into space. It moves downward with an increasing velocity according to the constant acceleration of gravity following a flight path the shape of a parabola. At the end of ½ second the object will have dropped 4 feet ($s = \tfrac{1}{2}at^2$) and be at point B. At the end of 1 second it will have dropped a total of 16 feet and be at point C (see Table 10–1).

Since this type of projectile flight has both horizontal and vertical velocity imparted to it initially, its flight will be determined by the nature of each of these components (Figure 10–15). The vertical flight of the object is the resultant of the imparted upward vertical velocity and the downward acceleration due to gravity (32 ft/sec² or 9.8 m/sec²). The resultant vertical velocity is a vector quantity which diminishes in amount until it reaches zero at the high point. It then continues to increase in

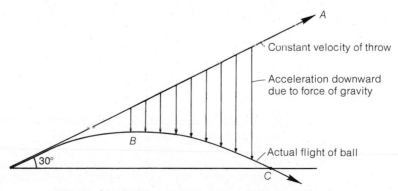

Figure 10–14   Effect of gravity on the flight of a projectile.

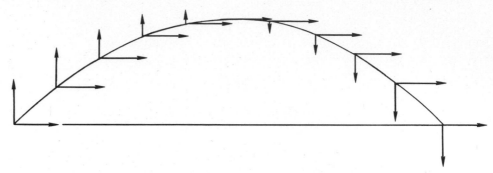

Figure 10–15 Magnitude of horizontal and vertical velocities during projectile flight.

the opposite direction until it is equal in amount but opposite in direction to its release value at the point when it lands at the same level as the release. The horizontal flight is governed only by the horizontal velocity of the projection and is shown in Figure 10–15 as a vector of constant length throughout the flight. Unlike the vertical velocity, the horizontal velocity remains constant because no other horizontal force is introduced to alter it (air resistance excluded). Therefore, the horizontal distance covered is the product of the horizontal velocity and the time in flight.

Optimum Angle of Flight

It has been shown that the horizontal distance that an object will travel in space depends upon both its horizontal velocity and the length of time that the object is in flight. The latter depends upon the height of its high point and that in turn is governed by the vertical velocity imparted to the object at release. Thus the horizontal distance an object will travel depends upon both the horizontal and vertical components of velocity that the projectile has at the initiation of flight. The size of these components depends upon the projection velocity and the projection angle. In Figure 10–16, the initial projection velocity of each projectile is the same, but Flight B has a projection angle twice that of Flight A. From the diagram it can be seen that the horizontal velocity component for Flight A is greater than its vertical component and that it is also greater than the horizontal velocity component for B. In contrast, the vertical velocity of B is greater than its horizontal velocity as well as the vertical velocity of A.

This can be shown mathematically using right triangle relationships:

Example

FLIGHT A	FLIGHT B
Given: Initial velocity 80 ft/sec	80 ft/sec
Angle of release 30°	60°

Find: Horizontal velocity 80 × cos 30° =   80 × cos 60° =
80 × .866 = $\boxed{69.3 \text{ ft/sec}}$ 80 × 0.50 = $\boxed{40 \text{ ft/sec}}$
Find: Vertical velocity 80 × sin 30°   80 × sin 60° =
80 × 0.50 = $\boxed{40 \text{ ft/sec}}$ 80 × 0.866 = $\boxed{69.3 \text{ ft/sec}}$

A simple experiment with a garden hose demonstrates that a stream of water projected vertically—i.e., at 90 degrees—will go higher than a stream projected at any other angle and drops from that stream will remain in the air longer. This stream has no horizontal velocity and therefore no horizontal distance is covered. A stream

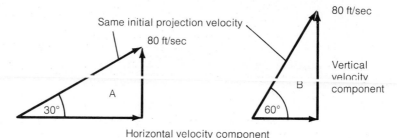

Figure 10–16 Effect of projection angle upon the magnitude of horizontal and vertical velocity components. As the angle decreases, the horizontal component increases and the vertical component decreases.

projected at 0 degrees at ground level has no vertical velocity component but consists entirely of horizontal velocity. The stream will not travel any vertical distance, but neither will it travel any horizontal distance in space in spite of its horizontal velocity. Vertical distance is needed for time in flight and this stream has none. If one were to experiment with other hose nozzle angles between 0° and 90° it would soon become apparent that different angles of projection produce different trajectories for the water stream, and that there is a pattern in the relationship between the angles and the vertical and horizontal distances of the flight paths. In Figure 10–17 Paths A and B show the least amount of horizontal displacement and, although the amount of horizontal displacement for both is the same, the vertical displacements are quite different. The angle of elevation for A is the complement of the angle for B (90° − B). This is also true for C and D. The angle for C is 60 degrees and for D it is 30 degrees. Either elevation angle will result in the same landing spot, but Flight D will go *higher* and take *longer* to land. Any complementary angles of projection produce the same horizontal displacements, but the vertical displacements resulting from the larger of the two angles will always be greater. The relationships are such that the greater the difference between the two angles, the greater is the vertical difference between the high points of their corresponding trajectories. Path E shows the flight when the initial angle is 45 degrees, the angle at which the vertical and horizontal components are equal. This angle represents the best compromise between maximum time in the air and maximum horizontal velocity, and therefore is theoretically the optimum angle for greatest horizontal distance.

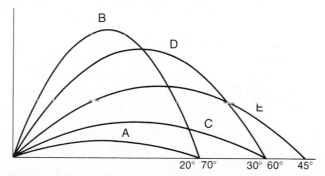

Figure 10–17 The angle of projection influences the horizontal and vertical distance covered by a projectile. Complementary angles of projection produce the same horizontal displacement.

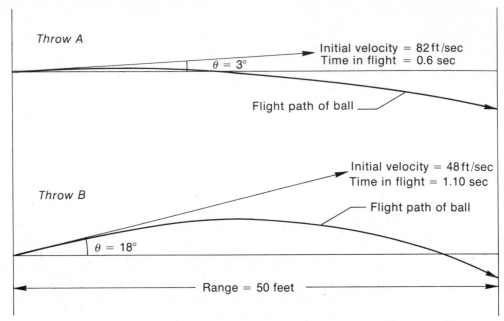

Figure 10–18 Comparison of flight paths of balls thrown with different initial velocities.

The optimum angle of flight depends upon many factors, including the purpose of the trajectory. Tennis lobs and high football punts are examples of Flights B or D and are used when extra time is desired. On the other hand, the longer an object is in the air, the greater the time for air and wind resistance to alter the flight. Where this is a detriment, flight patterns such as A or C should be selected. Moreover there are many occasions when the speed with which the object gets from A to B is extremely important. Base throwing in baseball is an example. The flatter the trajectory the faster the ball will reach its destination provided, of course, that its horizontal velocity is sufficiently great to get it to its destination before gravity causes it to drop too much. Figure 10–18 shows the trajectories of two balls thrown at a spot on a wall 50 feet away. Each ball was thrown as "hard and as fast" as the thrower was capable of throwing. Throw A reached the wall in .61 second while Throw B took 1.10 seconds. The velocity of the throw for A was 82 ft/sec and for B it was 48 ft/sec. The release angle for A was 3 degrees; for B it was 18 degrees.

Three factors control the range of a projectile: the angle, the speed of the release, and the height of release. As has already been pointed out the theoretical optimum angle for maximum horizontal distance is 45°. This is true, however, only when air resistance is discounted and the release and landing occur at the same level. If the landing is lower than the release, such as in shot-putting or throwing the hammer, an angle less than 45° is needed. How much less depends upon two factors. The first is the amount of difference between release and landing level. The greater this difference, the more the optimum angle must be decreased. The second factor is the initial velocity. All other things being equal, the greater the initial velocity the less the optimum angle needs to be decreased from 45°. Table 10–2 shows the relationships among speed, height, and angle as they affect the horizontal range in shot-putting.

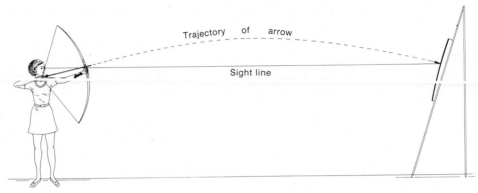

Figure 10–19 The force of gravity affects the flight of an arrow. An archer must account for this effect when aiming.

The characteristics of a projectile flight also affect the way one must aim for accuracy. A baseball pitcher must account for gravity by aiming at a point above the batter's head in order to compensate for gravity. In target archery there is only one distance away from the target where an archer uses point blank aim. At all other distances the arrow tip is aimed either above or below the target (Figure 10–19).

After reading this discussion of projectiles it should be apparent to the reader that how far one can throw a ball depends upon both the velocity one is capable of imparting to the ball and the angle of release. A person may execute a short throw because of a poor angle choice or because of inability to impart speed to the ball. Since alterations in angle are readily changed, it would seem that a measure of speed of the throw would be a better measure of skill than distance thrown. Improvements in

TABLE 10–2 Variation of Optimum Angle With Height and Speed of Release*

HEIGHT OF RELEASE	SPEED OF RELEASE					
	28 ft/sec	32 ft/sec	36 ft/sec	40 ft/sec	44 ft/sec	48 ft/sec
8 ft 0 in	38° (31.34 ft)	39° (38.99 ft)	40° (47.58 ft)	41° (57.13 ft)	42° (67.65 ft)	42° (79.15 ft)
7 ft 6 in	38° (30.95 ft)	39° (38.58 ft)	40° (47.15 ft)	41° (56.69 ft)	42° (67.21 ft)	42° (78.69 ft)
7 ft 0 in	39° (30.55 ft)	40° (38.16 ft)	41° (46.73 ft)	41° (56.25 ft)	42° (66.76 ft)	42° (78.23 ft)
6 ft 6 in	39° (30.16 ft)	40° (37.75 ft)	41° (46.29 ft)	42° (55.81 ft)	42° (66.31 ft)	43° (77.78 ft)

*The distance obtained by the indicated combinations of speed of release, height of release, and optimum angle are shown in parentheses. These distances do not include the extra distance (approximately 1 foot) that the shot is in advance of the inside edge of the stop board at the instant of release. (From Hay, 1978.)

throwing ability then would be noted by increases of speed of release. Cooper and Glassow (1976) present a method for determining the speed of a throw when the time of flight, range, release height, and landing height are known.

Angular Kinematics

Angular kinematics is very similar to linear kinematics because it is also concerned with displacement, velocity, and acceleration. The important difference is that the displacement, velocity, and acceleration are related to rotatory rather than to linear motion and, although the equations used to show the relationships among these quantities are quite similar to those used in linear motion, the units used to describe them are different (Table 10–3).

Angular Displacement

The human skeleton is made up of a system of levers that by definition are rigid bars that rotate about fixed points when force is applied. When any object acting as a rigid bar moves in an arc about an axis, the movement is called rotatory or angular motion. An attempt to describe angular motion in linear units presents real problems. As an object moves in an arc, the linear displacement of particles spaced along that lever varies. Particles nearer the axis have a displacement in inches, meters, feet, or centimeters that is less than those farther away. For example, in the underarm throw pattern the hand moves through a greater distance than the wrist and the wrist a greater distance than the elbow. Rotatory motion needs rotatory units to describe it. As might be expected, these units relate to the units of a circle and the fact that the circumference of a circle, C, is equal to $2\pi r$, where r is the radius and π is a constant value of 3.1416.

TABLE 10–3 Relationships Between Rotatory and Linear Motion

	LINEAR	ROTATORY
Symbols		
Displacement	s	θ
Velocity	$v, u, \bar{v}$	$\omega_v, \omega_u, \bar{\omega}$
Acceleration	$a, \bar{a}$	$\alpha, \bar{\alpha}$
Time	t	t
Equations		
Displacement	$s = u + \frac{1}{2}at^2$	$\theta = \omega_u + \frac{1}{2}\alpha t^2$
Velocity	$v = u + at$	$\omega_v = \omega_u + \alpha t$
	$v^2 = u^2 + 2as$	$\omega_1^2 = \omega_0^2 + 2\alpha\theta$
Acceleration	$a = \frac{v-u}{t}$	$\alpha = \frac{\omega_v - \omega_u}{t}$
Linear and Angular Conversions		
Displacement	$s = \theta r$	$\theta = \frac{s}{r}$
Velocity	$\bar{v} = \bar{\omega} r$	$\bar{\omega} = \frac{\bar{v}}{r}$
Acceleration	$a = \alpha r$	$\alpha = \frac{a}{r}$

There are three interchangeable rotatory or angular units of displacement: degrees, revolutions, and radians. One radian is the same as 57.3 degrees and one full revolution is the same as 360 degrees or 2π radians of displacement. The word revolution is not stated, but it is understood when we say that a diver executed a 1½ somersault tuck. The dive could also be described as a tuck somersault of 540 (360 + 180) degrees or 3π radians. Degrees are used most frequently in the measurement of angles, but radians, the term favored by engineers and physicists, are the units most often required in equations of angular motion. The symbol for angular displacement is the Greek letter θ (theta).*

Angular Velocity

The rate of rotatory displacement is called angular velocity, symbolized as ω (omega). Angular velocity is equal to the angle through which the radius turns divided by the time it takes for the displacement:

$$\overline{\omega} = \frac{\theta}{t}$$

It is expressed as degrees/second, radians/second, or revolutions/second. A softball pitcher who moves the arm through an arc of 140 degrees in 0.1 second has an average angular velocity of 1400 degrees per second. This could also be expressed as 3.88 revolutions per second or 24.43 radians/second. This velocity is called average velocity because film studies of pitchers show that the angular displacement during the execution of the skill is not uniform, and a velocity such as this represents the average velocity over the time span through which the displacement is measured. As with linear movements, most angular human movements are likely to be variable and not uniform. The longer the time span through which the displacement is measured the more variability is averaged. Thus, if one is interested in the velocity at a specific instant in a skill, the displacement must be measured over an extremely small time span. Figure 10–20 shows variations in displacement during the execution of the golf drive. When the total angular displacement of the golf club was measured from the beginning of the downswing to the point of contact with the ball and divided by the time it took for the swing, the average velocity of the club was 2148 degrees/sec (37.5 rad/sec). The "instant" velocity at A, however, was 1432 degrees/sec, and at B it was 2864 degrees/sec.

Angular Acceleration

In the discussion of linear velocity, a change in velocity was called acceleration. The same is true for changes in angular velocity. Angular acceleration α (alpha) is the rate of change of angular velocity and is expressed in equation form as:

$$\alpha = \frac{\omega_v - \omega_u}{t}$$

where ω_v is final velocity, ω_u is initial velocity, and t is time. If, in Figure 10–20, the angular velocity is 25 rad/sec at A and 50 rad/sec at B and the time lapse between A and B is 0.11 seconds, the angular acceleration between A and B is 241 rad/sec/sec. This value for α indicating that the velocity increased 241 radians per second each second would be true, of course, only if the velocity increased at a uniform rate.

---

*For a review of the geometry of circles and an additional explanation of degrees, radians, and revolutions, see Appendix F, Part 5.

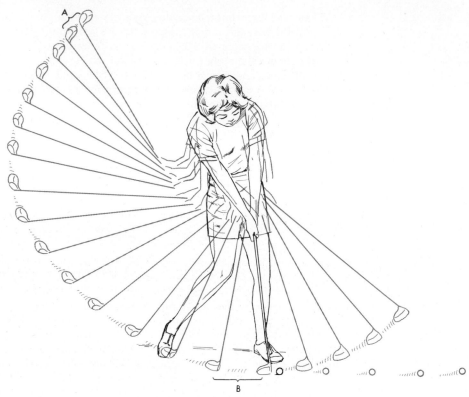

Figure 10–20 Variations in angular displacement of golf club over equal time intervals during the execution of a golf drive. (Drawn from motion picture film tracing.)

Otherwise this value has to be considered as an average of accelerations that may have been higher or lower during the time period studied.

Relationship Between Linear and Angular Motion

The description of angular motion in terms of displacement, velocity, and acceleration can tell us a great deal about human movements, but nothing in such a description accounts for or shows the effect of the length of the radius on the outcomes of the movements. We know that, all other things being equal, a baseball hit in the middle of a bat will not go as far as one hit at the end, that a ball hit by a tennis racket as an extension of the arm will travel farther than a ball hit with the hand, and that a golf driver will cause a struck ball to travel farther than a nine iron. In each instance greater force is imparted to the struck object because the radius of the striking implement (distance between axis and point of contact) is longer and greater linear velocity is generated at its end. As can be seen in Figure 10–21, Lever A is shorter than B, and B is shorter than C. If all three levers are moved through the same angular distance in the same amount of time, it is apparent that the end of Lever A would move with less speed than would the end of either B or C. All three levers have the same *angular velocity*, but linear velocity of the circular motion at the end of each lever is proportional to the length of the lever. An object moved at the end of a long radius will have a greater linear velocity than one moved at the end of a short radius, *if*

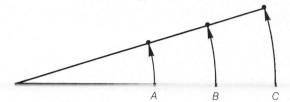

Figure 10–21 Lever A < B < C. Although the angular displacement for all three levers is the same, the linear displacement at the end of the longer levers is greater than that at the end of the shorter levers.

the angular velocity is kept constant. *The longer the radius, the greater is the linear velocity.* Thus it is to the advantage of a performer to use as long a lever as possible to impart linear velocity to an object if the long lever length does not cause too great a sacrifice in angular velocity. The longer the lever the more effort it takes to swing it. Therefore, the optimum length of the lever for a person depends upon the individual's ability to maintain angular velocity. A child who cannot handle the weight of a long radius is better off with a shortened implement that can be controlled and swung rapidly, whereas a strong adult profits by using a longer radius.

If the reverse occurs—that is, if the linear velocity is kept constant—an increase in radius will result in a decrease in angular velocity. Once an object is engaged in rotatory motion, the linear velocity at the end of the radius stays the same due to the conservation of momentum. The radius of rotation for a pike somersault dive is longer than that for a tuck somersault, and the radius for a layout somersault is longer than that for a pike somersault. If one starts a dive in an open position and then tucks tightly, the radius of rotation decreases but, because the linear velocity does not change, the angular velocity increases. The same situation occurs when a figure skater rotating slowly about a vertical axis with arms and one leg out to the side brings the arms and leg close to the axis. The radius decreases and the angular velocity increases. To slow down, the skater again reaches out with arms and leg. Figure 10–22 shows the effect of shortening the radius while maintaining a constant linear velocity at the end of the radius. *Shortening the radius will increase the angular velocity and lengthening it will decrease the angular velocity.* Points a and b on Radii A and B have moved through the same linear distance, but the angular displacement for A is greater than that for B. If the displacements of a and b each take place in the same amount of time, the linear velocities will be equal, but the angular velocity for A will be greater than that of B.

The relationship which exists between the angular velocity of an object moving in a rotatory fashion and the linear velocity at the end of its radius is expressed by the equation

$$\overline{v} = \omega\, r$$

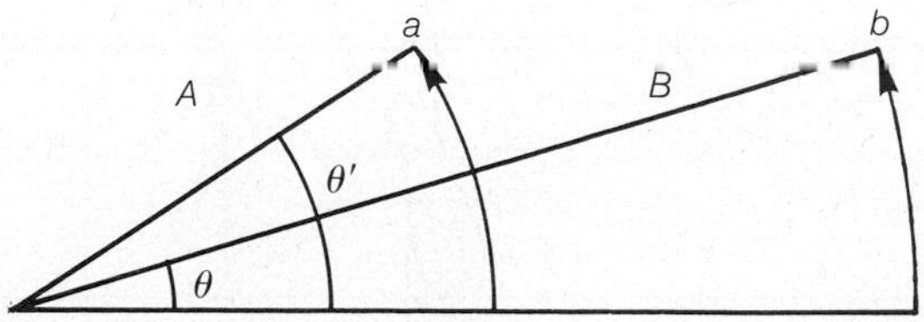

Figure 10–22 Increasing the length of the radius decreases the angular velocity when the linear velocity remains constant.

To use the equation in this form, ω must be expressed in radians. If the angular velocity is expressed in degrees/second, the equation becomes

$$\bar{v} = \frac{\omega r}{57.3}$$

Either form of the equation shows the direct proportionality that exists between linear velocity and the radius. For any given angular velocity, the linear velocity is proportional to the radius. If the radius doubles, the linear velocity does likewise. And for any given linear velocity, the angular velocity is inversely proportional to the radius. If the radius doubles, the angular velocity decreases by half. To achieve higher linear velocities at the end of levers, the motions must be done with longer levers or higher angular velocities (Figure 10–23).

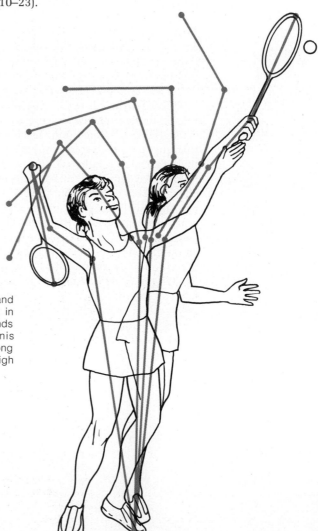

Figure 10–23 Long levers and high angular velocities result in high linear velocities at the ends of the levers. Thus the tennis racket, an extension of a long body lever, is able to impart high linear velocity to the ball.

Laboratory Experiences

1. An Olympic skater who participated in the men's speed skating events had the following times: 1500 m in 2 min 2.96 sec; 5000 m in 7 min 23.61 sec; and 10,000 m in 15 min 1.35 sec. What was his average speed for each of these events?

2. Using the concept of acceleration explain how a swimmer can have a better time for a 100-m race in a 25-m pool than in a 100-m pool.

3. How much time will a batter have to decide to swing at a pitch and still hit it under these circumstances?
   a. The pitcher throws the ball at 80 mph.
   b. The distance from the ball release to the plate is 56 ft.
   c. It takes the batter .30 second to get the bat to the desired contact point.

4. With the help of several classmates prepare a displacement-time graph and a velocity-time graph for your performance on the 50- or 100-yard dash. Class members should be spaced at 5-yard intervals along your running path, each with a stopwatch. On the signal for you to go, each timer will start the watch and stop it when you pass that timer's position. Prepare a table with the following data for each run:
   a. Distance intervals.
   b. Times recorded at each interval.
   c. Times over each 5-yard interval (subtract adjacent times).
   d. Average velocity over each 5-yard interval $\left(\bar{v} = \dfrac{s}{t} = \dfrac{15}{t_2 - t_1}\right)$.

   For each set of data prepare a displacement-time graph and a velocity time graph for the whole run. Describe your run in terms of displacement, velocity, and acceleration. Compare your graphs with other members of the group, and note any differences.

5. An arrow shot straight up into the air reached a height of 75 m. With what velocity did it leave the bow? How long was it in the air?

6. Place one coin near the edge of a table and another on the end of a ruler, as shown in the diagram. While pressing the center of the ruler to the table with an index finger, strike one end of it in the direction indicated so that both coins land on the ground. Diagram the path of each. Which hits the floor first? Explain.

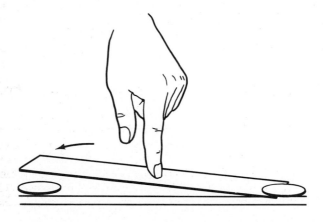

7. Throw a ball so that it is projected vertically upward. Catch it at the same height it was released. Have a partner measure the time the ball is in the air—i.e., from the time of release to the time the ball lands in your hand. Determine the velocity of the ball at the moment of release and the distance the ball traveled before it started its descent. Graph the flight of the ball on a piece of graph paper.

8. While walking along at a constant speed, project a ball vertically into the air. If you continue to walk without changing your speed or direction, where will the ball land? Explain. Draw a diagram of the ball's flight indicating the forces acting on it.

9. Assume that you are able to throw a ball with a velocity of 80 ft/sec and at an angle of 45 degrees with the horizontal. If it is caught at the same height from the ground at which it was released, neglecting air resistance, how far will it go? How long will it be in flight? Repeat with a 30-degree angle of release. How would these values change if the landing height were lowered?

10. Using Figure 10–3 determine the angular velocity of the lower leg at the knee joint at the beginning of the force phase and at the moment of foot contact with the ball. The time between each stick figure tracing is .0156 second. What is the linear velocity at the ankle at the moment of contact if the lower leg is 16 inches (knee joint to ankle joint)?

References

Basford, L. 1966. *The science of movement.* London: Samson Low, Marston.

Cooper, J. M., and Glassow, R. B. 1976. *Kinesiology.* 4th ed. St. Louis: C. V. Mosby.

Dull, C. E., Metcalfe, H. C., and Williams, J. E. 1963. *Modern physics.* New York: Holt, Rinehart and Winston.

Dyson, G. 1970. *The mechanics of athletics.* 5th ed. London: University of London Press.

Guidelines and standards for undergraduate kinesiology. Prepared by a task force of the Kinesiology Academy, consisting of K. Luttgens, Chair, A. Atwater, R. Burke, C. Dillman, and J. Hay. *J. Phys. Educ. Rec.* 51:19–21, 1980.

Hay, J. G. 1978. *The biomechanics of sports techniques.* 2d ed. Englewood Cliffs, N.J.: Prentice-Hall.

Jensen, C. R., and Schultz, G. W. 1970. *Applied kinesiology,* New York: McGraw-Hill.

Kelley, D. 1971. *Kinesiology—fundamentals of motion description.* Englewood Cliffs, N.J.: Prentice-Hall.

LeVeau, B. 1977. *Williams and Lissner: Biomechanics of human motion.* 2d ed. Philadelphia: W. B. Saunders.

McCloy, C. H. 1960. The mechanical analysis of motor skills. In *Science and medicine of exercise and sports,* ed. W. R. Johnson. New York: Harper & Row, pp. 54–64.

Miller, D. L., and Nelson, R. C. 1973. *Biomechanics of sport.* Philadelphia: Lea & Febiger.

Mortimer, E. M. 1951. Basketball shooting. *Res. Q. Am. Assoc. Health Phys. Educ. Rec.* 22:234–43.

Northrip, J., Logan G., and McKinney, W. 1979. *Biomechanic analysis of sport.* 2d ed. Dubuque, Iowa: William C. Brown.

Ruchlis, H. 1958. *Orbit: A picture story of force and motion.* New York: Harper & Row.

The Conditions of Linear Motion

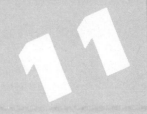

Objectives

At the conclusion of this chapter, the student should be able to:

1. Name, define, and use the following terms properly as they apply to linear motion: force, inertia, mass, weight, momentum, and impulse.

2. Explain what is meant by the terms magnitude, direction, and point of application of force and use these terms properly as they apply to internal and external forces.

3. Explain the effect of specified changes in the magnitude, direction, and point of application of force on the motion state of a body.

4. Define and give examples of the terms linear forces, concurrent forces, and parallel forces.

5. Determine the magnitude, direction, and point of application of muscle forces in hypothetical situations where specific muscles are considered in isolation.

6. State Newton's laws as they apply to linear motion.

7. Explain the cause and effect relationship between the forces responsible for linear motion and the objects experiencing the motion.

8. Name and define the basic external forces responsible for modifying motion: weight, normal reaction, friction, elasticity, buoyancy, drag, and lift.

9. Draw and analyze simple two-dimensional free-body diagrams in which all applicable external forces are properly accounted for.

10. Explain the work-energy relationship as it applies to a body experiencing linear motion.

11. Define and use properly the terms work, power, kinetic energy, and potential energy.

The Nature of Force

Objects start moving when they are pushed or pulled—that is, when some type of force acts on them. Forces produce motion, stop motion, and prevent motion. They may increase speed, decrease speed, or cause objects to change direction. They may push or pull to cause motion or produce a net effect so that bodies remain stationary. *Force is defined as that which pushes or pulls through direct mechanical contact or through the force of gravity to alter the motion of an object.* It is the effect that one body has on another.

The action of a force may be internal or external. Internal forces are defined as forces exerted by bodies on other bodies within a defined system, whereas external forces are those exerted by bodies within an arbitrarily specified system on bodies outside of the specified system. Internal forces cause differences in body shape and external forces cause displacement of the body. In kinesiology, internal forces are usually classified as muscle forces that act on the various structures of the body and external forces are those outside the body. The best known external force is weight, or gravitational force. Wind or water resistance forces, friction, or forces due to other objects acting on the body are also external forces.

Aspects of Force

How a force affects a body is determined by the size or **magnitude** of the force, the **direction** in which the force is acting, and the exact point at which the force is **applied** to the object. In order to describe force fully, all three of these characteristics must be identified and taken into account. A change in any one of them alters the nature of the motion. Two 50-pound forces applied in the same direction and in line with the center of an object will result in linear motion. The same forces also applied in the same direction but off center will cause rotatory motion. Finally, no motion will occur if these forces are applied at the same point but in opposite directions.

Magnitude, direction, and point of application are explained in the following sections as they relate to the external force of gravity and to internal muscular force.

MAGNITUDE   The force of gravity is the external force with which the human body must contend in all movement experience. It is the force that gives bodies weight, and it is measured in terms of the body's weight. When one holds a ball in the hand, the pull of gravity is felt as the weight of the ball. The ball stays in the hand as long as an equal and opposite force acting between the hand and the ball balances the downward gravitational force. In this example the equal and opposite force is muscular. When the opposing force is removed, the ball drops and gravity's pull is apparent in the downward motion of the ball. The weight of the ball is the **magnitude** of the force of gravity acting on the ball.

The magnitude of force that a body can exert varies with its location. The farther away an object is from the earth's center, the less gravitational pull it has and therefore the less weight. The equation for weight is $W = mg$, where m is the mass or quantity of matter of the object and g is the accelerative rate of gravity, accepted as 32 ft/sec² (9.8 km/sec/sec). The basic unit of force (weight) in the English system is the pound and in the metric system it is the newton (see Table 9–1). The pound is defined as the weight of a standard pound at sea level and at 45 degrees latitude. A newton is the force needed to lift a mass of 0.102 kilogram under the same conditions.

The magnitude of muscular force is in direct proportion to the number and size of the fibers in the muscle that is contracting. If muscles contracted individually, it would be a relatively easy matter to measure the force exerted by each one in a given movement. Since they normally act in groups, however, their force or strength is measured collectively. It is customary to measure maximum muscular strength by performing a simple movement against the resistance of a dynamometer, spring balance, or similar instrument. The instrument thus serves as the resistance to an anatomical lever whose force is provided by a group of muscles that act as a functional team to produce the movement of the lever. Among the muscle groups that are frequently measured by this method are the finger flexors (grip strength), elbow flexors, and knee extensors.

Although there is no way of determining the amount of force exerted by a single muscle in the living body, its potential strength can be calculated from its measurements, its internal structure, and the approximate number of pounds (or kilograms) that the average human muscle is known to exert per square inch (or centimeter). The muscle's external measurements and its internal structure form the basis for determining its physiological cross section, a term that refers to the perpendicular section of all the muscle's fibers. A study of the internal structure of various muscles reveals a variety of arrangements. In some muscles the fibers are arranged longitudinally, in some, in spindlelike fashion, in some, fanlike, and in some, featherlike (see page 34). Obviously a simple cross section of a penniform or bipenniform muscle will miss a large number of the fibers; hence a true cross section of the muscle's fibers is one that cuts across every fiber in the muscle. Figure 11–1 illustrates the method of measuring the physiological cross section of several types of muscles. The cross section does not reveal the actual number of fibers, to be sure, but it corresponds closely enough for us to use this measurement in estimating the muscle's potential force. The physiological cross section is found by adding the lengths of the lines that cut perpendicularly across the fibers and multiplying their sum by the average thickness of the muscle. Such measurements can, of course, only be made on dissected muscles, but in the living body they can be roughly estimated from the approximate circumference and length of the muscle belly and from a knowledge of the muscle's internal structure. Suppose a penniform muscle is 7 inches long, exclusive of its tendons, and its average thickness is ¾ of an inch. Suppose further that it takes three lines, measuring

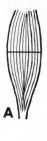
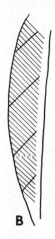
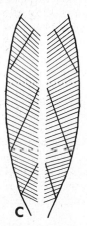

Figure 11–1 Method of measuring the physiological cross section of three types of muscles. *A*, A fusiform or spindle muscle. *B*, A penniform muscle. *C*, A bipenniform muscle.

respectively 4, 5, and 3 inches, to cut perpendicularly across the fibers. The physiological cross section of such a muscle is ¾ (4 + 5 + 3) = ¾ × 12 = 9 square inches.

The amount of force that the average human muscle can exert has been determined by several experiments. Fick (1910, 1929), one of the early investigators, found that human muscles exerted a force of 6 to 10 kilograms per square centimeter of their physiological cross section. This is approximately 85 to 141 pounds per square inch. Recklinghausen, according to Steindler (1970), concluded from his experimentation that human muscles exerted only 3.6 kilograms per square centimeter (approximately 51 pounds per square inch) of cross section. It is assumed that these two investigators used male subjects. A more recent investigator, Morris (1948), found that the muscles of male subjects exerted 9.2 kilograms per square centimeter (130 pounds per square inch), and of female subjects 7.1 kilograms per square centimeter (101 pounds per square inch). Because of the wide range of figures presented to date, further investigation of this matter would seem desirable. A study of the effect of training on muscular force per unit of cross section would also be of interest. If 95 pounds per square inch is arbitrarily selected as the force that an average human muscle can exert, the hypothetical muscle described above, having a physiological cross section of 9 square inches, would have a potential force of 9 × 95, or 855 pounds.

POINT OF APPLICATION   The point of application of a force is that point at which the force is applied to an object. Where gravity is concerned this point is always through the center of gravity of an object. For practical purposes it may be assumed that the point of application of muscular force is the center of the muscle's attachment to the bony lever. This usually corresponds to the muscle's insertion or distal attachment. Technically, however, it is the point of intersection between the line of force and the *mechanical axis* of the bone or segment serving as the anatomical lever. This axis does not necessarily pass lengthwise through the shaft of the bony lever. If the bone bends or if the articulating process projects at an angle from the shaft, the greater part of the axis may lie completely outside the shaft, as in the case of the femur (see Figure 1–2). *The mechanical axis of a bone or segment is a straight line that connects the midpoint of the joint at one end with the midpoint of the joint at the other end or, in the case of a terminal segment, with its distal end.*

DIRECTION   The direction of a force is along its action line. Because the force of gravity pulls all objects toward the earth's center, the direction of gravitational forces is vertically downward. The force of gravity acting on an object would be represented as a downward directed vector starting at the center of gravity of the object.

The direction of muscular force is represented by the direction of the muscle's line of pull. This direction is identified by the muscle's angle of pull that is bounded by the muscle's line of pull and the portion of the mechanical axis that lies between the point of application and the fulcrum. Figure 11–2A shows a muscle (the biceps) applying its force to a lever (the radius) at an angle of 30 degrees, while Figures 11–2B and C illustrate other angles of pull.

Resolution of Forces   Since force has the qualities of both magnitude and direction, it is a vector quantity. Graphically, the magnitude of the force is represented by the length of the vector line. The point of application of the force is the point where the force vector starts, and the direction of the force is always represented as a pull away from the point of applica-

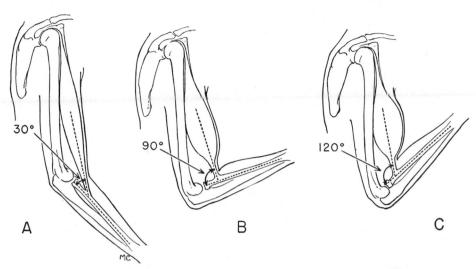

Figure 11-2 Angles of muscle pull, *A,* An angle less than 45 degrees . *B,* An angle of 90 degrees . *C,*An angle greater than 90 degrees .

tion. The vector line represents the line of force, and the arrowhead indicates the direction of the force application (Figure 11–3).

ANGLE OF PULL   As with any vector, a force may be resolved into a vertical and a horizontal component, and the relative size of these components depends upon the angle at which the force is applied. Where muscles are involved, the size of a muscles's angle of pull changes with every degree of joint motion and consequently so do the sizes of the horizontal and vertical components. These changes have a direct bearing on the effectiveness of the muscle's pulling force in moving the bony lever. The larger the angle between 0 degrees and 90 degrees the greater the vertical component and the less the horizontal component.

The vertical component of muscle pull is always perpendicular to the lever and is called the rotatory component. It is that part of the force that moves the lever. The horizontal component is parallel to the lever and is the nonrotatory component. It does not contribute to the lever's movement. The angle of pull of most muscles in the resting position is less than a right angle and it usually remains so throughout the movement (Figure 11–2A). This means that the nonrotatory component of force is directed toward the fulcrum, which gives it a stabilizing effect. By pulling the bone lengthwise toward the joint it helps to maintain the integrity of the joint. Under most circumstances, therefore, muscular force has two simultaneous functions—movement and stabilization. In the latter capacity it supplements the ligaments, an excellent example of the body's efficiency, since muscles perform this stabilizing function only during the period when the segment is moving, at which time the integrity of the joint may be threatened.

Occasionally the angle of pull becomes greater than a right angle, which means that the nonrotatory component of force is directed away from the fulcrum and is therefore a dislocating component. This does not happen in many instances, however,

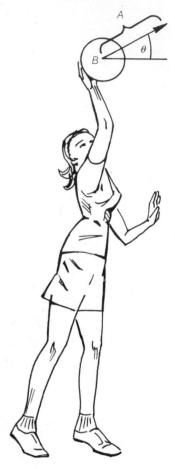

Figure 11–3 Graphic representation of a force vector. The magnitude of the force is the vector line, *A;* the point of application is the beginning of the vector, *B;* and the direction of the vector is represented by the arrowhead and the angle, *θ*. (Drawn from motion picture film tracing.)

and, when it does, the muscle is close to the limit of its shortening range and is therefore not exerting much force (Figure 11–2C).

When the angle of pull is 90 degrees, the force is completely rotatory. When it is 45 degrees the rotatory and stabilizing components are equal. Since the angle of pull usually remains less than 45 degrees, more of the muscle's force serves to stabilize the joint than to move the lever. In fact, there are some muscles whose angles of pull are always so small that their contribution to motion would seem to be negligible. This appears to be true of the coracobrachialis and the subclavius muscles. It is interesting to note that the upper extremity is frequently called upon to perform violent, powerful movements, as well as to support the body weight in suspension. The joints which bear the brunt of this violence and strain are the shoulder and sternoclavicular joints. They might well become dislocated more easily than they do were it not for the coracobrachialis and the subclavius muscles, which pull the bones lengthwise toward their proximal joints and thus serve to stabilize these joints.

The effect the angle of pull has upon the rotatory force of a muscle for a given angle is demonstrated in the following problem. The solution clearly shows an increase in rotatory force with each increase in angle size.

Example:

Muscle M exerts a force of 100 pounds at insertion and is pulling at an angle of 30 degrees. How much of its force is rotatory? stabilizing? How do these values change when the angle of pull is 10 degrees? 75 degrees? (See Figure 11–4.)

Solution:

ANGLE OF PULL OF 30°

Construct a right triangle where $\sin 30° = \dfrac{A}{100}$.

Rotatory component equals $100 \times \sin 30° = 50$ lb
Stabilizing component equals $100 \times \cos 30° = 86.6$ lb

ANGLE OF PULL OF 10°

Construct a right triangle where $\sin 10° = \dfrac{A}{100}$.

Rotatory component A equals $100 \times \sin 10° = 17.36$ lb
Stabilizing component B equals $100 \times \cos 10° = 98.48$ lb

ANGLE OF PULL OF 75°

Construct a right triangle where $\sin 75° = \dfrac{A}{100}$.

Rotatory component equals $100 \times \sin 75° = 96.59$ lb
Stabilizing component equals $100 \times \cos 75° = 25.88$ lb

ANATOMICAL PULLEY   The small angle of pull that most muscles have when in their normal resting position has already been noted. Were it not for anatomical devices that serve as fixed single pulleys some muscles would probably be unable to effect any movement whatsoever. The anatomical pulley serves the same purpose as the mechanical fixed single pulley, that of changing the direction of force by changing the angle of pull of the muscle providing the force. For instance, the angle of pull of

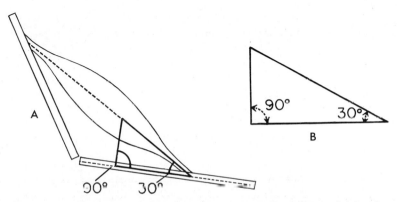

Figure 11–4   Method of constructing a right triangle for the purpose of determining the components of muscular force by the trigonometric method. Note that the hypotenuse coincides with a portion of the muscle's line of pull, and the side adjacent coincides with the mechanical axis of the bone into which the muscle is inserted.

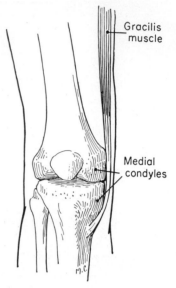

Figure 11–5   The medial condyles at the knee joint serving as a pulley to increase the angle of pull of the gracilis tendon.

the gracilis is increased by means of the bulging medial condyles both above and below the knee joint over which the tendon passes before it attaches to the tibia (Figure 11–5). The patella serves the same purpose for the quadriceps by increasing its angle of pull as it crosses the front of the knee (Figure 11–6). A pulley changing the angle of pull so that it changes the nature of the movement is illustrated by the peroneus longus muscle, which, by passing behind the lateral malleolus before it turns under the foot to attach to the first cuneiform and base of the first metatarsal bone, plantar flexes the foot at the ankle (Figure 11–7). If it passed in front of the malleolus its angle of pull would be shifted in front of the ankle joint, and this would cause it to dorsiflex the foot. In this example the lateral malleolus serves as the "fixed pulley."

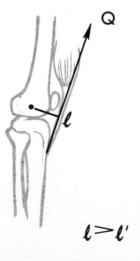

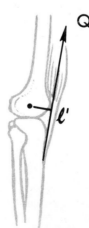

$\ell > \ell'$

Figure 11–6   By increasing the angle of pull the patella increases the rotatory force component of the quadriceps femoris. (From Williams, M., and Lissner, H. R.: *Biomechanics of human motion.* Philadelphia: W. B. Saunders, 1962.)

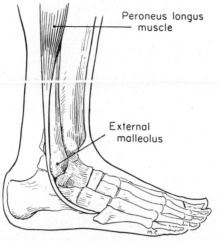

Peroneus longus
muscle

External
malleolus

Figure 11–7 The external malleolus serving as a pulley for the peroneus longus tendon.

RESOLUTION OF EXTERNAL FORCE The resolution of a single external force into component forces acting at right angles to each other is accomplished in the same manner as that explained for muscular forces, and would be used when the force is applied at an oblique angle. If, instead of giving a piece of furniture a horizontal push, one pushes it by standing close to it with the arms held at a forward-downward slant, only part of the force will push the table forward (Figure 11–8). The force is applied to the table at an oblique angle and thus has both a vertical and a horizontal component. Whether or not the table moves forward depends upon the amount of the total force applied in the horizontal direction. If sufficient, only the horizontal component of

Figure 11–8 The diagonal pushing force (*R*) consists of a horizontal and a vertical component. Only the horizontal component (*X*) serves to overcome the table's resistance to being moved. The vertical component (*Y*) adds to the resistance. (Drawn from a photograph.)

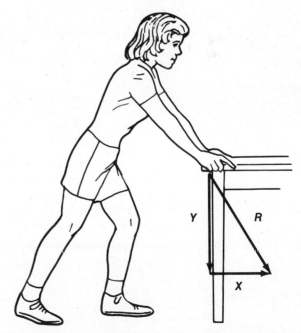

force will overcome the table's resistance to move. The downward component merely pushes the table against the floor and increases the friction between the floor and the table. The closer one can come to applying all of the available force in the desired direction of movement the more efficient will be the action. Another example of this principle is demonstrated in pulling actions. If a child's sled or cart is drawn by too short a rope, there will be a relatively large lifting component and a small forward pulling component. Since the purpose is to pull the cart horizontally, it is more efficient to use a long rope because this gives a relatively greater horizontal or pulling component.

Composite Effects of Two or More Forces

Frequently two or more forces are applied to the same object. A canoe may be acted upon by both the wind and the paddler, one force tending to send the canoe north and the other east. While in flight a punted ball's path is the result of the force imparted to it by the kicker, the downward force of gravity, and the force of the wind, if any. In the body it is rarely, if ever, the case that an individual muscle acts by itself. For example, there are at least four muscles that may act in flexion of the forearm, and more than five that contribute to flexion of the leg at the knee joint. The effect that composite forces have on the human body to cause or modify motion may be classified according to their direction and application as *linear, concurrent, or parallel.*

LINEAR FORCES   Forces applied in the same direction along the same action line are called *linear* forces. If a horizontal push is applied to a piece of furniture and the push is applied in line with the object's center of gravity, the object will move forward in a horizontal direction, providing of course that there is no additional conflicting force or resistance. If another force is applied to the furniture in line with and in the same direction as the first force, the resultant of the two forces has a value equal to the sum of the two forces ($a + b = c$).

Similarly, if the forces act in opposite directions, the resultant still equals the algebraic sum of the two forces ($a + (-b) = c$). This might be the case in a tug of war.

Examples of more than one force applied at the same point and acting in identical directions in the body are rare. Possibly there are two such examples, the gastrocnemius and the soleus acting at the ankle joint, and the psoas and the iliacus acting at the hip joint. In each of these examples, it will be noted that the two muscles have a common tendon for their distal attachments.

CONCURRENT FORCES   Forces acting at one point but at different angles are called *concurrent* forces. Several football players opposing each other in a blocking situation furnish opposing forces that may be considered as acting at one point (Figure 11–9). The resultant outcome of the blocking is found using the method known as the combination of vectors described in Chapter 9. This method assumes a common point of application. While this situation is common externally, it is not true of the majority of muscles that act on the same bone. Very few muscles have a common point of

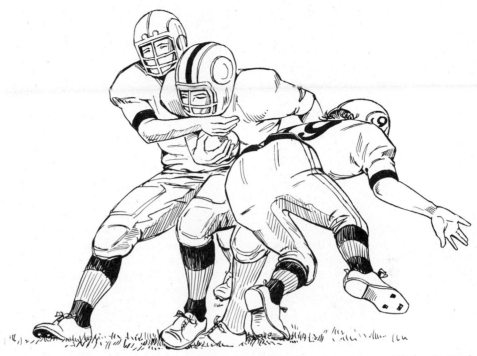

Figure 11–9 Opposing forces acting at one point but at different angles are called concurrent forces.

attachment. Nevertheless, the principle of finding the composite effect of two or more forces, with respect to magnitude and direction, is as true for forces acting on body segments as for forces acting on external objects. The important thing to remember is that the resultant magnitude of two or more concurrent forces is not their arithmetic sum, and the resultant direction of two concurrent forces is not halfway between them unless the two forces are of equal magnitude. *The resultant of two or more concurrent forces depends upon both the magnitude of each force and the angle of application— i.e., the direction of each force.*

PARALLEL FORCES In addition to linear forces, in which all forces occur along the same action line, and concurrent forces, in which forces acting at different angles are applied at the same point, another situation exists in which forces not in the same action line but *parallel* to each other act at different points on a body. The two students in Figure 11–10 are carrying a weight between them. Each one exerts an upward force on an end while the weight exerts a downward force between them. There are three parallel forces here, two in one direction and the third in an opposite direction. All three forces are acting on the same object but at different points. Another example of this situation would be that of holding a 10-pound weight in the hand when the forearm is flexed so that the angle of pull of the biceps is 90 degrees. The force of gravity may be represented as acting at two different points to push the forearm and the weight down while the force of the biceps acting in the opposite direction at another point pulls the forearm up. All three of these forces are parallel to each other but act at different points (Figure 11–11).

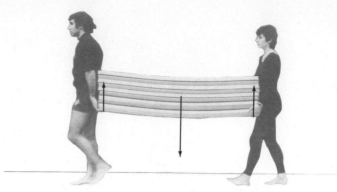

Figure 11-10 Examples of parallel forces. The mats exert a downward force while both carriers exert parallel forces upward.

The effect parallel forces have on the object they act upon depends on the magnitude, direction, and application point of each force. Parallel forces may act in the same or opposite directions. They may be balanced and cause no motion or they may cause linear or rotatory motion. When parallel forces act on an object, their relationship to the object's fixed axis or to its center of gravity, if it can move freely, determines the resultant action. In the case of the weight (mats) held at opposite ends by two students, the mats will remain balanced and motionless if all the forces about the center of gravity are balanced. The mats will move upward in a linear fashion if the students exert equal parallel forces upward that are greater than the downward force of the weight, and they will move in a rotatory fashion about their center of gravity if the students exert equal and opposite parallel forces. Other examples of parallel forces are shown in Figure 11-12.

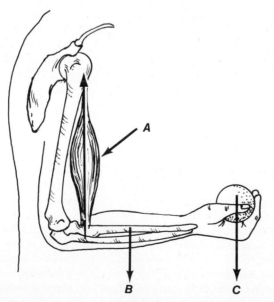

Figure 11-11 Example of parallel forces in equilibrium. The force of the biceps (A) balances the opposite force of gravity acting on the forearm at its center of gravity and on the weight held in the hand.

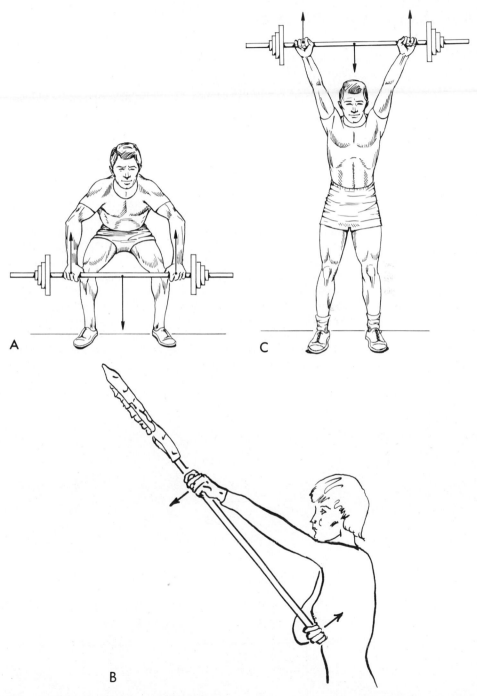

Figure 11–12 Example of parallel forces producing *A*, linear motion, *B*, rotatory motion, and *C*, no motion. (*A* and *C* drawn from motion picture film tracing; *B* drawn from photograph.)

Newton's Laws of Motion

The fact that motion is related to force in a precise manner was observed by Sir Isaac Newton in the seventeenth century. He formulated three Laws of Motion that explain why objects move as they do. Although all of these laws cannot be proved on earth even in ideal experimental situations, they are accepted as universal truths to explain the effects of force.

Law of Inertia   Newton's first Law of Motion states that **a body continues in its state of rest or of uniform motion unless an unbalanced force acts on it.** This means that an object at rest remains at rest, and one in motion will continue at a constant speed in a straight line unless acted on by a force. In effect, it identifies the conditions under which there is no external force. The fact that objects at rest need a force to move them seems obvious, but the need for force to slow or stop an object in motion is not always as apparent. We have all seen moving objects come to rest of their own accord, or what seems to be their own accord, but, in fact, other forces in the form of friction or air resistance caused the change in velocity. The tendency for a body to stay in motion for long periods of time is possible to observe more clearly in laboratory conditions where the effects of friction and air resistance can be minimized but, nevertheless, numerous examples of Newton's first law can still be observed in sport and everyday experiences. Base runners in baseball know it takes force to change velocity suddenly in order to avoid overrunning a base. Skiers continue into space if they traverse a hill or mogul at high speed (Figure 11–13). And everyone at sometime or other has exper-

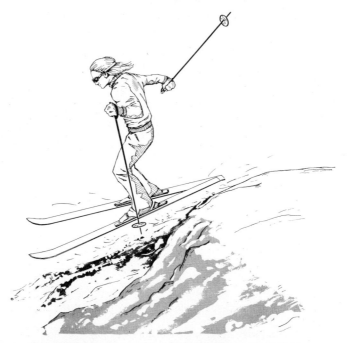

Figure 11–13   An example of Newton's first Law of Motion.

ienced the sometimes frightening situation of continuing forward when the vehicle in which the person is riding stops suddenly.

The property of an object that causes it to remain in its state of either rest or motion is called its *inertia*. Because of *inertia*, force is needed to change the velocity of an object. The amount of force needed to alter the object's velocity is directly related to the amount of inertia it has. The measure of inertia in a body is its mass—i.e., the quantity of matter it possesses. The greater the mass of an object, the greater its inertia. A medicine ball obviously has greater inertia than does a volleyball. A tennis racket has greater inertia than a badminton racket, and a baseball more than a whiffle ball.

Law of Acceleration

The second Law of Motion concerns acceleration and momentum, and it tells how the quantities of force, mass, and acceleration are related and how to measure force when it exists. The law states that **the acceleration of an object is directly proportional to the force causing it, is in the same direction as the force, and is inversely proportional to the mass of the object.** It is quite easy to show that change in velocity (acceleration) of an object is proportional to the force and in the direction of the force. The velocity of a pitched ball reflects the force with which it is thrown, and it moves in the direction of the line of force at the moment of release. Similarly it takes less braking force to stop a baseball moving at 10 feet per second than it does to stop a pitch of 100 feet per second. In both instances the change in velocity is directly proportional to the amount of force and is in the direction of the force. The mass of the ball is a measure of its inertia, and the greater the inertia the more force it takes to change the object's velocity. Thus, acceleration is inversely proportional to mass. A bowling ball requires more force to put it in motion than a playground ball, and the same is true for stopping it.

The relationships among force, acceleration, and mass, when combined and stated symbolically, become

$$a \propto \frac{F}{m} \quad \text{or} \quad F \propto ma$$

By defining terms, physicists have assigned values to units of force, mass, and acceleration so that an equals sign may be substituted for the proportion sign, and Newton's second law may be expressed in equation form as

$$F = ma$$

For this to be possible the force unit is the pound when acceleration is in feet/second/second and mass is in slugs. When acceleration is in meters/second/second and mass is in kilograms, force is expressed in newtons (see Table 9–1).

With this equation it is now possible to determine the force needed to produce a given linear acceleration of a body if the weight of the body is known. Since we know that $m = \frac{w}{g}$, the equation for force, $F = ma$, can be written as $F = \frac{w}{g} \times a$. For example, the force needed to accelerate a 160-pound object, 2 ft/sec^2 is $\frac{160}{32} \times 2$ or 10 pounds.

IMPULSE   The product of a force and the time over which it acts is called *impulse*. In Newton's second Law of Motion the time during which the force occurs must be considered, in addition to the magnitude of the force. One way of writing the impulse equation is

$$Ft = m(v - u)$$

That is, impulse is equal to the product of the mass of an object and its change in velocity. The equation is obtained by substituting the value for acceleration, $\dfrac{v - u}{t}$ in the equation $F = ma$, which then becomes $F = m\dfrac{(v - u)}{t}$. Transposed, the equation takes the form $Ft = m(v - u)$. From this form of the equation it should be apparent that the force required to produce a given change of velocity in a given time period is proportional to the mass. It is also easy to see that as the change in velocity of an object of *given mass* increases, so must the impulse increase proportionately. Conversely, if either force or time is increased, the change in velocity must also increase. Doubling either the force or time over which a force is applied will double the velocity change.

The importance of creating as large an impulse as possible is evident in the skillful execution of many sports techniques. A baseball pitcher uses a form that allows the longest time over which to apply the force to the ball before releasing it. This same long wind-up is seen in the technique used by hammer throwers, discus throwers, and shot-putters. In each instance the performer accelerates the object to be thrown as much as possible by generating as much force as strength permits and by using body segment adjustments that increase the time over which the force can be applied (Figure 11–14).

The impulse relationship also shows that force cannot be generated to cause a change in velocity unless time is available over which the force is applied. This helps to explain the value of the follow-through in throwing and striking objects. Although the follow-through does not affect the flight of the object once the object has left the throwing or striking implement, it does help to ensure that the missile will stay in

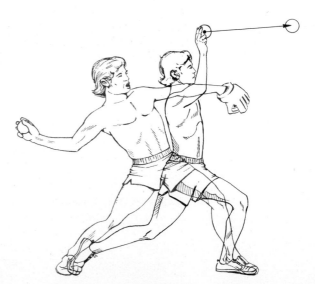

Figure 11–14 Example of impulse generation. (Drawn from motion picture film tracing.)

contact with the implement that is imparting force to it for as long as possible. The ball is actually carried along by the foot, golf club, or the tennis racket, and the longer the time that the force of the implement can be applied to the ball the greater will be the change in velocity in the ball.

MOMENTUM   The impulse equation is also written as

$$Ft = mv - mu$$

The product of mass and velocity (mv or mu) is momentum, and any change in momentum is equal to the impulse that produces it. Momentum is a quantity of motion that may be increased or decreased by increasing or decreasing either the mass or the velocity. The shot-putter who is able to push the shot with a greater speed than the opponent will cause the shot to have greater momentum at the moment of release. And, even though his mass is less, a smaller tackler may "take out" a larger opponent in football if his faster speed is sufficient to afford him a larger momentum than the person he tackles. Similarly, heavier bowling balls released with the same speed as lighter balls have greater momentum, and a heavier tennis racket will strike a tennis ball with greater momentum and cause a greater change in momentum in the tennis ball than will a lighter racket.

An increase in momentum occurs when the force is applied in the direction of the motion. Force applied in the opposite direction produces a slowing down or decrease in momentum. This is what happens when one catches a fast ball or lands from a jump. In both instances relatively large momentums are reduced to zero and large impulses occur. The momentum of the ball is large because of its large velocity and the momentum of the jumper is great because of a large mass. Looking again at the impulse equation, $Ft = mv - mu$, it can be seen that a short stopping time will require a large stopping force and that an increase in stopping time will reduce the amount of stopping force needed to change the momentum of the object to zero. This is why it is necessary to increase the stopping time by "giving" when catching the ball or when landing from a jump or fall. Without the "give" the impulse will not be enough, the momentum will not decrease to zero, and the ball will not be caught, or the momentum will reach zero but the force will be so great that injury in the form of damaged bones and joints may result. A 5-pound force falling for 5 seconds has the same impulse as a 25-pound force falling for 1 second.

Law of Reaction   The third Law of Motion considers the way forces act against each other. A book lying on a table (Figure 11–15) exerts a downward force on the table, and because the book is stationary, another equal and opposite force must be acting on the book. Newton's first law states that unbalanced forces produce motion. Since we have no motion here, we must have a balanced force system. The downward force of the book on the table is balanced by an upward force of the table on the book. The same is true when a person walks across a floor. The feet push back against the floor with the same magnitude as the floor pushes forward against the feet. Without the forward push of the floor against the feet, forward progress would not be possible. Notice how the front part of the foot in the footprint in Figure 11–16 makes a deeper impression in the front than the rear. In order to accelerate forward, the walker has to push backward. For this reason runners push against starting blocks at the beginning of a race so that a strong forward reaction push can be received from the blocks. In each of these instances, forces of equal magnitude are exerted in opposite directions. One force is called the

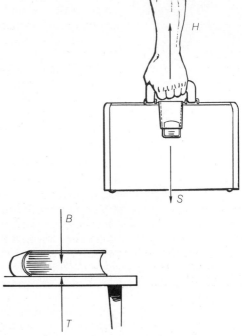

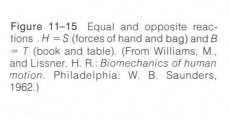

Figure 11–15 Equal and opposite reactions . *H* = *S* (forces of hand and bag) and *B* = *T* (book and table). (From Williams, M., and Lissner, H. R.: *Biomechanics of human motion*. Philadelphia: W. B. Saunders, 1962.)

action force and the other is the reaction force. Newton's third Law of Motion states that **for every action there is an equal and opposite reaction.** Whenever one body exerts a force upon a second body, the second exerts an equal and opposite force upon the first. This is the reason one makes less progress in walking on wet ice or in walking on soft sand than on firm, nonslippery surfaces. Because of a lack of friction between the feet and the supporting surface, the foot's force pushing back against the ice or sand is diminished, and therefore the ice or sand pushes the body forward with less force. To overcome the lack of friction, players engaged in activities involving quick starts, stops, and directional changes wear shoes with special cleats. The cleats

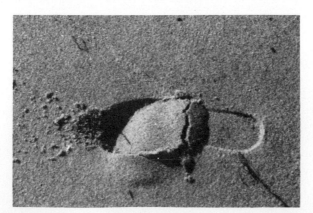

Figure 11–16 In order to accelerate forward, a walker must push backward. Notice how the front part of the footprint is more deeply depressed than the rear.

allow the player to dig in and push without slippage or loss of force. The maximum equal and opposite reaction then pushes the player in the desired direction. Consider the problem of trying to walk on ice with ball bearings attached to the shoe soles.

Action and reaction show up in countless ways when objects are in motion. When a boat is rowed the oars exert a force against the water and the water pushes against the oars with an equal and opposite reaction, causing the boat to be pushed forward as the force is transferred from the oar to the boat through the oarlock. The force of a volleyball can be felt pushing back against the hand as it is served with a forward force. A similar force is observed when a gun is shot or an arrow is released from a bow. The recoil of the gun or bow is due to the reaction force of the bullet or arrow to the action force of the gun or bow.

CONSERVATION OF MOMENTUM   When an object is set in motion by a force, the momentum (mv) of the object is changed. Since the force that causes this change in momentum must have an equal and opposite force, another equal and opposite momentum change must occur in the object producing the reactive force. The time the objects are in contact with each other would also be equal, and therefore the impulses (Ft) would be equal. This means that $m_1v_1 - m_1u_1 = m_2v_2 - m_2u_2$. This principle is summarized in the Law of Conservation of Momentum, which states that **in any system where forces act on each other the momentum is constant.** Thus, if an impact or action between objects occurs, the momentums before impact must equal the momentums after the impact, provided, of course, that no momentum is lost through friction or other forces. The momentum of a golf ball changes from zero to a larger quantity after it is struck by a club (Figure 11–17). Neglecting air resistance and friction, the momentum of the club will also change so that the momentum of ball and

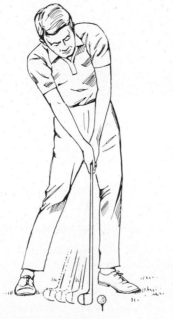

Figure 11–17   Momentum of club and ball before impact equals momentum of club and ball after impact. (Drawn from motion picture film tracing.)

club after impact will equal the momentum of ball and club before impact. This is proved by using the impulse equation.

$$m_b v_b - m_b u_b = m_c v_c - m_c u_c$$

where the subscript b refers to the ball and c to the club. Rearranged, this equation becomes

$$m_b u_b - m_c u_c = m_b v_b - m_c v_c$$

That is, the combined momentums before impact equal the combined momentums after impact. Momentum is conserved; none is lost.

The conservation of momentum may be easily apparent in some instances, whereas in others it is harder to visualize. When one steps out of a canoe onto a dock, the canoe is pushed back by the passenger as the passenger is pushed forward by the canoe. The change in momentum of the canoe backward ($m_1 v_1 - m_1 u_1$) will equal the change in momentum of the passenger forward ($m_2 v_2 - m_2 u_2$). Here the action-reaction relationship is evident in the movements of both the canoe and the person. But, if the same person steps off an ocean liner, the change in momentum of the ship is imperceptible yet it will still equal the change in momentum of the passenger. Because the mass of the ship is so great, its velocity is not apparent. In *both* instances, the change in the mass-velocity product of the passenger equals the change in the mass-velocity product of the boat (canoe or ship), and momentum is conserved. Incidentally, if the passenger disembarking from the canoe does not account for the backward acceleration of the canoe, the step toward the dock may be a wet one.

Forces That Modify Motion

There are modifying forces that are important to consider when studying the kinetics of linear motion. Francis (1976) has classified six of them into three categories:
1. **Weight**
2. **Contact Forces**
   a. Normal Reaction
   b. Friction
3. **Fluid Forces**
   a. Buoyancy
   b. Drag
   c. Lift

For purposes of discussion in this chapter, an additional category of elasticity and rebound has been added.

Weight

In what came to be known as the Law of Gravitation, Newton (remember the apple) was the first to point out that all bodies are attracted to each other in direct proportion to their masses and in inverse proportion to the square of the distance between them. The amount of this attraction between bodies on earth is negligible except for the attraction between the earth itself and the bodies on it. Because of the earth's huge mass, this attraction is quite noticeable. The force is called gravity, and it is measured

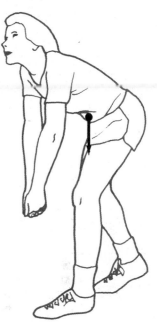

Figure 11–18 Gravitational force is measured as the weight of the body applied through the center of gravity of the body and directed toward the center of the earth.

as the weight of the body applied through the center of gravity of the body and directed toward the earth's axis (Figure 11–18). The closer a body is to the earth's center, the greater is the gravitational pull and, therefore, the more it weighs. When the body moves far enough away from the earth's center, such as to the moon, the decrease in the gravitational pull is apparent, as in the ease of giant leaps. The mass of the body is the same as on earth but the weight has decreased in proportion to the gravitational pull. The relation between weight, mass, and gravity is represented in equation form as $W = mg$. The force of weight must be considered in all motion analyses.

Contact Forces

NORMAL REACTION   As Newton's third law states, for every action there is an equal and opposite reaction. That is, the forces acting between two bodies are equal and acting in opposite directions. This implies that forces always exist in pairs. A gymnast hanging on the still rings pulls down on the rings as rings attached to the ropes pull up on the gymnast. Similarly the ropes pull on the supports as the supports pull on the ropes. A diver pushes down on the board and the board pushes back, or a hurdler pushes off the ground and the ground pushes back (Figure 11–19). Every time there is a push there has to be a push back. Without the reactive force there would be no motion.

FRICTION   Friction is the force that opposes efforts to slide or roll one body over another. Without friction it would be impossible to walk or run or do much of any kind of moving, but on the other hand it increases the difficulty of moving objects about with its deterrent effect. There are numerous examples in which we attempt to *increase* friction for more effective performance. The use of rubber-soled shoes on hardwood floors or wet decks, spikes on golf shoes, and cleats on football shoes

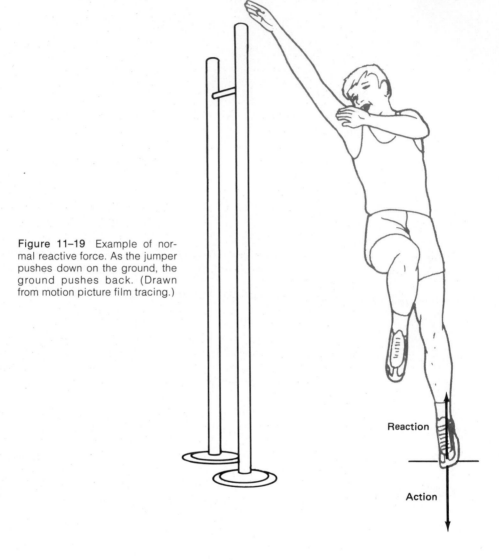

Figure 11–19 Example of normal reactive force. As the jumper pushes down on the ground, the ground pushes back. (Drawn from motion picture film tracing.)

Reaction

Action

improve friction with the supporting surface. Chalk on the gymnast's hands, golf gloves, and rubber grips on field hockey sticks are all used to decrease slipping. Even the surfaces of balls are designed to increase friction through irregularities such as the fuzz on the tennis ball or the dimples on a golf ball. Attempts to *decrease* friction are also evident in sports. The sole of one of a bowler's shoes is made to have little friction so that it can slide more easily in the approach. Sharp ice skates apply pressure on the ice and cause slight melting, thus making it easier for the skates to move across the ice. Ice covered with a slight film of water is more slippery than colder, drier ice. Skis are waxed, bicycles are greased, and roller skates have ball bearings, each for the purpose of minimizing the retardant effect of friction.

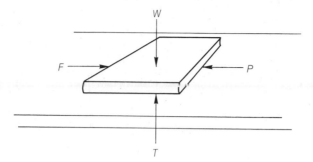

Figure 11–20 The coefficient of friction is the ratio between the force needed to overcome the friction, P, to the force holding the surfaces together, W.

The amount of friction between one surface and another depends upon the nature of the surfaces and the forces pressing them together. Generally speaking, smooth surfaces have less friction than rough surfaces but the area of surfaces in contact with each other does not affect friction. A footlocker pulled along on one end would take as much force to pull as one on its side. An empty footlocker, however, would take less force than one full of books. **Friction is proportional to the force pressing two surfaces together.**

The force of friction acts parallel to the surfaces that are sliding over each other and opposite to the direction of motion. In Figure 11–20 the book is pressing down on the table with a force, W, equal to its weight. The reactive force of the table, T, pushes up against the book. The force needed to put the book in motion is P. The force resisting the motion, F, is the force due to friction. F equals in magnitude the force P attempting to move the book. The ratio of the force needed to overcome the friction, P, to the force holding the surface together, W, is called the coefficient of friction, μ (mu).

$$\mu = \frac{P}{W}$$

This coefficient indicates the starting friction ratio for these two surfaces. It is an experimentally determined value that depends on the nature of the contact surfaces. Mu is a **constant** for any two given surfaces. The larger the coefficient the more the surfaces cling together. The smaller the coefficient the easier it is for the two surfaces to begin sliding over each other. A coefficient of 0.0 would indicate completely frictionless surfaces. The equation also shows that the coefficient of friction is totally dependent upon the force holding the surfaces together (W) and the force needed to slide one surface over the other (P). The coefficient will decrease as P decreases.

Friction is overcome by changing either the surface or the force. If one attempts to push an object forward with a force directed diagonally downward, the force holding the surfaces together is increased and so is the friction. Consequently, the effort needed to move the object increases proportionately. On the other hand, a force directed diagonally forward-upward would decrease the force holding the surfaces together, diminish the friction, and make the moving task somewhat easier.

Starting friction, the friction that resists the start of motion, is greater than sliding friction, the friction that resists continued motion. It takes less force to keep something sliding than it does to start it sliding. At low speeds friction usually decreases as speed increases, but at extremely rapid speeds friction increases proportionately until

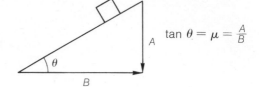

Figure 11–21   An inclined plane may be used to determine the coefficient of friction, μ, between two surfaces.

$$\tan \theta = \mu = \frac{A}{B}$$

the heat it generates causes the sliding surfaces to disintegrate. While sliding friction is less than starting friction, rolling friction is much less than sliding friction. The movement of heavier objects is much easier when they are put up on wheels. As with sliding friction, rolling friction varies with the nature of the surfaces and the magnitude of the force pushing the two surfaces together. Smooth, hard surfaces roll or are rolled upon more easily than soft, irregular surfaces. Field hockey players and golfers know this and must adjust their games to varying surfaces. Obviously, the rolling friction over thick, high, wet grass will be greater than that over a hard, dry, closely cropped surface.

The coefficient of friction between two objects may also be found by placing one object on the second and tilting the second until the first starts to slide. The tangent of the angle of the second object with the horizontal is the coefficient of friction (Figure 11–21). Bunn (1972) cited an interesting application of the use of μ with respect to the gripping power of basketball shoes. The amount of lean a player may safely take is

equal to the angle θ which the player makes with the vertical, whose tangent $= \frac{P}{W}$.

P is the amount of horizontal force needed to cause the feet to start sliding horizontally and W is the weight of the player (Figure 11–22). Shoes allowing a greater lean would certainly afford their wearers an advantage in the game. For this information to be of use to shoe manufacturers, however, a standard type floor surface would have to be determined.

Elasticity and Rebound

Objects that rebound from each other do so in a fairly predictable manner. The nature of a rebound is governed by the elasticity, mass, and velocity of the rebounding surfaces, the friction between the surfaces, and the angle with which one object contacts the second.

Any time two or more objects come into contact with each other some distortion or deformation occurs. Whether or not the distortion is permanent depends upon the elasticity of the interacting objects. Elasticity is the ability of an object to resist distorting influences and to return to its original size and shape when the distorting

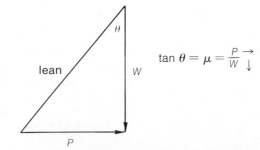

Figure 11–22   The amount of lean a basketball player can safely assume depends upon the friction between the floor and his shoes.

$$\tan \theta = \mu = \frac{P \rightarrow}{W \downarrow}$$

forces are removed. The force that acts on an object to distort it is called *stress*. The distortion that occurs is called *strain*, and is proportional to the stress causing it. Stress may take the form of tension, as in the stretching of a spring; compression, as in the squeezing of a tennis ball (Figure 11–23); flexion, such as the blending of a fencing foil; or torsion, as in the twisting of the spring. In all cases the object tends to resume its original shape when the stress is removed. If the stress is too large the elastic limit of the object is exceeded and permanent distortion occurs.

COEFFICIENT OF ELASTICITY   Substances vary in their resistance to distorting forces and in their ability to regain their original shape after being deformed. One usually thinks of a material such as rubber as being highly elastic since it yields easily to a distorting force and returns to its original shape. Actually, substances that are hard to distort and return perfectly to their original shape are more elastic. Gasses, liquids, highly tempered steel, and brass are examples. In comparing the elasticity of different substances, coefficients of elasticity are used. A *coefficient of elasticity* or *restitution* is defined as the stress divided by the strain. The coefficient of elasticity most commonly determined in sports activities is that caused in the compression of balls. If one drops a ball onto a hard surface like a floor, the coefficient of restitution may be determined by comparing the drop height with the bounce height in the equation

$$e = \sqrt{\frac{\text{bounce height}}{\text{drop height}}}$$

where e = coefficient of restitution or elasticity. The closer the coefficient approaches 1.0, the more perfect the elasticity. Rules require that a basketball should be inflated to rebound to a height of 49 to 54 inches at its top when its bottom is dropped from a height of 72 inches. For the maximum bounce height this is a coefficient of 0.781. In comparison, a volleyball dropped from the same height and inflated to 6 psi (pounds per square inch) rebounds to 51 inches and has a coefficient of 0.84. A tennis ball has a coefficient of 0.73 and a leather-covered softball one of 0.46.

The coefficient of restitution may also be found in another way. Because the Law of Conservation of Momentum states that the total momentum in any impact between the objects must remain the same, the momentum of one object may be reduced, but the momentum of the other will increase proportionately. Since the mass of neither object changes

$$e = \frac{V_2 - V_1}{U_1 - U_2}$$

where V_2 and V_1 are the velocities after impact and U_1 and U_2 are the velocities before impact.

ANGLE OF REBOUND   An elastic object dropped vertically onto a rebounding surface will compress uniformly on its underside and rebound vertically upward. An elastic object that strikes a rebounding surface obliquely will compress unevenly on the bottom and rebound at an oblique angle. The size of the angle compared to the striking angle depends upon the elasticity of the striking object and the friction between the two surfaces. The rebound of a perfectly elastic object is similar to the reflection of light: **the angle of incidence is equal to the angle of reflection** (Figure 11–24). Variations from this ideal are to be expected as the coefficient of restitution

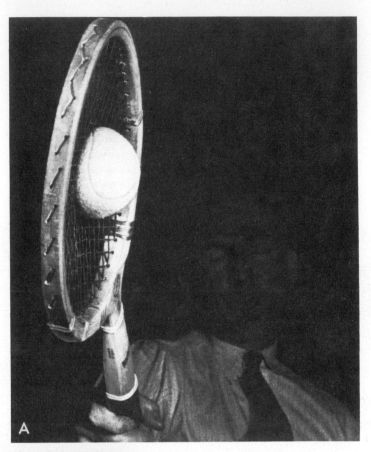

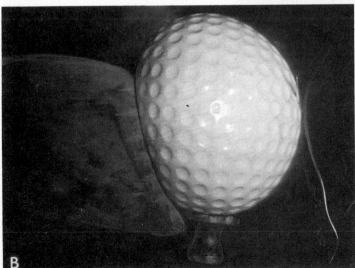

Figure 11–23   Compression of tennis ball (A) and golf ball (B) at moment of impact. (Courtesy of H. E. Edgerton.)

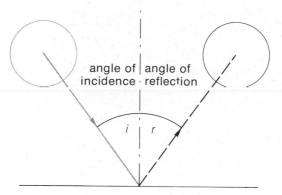

angle of | angle of
incidence · reflection

i *r*

Figure 11–24   The angle of incidence and the angle of reflection in oblique rebounds.

varies. Low coefficients will generally produce angles of reflection greater than angles of incidence. For example, an underinflated volleyball or basketball will rebound at an angle closer to the surface than it struck it. Friction also affects the angle. Whereas the coefficient of elasticity affects the vertical component of the rebound, friction will affect the horizontal component and decrease it. It is possible that a decreased horizontal component related to the coefficient of elasticity could occur in proportion to the decreased vertical velocity, so that although the resultant velocity of the rebound would be less than the initial velocity, the angle of reflection would equal the angle of incidence.

EFFECTS OF SPIN ON BOUNCE   Spin also influences rebounding angles. Balls thrown with top spin will rebound from horizontal surfaces lower and with more horizontal velocity than that with which they struck. They will tend to roll farther also, an action often desirable on long golf drives. Balls hitting a horizontal surface with back spin rebound at a higher bounce and are slower. Balls with back spin also roll for shorter distances than those with top or no spin. Because of the compression of the ball and the friction between it and the surface, a ball with no spin hitting the surface at an angle will develop some top spin on the rebound, and a ball hitting with top spin will develop greater top spin upon rebounding. With back spin, however, the spin may be completely stopped or reversed. A ball with side spin will rebound in the direction of the spin. A ball spinning or curving to the right will "kick" to the right upon rebounding and a left-spinning ball will do the reverse.

When spinning balls hit vertical surfaces, such as a basketball backboard or a squash court wall, they will respond in relation to the surface in the same manner as with horizontal surfaces. When the vertical surface is struck from below, a ball with no spin or top spin will have added spin on rebound, and the angle of reflection will be greater than the angle of incidence. With back spin the spin will stop or reverse and the angle of reflection will be less than the incidence angle. For this to be true, a back-spinning ball approaching a vertical wall from above must be regarded as moving with top spin in relation to the rebounding surface. Similarly, a top-spinning ball hitting the vertical surface from above is in actuality spinning backwards with respect to the rebounding surface.

When a spinning ball meets a forward moving object, as in tennis or table tennis, the ball will rebound in a direction that will be the resultant of the forces acting on it at impact. For example, a ball with top spin striking a stationary vertical surface head on will rebound upward. That same ball (with top spin) striking a moving vertical surface, like a tennis racket, will also rebound upward but not as much because the resultant rebound has a horizontal force component from the forward moving tennis racket. Nevertheless, the upward direction may be sufficient to send the ball out of bounds. To counteract the upward direction the racket face can be turned obliquely downward, thus adding a downward compensating force component as well as changing the spin of the ball.

The resultant force path of a rebounding ball is controlled by several factors. When one attempts to predict the direction of the rebound, the momentums of both the ball and the striking implement must be considered as well as the elasticity of the two objects, the spin of the ball, and the angle of impact. Awareness of these factors and the ways in which they affect play have numerous and valuable applications in sports such as handball, squash, racketball, table tennis, paddleball, and tennis.

Fluid Forces

Water and air are both fluids, and as such are subject to many of the same laws and principles. The fluid forces of buoyancy, drag, and lift apply in both mediums and have considerable effect upon the movements of the human body in many circumstances. A discus sails, a baseball curves, a volleyball "wobbles," and a shuttlecock drops because of contact with air currents. Sky jumpers and hang gliders control their flight paths by interacting with the air currents, while downhill racers, swimmers, and divers streamline their bodies to minimize the effect of fluid resistance.

BUOYANCY   If an adult female stands in shoulder deep water and abducts her arms as she lays her head back on the water's surface, most likely her feet will leave the bottom as her legs begin to rise. At some point between the vertical and horizontal, the swimmer will come to rest and she will be in a motionless back float. For this to occur an upward force must counterbalance the weight (force) of her body, acting vertically downward at her center of gravity. This upward force is called *buoyancy* and, according to *Archimedes' Principle*, the magnitude of this force is equal to the weight of water displaced by the floating body. Specifically, Archimedes' Principle states that **a solid body immersed in a liquid is buoyed up by a force equal to the weight of the liquid displaced.** This principle explains why some objects float and others do not, why some individuals float motionless like bobbing corks and why others struggle to keep their noses above water while attempting a back float. When a body is immersed in water, it will sink until the weight of the water it displaces equals the weight of the body. Sinking objects never do displace enough water to equal their body weight and eventually settle to the bottom. If such objects are weighed under water, they will be found to weigh less than when weighed in air. That difference in weight equals the weight of the water displaced and is the buoyant force acting on the immersed objects. Even a body which floats has some part of its volume beneath the surface, and thus displaces a volume of water. The weight of the water it displaces equals the *total* weight of the floating object. Any object stops sinking when the weight of the water it displaces equals its weight.

The ratio of body weight and the weight of an equal volume of water is called *specific gravity*. Objects that displace an amount of water equal in weight and volume to their weight and volume have a specific gravity of 1.0. Objects that displace a volume of water less than their volume have a specific gravity less than 1.0 and will float with some part above the surface. When the volume of water displaced weighs less than the weight of the object, the object will sink.

Human beings differ in specific gravity. Individuals with a greater proportion of fat will have a lower specific gravity than those with greater muscle mass and large bones. Men and children usually have higher specific gravities than women and consequently are poorer floaters. The position in which one floats is also determined by the distribution of muscle, bone, and fat within the body, since the specific gravity of the various body parts differs accordingly. Usually the legs have a high specific gravity and consequently are the part of the body that most often sinks during the back float. The thoracic region is the most buoyant part, having the lowest weight for its volume. A person can increase the buoyancy of this region by keeping the lungs inflated with air, thus increasing the ease of floating. Some few individuals have overall specific gravities greater than 1.0. It is impossible for these people to do a motionless float, for they are "sinkers." A practical way to determine whether a person is a floater or sinker is to have the person assume the tucked jellyfish float position with lungs inflated. If any portion of the individual's back is on or above the surface, the individual can learn to maintain a motionless floating position which, even though it may be more nearly vertical than supine, is still called a back float.

A floater has to be concerned with two forces, the downward force of the body's weight and the upward buoyancy of the water. When these forces act on the body so that their resultant is zero, the forces will be in equilibrium and the body will be in a motionless float. The downward force acts at the center of gravity of the body, a point somewhere in the pelvis. The buoyant force acts at the center of buoyancy of the body, a point that varies with individuals but is usually closer to the head than the center of gravity. If the body were of uniform density, the center of gravity and the center of buoyancy would coincide, but since the body has less mass toward the head, the center of buoyancy is usually higher in the body than the center of gravity. The center of buoyancy is the point where the center of gravity of the volume of displaced water would be if the water were placed in a vessel the shape and size of the floater's body. Because the water is of uniform density, its center of gravity will be in the direction of the greater volume—i.e., near the chest region. If the center of gravity and center of buoyancy are not in the same force line with each other, as shown in Figure 11–25A, the body will rotate in the direction of the forces until the forces are equal and opposite in line, direction, and magnitude. At this point the floater will be in a balanced float (Figure 11–25B). Individuals who float horizontally have the center of gravity and center of buoyancy in the same vertical line while in the horizontal position. These are usually individuals whose bodies contain a high percentage of fat.

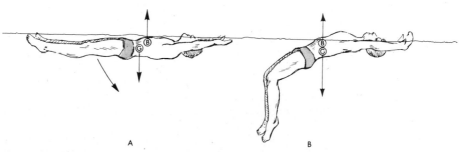

A   B

Figure 11–25   A balanced float occurs when the center of gravity and the center of buoyancy are in the same force line. G = downward force of body weight. B = upward force (buoyancy) of water.

Those floaters whose legs tend to drop when attempting the back float will have a balanced position somewhere between the horizontal and vertical at that point where the center of gravity and center of buoyancy are in the same vertical line.

The angle of the floating position with the horizontal may be decreased by making adjustments in the position of the body segments that move the center of gravity in closer alignment with the center of buoyancy. Raising the arms over the head, bending the knees, and flexing the wrists to bring the hands out of the water all contribute to moving the center of gravity closer to the head and thus closer to the center of buoyancy (Figure 11–25B).

LIFT AND DRAG   The fluid resistance to movement through water or air consists of two forces, **lift** and **drag.** When a body moves through a fluid the drag is the fluid force that opposes the forward motion of the body and reduces the body's speed. The lift force is perpendicular to the drag and causes the body to be lifted as it moves forward. If one were to place a hand in a moving stream of water or in the air stream of a circulating fan so that the hand is perpendicular to the path of the flow, considerable pressure would be felt on the hand as the fluid pushed against it. Turning the hand so that it is now horizontal to the fluid flow diminishes the pressure against the hand considerably. In fact very little, if any, pressure is felt, and it is quite easy to hold the hand in this position. A position halfway between these two—i.e., at 45 degrees to the flow direction—results in the feeling of some *uplift* pressure as well as backward pressure (Figure 11–26). The flat hand allows the layers of air or water to flow over it with little distortion, and only some small resistance or *drag* is evident at the leading edge of the hand. In contrast, the vertical hand has considerable pressure or drag on the front edge and, in addition, more resistance due to suction behind the hand as the displaced air goes around the hand and tries to fill in the vacuum behind.

The tilted hand experiences both lift and drag. The lift is due to a build-up of air pressure on the underside compared to the top side, and the drag comes from frictional or surface forces acting on the tilted hand as well as the drag resulting from its form. The ratio between lift and drag becomes extremely important in sports like discus throwing or ski jumping. Any changes in the angle of tilt or the air speed with respect to the object or body will produce a variation in lift and drag, and resultant differences in distance traveled by the object. The amount of lift and drag and the proportion of each depend upon a number of factors, including the density of the fluid, the shape and smoothness of the body moving through the fluid, the velocity of the fluid with respect to the body, and the temperature of the fluid. There are numerous examples of technique forms that attempt to minimize frontal drag by streamlining the shape and smoothing the surface texture. In all instances as little frontal surface as possible is presented. Skaters, skiers, bicyclists, and divers all assume positions that diminish the frontal surface area as much as possible. In addition they wear tight-fitting, smooth-textured clothing to assist in reducing drag. The optimum angle of body tilt for lift in almost all cases is greater than 0 degrees and less than 90 degrees.

AIR PATTERNS AND BALL SPIN   The air pattern that surrounds a moving object may be smooth or turbulent. Air passing around a smooth surface at slow speeds is usually smooth or laminar air, while high speeds and rough surfaces may cause laminar air to break up and become turbulent. Rotating balls act differently with respect to laminar flow than straight balls. A straight ball may cause laminar air to break up and become turbulent. This is likely to happen if the ball has an uneven or irregular surface or a

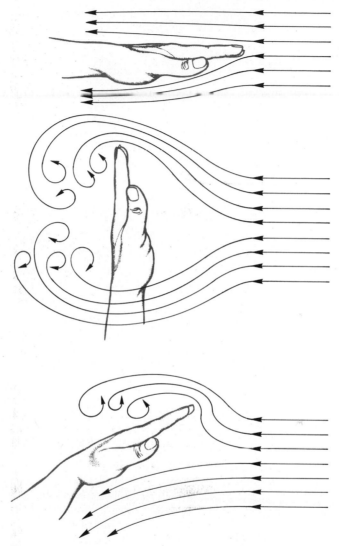

Figure 11–26   Patterns of air flow around an object vary with the shape of the frontal surface.

large surface area. The result is a wobbling or wavering such as is observed when a volleyball is served or thrown with no spin. A ball traveling at high speeds with no initial spin may also curve as a result of the laminar air becoming turbulent. This is often seen in baseball.

Bernouilli's Principle   An extremely important principle that applies to laminar air was discovered by Bernouilli. Simply stated, he determined that **the pressure in a moving fluid decreases as its speed increases.** A sheet of paper held by two corners will rise at its loose end if one blows over the surface of the paper. The air moving over the top of the paper is moving at a faster speed than the air under the paper. The

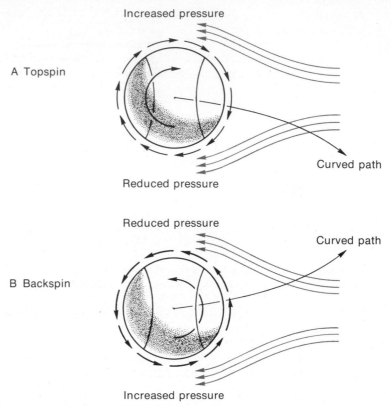

Increased pressure

A Topspin

Reduced pressure

Curved path

Reduced pressure

Curved path

B Backspin

Increased pressure

Figure 11–27   A spinning ball follows a curved path moving in the direction of least pressure. (The curve is exaggerated for clarity.)

pressure on top therefore is less, and the paper rises. Similarly, if one hangs two tennis balls on strings and then blows a stream of air between them, the balls will move closer to each other in the direction of the lowered pressure.

Bernouilli's principle applies for moving objects passing through a stationary fluid as well as for fluids passing stationary objects and, in addition to explaining why airplanes can fly, it also explains why balls with spin follow a curved path. This latter application of Bernouilli's principle is called the Magnus effect after the German physicist who first explained the phenomenon. A ball moving through the air will also move in the direction of least air pressure. As shown in Figure 11–27A, the ball spinning in a clockwise direction drags around a boundary layer of air. At the bottom of the ball this air current is moving in the same direction as the oncoming air. At the top, the boundary air is moving in the opposite direction. The air at the bottom is moving faster, and therefore the pressure is reduced. The air at the top moves more slowly and the pressure is increased. Thus the ball will move in a downward curve in the direction of least pressure. Viewed from the side this would be the behavior of a ball with top spin imparted to it. Balls with top spin drop sooner than balls with no spin. A ball with a counterclockwise or back spin will move in an upward curve and thus stay aloft longer than a ball with no spin (Figure 11–27B). Balls spinning about a vertical axis have side spin. Right spin causes the ball to curve to the right and occurs when the forward edge of the ball moves to the right. Left spin is the opposite.

The amount of air a ball drags around with it when spinning depends upon the surface of the ball and the speed of the spin. Rough or large surfaces, small mass, and a fast spin speed will all produce a more noticeable spin and curve deflection. The small mass of a table tennis ball, the fuzz on a tennis ball, and the seams on a baseball all enhance spin, an important element in each game's strategy. The deflection will also be more pronounced if the forward velocity is slow. This may occur because of little force imparted to the ball or a strong head wind. Spin on a ball may also smooth its flight by acting as a stabilizer. Like a gyroscope, a football or discus spinning around one axis resists spinning about another axis and therefore is less likely to tumble through the air.

Free-Body Diagrams

In analyzing any technique, the student should consider all the external forces by methodically accounting for the effect of each one on the body. To do this it is helpful to look at the body as if it were isolated from its surroundings. The isolated body is then considered to be a separate mechanical system whose boundaries have been defined. The isolation makes it easier to identify the forces and to represent them as vectors in a diagram of the body. This type of representation is called a *free-body diagram,* and can help to settle any doubts about the application and direction of the various forces acting on the body in any given time frame. The direction of each of the external forces and the point through which each acts are summarized in Table 11–1.

In Figure 11–28 the magnitude of each external force acting on the body is represented by the arrow length. The direction of the force is represented by the arrowhead, and the point of application is located at the arrow tail. The body is acted on by its weight (W) applied through the center of gravity, the reactive force (R) and the friction force (F), both applied at the point of contact with the ground, and the

TABLE 11–1 Direction and Point of Application of External Forces

FORCE	DIRECTION OF FORCE	POINT OF APPLICATION
Weight (W)	Downward (toward center of earth)	Center of gravity of body
Normal reaction (R)	Perpendicular to contact surface	Contact
Friction (F)	Along contact surface (perpendicular to normal reaction)	Contact
Buoyancy (B)	Upward	Center of buoyancy of body
Drag (D)	Opposite the direction of oncoming fluid flow	Center of gravity of body
Lift (L)	Perpendicular to drag	Center of gravity of body

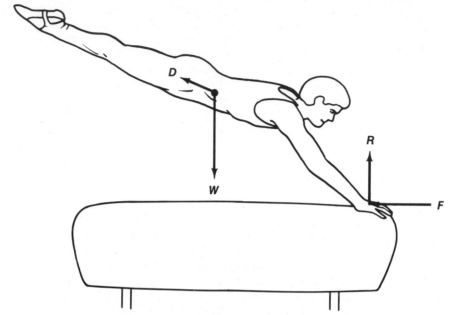

Figure 11–28 A free-body diagram showing the application and direction of the external forces acting on the vaulter: weight (*W*), normal reaction (*R*), friction (*F*), and drag (*D*).

drag force (*D*) directed through the center of gravity. In Figure 11–29, the forces acting on the body are weight (*W*), buoyancy (*B*), lift (*L*), and drag (*D*).

The importance of visualizing all the forces acting on the body relates to the fact that the state of motion or rest of a body depends upon the vector sum of all these forces. With a diagram, the forces that can be manipulated to alter the vector sum and

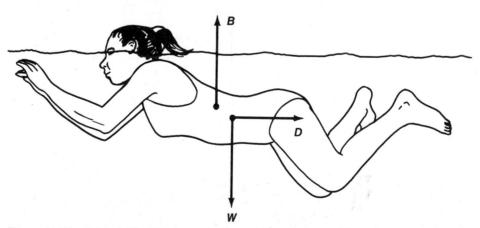

Figure 11–29 A free-body diagram showing the application and direction of external forces acting on the breast-stroke swimmer: buoyancy (*B*), weight (*W*), and drag (*D*). The more streamlined the body with respect to the flow, the less will be the drag.

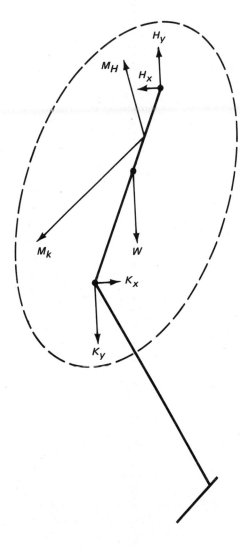

Figure 11–30 Free-body diagram of forces acting on a stationary thigh. Isolation of the limb is shown by the dotted line. Composite muscle forces are M_H and M_K. Reactive forces at the hip are H_y and H_x and at the knee are K_y and K_x. The weight force is W. (Adapted from Miller, D. I., and Nelson, R. C.: *Biomechanics of sport.* Philadelphia: Lea and Febiger, 1973.)

produce the desired outcome are more readily apparent. If the swimmer in Figure 11–29, for instance, wants to stress horizontal speed, attention should be paid to those factors that will maximize the propulsive force and minimize the opposing drag force, since little can be done to alter the weight and buoyancy forces.

Free-body diagrams are also used to show the forces acting on an isolated body segment. In Figure 11–30, the thigh has been isolated from the rest of the lower limb, and the forces acting on it are shown. The forces acting on the limb include the weight of the thigh (W), the resultant muscle force acting across the hip joint (M_H), the resultant muscle force acting across the knee joint (M_K), and the reactive force components acting across the hip joint (H_x and H_y) and knee joint (K_x and K_y). Students interested in more information on free-body diagrams are referred to Dempster (1961), Miller and Nelson (1973), or Plagenhoef (1971).

Work, Power, and Energy

Work

Simple machines such as the lever are devices designed to do work. In each instance the machine aids in the use of a force to overcome a resistance. When the resistance is overcome for a given distance, *work* is done. Mechanically speaking, **work is the product of the amount of force expended and the distance through which the force succeeds in overcoming a resistance it acts upon.** For work done in making a body move in a linear fashion this may be expressed as

$$W = Fs$$

where W stands for work, F for force, and s for the distance along which the force is applied. Units for expressing work are numerous because any force unit may be combined with any distance unit to form a work unit. In the English system the foot-pound is the most common work unit, while the joule is the most frequently used unit in the metric system. A joule is equivalent to $10^7 \times 1$ gram of force exerted through 1 centimeter.

In computing work, the distance, s, must always be measured in the direction in which the force acts, even though the object whose resistance is overcome may not be moving in the same direction. If one lifts a 20-pound suitcase from the floor to place it on a shelf 5 feet above the floor, the work accomplished is 100 foot-pounds. If, on the other hand, that same weight is lifted an equal distance upward but along a 10-foot inclined plane, the amount of work done is still 100 foot-pounds (Figure 11–31). The work done along the incline is the same as the work done to lift the weight to the height of the incline. The horizontal distance the suitcase moves is not included.

Work done in the same direction that the body moves is called **positive** work, whereas work done in the opposite direction is called **negative** work. When an individual does a deep knee bend, the extensor muscles of the leg contract eccentrically to resist the effect of gravity on the body. The body moves in a direction opposite to the upward force of the muscles, and thus negative or resistive work is performed by the muscles. In the return to standing from the knee bend position, the body moves in the same direction as the concentrically contracting extensors, and the work of the muscles is positive. The net work accomplished during the down and up movement of the knee bend is the vector sum of the positive and negative work. Negative forces resisting gravity perform less work over a given distance than positive forces overcoming gravity. For example, one performs more work walking up a mountain than walking back down.

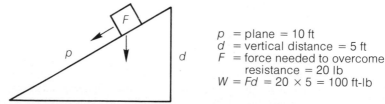

p = plane = 10 ft
d = vertical distance = 5 ft
F = force needed to overcome resistance = 20 lb
$W = Fd = 20 \times 5 = 100$ ft-lb

Figure 11–31 Work is the product of force needed to overcome a resistance and the direction over which the force is applied. The force lifting the 20-pound weight 5 vertical feet does 100 foot-pounds of work even though the 20 pounds are moved 10 feet along the plane.

When the exertion of effort produces no motion, such as might happen during a tug of war, no work is accomplished. Static contraction of muscles may be evident and considerable physiological effort may be expended but, in the strict mechanical sense, no work is being done. The physiological measure of such efforts is determined by obtaining the energy costs, which in turn are usually measured by computing the amount of oxygen consumed during the effort and converting it to calories per minute.

Theoretically, the mechanical work performed by an individual muscle can also be determined using the equation $W = Fs$. Suppose, for instance, that there is a rectangular muscle, 4 inches long and 1½ inches wide, that exerts 66 pounds of force as it turns a bony lever. Since the average muscle fiber shortens to one-half of its resting length and the fibers of a small rectangular muscle run the full length of the muscle, the force of the muscle in question is exerted over a distance of 2 inches (the amount of shortening, equal to one-half the resting length). Therefore, since $F = 66$ pounds and $s = 2$ inches, the muscle is performing 132 inch-pounds, or 11 foot-pounds, of work. In brief: $W = F$ (66 lb) $\times s$ (2/12 ft).

If the force of the muscle is not known it is computed from the muscle's cross section (see page 309). Assuming the muscle in question to be ½ inch thick and the force per square inch of cross section to be 90 pounds, the following steps are taken.

1. Find the muscle's cross section:
    Cross section = width × thickness.
    1.5 in × 0.5 in = 0.75 sq in (cross section)
2. Find the amount of force exerted by the muscle:
    Average force = 90 lb per sq in
    Cross section = 0.75 sq in
    $F = 90 \times 0.75 = 67.5$ lb
3. Find the amount of work performed by this muscle, first in inch-pounds, then in foot-pounds:
    $W = Fs$

    $W = 67.5 \text{ lb} \times 2 \text{ in} = \dfrac{135}{2} \times 2 = 135 \text{ in-lb}$

    $\dfrac{135}{12} = 11.25 \text{ ft-lb}$

For purposes of simplification the internal structure of the hypothetical muscle used in these examples was rectangular. This means that a simple geometric cross sectional measure could be used. For penniform and bipenniform muscles, however, it would be essential to determine the physiological cross section (see page 309). It must also be remembered that "s" in the work equation represents one-half the length of the average fiber in the muscle and that this may or may not coincide with the total length of the fleshy part of the muscle, depending upon its internal structure.

The number of pounds of force per square inch exerted by the average human muscle must be selected arbitrarily, depending upon whose research the student accepts.

A single equation for computing the work performed by a muscle whose average fiber length is known and whose physiological cross section (PCS) has been determined, is as follows:

$W = 90 \times PCS$ (in square inches) $\times$ ½ the length of the fibers (in inches)

This gives work in terms of inch-pounds. Since it is customary to measure work in terms of foot-pounds, the result should be divided by 12. The following equation includes this step:

$$W = \frac{90 \ (PCS \text{ in square inches})(\tfrac{1}{2} \text{ the fiber length in inches})}{12}$$

Power

Any measure of work does not account for the time involved in performing the work. When one lifts 200 pounds a distance of 3 feet, 600 foot-pounds of work is done regardless of the time it takes to do it. The *rate* at which work is done is called power, and may be expressed as

$$P = \frac{Fs}{t} \quad \text{or} \quad P = \frac{W}{t}$$

where P stands for power, W for work, and t for time. Since s/t is velocity, still another form for the power equation is $P = Fv$. Any form of the equation clearly points out that the machine or person who can perform more work in a given unit of time or who takes less time to do a specified amount of work is more powerful.

In the English system, power is expressed as ft-lb/sec or as horsepower (550 ft-lb/sec = 1 horsepower). The metric system unit is the watt, which is equivalent to one joule/second.

Energy

Energy is defined as the capacity to do work. A body is said to possess energy when it can perform work, and the energy that the body possesses is measured as the work accomplished. Energy may take numerous forms, and it is common for it to be converted from one form to another, although according to the Law of Conservation of Energy it can neither be created nor destroyed. Some forms which energy may take are heat, sound, light, electric, chemical, atomic, and mechanical. When a ball is hit with a bat, some of the mechanical energy is converted to sound and heat energy, but none of the energy is lost. **The total amount of energy possessed by a body or an isolated system remains constant.**

Potential energy and **kinetic energy** are two classifications of energy that have important implications in biomechanics. Potential energy is the capacity for doing work that a body has because of its position or configuration. A raised weight such as a diver standing on a platform, a bent bow, or a compressed spring all have potential energy. Measured in work units potential energy is the product of the force an object has and the distance over which it can act. The potential energy of a 150-pound diver whose center of gravity is 20 feet above the water surface is 3,000 foot-pounds. In this instance the appropriate form for the potential energy equation is

$$PE = mgh$$

where m is the mass of the body, g is the force of gravity, and h is the height between the diver's center of gravity and the water surface. The product of m and g (mg) is the same as the diver's weight.

The distance selected for h in the potential energy equation is established by choosing an arbitrary zero level. The potential energy of someone standing on a table 3 feet from the floor can be increased by boring a large hole in the floor directly in front of the table. The individual's potential for dropping farther is now greater because h is greater.

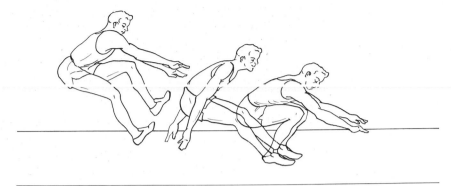

Figure 11–32 Effecting a gradual loss of kinetic energy by bending the knees upon landing from a jump.

The kinetic energy of a body is the energy due to its motion. The faster a body moves, the more kinetic energy it possesses. When a body stops moving the kinetic energy is lost. This is readily seen in the equation for kinetic energy

$$KE = \tfrac{1}{2} mv^2$$

where m is the mass of the object and v is its velocity. If v is zero, then KE is also zero.

Energy has been defined as the capacity to do work and, since energy can neither be created nor destroyed, the work done is equal to the kinetic energy acquired, or

$$Fs = \tfrac{1}{2} mv^2$$

This relationship is extremely helpful in explaining the value of "giving" when receiving the impetus of any moving object. In attempting to catch a fast-moving ball, one's chances of success are improved by increasing the distance used for stopping the ball's motion. The work of the kinetic energy against the hands depends upon the kinetic energy the ball possesses when it hits the hand. Whether that work consists of a large F and a small s or a small F and a large s depends upon the technique used by the catcher. As s increases in $Fs = \tfrac{1}{2} mv^2$, the force of the impact, F, must decrease. The skillful performer knows this and will decrease the possibility of injury and increase the chances of holding onto the ball with the choice of a small F and a large s. Achieving a gradual loss of kinetic energy is likewise advantageous when landing from a jump or a fall (Figure 11–32).

Energy is frequently transformed from kinetic into potential energy or conversely from potential to kinetic energy. The diver who jumps from a platform above the water immediately begins to lose potential energy in proportion to the gain in kinetic energy. At platform height all of the diver's energy is potential. At zero elevation all of the potential energy has been converted into an equivalent amount of kinetic energy. Barring no conversion of energy to other forms (heat, sound, and so forth) the potential energy at the top equals exactly the kinetic energy at the bottom.

The transformation from one energy state to another is interesting to note in a gymnast swinging on the flying rings. Like a pendulum, the swinger's energy is transformed from kinetic to potential on every swing. As the suspended body moves upward, the kinetic energy is continuously changed to potential energy, and the higher the swinger goes the greater the potential becomes for doing work on the downswing. At the top of the swing the conversion to potential energy is complete. Once more as the gymnast begins to fall kinetic energy again develops and becomes greatest at the bottom of the swing, when the speed is greatest and potential energy is zero. Theoretically the swinging should continue uninterrupted, but because of friction some energy is converted to heat and eventually the "pendulum" will come to rest.

Laboratory Experiences

Note: Assume that the muscles can exert a force of 100 pounds per square inch of cross section.

1. How much force can each of the following muscles exert?
    a. Muscle A, having a cross section of 2 square inches.
    b. Muscle B, having a cross section of 4 square inches.
    c. Muscle C, having a cross section of 13 square inches.

2. Find the approximate force of which the muscle shown in Figure 11–33 is capable. Assume that the diagram is drawn to scale, ½ inch being the equivalent of 1 inch. The muscle is 1 inch thick.

3. Estimate the cross section of your own biceps muscle. Approximately how much force should it be able to exert?

4. Approximately how much force should your triceps be able to exert?

5. In the diagram of the biceps muscle in Figure 11–34, find the size of the angle of pull.

6. Place a book on a table and stand a small bottle on top of it. Pull the book toward you with a quick jerk. Note the action of the bottle. Stand the bottle on the book again and pull the book across the table with a steady pull. How does the bottle move? Now pull the book and stop it suddenly. Explain the action of the bottle in all three instances.

7. Hit a softball with a bat from a tee, from a self-toss, and from a pitch. Which hit goes the farthest? Explain.

8. Lie on your back in the water with your arms over your head. Raise your legs by flexing your hips. What happens to your arms and trunk? Explain. Devise another experiment which demonstrates the same principle.

9. While both of you have on ice skates or roller skates, stand facing someone whose weight is the same as yours. Push against each other. Observe and compare the distance and velocity each of you moves. Repeat the procedure with someone who weighs considerably more or less than you do. Explain the difference between the two performances.

10. Place a long wide board on some rollers (pencils, dowels, or pipes) so that there is very little friction between the board and the floor. Carefully step on the board and attempt to walk

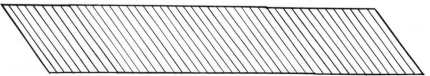

Figure 11–33   What is the approximate force that this muscle can exert? (Scale ½ inch = 1 inch).

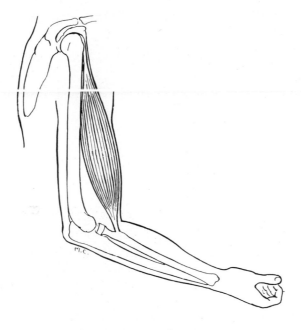

Figure 11–34 The forearm as a lever with the biceps providing the force.

normally along it. What happens to you? to the board? Take the board off the rollers and place it on the floor. Walk along it. Explain the reason for the differences in the behavior of the board and your ability to walk along it. The use of spotters is advised for this exercise.

11. Determine the coefficient of restitution for each of the following objects dropped from a height of 72 inches onto a wooden floor:
    a. Hockey ball.
    b. Lacrosse ball.
    c. Golf ball.
    d. Soccer ball.
    e. Baseball.
    Repeat the calculations for the above objects rebounding from concrete, from asphalt tile, from artificial turf, and from a tumbling mat.

12. Using a tennis racket or a paddle, impart top spin, back spin, no spin, and side spin to a ball. Note the effect on the velocity and angle of reflection when the ball rebounds from a horizontal surface, from a vertical surface when struck from above, and from a vertical surface when struck from below.

13. Assume a back-lying position in the water with your arms at your sides. Note and explain any shift in body position. Slide your arms from your sides to a side horizontal position, keeping them close to and parallel to the surface of the water. What effect does this have on body position? Continue moving your arms until they are overhead. Next flex the wrists so the hands are out of the water. Finally, flex the legs at the knees. Explain the effect of these last three moves upon your position in the water.

14. Record the body weight for each of five subjects. Using a stopwatch, record the time necessary for each subject to run up two flights of stairs. Determine the vertical distance from the bottom of the first flight to the top of the second flight. Calculate the work done by each subject and the power of each. Complete the chart on the next page.

SUBJECT	WEIGHT	TIME	WORK	POWER
1.				
2.				
3.				
4.				
5.				

a. Which subjects did the most work? Why?

b. Did those who did the most work have the most power? Explain.

c. If power is an important part of an event how should an athlete train for it?

References

Barham, J. 1978. *Mechanical kinesiology.* St. Louis: C. V. Mosby.

Basford, L. 1966. *The restlessness of matter.* London: Sampson Low, Marston.

Basford, L. 1966. *The science of movement.* London: Sampson Low, Marston.

Broer, M., and Zernicke, R. 1979. *Efficiency of human movement.* 4th ed. Philadelphia, W. B. Saunders.

Bunn, J. W. 1972. *Scientific principles of coaching.* 2d ed. Englewood Cliffs, N.J.: Prentice-Hall.

Cooper, J. M., and Glassow, R. B. 1972. *Kinesiology.* 3d ed. St. Louis: C. V. Mosby.

Cureton, T. K. 1939. Elementary principles and techniques of cinematographic analysis. *Res. Q. Am. Assoc. Health Phys. Educ. Rec.* 10:3–24.

Dempster, W. T. 1961. Free-body diagrams as an approach to the mechanics of human posture and motion. In *Biomechanical studies of the musculo-skeletal system,* ed. F. G. Evans. Springfield, Ill.: Charles C Thomas, pp. 81–135.

Dyson, G. 1970. *The mechanics of athletes.* 5th ed. London: University of London Press.

Fick, R. 1910. Handbuch der Anatomie and Mechanik der Gelenke. Jena: G. Fischer.

Fick, R. 1929. Review of literature on mechanics of joints and muscles. *Z. Orthop. Chir.* 51:320–37.

Francis, P. R. 1976. *Kinesiology newsletter, summer, 1976.* Ames, Iowa: Iowa State University.

Gardner, R., and Webster, D. 1978. *Moving right along.* Garden City, N.Y.: Doubleday.

Hay, J. G. 1978. *The biomechanics of sports techniques.* 2d ed. Englewood Cliffs, N.J.: Prentice-Hall.

Miller, D. I., and Nelson, R. C. 1973. *Biomechanics of sport.* Philadelphia: Lea & Febiger.

Morris, C. B. 1948. The measurement of the strength of muscle relative to the cross section. *Res. Q. Am. Assoc. Health Phys. Educ. Rec.* 19:295–303.

Plagenhoef, S. C. 1971. *Patterns of human motion.* Englewood Cliffs, N.J.: Prentice-Hall.

Steindler, A. 1970. *Kinesiology of the human body.* Springfield, Ill.: Charles C Thomas.

Tricker, R. A. R., and Tricker, B. J. K. 1967. *The science of movement.* New York: American Elsevier.

Williams, M., and Lissner, H. R. 1962. *Biomechanics of human motion.* Philadelphia: W. B. Saunders.

The Conditions of Rotatory Motion

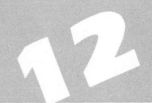

Objectives

At the conclusion of this chapter the student should be able to:

1. Name, define, and use the following terms properly as they relate to rotatory motion: eccentric force, moment, torque, couple, lever, moment of inertia, and angular momentum.
2. Solve simple lever and torque problems involving the human body and the implements it uses.
3. Demonstrate an understanding of the effective selection of levers by relating speed, range of motion, and mechanical advantage to the properties of given lever systems.
4. Explain the analogous kinetic relationships that exist between linear and rotatory motion.
5. State Newton's Laws of Motion as they apply to rotatory motion.
6. Explain the cause and effect relationship between the forces responsible for rotatory motion and the objects experiencing the motion.
7. Define centripetal and centrifugal force, and explain the relationships that exist between these forces and the factors influencing them.

Rotatory Force

Eccentric Force

The student already knows that the effect forces have on an object depends upon the magnitude, point of application, and direction of each force. When force is applied in line with a freely moving object's center of gravity, linear motion occurs. When the direction of force is not in line a combination of rotatory and translatory motion is likely to occur. This relationship between force application and direction and the resulting motion is apparent when a book is pushed along a table. Linear motion occurs when sufficient force is applied in line with the book's center of gravity, and a combination of linear and rotatory motion results from a force directed left or right of center. Similarly, an object with a fixed axis, like a door or one of the body's limbs, ro-

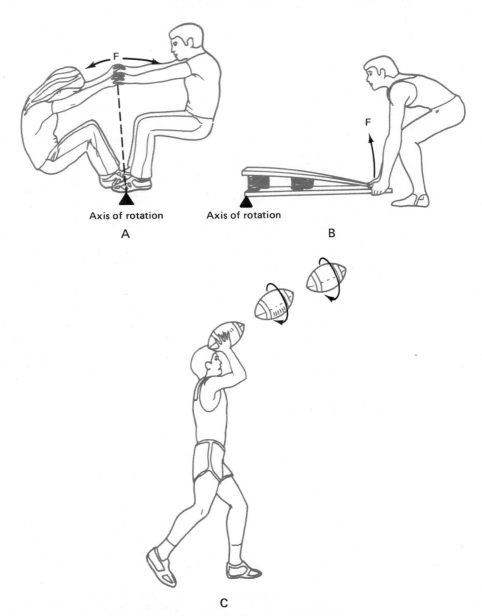

Figure 12–1   Examples of the application of eccentric force.

tates when the force is applied "off center" but does not rotate when the force is in line with the axis of rotation. In the latter instance translatory motion will occur if the force is adequate. A force whose direction is not in line with the center of gravity of a freely moving object or the center of rotation of an object with a fixed axis of rotation is called an **eccentric** force. There must be an eccentric force for rotation to occur. Some examples of the application of eccentric force are shown in Figure 12–1.

Torque and Moments

The turning effect of a force is called the *torque,* or *moment of force.* **The torque about any point equals the product of the force magnitude and its perpendicular distance from the direction of force to the point or axis of rotation.** The perpendicular distance is called the *moment arm* or *torque arm.* Neglecting the weight of the arm, the torque or turning effect caused by a 5-pound weight held in the hand with the forearm horizontally flexed at the elbow joint is the product of the weight times its perpendicular distance or moment arm length from the elbow joint. If this distance is 1 foot, the amount of torque or downward turning force is 5 foot-pounds. To keep the arm motionless in this position the elbow flexors must exert an equal and opposite torque or upward-directed turning force of 5 foot-pounds.

Since a moment is the product of force and moment arm length, it may be increased or decreased by increasing or decreasing either the force or the moment arm length. A small weight a given distance away from the turning point will have a smaller torque or moment than a large weight equidistant from the axis. If, however, the moment arm for the larger weight is shortened by moving it closer to the axis, the torque for both weights could be equal. This is why the force of the elbow flexors needed to maintain the forearm in a horizontal position is less when the 5-pound weight held in the hand is moved closer to the elbow. For the same reason it also takes less effort to move the forearm upward in a rotatory fashion about the elbow joint when the weight is closer to the elbow. The weight has not changed its mass and neither has the arm. The only factor that has changed is the distance between the weight and the elbow. The farther from the axis a force is applied, the greater is its turning effect (torque) and the greater is the effort needed to resist the turning.

It is important to emphasize that the torque arm is the *perpendicular* distance from the direction of force to the axis of rotation. In the example just given the torque arm length was the same as the length of the forearm because the horizontal forearm was perpendicular to the vertical direction of the force, and therefore the forearm length was equal to the perpendicular distance from the force direction to the axis. If the arm were in some position other than the horizontal, its length would no longer be equal to the moment arm distance between the force direction and axis. Suppose the forearm's position is shifted from the horizontal to one of 45 degrees of flexion with the horizontal. Now the force line of the weight is not at right angles to the forearm (Figure 12–2). This means that the length of the moment arm is no longer the length of the forearm because, by definition, the moment arm is the perpendicular distance from the direction or line of force to the axis of motion. The moment arm now is considerably shorter. Using trigonometric relations we find that the moment arm length is .707 feet. Consequently, the torque decreases from 5 foot-pounds to 3.5 foot-pounds, and the amount of muscular effort needed to counteract this downward force decreases proportionately.

In the human body the mass or weight of a segment cannot be altered instantaneously. Therefore the torque of a segment due to gravitational force can only be changed by changing the length of the moment arm in relation to the axis. This is

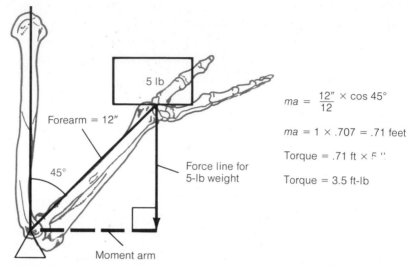

$$ma = \frac{12''}{12} \times \cos 45°$$

$$ma = 1 \times .707 = .71 \text{ feet}$$

$$\text{Torque} = .71 \text{ ft} \times 5 \text{''}$$

$$\text{Torque} = 3.5 \text{ ft-lb}$$

Figure 12–2 The torque of the 5-pound weight about the elbow joint is the product of the weight and the perpendicular distance from the force line of the weight to the axis of rotation (elbow joint).

done by moving a body segment so that the force line of the weight is closer to or farther from the axis. The effect of doing this is quite apparent in the stages of the sit-up. Compare the gravitational torque on the trunk when the trunk is just leaving the floor with the torque when the trunk is at a 30-degree angle from the floor (Figure 12–3).

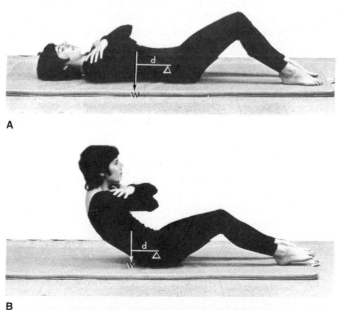

Figure 12–3 Gravitational torque (d) decreases in going from *A* to *B* as the force line moves closer to the axis. The torque is zero at 90°.

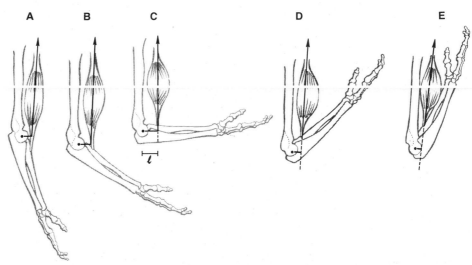

Figure 12–4 The biceps at various points of elbow flexion, showing variations in the moment arm. (From LeVeau, B.: *Williams and Lissner: Biomechanics of human motion.* 2nd ed. Philadelphia: W. B. Saunders, 1977.)

Muscle forces also exert torque on rotating segments. The amount of torque depends upon both the magnitude of the muscle force and the moment arm length. Unlike gravitational torque, each of these factors can be altered. The moment arm length depends upon the point of insertion of the muscle and the position of the body segment at any point in a given motion. Figure 12–4 shows how the moment arm of the biceps changes for every change of arm position during elbow flexion. The magnitude of the force of the muscle contributing to the torque changes also as its length, tension, and angle of pull change.

The important thing to remember from this discussion is that the turning effect or torque produced on objects free to rotate depends upon two factors, the magnitude of the applied force and the perpendicular distance from the force direction to the axis. Change in turning effect occurs when either of these factors is altered. Shortening the moment arm distance or decreasing the force magnitude will decrease the torque. Lengthening the moment arm or increasing the force magnitude will increase the turning effect and consequently the effort necessary to resist it.

Summation of Moments

The sum of two or more moments may result in no motion, linear motion, or rotatory motion. When eccentric parallel forces are applied in the same direction on opposite sides of the center of rotation of an object either no motion or linear motion will occur. An example of no motion is two children balanced on a seesaw. When the parallel forces are adequate to overcome the resistance of the object, linear motion will occur. This could be the situation with paddlers in a canoe, with one paddling on the port side and the other on the starboard side. When equal and opposite parallel forces are exerted on opposite sides of the axis of rotation, rotatory motion will occur. The effect of equal parallel forces acting in opposite directions is called a *couple* or *force couple*. An example of this type of movement is steering a car or boat when both hands are used on opposite sides of the wheel (Figure 12–5). Another example is that of turning in a rowboat by simultaneously pulling on the handle of one oar while pushing on the handle of the other.

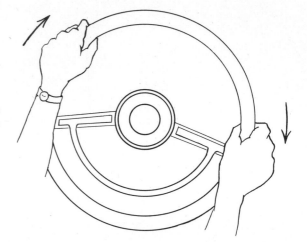

Figure 12–5 When one steers with two hands, the hands act as a force couple.

There are many examples in the human body in which two muscles rotate a bone by acting cooperatively as a force couple; for instance, trapezius II and the lower portion of serratus anterior are a force couple, rotating the scapula upward. Trapezius II and IV, acting on the two extremities of the spine of the scapula, similarly serve as a force couple to help rotate the scapula upward, as do the oblique abdominals in acting to rotate the trunk (Figure 12–6).

PRINCIPLE OF MOMENTS   It is common for more than one moment to act on a body at any given time. The resultant effect of these moments is expressed in the principle of the summation of moments, which states that the **resultant moment of a force system must be equal to the sum of the moments of the individual forces of the system about the same point.** Because moments are vector quantities the summation must consider both magnitude and direction. The direction of rotation is expressed either as clockwise or counterclockwise direction. Clockwise moments are usually labeled as negative and counterclockwise moments as positive. Their signs must be accounted for when they are summed.

When the sum of counterclockwise moments equals the sum of clockwise moments no turning will occur. This idea may also be expressed by stating that rotation will be absent when the sum of the moments of all forces about any point or axis equals zero. When the sum of clockwise moments does not equal the sum of the counterclockwise moments, the resultant turning effect (torque) will be the difference between the two opposing forces and in the direction of the larger.

In Figure 12–7 all the forces are applied perpendicular to the lever. Force *A* is 1.15 m from the axis and *B* is 3 m away. Both *A* and *B* are clockwise forces. Force *C* is a counterclockwise force that also is 3 m away from the axis. The sum of these force moments produces a resultant torque of 22.5 Newton-meters in a clockwise direction about the center of rotation.

When an eccentric force is applied at an angle to the lever other than 90 degrees,

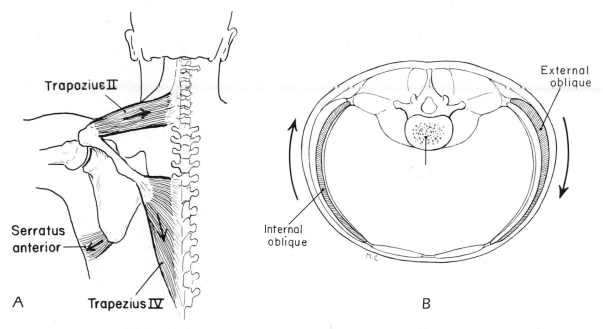

Figure 12–6 *A,* Two force couples acting on the scapula to rotate it upward. (Trapezius II and lower serratus anterior are an excellent example. Trapezius II and the lower fibers of IV also tend to act as a force couple although their pulls are not in opposite directions. *B,* A cross section of the trunk in which the oblique abdominal muscles act as a force couple to rotate the trunk.

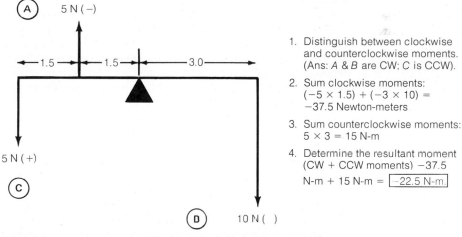

1. Distinguish between clockwise and counterclockwise moments. (Ans: *A & B* are CW; *C* is CCW).

2. Sum clockwise moments: $(-5 \times 1.5) + (-3 \times 10) = -37.5$ Newton-meters

3. Sum counterclockwise moments: $5 \times 3 = 15$ N-m

4. Determine the resultant moment (CW + CCW moments) -37.5 N-m + 15 N-m = $\boxed{-22.5 \text{ N-m.}}$

Figure 12–7 Summation of moments. The resultant moment about a point is equal to the sum of the moments of the individual forces about the same point. Clockwise moments are negative, and counterclockwise moments are positive. The sum of the moments about the fulcrum on this diagram is 22.5 Newton-meters in a clockwise direction.

the moment arm is not along the lever line. Before the moment can be found, the length of the moment arm must be determined. This can be done using trigonometric functions. An example of this procedure is shown in the following problem.

> What muscular force F pulling at an angle of 25 degrees would be required to keep the abducted arm in a position of 20 degrees with the horizontal? The muscle inserts 4 inches from the shoulder joint. The arm weighs 13 pounds and its center of gravity is located 12 inches from the shoulder. A 10-pound weight is held in the hand 23 inches from the shoulder joint. *Note:* For the arm to be held stationary the sum of the counterclockwise moments must equal the clockwise moments (ΣCCW = ΣCW). (See Figure 12–8 for solution.)

The Lever

A simple machine that operates according to the principle of moments is the *lever*. A lever is a rigid bar that can rotate about a fixed point when a force is applied to overcome a resistance. When they move, levers serve two important functions. They are used either to overcome a larger resistance than the effort applied or to increase the distance a resistance can be moved through use of an effort greater than the resistance. When there is no motion, the effort turning effect (torque) equals the resistance turning effect (torque) and the lever system is said to be balanced.

External Levers

We use levers every day of our lives. In the kitchen the old-fashioned hand can opener, nut pick, punch can opener, and bottle opener or lid pry are all examples of simple levers. Likewise, in the workshop or about the house and grounds the tack lifter, crowbar, pinch bar, and wheelbarrow are levers. What do these implements have in common? Even though their shapes vary and their structures differ in complexity, each of these is a rigid bar. When a force is applied to one of them, it turns about a fixed point known as a *fulcrum,* and it overcomes a resistance that may, in some cases, be no more than its own weight. All the levers mentioned are designed for the purpose of using a relatively small force to overcome a relatively large resistance. In levers such as these the range of movement of the resistance is relatively slight, while the range of movement of the effort is large. The tack lifter, for instance, lifts the tack only a fraction of an inch, while the handle moves through a much larger distance. In other words, the power to overcome a considerable resistance is gained at the expense of range of motion.

The striking implements used in sports are levers that do the opposite of this. The golf club, for instance, is used for gaining range of motion at the expense of force. The length of the shaft enables the club head to travel through a large arc of motion, but it is used to overcome the relatively slight resistance of the weight of the club itself. Tennis and squash rackets, baseball bats, hockey sticks, and fencing foils are other examples of levers used for the purpose of gaining distance at the expense of force. These levers do not save the strength of the user, as do the household levers mentioned, but they increase the user's range and speed of movement. By striking a ball with a racket, for instance, the striker can impart more speed to it and send it a greater distance than could be done by striking it with the hand. This is because the head of the racket travels a greater distance, and therefore at a greater speed, than the hand alone is able to do.

**How much muscle force is needed
to hold the arm and 10-lb weight
in this position?**

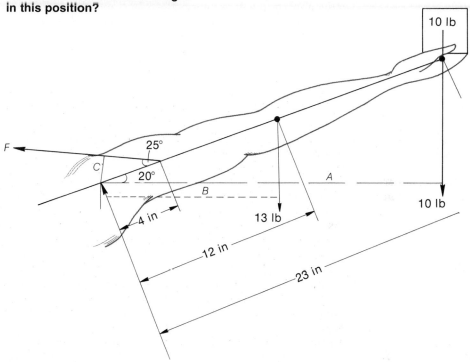

Solution

▲ = axis
F = force of muscle
A = moment arm for 10-lb weight

B = moment arm for 13-lb arm
C = moment arm for F

To balance, clockwise moments must equal counterclockwise moments.

1. *Clockwise moments*
   a. 10 lb × A = 10 × 23 cos 20°
   b. 13 lb × B = 13 × 12 cos 20°
2. *Counterclockwise moments*
   a. F × C = F × 4 sin 25°
3. CW = CCW
   F × C = (10 × A) + (13 × B)

4. 230 cos 20° + 156 cos 20° = 4 sin 25° × F
5. $F = \dfrac{230 \cos 20° + 156 \cos 20°}{4 \sin 25°}$
6. $F = \dfrac{(230 \times .940) + (156 \times .940)}{4 \times .422}$

   $F = \dfrac{362}{1.69} = 215 \text{ lb}$

Figure 12–8 Summation of force moments using trigonometric functions. The amount of muscle force needed to counteract the force of gravity in this example is 215 pounds.

A still different kind of lever is seen in the seesaw on the playground, the scales in the laboratory, and the yoke used for carrying balanced loads across the shoulders. These levers gain neither force nor distance, but provide for a balancing of weights. If the loads are equal, they will balance each other when they are equidistant from the fulcrum. If they are unequal, they will balance only if the heavier load is placed closer to the fulcrum. There is an exact relationship between the magnitude of the weights and their respective distances from the fulcrum so that when the torques are summed, the resultant is zero.

This kind of lever may also be used to balance a force and a load. The skier carrying skis over one shoulder, balanced by a hand holding the other end, is an example. The amount of effort exerted by the hand depends upon what portion of the ski is in contact with the shoulder. If the weight of the skis is evenly distributed on each side of the shoulder, the hand needs to exert little or no effort.

Anatomical Levers

But where in the human body do we have anything even faintly resembling a punch can opener, hockey stick, or seesaw? When we recognize each of these levers as a rigid bar that turns about a fulcrum when force is applied to it, it is then apparent that nearly every bone in the skeleton can be looked upon as a lever. The bone itself serves as the rigid bar, the joint as the fulcrum, and the contracting muscles as the force. A large segment of the body, such as the trunk, the upper extremity, or the lower extremity, can likewise act as a single lever if it is used as a rigid unit. When the entire arm is raised sideward, for instance, it is acting as a simple lever. The center of motion in the shoulder joint serves as the fulcrum. The effort is supplied mainly by the deltoid muscle and the resistance in this instance is the weight of the arm itself. The point at which the effort is applied to the lever is approximately the point at which the deltoid inserts into the humerus, and the point at which the resistance is applied is the center of gravity of the extended arm. If a weight is held in the hand, the resistance point is then the center of gravity of the arm plus its load and is located closer to the hand than before. If a relatively heavy weight is lifted, for practical purposes the weight of the arm may be disregarded and the resistance point may be assumed to be the center of the object's point of contact with the hand.

Anatomical levers do not necessarily resemble bars. The skull, shoulder blade, and vertebrae are notable exceptions to the definition. The resistance point, also, may be difficult to identify, especially in the seesaw type of lever. It is not always easy to tell whether the resistance is the weight of the lever itself or is the resistance afforded by antagonistic muscles and fasciae that are put on a steadily increasing stretch as the movement progresses. For instance, when the head is turned easily to the left, the resistance point may be regarded as the center of gravity of the head. We can only guess at the approximate location of this. If the turning of the head is resisted by the pressure of someone's hand against the left side of the chin the resistance point is the midpoint of the contact area. If the head is turned without external resistance but is forced to the limit of motion, resistance to the movement is afforded by the antagonistic rotators, and possibly by the ligaments and fasciae. The resistance *point* in such a case is the midpoint of the area over which these resisting forces act on the head. As in the first example, the location of this point can only be estimated.

Classification of Levers

In the examples cited, three points on the lever have been identified: the point about which it turns, the point at which effort is applied to it, and the point at which the resistance to its movement is applied or concentrated. Since there are three points, there

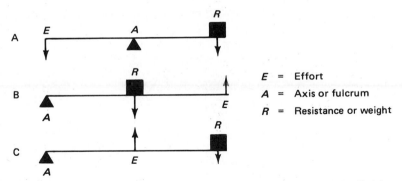

Figure 12–9   Levers. *A*, A lever of the first class. *B*, A lever of the second class. *C*, A lever of the third class.

are three possible arrangements of these points. Any one of the three may be situated between the other two. The arrangement of these three points provides the basis for the classification of levers.

1. In a first class lever the fulcrum lies between the effort and resistance points (Figure 12–9A).
2. In a second class lever the resistance point lies between the fulcrum and the effort point (Figure 12–9B).
3. In a third class lever the effort lies between the fulcrum and the resistance point (Figure 12–9C).

FIRST CLASS LEVERS   Examples of external first class levers are the seesaw, balance scale, crowbar, scissors, and automobile jack.

The head, tipping forward and backward, is a good example of a first class lever in the body (Figure 12–10). To be sure, it is a sphere rather than a bar, and the axis of motion would seem to be an imaginary one located in the frontal plane approximately between the ears. The effort is supplied by the extensors of the head, notably the splenius and upper portions of the semispinalis, and is applied to the head at the base of the skull. The resistance to the movement is furnished by the weight of the head itself, together with the tension of the antagonistic muscles and fasciae, as the limit of motion is approached. The center of concentration of the resistance is difficult to determine. If the head is acting like a seesaw, the resistance would seem to be centered in the front half of the head for hyperextension. Additional resistance is provided by the tension of opposing muscles and ligaments, the resistance point being the point at which the various resistance forces are concentrated.

Another first class lever is seen in the foot when it is not being used for weight-bearing, as when the knees are crossed in the sitting position. As the soleus pulls upward on the heel, the foot plantar flexes at the ankle joint where the fulcrum is situated. The resistance seems to be provided by the tonus of the dorsiflexor muscles. The weight of the foot apparently is not a factor here, since the foot has already relaxed into a position of partial plantar flexion. The picture would be changed, however, if the person were lying face down with the leg bent at the knee and the lower leg extended vertically upward. If the foot were then plantar flexed, the weight of the foot would be a factor in the resistance.

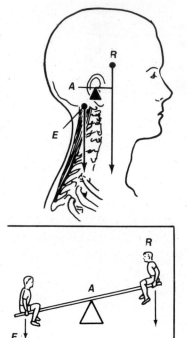

Figure 12–10   The head acting as a first class lever like the seesaw. *A* = The approximate position of the axis or fulcrum; *E* = the point where the force is applied; *R* = the approximate point where the resistance is concentrated.

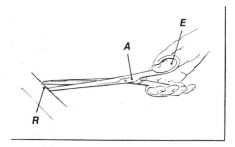

Figure 12–11   The forearm acting as a first class lever, similar to a pair of paper shears.

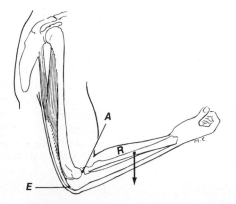

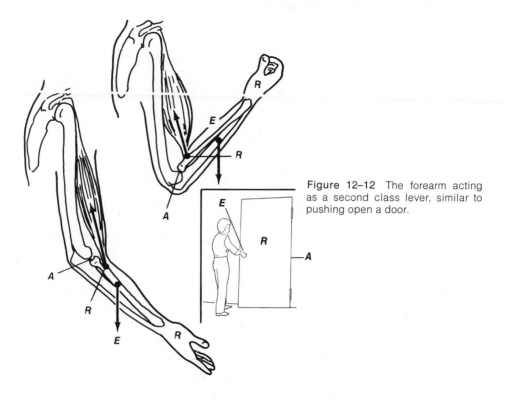

Figure 12–12 The forearm acting as a second class lever, similar to pushing open a door.

The forearm is another example of a first class lever *when it is being extended by the triceps muscle against a resistance* (Figure 12–11). The fulcrum is situated at the elbow joint, the effort is applied at the olecranon process, and the resistance point is located at the forearm's center of gravity when no external resistance is present, and at the hand when the latter is pushing against an external resistance. Internal resistance does not appear to be a factor in this movement.

SECOND CLASS LEVERS   Examples of external second class levers are the wheelbarrow, door (effort applied at the knob), and nutcracker. Whether or not there are any second class levers in the body seems to be a controversial matter among anatomists and kinesiologists. Some claim that when the foot is being plantar flexed in a weight-bearing position, as when rising on the toes, it is a second class lever. The fulcrum is said to be at the point of contact with the ground, the effort point at the heel where the tendon of Achilles attaches and the resistance at the ankle joint where the weight of the body is transferred to the foot. Another second class lever might be the forearm if it were being flexed by the brachioradialis alone, but this could occur only if the other flexors were paralyzed.

There are numerous second class levers involving body segments if those actions where gravity supplies the effort for the movement and muscles control or resist the movement through eccentric contraction are included. The forearm in slow downward extension is an example. The fulcrum is at the elbow joint, the effort may be considered to be applied at the insertion of the elbow flexor, which for this example is

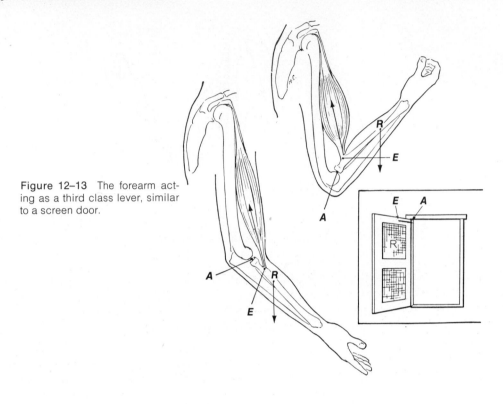

Figure 12–13 The forearm acting as a third class lever, similar to a screen door.

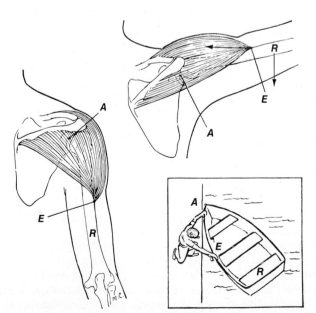

Figure 12–14 The humerus acting as a third class lever, somewhat like a boat being pulled alongside the dock.

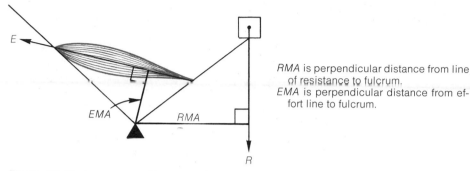

RMA is perpendicular distance from line of resistance to fulcrum.
EMA is perpendicular distance from effort line to fulcrum.

Figure 12–15 Lever arms, like moment arms, are the perpendicular distance between the fulcrum and the force line.

considered to be the brachialis. The brachialis through eccentric contraction resists the downward-directed weight of the arm (Figure 12–12). Another example is the slow lowering of the leg at the knee from an extended to a flexed position. The fulcrum is at the knee joint, the effort is the lower leg applied at its center of gravity, and the resistance is the eccentric contraction of the quadriceps at its point of insertion on the tibial tuberosity.

THIRD CLASS LEVERS There are not too many examples of external third class levers. One example is a screen door with a spring closing. There are, however, many examples of anatomical third class levers, since most body segments that are moved by muscular effort fall into this class. The forearm is a good example of a third class lever when it is being flexed by the biceps and the brachialis (Figure 12–13). Another third class lever is seen in the example cited earlier, namely, the arm as it is raised sideward-upward by the deltoid muscle (Figure 12–14).

Lever Arms

Lever arms are commonly defined as the portion of the lever between the fulcrum and the force points. The effort arm is the distance between the fulcrum and the effort point, and the resistance arm is the distance between the fulcrum and the resistance point. These definitions are valid, however, only when the effort and resistance are applied at right angles to the lever. When the effort and resistance are applied at some angle other than 90 degrees to the lever, these definitions are inaccurate. A better definition of a lever arm that applies regardless of the angle of force application is one synonymous to that of a moment arm. Indeed, a lever arm is a moment arm. In a lever the perpendicular distance between the fulcrum and line of force of the effort is the *effort moment arm (EMA)* or *effort arm.* Similarly, the perpendicular distance between the fulcrum and the line of resistance force is the *resistance moment arm (RMA)* or *resistance arm.* In Figure 12–15, *EMA* is the effort arm and *RMA* is the resistance arm.

The Principle of Levers

A lever of any class will balance when the product of the effort and the effort arm equals the product of the resistance and the resistance arm. This is known as the *principle of levers.* It enables us to calculate the amount of effort needed to balance a known resistance by means of a known lever or to calculate the point at which to

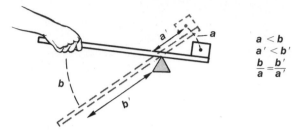

Figure 12–16 The range of motion increases as the lever arm length increases.

place the fulcrum in order to balance a known resistance with a given effort. If any three of the four values are known, the remaining one can be calculated by using the following equation:

$$E \times EMA = R \times RMA$$

(effort times effort arm equals resistance times resistance arm)

This equation restates a principle already studied under the summation of moments. When the force moments in one direction equal the force moments in the opposite direction, equilibrium exists. $E \times EMA$ is a force moment, as is $R \times RMA$. When applied to Figure 12–15, this means that it will be possible to balance the weight in the hand when the product of the weight and the perpendicular distance from its direction to the fulcrum ($R \times RMA$) equals the product of the muscle effort and the perpendicular distance from its direction to the fulcrum ($E \times EMA$).

The lever equation also shows the importance of lever arm lengths in determining the amount of effort needed to balance a given resistance. If EMA is lengthened while $R \times RMA$ remains constant, the amount of effort needed to balance the lever must decrease, but if, on the other hand, RMA is increased, the amount of effort must increase. For this reason, second class levers require less effort to balance or move heavier resistances, while third class levers require more effort than the resistance they must balance or move (Figures 12–13 and 12–14). The first class lever may have either a longer EMA or RMA, depending upon the placement of the fulcrum (Figures 12–10 and 12–11).

Figure 12–17 Comparison of a long and a short lever turning the same number of degrees. It takes B the same amount of time to reach B' that it takes C to reach C'.

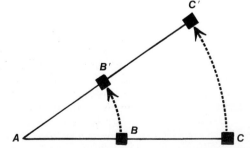

A lever whose effort arm is the longer of the two, whether it be a first or second class lever, is said to favor *force*. Less effort is required to overcome a resistance with this kind of lever than it would take to overcome the same resistance without the aid of the lever. This advantage is gained at the expense of speed and range of movement. The heavier resistance will always move through a smaller distance than the effort (Figure 12–16). Conversely, a lever whose resistance arm is longer, whether it be a first or a third class lever, is said to favor speed and distance. However, more effort is required to move it than would be the case if the relative lengths of the effort and resistance arms were reversed. Furthermore, an object of negligible weight can be moved a greater distance and more rapidly by this kind of lever than it could be without the aid of the lever.

Relation of Speed to Range in Movements of Levers

The reader will have noticed that in the foregoing discussion of levers the terms "speed" and "range" were usually linked together. There is a reason for this. In angular movements speed and range are interdependent. For instance, if two third class levers of different lengths each move through a 40-degree angle at the same angular velocity, the tip of the longer lever will be traveling a greater distance or range than the tip of the shorter lever. Since it covers this distance in the same time that it takes the tip of the shorter lever to travel the shorter distance, the former must be moving faster than the latter. This is easily seen if the shorter lever is superimposed on the longer, as in Figure 12–17. Here the shorter lever, *AB*, has been superimposed on the longer lever, *AC*. The levers are moving from the horizontal position to the diagonal one. Since the point *C* travels to its new position, *C'*, in the same time that it takes *B* to travel to *B'*, point *C* must obviously be moving farther and faster than point *B*.

With few exceptions, the effort arm in skeletal levers is shorter than the resistance arm. Thus, anatomical levers tend to favor speed and range of movement at the expense of effort. Examples of this preference are seen in the throwing of a baseball or the kicking of a soccer ball. The hand in the one case and the foot in the other travel through a relatively long distance at considerable speed. Both these movements require strong muscular action, in spite of the fact that the balls are relatively light in weight. This type of leverage is the reverse of the kind usually seen in mechanical implements such as the crowbar and the automobile jack, both of which are used to move heavy weights a relatively short distance. Sports implements that may serve as levers in themselves or as artificial extensions of the human arm also favor speed and range of movement. Frequently the sport implement, arm, and a large part of the rest of the body act together as a system of levers. In batting a baseball, for instance, the trunk forms one lever, the upper arms another, the forearms another, and the hands and bat still another. This use of multiple leverage is for the purpose of building up speed at the tip of the bat, because the greater this speed, the greater the force that can be imparted to the ball.

Selection of Levers

Skill in motor performance depends upon the effective selection and use of levers, both internal and external. Long golf clubs are selected for distance and shorter clubs for accuracy at close range. Heavy baseball bats are chosen by those with the strength to swing them, while children are often taught tennis with short-handled rackets. In most instances external levers are designed for a specific purpose and are selected accordingly. The levers of the human body, on the other hand, are not designed for

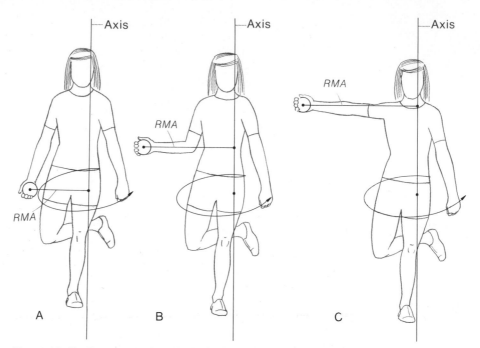

Figure 12–18 The length of the *RMA* determines the linear velocity at the end of the lever. In the positions pictured, when the pelvis rotates to the left, the linear velocity of the ball is least in *A* and most in *C*. The movement occurs at the left hip and results in the lower extremity's being medially rotated, relative to the pelvis.

one action or purpose. Body parts or segments may be held in numerous positions for any given joint action and thus provide a great variety of lever arrangements. Consequently, skill depends upon the right choice of joint axis, joint action, and moment arm length. In all three instances in Figure 12–18, the ball in the hand is carried forward by virtue of the counterclockwise (as seen from above) rotation of the pelvis that takes place at the left hip joint. The pelvis carries the trunk with it but no movement occurs in any joint other than the left hip. In all three positions the resistance moment arm for the action is the perpendicular distance between the hip axis and the line of action of the resistance (the ball). However, the resistance moment arm is a different length in each situation. It is smallest in *A* and largest in *C*. Consequently the linear velocity of the ball is largest in *C* and smallest in *A* when the angular velocity is the same in each instance. (See Figure 12–17.) Similarly, if flexion of the shoulder is the joint action, the position of the arm that will provide the greatest linear velocity to the object in the hand at the moment of release is one in which the elbow is extended and the arm is perpendicular to the desired direction of flight (Figure 12–19).

It is not always desirable to choose the longest lever, however. The positioning of body parts to form short levers enhances the angular velocity of the levers while sacrificing linear speed and range of motion at the end of the lever. And, while forming the longest possible lever can increase speed and range of motion at the end of the lever, the strength needed to maintain the desired angular velocity increases as the lever lengthens. This is why the tennis player may flex the elbow in the forehand drive or the batter may "choke up" when swinging a heavy bat.

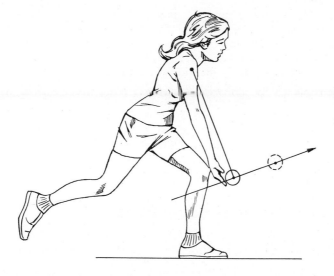

Figure 12–19 A straight arm perpendicular to the desired line of flight provides the greatest linear velocity to the ball when the joint action is shoulder flexion.

Mechanical Advantage of Levers

Machines are judged good if they are efficient, poor if they are inefficient. How is the efficiency of a machine measured? Since the machines used in industry and in the workshop are usually for the purpose of magnifying force, it is customary to measure their efficiency in terms of their *mechanical advantage*, in other words, their ability to magnify force. Another way of expressing this ability is to state the "output" of the machine relative to its "input." In levers this is the ratio between the effort applied to the lever and the resistance overcome by the lever. It may be expressed in terms of the equation: mechanical advantage equals the ratio of the resistance overcome to the effort applied, or, simply,

$$MA = \frac{R}{E}$$

Since the balanced lever equation may also be expressed as

$$\frac{R}{E} = \frac{EA}{RA}$$

it is seen that the mechanical advantage may be expressed in terms of the ratio of the effort arm to the resistance arm. Hence, if

$$MA = \frac{R}{E}$$

it also holds that

$$MA = \frac{EA}{RA}$$

When a muscle is said to have poor leverage it means that it has poor mechanical advantage. In other words, the effort arm of the lever upon which it is acting is short compared with the resistance arm.

Identification and Analysis of Levers

Figures 12–10 to 12–14 depict certain anatomical levers and their mechanical counterparts. These should enable the student to understand the principle of leverage as it applies in the human body and to see how the anatomical levers compare with the levers of everyday life. For each of these levers and for every lever that the student observes, these questions should be answered: (1) What are the locations of the fulcrum, effort point, and resistance point? (2) At what angle is the effort applied to the lever? (3) At what angle is the resistance applied to the lever? (4) What is the effort arm of the lever? (5) What is the resistance arm of the lever? (6) What are the relative lengths of the effort and resistance arms? (7) What kind of movement does this lever favor? (8) What is the mechanical advantage? (9) What class of lever is this?

Newton's Laws and Rotational Equivalents

When applied to rotatory motion Newton's Laws of Motion may be stated as follows:

1. A body continues in a state of rest or uniform rotation about its axis unless acted upon by an external torque.
2. The acceleration of a rotating body is directly proportional to the torque causing it, is in the same direction as the torque, and is inversely proportional to the moment of inertia of the body.
3. When a torque is applied by one body to another the second body will exert an equal and opposite torque on the first.

The laws themselves are analogous to those stated for linear motion. In order to comprehend their application to rotatory motion, however, an understanding of the rotatory equivalents of linear mass, momentum, and force is necessary. These parallel relationships between linear motion and rotatory motion quantities become quite apparent when presented side by side, as in Table 12–1.

TABLE 12–1 Analogous Quantities in Linear and Rotatory Motion

UNIT	LINEAR MOTION	ROTATORY MOTION
Distance	s	θ (theta)
Velocity	v	ω (omega)
Acceleration	a	α (alpha)
Mass	m	I (moment of inertia)
Force	F	L (torque)
Force equation	$F = ma$	$L = I\alpha$
Momentum	mv	$I\omega$
Impulse	Ft	Lt
Work	Fs	$L\theta$
Power	Fv	$S\omega$
Kinetic energy	$\frac{1}{2}mv^2$	$\frac{1}{2}I\omega^2$

Moment of Inertia

In the preceding discussion of Newton's laws, the quality of a body to resist change in its state of motion was identified as inertia. The inertia of a body with respect to linear motion was shown to be directly proportional to the mass of the object. The heavier an object the more force it takes to start it moving and the more force required to stop it. This is also true in rotatory motion. Once they are set in motion, spinning bodies tend to keep spinning. As with linear motion, the amount of force needed to start or stop a spinning object is related to its mass: the heavier the object, the more effort required to start or stop it rotating. However, there is an additional factor to be considered. The hammer thrower knows that it takes more effort to start the weight moving in a circular fashion at the end of the wire than it does to start it moving in a linear fashion. It is also true that once the hammer is moving in a circular fashion it is more difficult to slow it down than if it were moving in a straight line. Therefore it seems that the hammer's inertia is greater when moving in an angular pattern than when moving in a linear path. Since the mass of the hammer does not change, this increase in inertia must be due to some other element. In the same way that the torque causing rotatory motion is dependent upon the magnitude of force and the distance from the line of action of the force to the axis, the inertia of a rotatory body is affected by both the mass and the distance between the mass and axis of rotation. A ball rotating on the end of a long string is harder to stop and start than one on a short string. As the distance between the axis and the mass increases, the inertia increases. Thus, the size of the angular inertia, called the moment of inertia, I, depends upon both the quantity of the rotating mass and its distribution around the axis of rotation. The exact nature of this relationship is shown in the equation for the moment of inertia.

$$I = \Sigma mr^2$$

where m is the mass of a particle in the rotating body and r is the perpendicular distance between the mass particle and the axis of rotation. Thus the moment of inertia of an object is the sum of the mass of each of the particles multiplied by the square of the distance to the axis (Figure 12–20). If the mass of an object is concentrated close to the axis of rotation, the object is easier to turn because the radius for each particle is less, thus making I less. Conversely, if the mass is concentrated farther away from the axis, I becomes greater and the rotating body will require more force to start or stop it.

In the human body the mass distribution may be altered by changing the body position, thereby changing the moment of inertia. A runner is able to move the

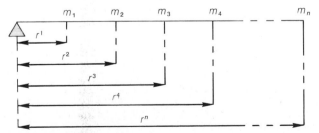

$I = \Sigma\, mr^2$
I = moment of inertia
m = mass particle
r = perpendicular distance of m from axis (▲)

Figure 12–20   The moment of inertia about an axis is the sum of the mass particles multiplied by the square of the distance of each particle from the axis. $(I = \Sigma\, mr^2)$

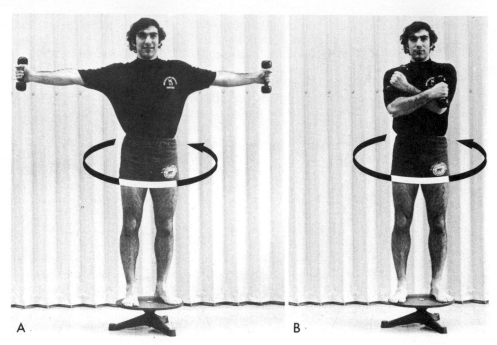

Figure 12–21   The moment of inertia about an axis decreases when the mass is concentrated close to the axis of rotation. The moment of inertia in *A* is greater than that in *B*.

recovery leg forward more rapidly when it is in a flexed position than when it is extended. The mass of the leg is the same in both instances, but it is closer to the axis when the leg is flexed and the moment of inertia is less. Using data for average mass proportions of body segments and the location of the center of gravity of each segment, Dyson (1970) estimated that a person standing on a frictionless turntable with arms outstretched to the side has a moment of inertia three times greater than when the arms are at the side (Figure 12–21). When a person lies horizontally on the table, with the arms at the sides and the vertical axis passing through the center of gravity, *I* becomes 14 times greater. The moment of inertia of the body is least about a vertical axis passing through the center of gravity when the arms are raised and held close to the head, and greatest when the body is in a fully extended position rotating about the hands, as in the giant swing on the high bar.

Using a method similar to finding the center of gravity of the body by the segmental method (see Chapter 13, p. 399), Hay (1978) reported the moment of inertia of the human body in some common rotating positions. In the tuck position, *I* about the body's center of gravity was 2.58 slug-ft², in the pike position it was 4.89 slug-ft², and in the layout 11.15 slug-ft². The moment of inertia about the hands of the giant swing position was 60.90 slug-ft². These figures verify that inertia to rotation increases as the mass is distributed farther away from the axis.

When one is interested in the moment of inertia of a specific body segment, it is usually taken about the center of the joint serving as the axis, although other axes may be chosen. If another axis is selected, such as the center of gravity of the segment, *I* will change accordingly because values of r will be different in the equation $I = \Sigma mr^2$.

Acceleration of Rotating Bodies

The equation for Newton's second Law of Motion when applied to linear motion was shown to be $F = ma$. The rotational equivalent is $L = I\alpha$—that is, the rotatory force or torque (L) is equal to the product of the moment of inertia (I) of the rotating object and the angular acceleration (α).

The fact that this rotatory equation for force is equivalent to the linear equation is easily proved. If both sides of the equation $F = ma$ are multiplied by r, we have $Fr = mra$. Since Fr equals torque and $a = \alpha r$, the equation can next be written as $L = mr^2\alpha$. And, since mr^2 is equivalent to I, the equation can take the same form as its linear counterpart—i.e., $L = I\alpha$ (Table 12–1). The rotatory equivalent of linear force is torque, the rotatory equivalent of mass is the moment of inertia, and the rotatory equivalent of linear acceleration is angular acceleration. With a little transposing of the equation it becomes apparent how the rotatory equivalent of Newton's second Law of Motion states that the change in rotatory velocity (α) is directly proportional to the torque (L) and inversely proportional to the moment of inertia (I)—that is, $\alpha = \dfrac{L}{I}$.

ANGULAR MOMENTUM   Momentum is a measure of the force needed to start or stop motion. Objects undergoing angular motion have momentum in the same fashion as objects engaged in linear motion. Linear momentum is the product of mass and velocity. Angular momentum is the product of the angular equivalents of mass and velocity—that is, the moment of inertia, I, and angular velocity, ω.

$$\text{linear momentum} = mv$$

$$\text{angular momentum} = I\omega$$

The momentum of a skater skating in a straight line is mv. The momentum of the skater spinning is $I\omega$.

Angular momentum can be increased or decreased by increasing or decreasing either the angular velocity or the moment of inertia. A heavy bat-swing with the same velocity as a light bat-swing has greater angular momentum. However, increasing the velocity-swing of the lighter bat could produce an angular momentum equal to or greater than that of the heavier bat. Similarly, the angular momentum of a kicking leg can be increased by increasing its angular velocity. Conversely, it will decrease if the leg is flexed at the knee (thus decreasing the moment of inertia) while keeping the velocity constant.

CONSERVATION OF ANGULAR MOMENTUM   Newton's first law as applied to rotatory motion can also be stated in terms related to momentum. Worded thus it states that the total angular momentum of a rotating body will remain constant unless acted upon by external torques. This is why the law is also known as the Law of Conservation of Angular Momentum. Like linear momentum, angular momentum is conserved. Once a spinning body is in motion its angular momentum will not alter, provided, of course, that no outside forces are introduced. Divers, trampolinists, dancers, and any other rotating performers all make use of the conservation of angular momentum to control the speed of bodily spin. A skater starts to spin with the arms outstretched. After spinning slowly in this position, the skater brings the arms in close to the body and immediately begins to spin rapidly. The increase in angular velocity occurs with no effort on the skater's part. By bringing the arms in closer to the axis of rotation the moment of inertia is decreased about that axis and, since the

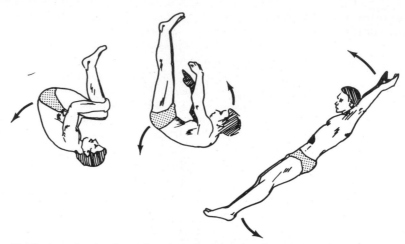

Figure 12–22 Lengthening the radius of rotation increases the moment of inertia and decreases the angular velocity. The angular momentum of the rotating diver is conserved. (Drawn from motion picture film tracing.)

angular momentum must remain constant, a decrease in I produces an increase in ω. Increasing I by stretching the arms and perhaps a leg out to the side will again slow down the skater. A diver performing a tuck somersault can control the speed of rotation by changing the tightness of the tuck, thus changing the moment of inertia. If the diver thinks the entry into the water will be spoiled because of too rapid a rotation, the I can be increased and the angular velocity decreased proportionately by "opening up" or loosening the tuck (Figure 12–22).

Action and Reaction

As previously explained, the force for angular motion is torque. For every torque exerted by one body on a second body, there is another torque equal in magnitude and opposite in direction exerted by the second body on the first. This is Newton's third Law of Motion as applied to angular movement. A force that causes a change in angular momentum must have an equal and opposite force creating an equal and opposite momentum change. In other words, angular momentum is conserved. When one jumps straight up from a trampoline bed with arms stretched upward and then swings the legs forward and up, the body will jackknife at the hips. The torque acting on the legs results in an equal and opposite torque acting on the rest of the body. A change in angular velocity is observed in both body segments, although that in the trunk segment is less because I is greater. Another jump upward followed by a sharp flexion of the wrists only will also produce an equal and opposite torque upon the rest of the body. However, in this case the change in angular velocity of the arms and trunk resulting in forward upward motion will be barely visible. I for the arms and trunk is so large compared to I for the hands that the opposite rotation will be very slight. The angular velocity of the two moving parts is inversely proportional to their moments of inertia about the axis of motion (the wrist joint in the example just given). Axes for such actions may be in any plane but the reactions must be in the same or parallel planes. The arms swinging horizontally across in front of the trunk will produce an opposite action of the rest of the body in the transverse plane (Figure 12–23). Movement of one arm downward in the frontal plane produces an equal and opposite action of the rest of the body in the frontal plane. This is the movement that

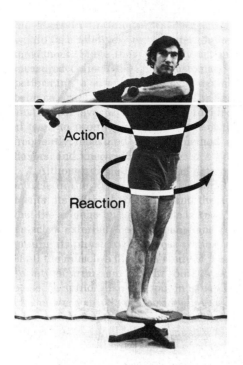

Figure 12–23 Angular action and reaction. As the arms swing across the body in one direction, an equal and opposite reaction occurs in the rest of the body.

may be used to regain balance on a beam or tightrope. If one falls to the left, a downward movement of the left arm produces a reaction of the rest of the body to the right and hopefully prevents a fall.

The equation describing this action-reaction relationship may be written as

$$I_1(\omega_{v_1} - \omega_{u_1}) = I_2(\omega_{v_2} - \omega_{u_2})$$

Any changes in the moments of inertia of the two bodies (I_1 and I_2) or of their respective velocities (ω_1 and ω_2) will produce equal and opposite momentum changes so that $I_1(\omega_{v_1} - \omega_{u_1})$ and $I_2(\omega_{r_2} - \omega_{u_2})$ continues to be equal and opposite.

Sometimes action and reaction to specific body parts is not desired and should be controlled. This can be done by substitution or absorption of the undesired action. In running, the rotation of the pelvis and legs about a vertical axis produces an undesired reaction of the upper trunk in the opposite direction if it is not compensated in some fashion. To prevent this, the arms move in opposition to the legs to "absorb" the reaction by producing a counter twist that cancels out the reaction of the body to the leg action. The faster one moves or the more massive the legs, the more vigorous must be the arm action. The arms are used in the same fashion to prevent undesired trunk reaction to leg action in hurdling, diving, and jumping.

Transfer of Momentum

Because of the Law of Conservation of Momentum, angular momentum may be transferred from one body or body part to another as the total angular momentum remains unaltered. In the suspended balls shown in Figure 12–24, the sudden checking of motion in Ball A produces a comparable action in Ball E. Similarly, the checking of simultaneous motion in A and B produces equal momentum in D and E. Examples of transfer of angular momentum in movement patterns are numerous. As a

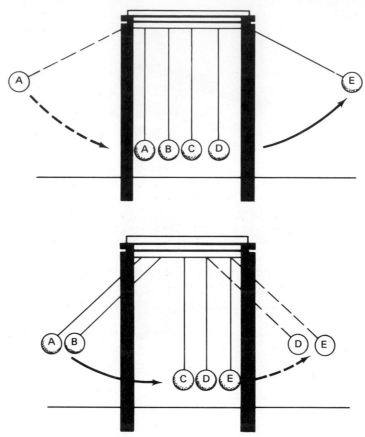

Figure 12–24 Example of conservation of angular momentum resulting in transfer of angular momentum from one body to another.

back diver leaves the board, the arms are swung upward until the motion is checked by the limitation of range of motion in the shoulder joint. The checked momentum transfers to the body and increases its angular momentum, thus helping to turn the body in the air. In the racing dive, the angular momentum of the diver's arms is also transferred to the body as the diver stops the upward movement of the arms in the forward reach, and in a jump twist the dancer transfers twisting momentum from the upper arms and trunk to the legs as the feet leave the ground. In each of these instances the body is in contact with the ground while the momentum is developing. Otherwise, an equal and opposite reaction, rather than a transfer, would occur. The effect that the transfer of angular momentum has on unsupported bodies is discussed in Chapter 17.

Angular momentum can be transferred or converted into linear momentum, or the reverse can occur. The angular momentum of the hammer becomes linear momentum when it is released. Conversely, a ball that hits the ground with no spin but rebounds spinning has had some of its linear momentum converted to angular momentum. Similarly, a long jumper's linear momentum most often is partially converted to angular momentum at the takeoff. Those who advanced the somersault technique for long jumping thought that as long as the angular momentum existed, it should be used to advantage. Unfortunately there were too many disadvantages, and the style is no longer legal. The hitch kick technique that most good jumpers currently use provides the necessary "opposite" reaction to minimize the undesired forward rotation "action" of the trunk while putting the feet in an optimum landing position.

Centripetal and Centrifugal Forces

A weight whirling around on the end of a string is engaged in linear motion of the circular type (see p. 281) while the string itself is undergoing rotatory motion about an axis. If one lets go of the string both the string and weight fly off and experience linear motion. This is expected, since according to Newton's first law a moving body left alone travels uniformly in a straight line. To make that body leave the straight path requires application of an additional force. In the case of the weight on the string the force has to be applied in a manner that will cause the weight to change direction and move in a circular path about the axis. This force is called *centripetal force*. Is is a constant center-seeking force that acts to move an object tangent (at right angles) to the direction in which it is moving at any instant, thus causing it to move in a circular path.

The centripetal force acting on the weight is an external force that is applied by the finger through the string to the weight. The finger, in turn, must have a force pulling on it since, according to Newton's third law, if one body exerts a force on the second body, that body will reciprocate with an equal and opposite force on the first body. This outward-pulling force is called *centrifugal* (center-fleeing) force, and is felt in the tension exerted on the finger by the string attached to the circling object. Centrifugal force is equal in magnitude to centripetal force. If centripetal force ceases there is no longer an inward pull on the object and the latter then flies off at a tangent to the direction in which it was moving at the instant the force stopped. Without centripetal force, there will be no centrifugal reaction, and the object will once more travel uniformly in a straight line.

Even though the speed of a whirling object is constant, its direction changes continually—that is, there is a constant change in velocity. This, in effect, is the same as saying that the weight is uniformly accelerating since, by definition, acceleration is the rate of change of velocity. The amount of acceleration that a whirling object possesses increases with the speed with which it is orbiting and decreases with the distance from the axis to the object. This relationship is represented in equation form as $a = v^2/r$. The substitution of this value for acceleration in the equation obtained from Newton's second Law of Motion, $F = ma$, results in the equation for centripetal force:

$$F_c = \frac{mv^2}{r}$$

The equation for centrifugal force is the same, since it is equal in magnitude and opposite in direction to centripetal force.

From the equation it can be seen that the amount of centripetal force necessary to keep an object moving in a circular path is proportional to its mass and the square of

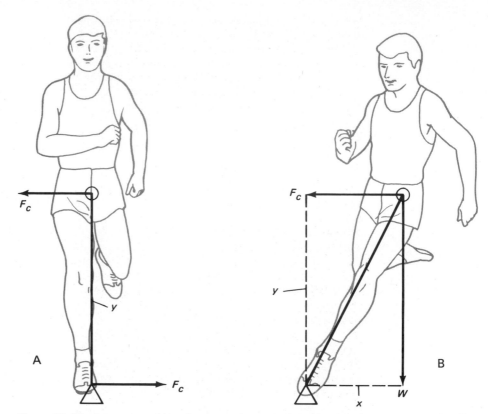

Figure 12–25   A runner must lean in when going around a corner to balance an outward pulling torque ($F_c y$). The outward pulling torque ($F_c y$) will topple the runner unless it is counterbalanced by an opposite torque (W_x) so that $F_c y = W_x$.

its velocity and inversely proportional to its radius. Doubling the mass doubles the centripetal force, while doubling the radius decreases it by half. Changes in velocity have an even greater impact and are more dramatic. Doubling the velocity along the curve increases the centripetal force fourfold, and decreasing the velocity by one-half decreases to one-fourth the force needed to keep the object in orbit.

When runners or bicyclists negotiate corners with any appreciable speed they lean into the curve. If they did not, they would tend to topple outward. In the same manner that centripetal force was exerted by the finger on the weight at the end of the string, the ground exerts centripetal force on the body of the runner through the feet and on the body of the cyclist through the bicycle wheel. While the centrifugal force tends to pull horizontally inward toward the center of the circle from the contact point with the ground, it tends to cause the rest of the body to fall outward because it creates a torque by exerting a force that is not in line with the center of gravity of the body. In Figure 12–25A, this outward rotating torque, $F_c y$, is shown as the product of the centripetal-centrifugal force and the distance between the center of gravity of the runner and the axis of rotation about the foot. When one leans in, an opposite reacting force moment is created, also about the feet, and is equal to the product of the weight and the perpendicular distance from the direction of weight to the axis. In Figure 12–

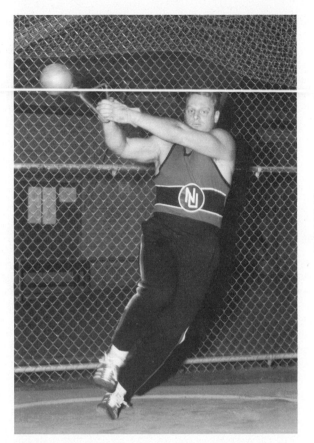

Figure 12–26 Centripetal-centrifugal forces operating in weight event. (Boris Djerassi, A.A.U. and N.C.A.A. Hammer Throw Champion, 1975. Photograph courtesy of Northeastern University.)

25B the torque due to the lean (W_x) balances the opposite acting torque due to centripetal force, so that $F_c y = W_x$. This relationship demonstrates that as F_c increases, the amount of lean will also have to increase. As this occurs, x increases, y decreases, and W, of course, remains the same. It also shows that the lower the center of gravity of a body negotiating a curve the smaller will be the outward rotating force because the moment arm, y, will be less.

Where speeds are too great or radii too small for participants to negotiate curves successfully, the track may be banked. The amount of banking is determined for the particular radius and the average expected velocity so that the performer may remain perpendicular to the surface while rounding the curve. As might be expected, the greater the anticipated velocity for negotiating the curve, or the smaller the radius of the turn, the more the track must be banked.

Centripetal–centrifugal forces are evident in many instances where the body imparts force to an external object. Overarm, sidearm, or underarm throwing patterns all involve the application of force to the object to be thrown in order to keep it moving in a circular path for all or part of the time before it is released. As soon as the object is released its inertia causes it to move in a straight line. In the hammer throw (Figure 12–26), the thrower transmits force to the head of the hammer along the flexible wire. This is centripetal force directed inward toward the axis of rotation. As the performer increases the speed of his rotation the velocity of the hammer increases, and the increased centripetal force the thrower must exert is proportional to the square of the velocity. The outward pulling centrifugal force increases accordingly on the thrower, and he must adjust by leaning back or be pulled off balance. A hammer thrower needs considerable strength to resist centrifugal force. This is also true with discus throwers who generate considerable centripetal force during the turn prior to delivery, or baseball pitchers whose elbows are subject to great forces because of the tremendous speed with which the forearm is whipped forward in the pitch. Another instance where centripetal force is an important factor is in all swinging activities in gymnastics. Cureton (1939) found that, although the centrifugal force acting on a 160-pound gymnast was only 121.2 pounds at the top of a giant swing, it was 789.2 pounds at the bottom of the swing.

Laboratory Experiences

1. For each of the following anatomical levers estimate the approximate length of the effort moment arm—i.e., the perpendicular distance. Refer to anatomical illustrations or to a muscle mannequin to help you estimate the angle of pull of the muscles. Unless otherwise stated, assume that the segments are in their normal resting position. (*Hint:* Use the mechanical axis of the segment for the lever.)
   a. The forearm lever with the biceps providing the effort.
   b. The upper arm lever with the middle deltoid providing the effort.
   c. The upper arm lever in the side-horizontal position with the entire pectoralis major providing the effort. (*Hint:* Which view would show you the angle of pull for this movement, facing the subject or looking down from above?)
   d. Same lever as in c, with the anterior deltoid providing the effort.

2. Referring to the diagrams in Figure 12–4 assume that a weight is suspended from the wrist. Find the resistance moment arm of the forearm lever in positions B, D, and E. Consider that the scale for these diagrams is 2 cm = 25 cm.

3. Assume that a muscle having a force of 300 pounds is pulling at an angle of 75 degrees. Find the components of the force: (a) by the trigonometric method; (b) by the graphic method.

4. Assuming that the weight used in Question 2 is 8 pounds, determine the rotatory and nonrotatory components of the weight: (a) by the trigonometric method; (b) by the graphic method.

5. Referring to Figure 6–14, make a tracing of the femur and the adductor longus muscle. Draw a straight line to represent the mechanical axis of the femur and another to represent the muscle's line of pull (connecting the midpoints of the proximal and distal attachments).
   a. Using a protractor, measure the angle of pull—i.e., the angle facing the hip joint—formed by the intersection of the muscle's line of pull with the bone's mechanical axis.
   b. Measure the effort moment arm of the lever—i.e., the perpendicular distance from the fulcrum (center of hip joint) to the muscle's line of pull. To convert this to a realistic figure use the scale 1 cm = 1 in.
   c. Assuming the muscle's total force to be 250 pounds, calculate the moment of force (i.e., the torque) of the lever.
   d. Calculate the rotatory and the nonrotatory components of force.

6. Place a pole across the back of a chair, hang a pail or basket containing a 5-pound weight on one end, and hold the other end of the pole. Now adjust the pole so that it becomes increasingly difficult to balance the weight of the pail with one hand. Stop when you reach the point where you are barely able to lift the pail by pushing down on the opposite end of the pole. Have an assistant measure the effort arm and the resistance arm of the lever. Without shifting the position of your hand, draw the pole toward you until you can easily lift the pail by pushing down on the opposite end of the pole with one finger. Again, have an assistant measure the effort and resistance arms of the lever. What do you conclude concerning the relative length of two arms? In which case does the pail move through the greater distance? What do you conclude about the relationship between the effort required to move an object by leverage and the distance that the object is moved?

7. Balance a pole across the back of a chair, hanging a 5-pound weight at each end. Let one of these represent the effort and the other the resistance. The effort arm and the resistance arm should be exactly equal if the pole is symmetrical. Now add 5 more pounds at another point on the resistance end and adjust the pole until it balances. Measure the effort and resistance moment arms. What do you conclude about:
   a. The relationship between the resistance and the resistance arm? between the effort and the effort arm?
   b. The relationship between the resistance and the resistance arm, given a changing resistance and a constant effort?

8. Compute the amount of effort necessary to lift a resistance of 20 pounds with a 6-foot, first class lever whose fulcrum is located 2 feet from the point at which the weight is attached, and 4 feet from the point at which the effort is applied. Assume that both the effort and the resistance are applied at right angles to the lever.

9. Where would the fulcrum have to be located in the above-mentioned 6-foot first class lever if there were only 5 pounds of effort available to balance the 20-pound weight? Determine this by experiment. Check your answer by the algebraic method.

10. For each of the anatomical levers listed below identify the class of lever represented; identify the fulcrum, effort point, and resistance point; and name the kind of movement favored by this type of lever.
    a. Leg being flexed at knee by hamstrings.
    b. Leg being extended at knee by quadriceps femoris.
    c. Pelvis being tilted to right by left quadriceps lumborum.
    d. Clavicle being elevated by trapezius I.
    e. Lower extremity being abducted by gluteus medius.
    f. From supine lying position, lower extremities being raised by hip flexors.
    g. From supine lying position, trunk being raised by hip flexors.

11. Perform the following paired movements, noting the difference in the effort needed. Diagram and explain the reasons for the difference.
    a. A push-up from the toes and a push-up from the knees.
    b. A sit-up with hands on the thighs and a sit-up with a 5-pound weight held behind the head.
    c. A 5-pound weight held in the hand with the arm outstretched horizontally sideward and a 5-pound weight suspended from the elbow crotch when the arm is outstretched sideward.

12. Explain the difference in effort needed to hold the body levers in Question 11a, b, c, at a 10-degree angle with the horizontal compared with holding them at a 30-degree angle; a 45-degree angle.

13. What muscular effort, E, pulling at an angle of 80 degrees would be required to keep the lower leg in a position of 10 degrees with the horizontal? The muscle inserts 3 inches from the

knee joint. The lower leg and foot weighs 8 pounds and its center of gravity is located 7 inches from the knee joint. A 10-pound weight is hung from the ankle 13 inches from the knee joint.

14. A gymnast weighing 56 kg attempts a handstand on the balance beam. Her center of gravity is 1 meter above the beam. What is the moment of force tending to pull her over if her center of gravity moves 3 cm ahead of the center of her support? 15 cm ahead?

15. Perform a vertical jump with and without the use of your arms. Have someone compare the height of the two jumps by noting the level of the top of your head. A chart with numbered horizontal lines on the wall behind you will help in scoring. The observer's eyes should be at the level of the top of your head at the peak of the jump. Repeat several times and compare your results with those of others doing the same experiment. Explain the results.

16. Stand on a frictionless turntable or sit on a swivel stool. Hold a 5-pound weight in each hand and hold the arms out to the side. Have a partner spin you around. Alternately bring your hands into your shoulders and move them out to the side. Explain the changes in your angular velocity.

17. Stand on a frictionless turntable or sit on a swivel stool. Determine how you can rotate yourself moving just your arms. Explain why your arm motions make the rotation possible.

18. Firmly tape equal length chains of small rubber bands to a golf ball and a ping-pong ball.
    a. Holding the end of the elastic, swing the golf ball around in a circle. Repeat with the lighter ball, swinging it with the same speed as the heavier ball.
    b. Swing the ping-pong ball at different speeds.
    c. Swing the ping-pong ball with one-half the radius length; one-fourth. What does this experiment tell about the relationship of mass, velocity, and radius to centripetal force? How can you tell whether or not the centripetal force is increasing or decreasing?

References

Basford, L. 1966. *The restlessness of matter.* London: Sampson Low, Marston.

Basford, L. 1966. *The science of movement.* London: Sampson Low, Marston.

Broer, M., and Zernicke, R. 1979. *Efficiency of human movement.* 4th ed. Philadelphia: W. B. Saunders.

Bunn, J. W. 1972. *Scientific principles of coaching.* 2d ed. Englewood Cliffs, N.J.: Prentice-Hall.

Cooper, J. M., and Glassow, R. B. 1976. *Kinesiology.* 4th ed. St. Louis: C. V. Mosby.

Cureton, T. K. 1939. Elementary principles and techniques of cinematographic analysis. *Res. Q. Am. Assoc. Health Phys. Educ. Rec.* 10:3–24.

Dull, C. E., Metcalfe, H. C., and Williams, J. E. 1963. *Modern physics.* New York: Holt, Rinehart, and Winston.

Dyson, G. 1970. *The mechanics of athletics.* 5th ed. London: University of London Press.

Fick, R. 1929. Review of literature on mechanics of joints and muscles. *Z. Orthop. Chir.* 51:320–37.

Gardner, R., and Webster, D. 1978. *Moving right along.* Garden City, N.Y.: Doubleday.

Hay, J. G. 1978. *The biomechanics of sports techniques.* 2d ed. Englewood Cliffs, N.J.: Prentice-Hall.

LeVeau, B. 1977. *Williams and Lissner: Biomechanics of human motion.* 2d ed. Philadelphia: W. B. Saunders.

Miller, D. I., and Nelson, R. C. 1973. *Biomechanics of sport.* Philadelphia: Lea & Febiger.

Tricker, R. A. R., and Tricker, B. J. K. 1967. *The science of movement.* New York: American Elsevier.

The Center of Gravity and Stability

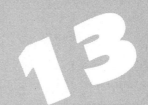

Objectives

At the conclusion of this chapter, the student should be able to:

1. Define the term *center of gravity*, and explain the basis for its location in the human body.
2. Estimate the location of the center of gravity of individuals in any position.
3. State the principles of equilibrium, and explain and demonstrate applications of each.
4. Locate the center of gravity of an individual using either the reaction board or segmental method.

Center of Gravity

Definition of Center of Gravity

The center of gravity of a body is sometimes described as its balance or pivot point. A simple experiment to locate the pivot point consists of suspending an irregularly shaped object by a string and letting it hang until it ceases to move. A vertical line is then drawn on the object from its point of suspension as a continuation of the string. The object is then suspended from another point, and the vertical continuation line is drawn again (Figure 13–1). This procedure is repeated once more. The point G where the three lines intersect is the center of gravity of the object. If the object is suspended from G it will hang in whatever position it is placed, as if the weight of the object were all concentrated at this point. It is for this reason that the center of gravity is sometimes defined as the point where all of the weight of the object is concentrated. More accurately, it is the point where the weight of the body may be said to act.

The ability to locate the center of gravity of a body is based on the knowledge of what it takes for a system to be balanced, or in equilibrium. There are two conditions that must be met:

1. All the linear forces acting on the body must be balanced.
2. All the rotatory forces (torques) must be balanced.

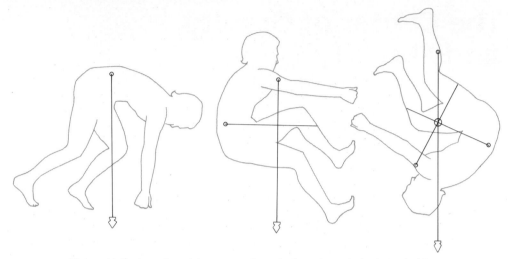

Figure 13–1   Location of the center of gravity in an irregularly shaped object.

Another way of expressing these necessary conditions for equilibrium is to say that the sum of all the forces acting on the body must equal zero. If there is a downward directed linear force there must be an equal upward force so that the vector sum of these forces equals zero. If there is a negative clockwise torque it must be canceled out by a positive counterclockwise torque of equal magnitude.

The performer's body in Figure 13–2 is being acted upon by gravity, as is each segment and every particle of the body. The downward directed force of each particle is equal to its weight and is parallel to the force of every other particle. If summed, the weight of the particles equals the weight of the performer, and the point where the total weight (force) is applied is the point where all of the individual particle weights (forces) are in equilibrium, or are balanced. This theoretical point is the center of gravity and can be located by using the principle of moments (see p. 354). It is the point where the sum of the particle torques on one side of an axis equals the sum of the particle torques on the other side. The sum of the torques about the y axis equals zero and, in addition, the sum of the torques about the x and z axes also equals zero.

The location of the center of gravity of any object remains fixed as long as the body does not change shape. In rigid bodies of homogeneous mass, the center of gravity is at the geometric center. Where the density of a rigid body varies, the center of gravity is not at the geometric center but is shifted toward the more weighted section. If an object's shape or position changes, the location of the center of gravity will also change. This happens in the human body (Figure 13–3). It is a segmented structure, capable of numerous positions, and the location of its center of gravity changes accordingly. This is an important consideration in the execution of sports skills. The evolution of the technique for the high jump shows how the change of placement of the center of gravity in the body increased the height of the bar over which the jumper could project himself (Figure 13–4). As one changes the relationship of the body segments to each other, the center of gravity may even be located completely outside of the body itself.

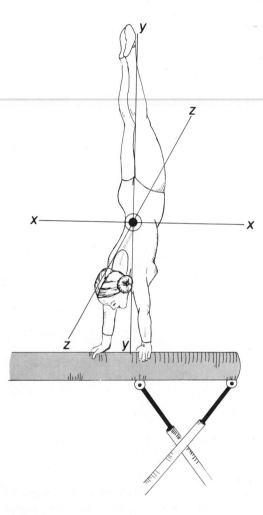

Figure 13–2 The center of gravity of a body is the point where all forces acting on the body equal zero. In this illustration it is represented as the intersection of the x, y, and z axes. It may be located by application of the principle of moments.

Figure 13–3 A shift in segment configuration results in a relocation of the body's center of gravity. (Drawn from motion picture film tracing.)

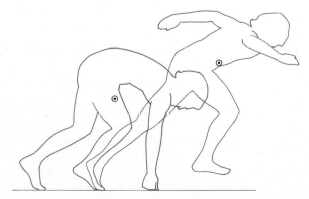

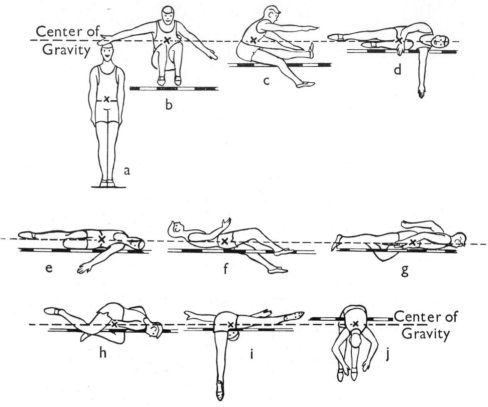

Figure 13–4 Effect of shift in center of gravity on high jump performance. (From Dyson, G. H. G.: *The mechanics of athletics.* London: University of London Press, 1970.)

Placement of Center of Gravity in Humans

The location of the center of gravity of a human being in the normal standing position varies with body build, age, and sex. A number of experiments relating to the center of gravity were made by Hellebrandt (1942) at the University of Wisconsin. She found the height of the center of gravity in women to be 55 percent of their standing height. In other studies, Croskey et al. (1922) found the center of gravity in men to be 56.18 percent of their height and, in women, 55.44 percent. They also found that the height of the center of gravity was considerably more variable in women than in men. They found no correlation between the height of the center of gravity and body weight or height.

In a series of studies on the relation of age to the height of the center of gravity, Palmer (1944) found that the latter maintained a fairly constant ratio to the height of the individual at all ages, ranging from 55 to 59 percent. From the age of 6 fetal months to 70 years the center of gravity was found to descend gradually from the level of the seventh thoracic vertebra to the level of the first sacral segment. Swearingen et al. (1969) substantiated these results in their studies of the center of gravity of infants. In addition they found that the height of the center of gravity above the crotch remains more or less constant at 6 inches throughout life.

Hellebrandt (1942) also studied the way in which the body sways when a person attempts to stand still, and observed that although the center of gravity of the body as a whole shifts constantly during relaxed and effortless standing, the patterns formed by a trajectory of the shifting center of weight and the mean position of the vertical projection of their theoretical point (i.e., the line of gravity) are relatively constant. She found that the average area of maximal sway for a group of men and women was only 4.09 square centimeters, and that the differences between the men and the women were not statistically significant. It was noted that, although the line of gravity intersected the base of support close to its center, in the majority of subjects it was slightly to the left and behind the exact center. In a study on the influence of shoes on the position of the center of gravity, Hellebrandt found that shoes with low and moderate heels had a negligible effect upon postural stability and the position of the line of gravity, but that high-heeled shoes tended to cause a forward shifting of the line of gravity and to increase the amount of swaying, apparently indicating a decrease in stability.

Stability and Equilibrium

All objects at rest are in equilibrium. All of the forces acting on them are balanced; the sum of all linear forces equals zero and the sum of all torques equals zero. However, all objects at rest are not equally stable. If the position of an object is slightly altered and the object tends to return to its original position, the object is in *stable* equilibrium. **Stable equilibrium** occurs when an object is placed in such a fashion that an effort to disturb it would require its center of gravity to be raised. Thus it would tend to fall back in place (Figure 13–5A). The more its center of gravity has to be raised to upend it, the more stable it is. A brick on its side is more stable than one on end because its center of gravity needs to be raised higher to upend it. The wrestler and defensive lineman both know the value of shifting body position to increase stability by lowering the center of gravity. In fact, if for any reason the equilibrium is too precarious, assuming a crouching, kneeling, or sitting position will lower the center of gravity and increase stability.

Unstable **equilibrium** exists when it takes only a slight push to destroy it. This is the situation when the center of gravity of the object drops to a lower point when the object is tilted (Figure 13–5B). A pencil on end or a tightrope walker displays unstable equilibrium because the center of gravity is bound to be lowered if either loses its balance. Swimmers standing on the starting block poised for the start of a race or sprint runners at the start of their race are in unstable equilibrium, as are toe dancers on point or balance beam performers. In each instance the center of gravity will be lowered if the individual is disturbed so that rotation occurs around the point of support.

The third classification of equilibrium is called *neutral* **equilibrium,** and exists when an object's center of gravity is neither raised nor lowered when it is disturbed (Figure 13–5C). A ball lying on a table is in neutral equilibrium. Objects in neutral equilibrium will come to rest in any position without a change in level of the center of gravity. Upon receiving a slight push such objects neither fall backward nor forward.

Because humans ordinarily hold themselves in an upright position and because the effect of gravity is always in operation on this earth, the problems of stability are

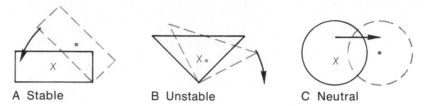

A Stable   B Unstable   C Neutral

Figure 13–5   Types of equilibrium.

ever present. Probably the only time the human body is not adjusting itself in response to gravitational force is when it is in a position of complete repose. Either consciously or unconsciously, humans spend most of their waking hours adjusting their positions to the type of equilibrium best suited to the task.

Factors Affecting Stability

The ability to maintain one's balance under unfavorable circumstances is recognized as one of the basic motor skills. Standing on tiptoe or on one foot without losing one's balance or maintaining a headstand or a handstand for an appreciable length of time is such a skill. These particular feats are examples of static balance, and the mark of skill is to accomplish them with a minimum of motion. Familiarity with the following factors affecting the stability of a performer's equilibrium state should make analysis of the balance problem easier, and may suggest means for improvement of the skill with which the technique is executed.

Relation of the Line of Gravity to the Base of Support

An object retains its equilibrium only so long as its line of gravity falls within its base of support. When the force that the body is resisting is the downward force of gravity, the nearer the line of gravity to the *center* of the base of support, the greater the stability (Figure 13–6) and, conversely, the nearer the line of gravity to the *margin* of the base of support, the more precarious the equilibrium (Figure 13–7). Once it passes beyond the margin, stability is lost and a new base must be established. It is this factor that constitutes the major problem in some modern dance techniques, balance stunts, walking a tightrope, and building pyramids. For developing the neuromuscular control necessary for acquiring such skills as these, there is no substitute for repeated practice. There are, however, a few devices that help to keep the center of gravity centered over the base of support. One of these we do almost unconsciously. If we carry a heavy weight at one side of the body (e.g., a suitcase or a pail of water), *this constitutes a unilateral* load which, if uncompensated, would shift the center of gravity to that side, bringing it dangerously close to the margin of the base of support. By raising the opposite arm sideways, by bending or leaning to the opposite side, or by a combination of these, we counterbalance the external load and keep the line of gravity close to the center of the base of support (Figures 13–8 and 13–9). Another application of the principle of keeping the line of gravity over the center of the base of support is seen in the tightrope walker who carries a balancing pole or, to a lesser degree, in the gymnast walking on a balance beam with arms extended sideward.

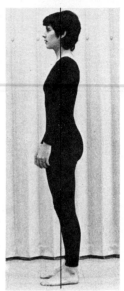

Figure 13–6 Position of the body in which the line of gravity falls approximately through the center of the base of support. This is a stable position.

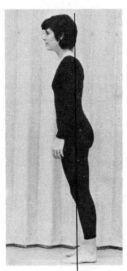

Figure 13–7 Position of the body in which the line of gravity falls near the anterior margin of the base of support. This position is less stable than the one shown in Figure 13–6.

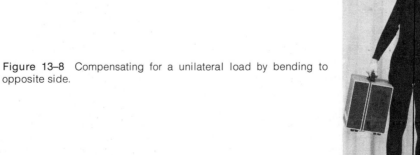

Figure 13–8 Compensating for a unilateral load by bending to opposite side.

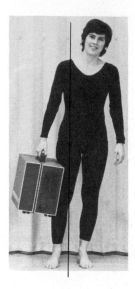

Figure 13–9 Compensation for a unilateral load by inclining the entire body to the opposite side.

When the external force acting on a body is a lateral one, stability is increased if the line of gravity is placed so that it will continue to remain over the base even when forced to move by the external force. Leaning into the wind (Figure 13–10) or pushing a heavy chest are examples where the line of gravity should be close to the edge of the base of support nearest the oncoming force. Pulling in a tug of war is an example of having the gravity line near the edge of the base of support farthest away from the external force. When one is not certain from which direction an external force may be applied, equilibrium is most stable when the line of gravity is in the center of the base of support.

There are also occasions in movement activities when a person may wish to place the line of gravity so that the equilibrium is unstable. Swimmers and runners waiting for the·start of a race assume a position in which the line of gravity is as close to the front edge as possible, since they wish to lose balance rapidly.

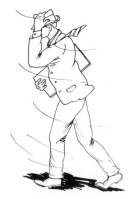

Figure 13–10   Leaning into the wind to balance the effect of its force on the body.

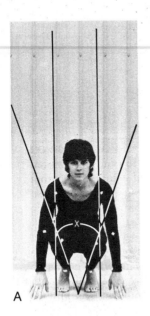
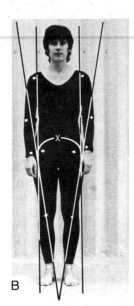
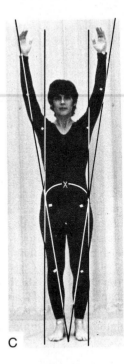

Figure 13–11   The height of the center of gravity changes with a change in body position. X = center of gravity. As the center of activity moves closer to the base of support more angular displacement of the center of gravity can occur before it goes beyond the base of support. The angle in A is greater than that in B and the angle in B is greater than that in C. Thus, A > B > C with respect to lateral stability.

Height of the Center of Gravity

Ordinarily, the center of gravity in an adult human is located approximately at the level of the upper third of the sacrum, but *only* during the normal standing position. If the arms are raised or if a weight is carried above waist level, the center of gravity shifts to a higher position and it becomes more difficult to maintain one's equilibrium. Activities and stunts such as walking on stilts, canoeing, and balancing a weight on the head are difficult or dangerous because of the relatively high center of gravity. Lowering the center of gravity will increase the stability of the body because it allows greater angular displacement of the center of gravity within the bounds of the base of support (Figure 13–11).

Size and Shape of the Base of Support

It is obvious that a wide base of support adds to the stability of an object. In addition to the height of the center of gravity, much of the difficulty experienced in walking on a balance beam, railroad track, or tightrope, or in ice skating and toe dancing, is due to the narrow base of support. The problem is to keep the center of gravity over the base of support, a requisite for maintaining equilibrium. The wider the base, the easier this is.

The base of support includes the part of a body in contact with the supporting surface and the intervening area (Figure 13–12). In a person whose weight is supported entirely by the feet, the base of support includes the two feet and the space between. If the feet are separated, the base is widened and the equilibrium improved.

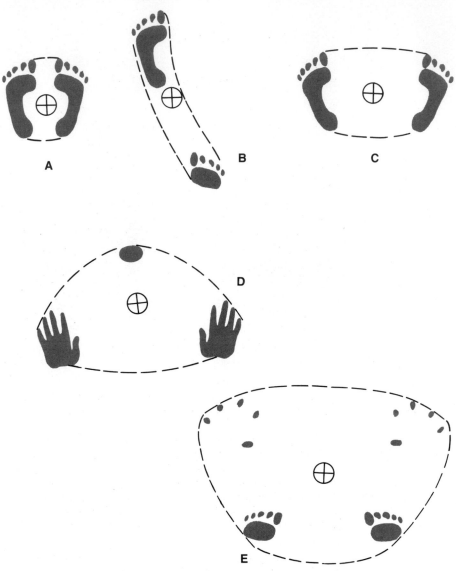

Figure 13–12   The base of support includes the part(s) of the body in contact with the supporting surface and the intervening area. What can you conclude about the stability of the base of support in these illustrations? In *A, B,* and *C,* the weight is supported by the feet; in *D,* it is supported by the forehead and hands during a headstand; in *E,* the weight is supported by the hands and feet while the body is in a squat position. Circled crosses indicate point of intersection of line of gravity with base of support.

The person supported by crutches in Figure 13–13A has a base of support that encompasses the area bounded by the feet and crutches. He will be more stable if he places the crutches forward, making a triangular base instead of a linear one. There is another factor, however, that must not be overlooked. If one takes a stride position that

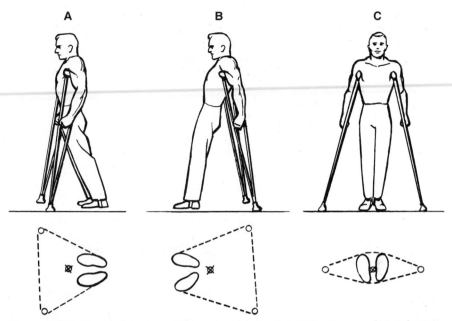

Figure 13–13 Bases of support with varying degrees of stability. Can you rank these from most stable to least stable? The subject in *A* and *B* is secure primarily in the anteroposterior direction; the position in *C* provides greater stability in the frontal plane than in the sagittal plane. (From Leveau, B.: *Williams and Lissner: Biomechanics of human motion.* 2nd ed. Philadelphia: W.B. Saunders, 1977.)

is wider than the breadth of the pelvis, the legs will assume a slanting position. This introduces a horizontal component of force that, if accompanied by insufficient friction between the feet and the supporting surface, as when standing on ice, obviously does not make for greater stability. In fact, the wider the stance, the less one can control the sliding of the feet. From this we see that we must observe *all* the principles that apply to a situation. Observance of only one may not bring the results expected.

In addition to the size of the base of support, the shape is also a factor in stability. To resist lateral external forces the base should be widened in the direction of the oncoming force. In Figure 13–13C the position provides great stability for lateral forces from the side but very little from the front or back. Where the forces are known to be coming from a forward-backward direction, as when catching a swift ball or spotting a performer in gymnastics, a forward-backward stance is recommended. A similar adjustment is made when one stands in a bus or a subway train. The tendency to be thrown backward when the vehicle starts up is resisted either by standing sideways with the feet in a moderately wide stance, or by facing forward and leaning forward with one foot placed forward. These automatic reactions to external forces are for one purpose only—namely, to enable one to keep the center of gravity over the base of support in spite of the disturbing lateral forces. When the direction of oncoming force cannot be predicted, a slight oblique stance is probably best.

Mass of the Body   The mass or weight of an object is a factor in equilibrium only when motion or an external force is involved. Then, as Newton's second law states, $F = ma$. The amount of force needed to effect a change in motion (acceleration) is proportional to the mass being moved. The greater the mass, the greater the stability. It is a matter of common observation that an empty cardboard carton is more likely to blow down the street than one filled with canned goods. Likewise, a 250-pound lineman is less likely to be brushed aside than one weighing 130 pounds. In all sports involving physical contact, the heavy, solid individual stands a better chance of keeping his or her footing than does the lightweight one. When all factors are considered, however, mass is less a factor in stability than are the location of the line of gravity and the height of the center of gravity.

Friction   Friction as a factor in stability has already been suggested in relation to the size of the base of support. It has even greater influence when the body is in motion or is being acted upon by an external force. Inadequate friction is what makes it difficult to keep one's equilibrium when walking on an icy pavement, particularly if a frisky dog tugs unexpectedly on its leash. When the supporting surface presents insufficient friction, the footgear can make up for it. The person who must walk on icy pavements can wear "creepers" on the shoes, the golfer and the field hockey player can wear cleats, and the gymnast and basketball player can wear rubber-soled shoes.

Segmentation   If, instead of being in one solid piece, an object consists of a series of segments placed one above the other, the problem of retaining its equilibrium is a multiple one. Maximum stability of a segmented body is assured when the centers of gravity of all the weight-bearing segments lie in a vertical line that is centered over the base of support. In a column of blocks, this means that each block must be centered over the block beneath. In a jointed column, as in the human body, one segment cannot slide off another, but it is quite possible for the segments to be united in a zigzag alignment. Such is all too often the case in human standing posture. In fact, the alignment of the body segments is a widely used criterion for judging standing posture. When the segments are aligned in a single vertical line, the posture is not only more pleasing in appearance to most of us, but there is less likelihood of strain to the joints and muscles. When one segment gets out of line, there is usually a compensatory disalignment of another segment in order to maintain a balanced position of the body as a whole. (In other words, for every "zig" there is a "zag.") At every point of angulation between segments there is uneven tension thrown on the ligaments and uneven tonus in opposing muscle groups. This causes fatigue, if not actual strain.

The addition of an external weight to the body, as when one carries books, babies, or suitcases, may be thought of as the addition of a segment. The additional segment will add mass to the body and change its stability somewhat. More important, though, is the effect on the height of the center of gravity and the location of the line of gravity. The center of gravity will be displaced in the direction of the added weight, and the line of gravity will shift accordingly. Its new location will be governed by the nature of compensation made to accommodate the additional weight (Figures 13–8 and 13–9).

Visual and Psychological Factors   Factors which belong in this category are less easily explained than the others but are familiar to everyone. The giddiness that many experience when walking close to an unprotected edge high above the ground or when crossing a swirling river on a foot bridge is a real detriment to one's equilibrium. Even if the supporting surface is entirely adequate, the sense of balance may be disturbed. A common means of preserving the balance, both in this type of situation and when walking on a narrow rail, is to fix the eyes on a stationary spot above or beyond the "danger area." This seems to facilitate neuromuscular control by reducing the disturbing stimuli.

Physiological Factors

Besides the visual and psychological factors there are also physiological factors related to the physical mechanism for equilibrium, namely, the semicircular canals. In addition to actual lesions of this mechanism, any disturbance of the general physical condition is likely to affect the sense of balance. Feelings of dizziness accompanying nausea or any form of debility reduce one's ability to resist other factors that threaten the equilibrium. These physiological factors are largely beyond our control. One principle that can be derived from them, however, is that it is better to avoid situations likely to threaten the equilibrium when there is a temporary physiological disturbance.

Principles of Stability

The principles of stability are stated here as simply and concisely as possible, and brief applications are suggested in each case.

Principle I

Other things being equal, the lower the center of gravity, the greater will be the body's stability.

APPLICATIONS

a. The easiest and safest pyramids for beginners are those in which the participants are on their hands and knees. This position provides for a lower center of gravity than the kneeling or standing position.

b. In canoeing the kneeling position represents a compromise position that combines the advantages of stability and ease of using the arms for paddling. Kneeling is preferable to sitting on the seat because the lowering of the center of gravity makes the position a more stable one. While it is less stable than sitting on the floor of the canoe, it is a more convenient position for paddling. A position frequently recommended is kneeling and sitting against a thwart or the edge of a seat.

c. A performer on a balance beam quickly squats when he or she feels as if balance is being lost.

d. A wrestler tries to remain as stable as possible by lowering the center of gravity.

Principle II

Greater stability is obtained if the base of support is widened in the direction of the line of force.

APPLICATIONS

a. This helps an individual to keep from being thrown off balance when punching with force, pushing a heavy object, or throwing a fast ball. It also enables the puncher to "put the full body weight behind the punch" because, with a relatively wide forward-backward stance, the weight can be shifted from the rear foot to the forward foot as the force is delivered.

b. In pushing and pulling heavy furniture the whole body can be put into the act without loss of balance.

c. When catching a fast-moving object such as a baseball, or a heavy one such as a medicine ball, widening the base in line with the direction of the force enables the catcher to "give" with the catch and, in this way, to provide a greater distance in which to reduce or stop the motion of the object. It also assures greater accuracy by reducing the likelihood of rebound.

d. The military "at ease" is more stable than the position of "attention."

e. Keeping one's balance when standing on a bus or train that is accelerating or decelerating is facilitated by widening the stance in the direction that the vehicle is moving—that is, in a forward-backward direction in relation to the vehicle.

Principle III

For maximum stability the line of gravity should intersect the base of support at a point that will allow the greatest range of movement within the area of the base in the direction of forces causing motion.

APPLICATIONS

a. A football player knowing he will be pushed from in front should lean forward so that he can "give" in a backward direction without losing his balance.

b. A person in a tug-of-war line leans backward in preparation for absorbing a strong forward pull from the opponent.

c. A tennis player anticipating the opponent's return will keep the line of gravity centered so that the center of gravity can be shifted quickly in any direction without loss of balance.

d. Dragging a heavy box forward on a high shelf and then lifting it down is an activity in the home to which this principle applies. Assuming a forward-backward stance and leaning forward for this act gives the individual a wider distance for receiving the weight of this forward-moving object. This decreases the likelihood of being thrown off balance when the box suddenly comes free of the shelf. It also enables one to take a step backward, which makes it easier to lower the box in front and to keep control of it. With a sideward stance one would be likely to be thrown off balance as the box comes free. There is also the danger of exerting so much horizontal force that, instead of lowering the box in front, the individual swings back overhead, hyperextending the spine and running the risk of straining the back.

e. Basketball and other team games involving running often require sudden reversals of direction. If the player tries to turn while the feet are close together the momentum is likely to throw the runner off balance. This can be prevented by spreading the feet to check the forward motion and leaning back so that the line of gravity will be toward the rear. The runner can then quickly pivot to reverse direction.

Principle IV

Other things being equal, the greater the mass of a body, the greater will be its stability.

APPLICATION In sports in which resistance to impact is a factor, heavy, solid individuals are more likely to maintain their equilibrium than lighter ones. This provides one basis for selecting linemen in football.

Principle V

Other things being equal, the most stable position of a vertical segmented body (such as a column of blocks or the erect human body) is one in which the center of gravity of each weight-bearing segment lies in a vertical line centered over the base of support or in which deviations in one direction are exactly balanced by deviations in the opposite direction.

APPLICATIONS

a. This applies to postural adjustments for achieving a pleasing, well-balanced alignment of the body segments, both with and without external loads.

b. In pyramid building and other balance stunts in which one person (or group of persons) supports the weight of another person or persons, the chief problem is one of either aligning or balancing the several centers of gravity over the center of the base of support.

Principle VI

Other things being equal, the greater the friction between the supporting surface and the parts of the body in contact with it, the more stable the body will be.

APPLICATION The wearing of cleats and rubber-soled shoes for sport activities not only aids in locomotion but also serves to increase one's stability in positions held momentarily between quick or forceful movements, as in basketball, fencing, football, field hockey, lacrosse, and other sports.

Principle VII

Other things being equal, a person has better balance in locomotion under difficult circumstances when the vision is focused on stationary objects rather than on disturbing stimuli.

APPLICATION Beginners learning to walk on a balance beam or to perform balance stunts, and others who for any reason have difficulty in keeping their balance, can minimize disturbing visual stimuli by fixing their eyes on a stationary spot in front of them, either at eye level or somewhat above eye level.

Principle VIII

There is a positive relationship between one's physical and emotional state and the ability to maintain balance under difficult circumstances.

APPLICATION Persons should not be permitted to attempt dangerous balance stunts or activities requiring expert balance ability when their physical or emotional health is impaired.

Principle IX

Regaining equilibrium is based on the same principles as maintaining it.

APPLICATIONS

a. After an unexpected loss of balance, such as when starting to fall or after receiving impetus when "off balance," equilibrium may be more quickly regained if a wide base of support is established and the center of gravity is lowered.

b. Upon landing from a downward jump, stability may be more readily regained if the weight is kept evenly distributed over both feet or over the hands and feet, and if a sufficiently wide base of support is provided.

c. Upon landing from a forward jump, the balance may be more readily regained if one lands with the weight forward and uses the hands, if necessary, in order to provide support in the direction of motion.

From this emphasis on stability it might seem that one should seek maximum stability in all situations. This is not true regarding certain stunts and gymnastic activities that are designed for the purpose of testing and developing body control under difficult circumstances. In many gymnastic vaults, for instance, "good form" stipulates that the performer land with the heels close, the knees separated, the arms extended sideward, and the trunk as erect as possible, while the knees bend slightly to assure a light landing. In teaching beginners it would seem wiser to postpone emphasis on form from the point of view of appearance and to stress good mechanics and safety.

Finding the Center of Gravity in the Human Body

The location of the center of gravity in humans is of interest to scientists in many areas. Anatomists, kinesiologists, orthopedists, physical therapists, space engineers, and equipment design engineers have all shown interest in methods of determining the location of the center of gravity. Earliest experiments located the center of gravity by balancing the body over a wedge. Various other methods have since been developed to estimate the location of the center of gravity, either at rest or in motion. Two of these procedures, easily replicated with a minimum of equipment, are described here.

Reaction Board Method

It is a fairly simple matter to find an estimate of the center of gravity of a motionless body using the *reaction board method*. Making use of the principle of moments, this procedure relies on the fact that the sum of the moments acting on a body in equilibrium is zero. Using this information the location of the gravitational line is found for each plane. The center of gravity of the body becomes the intersection of the values for each of these three planes. Directions for locating the center of gravity in three planes follow.

APPARATUS   (Figure 13–14)

1.   Scales: preferably either the Toledo or the spring balance type.
2.   A stool or block the same height as the platform of the scales.

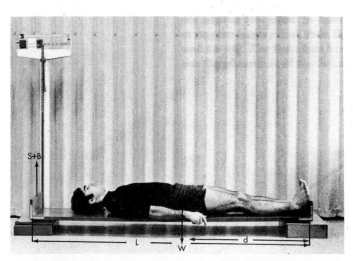

Figure 13–14   Reaction board method for locating the height of the center of gravity.

3. A board about 40 cm wide and 200 cm long. A knife edge should be attached to the underside of each end in such a way that when the board is placed in a horizontal position it will rest on the knife edges. For simplifying the calculations the distance from knife edge to knife edge should measure exactly 200 cm. The front edge of the board should be marked in centimeters. The board should be tested with a level to make certain it is horizontal.

DIRECTIONS   (Refer to Figure 13–14)

1. Find the subject's total weight.
2. Put one knife edge of board on scale platform and the other edge on box platform. Use a spirit level to make sure board is horizontal Note the reading on the scales. This is the partial weight of the board, **B.**
3. Have the subject lie supine on the board with the heels against the footrest at the end of the board away from the scales. The position the subject assumes should be as similar to the standing position as possible. Record the reading on the scales. This is the partial weight of the subject and scales (**S** + **B**).
4. For equilibrium to exist about the point **P,** the counterclockwise moments must equal the clockwise moments. If **W** is the total weight of the subject, **B,** the partial weight of the board, **S** + **B** the partial weight of the subject and board, **L** the length of the board, and **d** the perpendicular distance from P to W, then

$$d \times W = \left[(S + B) - B \right] L$$

(clockwise moments = counterclockwise moments).

Rearranged,

$$d = \frac{\left[(S + B) - B \right] L}{W}$$

The distance between the subject's feet and center of gravity is **d.** This is comparable to the distance between the ground and the center of gravity when the subject is standing, but must be viewed as an estimate because of shifts in body organs and tissues when lying down.

5. The percentage height of the center of gravity with respect to the subject's total height is found by dividing the value of **d** in the transverse plane (supine lying position) by the subject's total height and multiplying by 100.

$$percent = \frac{d \text{ in transverse plane}}{subject's \text{ height}} \times 100$$

6. To locate the center of gravity in the frontal or sagittal planes the procedure must be repeated with the subject standing on the board (preferably near the middle). For the sagittal plane, the subject stands with the side to the scales (Figure 13–15) and for the frontal plane location, the subject stands facing the scales. Use the same formula

$$d = \frac{\left[(S + B) - B \right] L}{W}$$

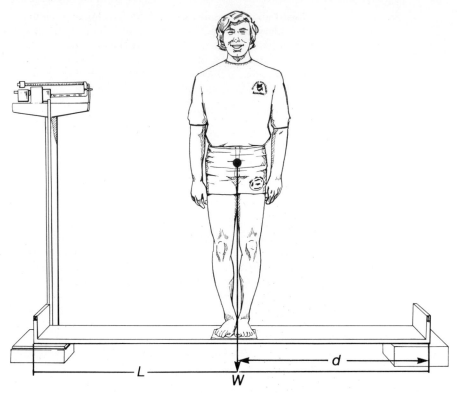

Figure 13–15   Reaction board method for locating the line of gravity in the sagittal plane.

to solve for *d.* The value of *d* represents the distance from the knife edge *P* to the plane in which the subject's center of gravity is located.

7. If it is desired to find the single point representing the spot where the line of gravity intersects the base of support, a piece of paper should be placed under the subject's feet for the side view measurement. The outline of the feet is traced on the paper. When the first *d* is found, the distance is measured and marked on both the left and right sides of the paper. The paper should then be removed and the points connected by a straight line. When the subject faces forward for the second measurement, the paper should be placed on the board so that the subject's feet will fit in the footprints. When the second *d* is found, the distance should be measured and marked on both edges of the paper, and the place where two lines intersect represents the approximate position of the point where the line of gravity strikes the base of support. This is a crude method of locating this point and is not strictly accurate since the subject may not be standing in exactly the same posture for both measurements. Furthermore, the element of swaying always introduces a source of error.

A modification of the reaction board method involves the use of a large triangular board supported by scales on two corners and a platform of equal height under the third corner (Waterland and Shambes, 1970). Each corner makes contact with its support through a pointed bolt. Again it is important that the board be horizontal. If this triangle is equilateral, the moments are taken about lines forming two sides of the triangle, and the perpendicular distance from each line to the center of gravity is determined as follows:

$$d_1 = \frac{\left[(S + B)_Y - B_Y\right] L}{W}$$

$$d_2 = \frac{\left[(S + B)_X - B_X\right] L}{W}$$

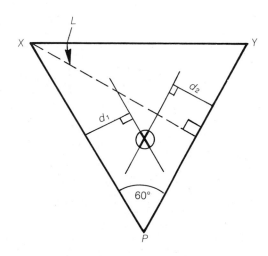

d_1 = distance between XP and center of gravity
d_2 = distance between YP and center of gravity
$(S + B)_X$ = partial weight of subject and board on scale X
$(S + B)_Y$ = partial weight of subject and board on scale Y
B_X = partial weight of board recorded on scale X
B_Y = partial weight of board recorded on scale Y
W = weight of subject
L = altitude of triangle (perpendicular distance from scale to line about which moment is being taken)

Segmental Method

Experiments using the reaction board are convincing in showing how the body automatically compensates for external loads and segmental adjustments. It is revealing also to see how the body adjusts for the sideward raising of an arm, the forward bending of the trunk, a briefcase carried in one hand, or a load of books carried on the hip. Such analysis, however, is limited to the body in a stationary position. The location of the center of gravity of someone in action requires the use of another method. A highly useful procedure is one called the *segmental method*. This technique makes use of a photograph of the subject and involves finding the location of the center of gravity of each of the body segments, the position of these individual gravity points with respect to arbitrarily placed x and y axes, and knowledge of the ratio between the individual segment weights and the total body weight.

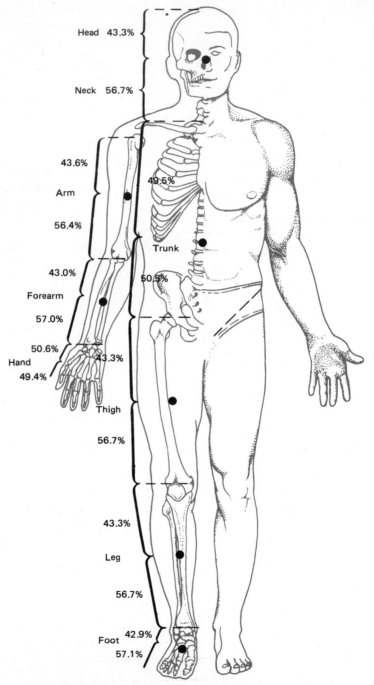

Figure 13–16   Joint centers and percentage distance of centers of gravity from joint centers. (Prepared from data presented in Dempster, W. T.: Space requirements of the seated operator. WADC Technical Report 55–159. Wright-Patterson Air Force Base, Ohio, 1955.)

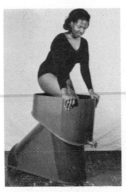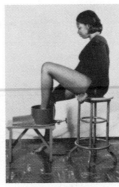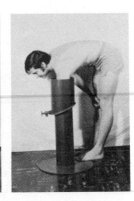

Figure 13–17   Immersion tanks for determination of segmental weights. Using segment landmarks as defined by Dempster, the segment is immersed in water. The displaced water is weighed and multiplied by the specific gravity of the segment to obtain the segmental weight. (From Gowitzke, B., and Milner, M.: *Understanding the scientific bases of human movement*. 2nd ed. Baltimore: Williams & Wilkins, 1980.)

Considerable research has been done to determine values for the proportionate weights of body segments and the locations of the segmental centers of gravity. These data have been obtained through the weighing and suspension of cadaver segments, determination of the weight of segments of living subjects through the amount of water displaced by the immersed segment, and through the formation of mathematical models. Probably the most commonly used data today are those of Dempster (1955). He weighed eight elderly male cadavers, dismembered them, weighed the segments, and determined the proportion of total weight for each segment. In addition he located the center of gravity and specific gravity for each segment. The percentage distance of segment centers of gravity from joint centers is shown in Figure 13–16.

The locations of segmental centers of gravity have not been determined in living subjects, but the weights of individual body segments of men and women have been calculated through the determination of the amount of water displaced by an individual segment (Figure 13–17). Using specific gravity data from Dempster and the volumetric displacement method, Plagenhoef (1971) reported body segment weights as percentages of total body weight for living college-age males, and quoted Kjeldsen as having obtained the same information for college-age females. These results are summarized in Table 13–1.

Unfortunately, when applied to women and children, calculations using Dempster's (1955) data have to be considered as rough estimates, since all of Dempster's work was done with male subjects. Use of the data with living adult males, however, is considered accurate even though much of the basic research was done on cadavers.

With information on the proportionate mass of body segments and the location of the center of gravity of each segment, the center of gravity of the whole body in any plane may now be determined by making use of the principle of moments. The sum of the moments of the individual segments about arbitrarily placed x and y axes will produce the location of the center of gravity of the whole body with respect to the x and y axes. This is because the total body weight acting at the center of mass is the resultant of the combined segment weights acting at their mass centers and the resul-

TABLE 13–1 Body Segment Percentages of Total Body Weight For Living Men and Women*

SEGMENTS	MEN	WOMEN
Hands	1.3	1.0
Forearms	3.8	3.1
Upper arms	6.6	6.0
Feet	2.9	2.4
Shanks	9.0	10.5
Thighs	21.0	23.0
Trunk (including head and neck)	55.4	54.0

*From data presented in Plagenhoef, 1971, pp. 25, 27.

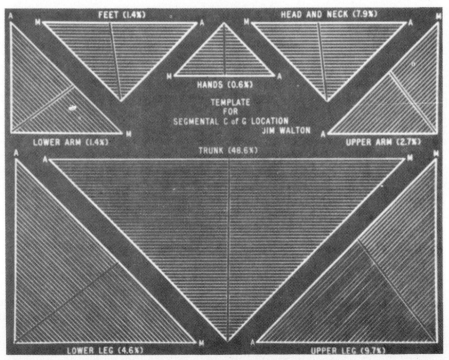

Figure 13–18   Walton template for use in segmental determination of center of gravity. (From Walton, J. S.: A template for locating segmental centers of gravity. *Res. Q. 41*:615–18, 1970.)

tant moment of the total body weight about the x, y axes is the sum of the individual segment moments about the same axes.

The segmental method for determining the center of gravity requires a considerable amount of measurement and calculation and therefore can be time consuming. The use of computer programs speeds up the process considerably, as does the use of digitizers or film analyzers with built-in x-y coordinate systems. When these technical aids are not available, the process may be simplified with an inexpensive device called the Walton template (Figure 13–18). The template makes use of the principle of similar triangles and eliminates the need to calculate the location of the mass center for each segment.

Directions for locating the center of gravity using the segmental method follow.

APPARATUS

1. Walton template, if available.*
2. Line drawing on graph paper taken from photographic image of subject (Figure 13–19).
3. Worksheet with Dempster proportions listed (Figure 13–20).

DIRECTIONS

1. The locations of the extremities of the individual segments must be marked according to the link boundaries shown in Figure 13–16. This will result in marks at the end of the second toe, ankle, knee, hip, knuckle III of the hand, wrist, shoulders, seventh cervical vertebra, and top of the head. Where these points are obscured by other body parts, an estimate must be made. The upper trunk mark is the seventh cervical, located slightly above the midpoint of the transverse line joining the shoulders. The lower trunk mark is the midpoint of the transverse line joining the hips.
2. The extremity limits are joined to form a stick figure consisting of 14 segments (Figure 13–19A).
3A. **With Walton template:** The appropriate triangle on the Walton template is placed over one of the body segment lines so that the proximal end of one of the triangle lines coincides with the proximal end of the body segment line, and the distal end of the same triangle line coincides with the distal end of the body segment. The center of mass of the segment is marked on the tracing by drawing a short line through the slot in the triangle. (The location of the slot in the triangle is positioned according to proportions given by Dempster.) This process is repeated for the remaining segments, selecting the appropriate triangle each time (Figure 13–19B).
3B. **Without template:** If the Walton template is not used, the mass center location for each segment length is found using the data provided in Figure 13–16, where centers of gravity are located as a percentage of the distance between segment end points. The amount of the percentage distance from one segment end point is multiplied by the picture-length of the segment. The resulting product is the distance from the selected end point to the center of gravity of the segment. The distance is measured from the end point, and the center of gravity is marked by a short slash mark intersecting the segment line.
4. x and y axes are drawn on the paper in any convenient location.

---

*Template dimensions can be found in Walton, 1970.

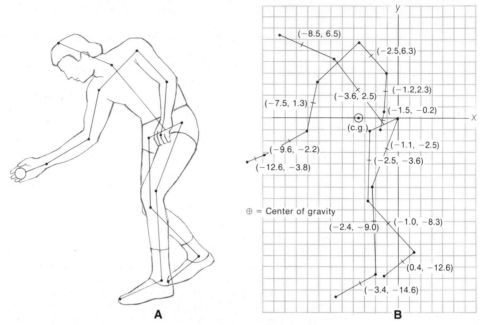

Figure 13–19   Segmental determination of the center of gravity. *A,* Location of body segments. *B,* The center of mass of each body segment is marked, and *x, y* coordinates are found using an arbitrarily placed *x, y* axis. With information on the proportionate mass of each body segment and the location of the center of mass of each segment, the center of gravity of the whole body may be determined using the principle of moments.

5.   The x, y coordinates for each of the 14 segment mass centers are determined and recorded on the diagram of the figure at the respective mass centers.

6.   A worksheet such as that shown in Figure 13–20 is used to record the x, y coordinate values and the moments of those segments about the x and y axes. *Note:* The positive and negative values of the x and y coordinates must be retained. The individual moments are the products (Col. 3) of the coordinate values (Col. 2) and their related body segment proportions (Col. 1).

7.   The algebraic sum of the x products represents the x coordinate of the total body's mass center, and the algebraic sum of the y products is the y coordinate. These values are located and marked on the tracing (Figure 13–19B).

This procedure has made it possible to locate the center of gravity of the handball player at the moment of contact with the ball. It must be remembered that this location is for one brief moment during the performance of the skill, and the position of the center of gravity will shift with body segment shifts. If more information is desired about the location of the center of gravity at other critical moments during the execution of the skill, this process should be repeated using appropriate line drawings of those critical moments. Although arduous, even with the use of a computer, the process is invaluable for those individuals who are in need of detailed analysis of dynamic skills.

Body Segment	Propor-tion of Body Wt.	x + or − Value	Products	y + or − Value	Products
1. Trunk	.486	−3.6	−1.75	2.5	1.22
2. Head & Neck	.079	−8.5	−0.67	6.5	0.51
3. R. Thigh	.097	−2.5	−0.24	−3.6	−0.35
4. R. Lower Leg	.045	−1.0	−0.05	−8.3	−0.37
5. R. Foot	.014	0.4	0.01	−12.6	−0.18
6. L. Thigh	.097	−1.1	−0.11	−2.5	−0.24
7. L. Lower Leg	.045	−2.4	−0.11	−9.0	−0.41
8. L. Foot	.014	−3.4	−0.05	−14.6	−0.20
9. R. Upper Arm	.027	−7.5	−0.20	1.3	0.04
10. R. Lower Arm	.014	−9.6	−0.13	−2.2	−0.03
11. R. Hand	.006	−12.6	−0.08	−3.8	−0.03
12. L. Upper Arm	.027	−2.5	0.07	6.3	0.17
13. L. Lower Arm	.014	−1.2	0.02	2.3	0.03
14. L. Hand	.006	−1.5	0.01	−0.2	−0.00
Total-Plus Products			0.01		1.97
Total-Minus Products			3.49		1.81
x - y Resultants (Larger-Smaller) product total			−3.48		0.16

x Coordinate = __−3.48__

y Coordinate = __+0.16__

Figure 13–20   Worksheet for locating the center of gravity using the segmental method.

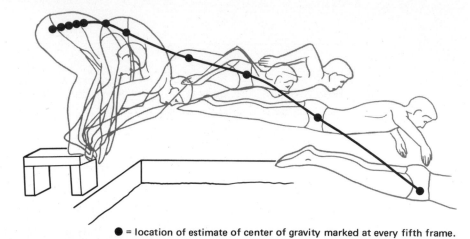

● = location of estimate of center of gravity marked at every fifth frame.

Figure 13–21   The iliac crest is used as an estimate of the location of the center of gravity of a swimmer during the execution of a racing dive. The tracking of the center of gravity of a dynamic skill is done through the use of tracings of individual motion picture frames.

Students who desire to trace the path of the center of gravity during the execution of a dynamic skill, but who do not need the accuracy of the segmental method, may find the placement of a dot on the iliac crest to be a useful estimate for the location of the body's center of gravity (Figure 13–21). This technique should be used with caution, however. It is important to remember that the center of gravity will deviate appreciably from this location in some body positions (Figures 13–2, 13–3, and 13–4).

Laboratory Experiences

1. a. Working with a partner, determine the position of your line of gravity using the reaction board method. Locate the point where this line intersects your base of support by marking it on a tracing of your feet.
   b. Determine the position of your line of gravity leaning as far forward as possible with the body in a straight line from the top of the head to the ankles. Repeat leaning as far backward as possible.
   c. Locate the line of gravity in the sagittal plane while leaning as far as possible to one side.
   d. Determine the height of your center of gravity with your arms at your side and then with them stretched over your head. What percent of your total height is your center of gravity? How does this compare with averages for your sex?
   e. Choose an original position with a small or unstable base of support. Locate the point where the line of gravity intersects the base of support.
2. Make a tracing on graph paper of a picture of a person engaged in a motor skill. Locate the center of gravity using the segmental method.
3. Walk on a low balance beam:
   a. Looking ahead at the wall.
   b. Looking at a person who is in front of the balance beam doing a vigorous exercise such as a jumping jack.

c. With your eyes blindfolded.

d. Walk along with a partner beside you. Without warning, the partner is to give you a slight but sudden sideward push. What measures do you take to maintain your balance? If you fail, explain why.

4. Build two columns of blocks, one with the blocks carefully centered one over the other, the second column with the blocks staggered but balanced. Grasping the lowest block of each column, slide the columns back and forth, changing the speed frequently and suddenly until the blocks tumble. Which column is the first to topple? Why?

References

Basford, L. 1966. *The science of movement.* London: Sampson Low, Marston.

Croskey, M. I., Dawson, P. M., Luessen, A. C., Marohn, I. E., and Wright, H. E. 1922. The height of the center of gravity in man. *Am. J. Physiol.* 61:171–85.

Cureton, T. K., and Wickens, J. S. 1935. The center of gravity of the human body in the antero-posterior plane and its relation to posture. Springfield College Suppl. to *Res. Q.* 6:93–105.

Dempster, W. T. 1955. *Space requirement of the seated operator.* Ohio: Wright-Patterson Air Force Base (WADC TR 55-199).

Dull, C. E., Metcalfe, H. C., and Williams, J. E. 1963. *Modern physics.* New York: Holt, Rinehart and Winston.

Gowitzke, B. A., and Milner, M. 1980. *Understanding the scientific basis of human movement.* 2d ed. Baltimore: Williams & Wilkins.

Hanavan, E. A. 1964. *A mathematical model of the human body.* Ohio: Wright-Patterson Air Force Base (AMRL-TR-64-102).

Hay, J. G. 1973. The center of gravity of the human body. In *Kinesiology III.* ed. Washington, D.C.: American Association of Health, Physical Education and Recreation.

Hellebrandt, F. A., Riddle, K. S., Larsen, E. M., and Fries, E. C. 1942. Gravitational influences on postural alignment. *Physiother. Rev.* 22:143–49.

Hellebrandt, F. A., and Franseen, E. B. 1943. Physiological study of vertical stance of man. *Physiol. Rev.* 23:220–25.

LeVeau, B. 1977. *Williams and Lissner: Biomechanics of human motion.* 2d ed. Philadelphia: W. B. Saunders.

Miller, D. I., and Nelson, R. C. 1973. *Biomechanics of sport.* Philadelphia: Lea & Febiger.

Palmer, C. E. 1944. Studies of the center of gravity in the human body. *Child Dev.* 15:99–180.

Plagenhoef, S. 1971. *Patterns of human motion: A cinematographic analysis.* Englewood Cliffs, N.J.: Prentice-Hall, pp. 25, 27.

Reynolds, E., and Lovett, R. W. 1909. Method of determining the position of the center of gravity in its relation to certain bony landmarks in the erect position. *Am. J. Physiol.* 24:286–93.

Swearingen, J. J., Braden, G. E., Badgley, J. M., and Wallace, T. F. 1969. *Determination of centers of gravity in children.* Washington, D.C.: Federal Aviation Administration, Report AM 69-22.

Walton, J. S. 1970. A template for locating segmental centers of gravity. *Res. Q.* 41:615–18.

Waterland, J. D., and Shambes, G. M. 1970. Biplane center of gravity procedure. *Percept. Mot. Skills.* 30:511–14.

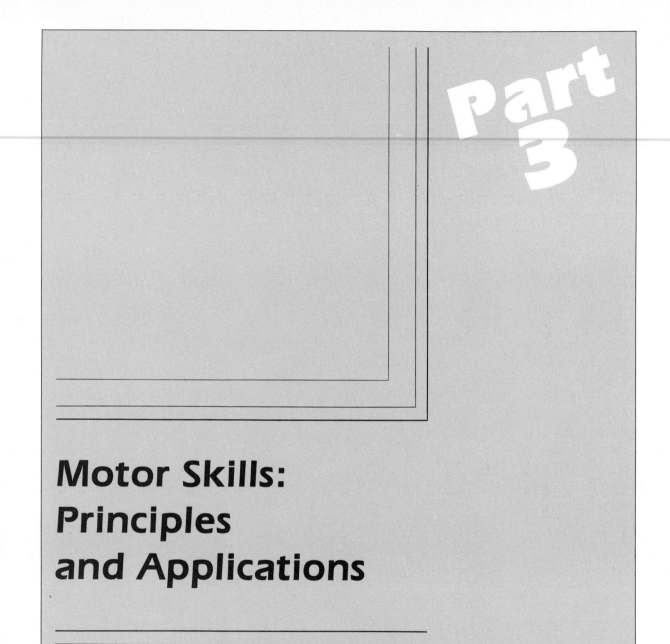

Part 3

Motor Skills:
Principles
and Applications

Introduction to Part 3

At the conclusion of Part Three students should be able to complete basic qualitative kinesiological analyses for all categories of skill classification. This means that they will have learned to describe movements accurately, evaluate performance according to anatomical and mechanical principles, and prescribe corrective actions when needed. As a consequence, they should be able to assume the responsibilities of teaching motor skills with a systematic and valid approach to the learning and improvement of performance.

Part Three opens with a chapter on approaches to the kinesiological analysis of motor skills. It contains a comprehensive outline of motor skills organized in accordance with the major objectives of these skills. These are the (1) maintenance of erect posture, (2) giving of impetus, both to one's own body and to external objects, and (3) receiving of impetus, both from one's own body and from external objects. The next six chapters, which follow this outline closely, include discussions of the different types of skills. They draw on both the anatomical and mechanical information found in Parts One and Two and present the principles that provide the basis for the successful performance of each skill.

This group of chapters is followed by a single chapter on exercises for special purposes. The exercises that are discussed fall into three general classifications: exercises for increasing the range of joint motion, exercises for developing muscle strength and endurance, and exercises for correcting posture faults. Inasmuch as the exercises incorporate several of the types of motor skills listed in the outline, this chapter does not fit into any one particular motor skill category, and for that reason it follows the chapters that are based on the outline.

The final chapter in Part Three is addressed particularly to those students who will soon be joining the ranks of instructors of motor skills. It discusses the implications of kinesiology for effective instruction of physical activities and presents different views concerning the value of teaching biomechanical principles to students as an aid to learning motor skills. Some investigators have found this practice beneficial, although others have not. As to the value of a sound knowledge of mechanical principles to the instructor, there can be no question. The increased understanding that this gives provides a scientific basis for selecting one particular technique in preference to another; it enables the diagnosis of individual needs and difficulties, it reveals basic similarities between motor skills in the same category and thus enables a clearer presentation of new activities that involve the same movement patterns as those with which the learner is already familiar; it enables the offering of pertinent suggestions with true insight. A thorough grasp of this subject adds immeasurably to the instructor's background. In short, the intelligent use of one's knowledge of kinesiology often makes all the difference between effective and ineffective teaching.

Approaches to the Kinesiological Analysis of Motor Skills

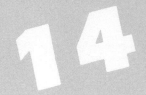

Objectives

At the conclusion of this chapter, the student should be able to:

1. Describe the major components of a kinesiological analysis.
2. Classify motor skills using the classification system presented.
3. Complete an anatomical description of a motor skill that requires motion in most joints and that has at least three phases.
4. Name at least three mechanical principles that apply to each subcategory in the classification system and which, if violated, will result in major performance errors.
5. Complete a qualitative kinesiological analysis of a simple motor skill performance of the student's own choosing.

Components of a Kinesiological Analysis

The teaching of motor skills, whether it takes place in the clinic or on the playing field, consists of presenting a skill and in knowing what points to emphasize. It also consists to a large extent of diagnosing difficulties, correcting errors, and eliminating actions that limit performance. In addition, the teacher of motor skills must be aware of the types of injuries that are likely to occur in a particular skill and how to prevent them. These tasks which, on the surface, may seem simple can indeed be quite complex if for no other reason than that motor skills themselves are complex. An effective aid in helping to understand the basic elements and requirements of a motor skill is a kinesiological analysis.

In the preceding chapters the anatomical components of human movement—the bones, the joints, the muscles, and the related portions of the nervous system—were presented, and both the anatomical and mechanical aspects of human motion were discussed. The basic movements of the body segments were described, and it was

Table 14–1   An Outline for a Kinesiological Analysis

A. Description of skill performance
   1. Name and primary purpose of performance
   2. Classification
   3. Brief word description of skill
B. Anatomical analysis
   1. Skeletal/joint actions
   2. Muscle participation
   3. Neuromuscular considerations
   4. Anatomical principles related to effective and safe performance
C. Mechanical analysis
   1. Underlying mechanics objective(s)
   2. Nature of motion and forces
      a. Motion type(s)
      b. Forces involved (enumerate and specify magnitude, application point, and angle)
   3. Identification of mechanical principles that apply, e.g., stability and equilibrium, momentum and impulse, muscle forces (joint torques), continuity of force application (timing), reaction, friction, conservation of momentum, kinematic principles
   4. Violation of principles
      a. Which application(s) of principles is (are) violated?
      b. What are the errors?
      c. What are the sources for error?
D. Prescription for improvement of performance: indicate how the performance should be changed so that the principles are no longer violated.

shown how observation of both anatomical and mechanical principles contributes to the efficient use of the body in the performance of motor skills. A kinesiological analysis applies this information in order to analyze and assess the effectiveness of a given motor performance. It consists of:

1. *Describing* a skill in a logical and systematic fashion by breaking it down into its constituent elements.
2. *Evaluating* the performance of the skill by determining if and how the related anatomical and mechanical principles have been violated.
3. *Prescribing* corrections based on an appropriate identification of the cause(s).

An outline of the basic components for the kinesiological analysis of a motor skill is presented in Table 14–1. The emphasis in this analysis is on a qualitative assessment of the performance, and may be conducted with the assistance of videotapes, motion pictures, or the naked eye. If no type of photographic record is available, the analyst must use a systematic approach to the observation of the performance. After scanning the whole performance, focusing on different aspects of the performance in repeated trials is essential, since it is virtually impossible to observe all important actions with a nonfocused single observation. Being familiar with the purpose of the skill and its classification helps to determine what to focus on in each repetition. For example, the purpose of the standing long jump is to cover as much horizontal distance as possible between the points of takeoff and landing (Figure 14–1). The body is projected into the air and, like any projectile, its direction and distance depend upon what happens at the point of projection. Therefore much attention in the observation should be directed to the force generation and angle at the moment of takeoff. The next most critical point is the landing, and the behavior of the body at

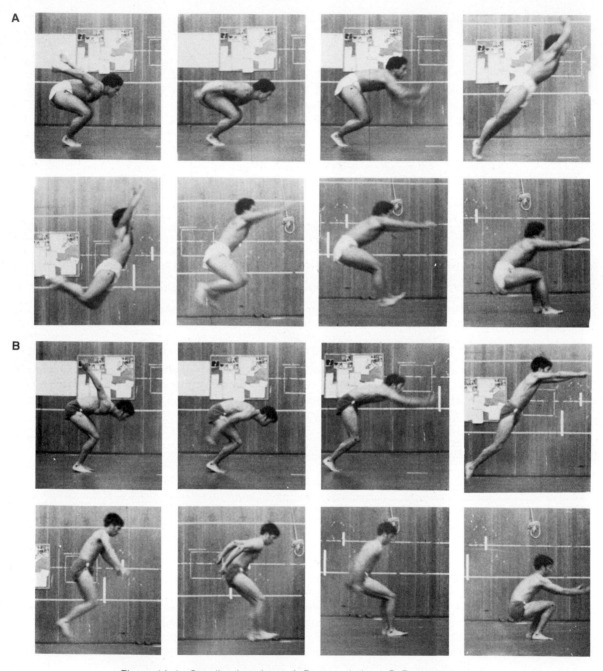

Figure 14–1 Standing long jump. *A*, Better technique. *B*, Poorer technique.

that instant should be scrutinized in subsequent observations. Each observation should also be directed to different parts of the body whose relative positions are known to be critical. It is known, for instance, that the thighs in good standing long jumpers are horizontal at the moment of landing.

Primary Purpose of Motor Skill

The first step in the analysis is to identify the primary purpose of the movement. Without a clear understanding of why the skill is being done, it is virtually impossible to evaluate its effectiveness. In this statement of purpose applicable references to accuracy, speed, form, or distance should be included. For example, in the 50-meter breast stroke, the purpose is to cover the course in the shortest amount of time. Speed is a major factor. The purpose of the tennis serve is to hit the ball into the opponent's service court in a manner that will make it difficult for the opponent to return it. To accomplish this both accuracy and speed are essential elements in the execution of the serve. In springboard dives, the purpose is to execute the dive according to a prescribed form, and neither speed nor accuracy is stressed, but appearance is. The purpose of putting in golf is to get the ball in the cup from a relatively short distance away. Accuracy is essential for accomplishing this aim.

Classification of Motor Skills

The undertaking of analysis assumes an organization of the factors and circumstances related to the area of investigation. Hence, in the field of motor skills, it is appropriate first to identify major categories and then the subdivisions to which the skills belong. This approach makes it possible to categorize the nature of a given motor skill with a fair degree of precision.

Many systems of classification have appeared in the literature. Although a review of these is of interest because of the different points of view they represent, it is unprofitable to spend time comparing their relative merits since a classification should be judged solely on the basis of its meaningfulness to those using it. The classification presented below has been of use to the authors as a basis for discussing the kinesiological aspects of human motion. It is based on three major divisions of motor skills according to their objectives, on the subcategories relating to the mediums in which they take place, and on the nature of the body's support (or lack of it, in some instances).

A SYSTEM FOR CLASSIFICATION OF MOTOR SKILLS

I. Maintaining erect posture

II. Giving impetus
    A. To one's own body
        1. Supported by the ground or other resistant surface
            a. Movements on a stationary or limited base
            b. Locomotion on foot, on wheels and blades, on hands, on hands and knees (or feet); rotatory locomotion
        2. Supported in suspension
            a. Swinging activities on trapeze, flying rings, or similar equipment
            b. Hand traveling on traveling rings or horizontal ladder
        3. Unsupported—i.e., projected into or falling through the air
            a. Diving
            b. Trampoline activities
            c. Acrobatics
        4. Supported by water
            a. Aquatic locomotion
                1. Swimming
                2. Boating
            b. Aquatic stunts

    B.   To external objects
        1.   Throwing with hand or implement
        2.   Pushing, pulling, thrusting, lifting
        3.   Striking, hitting, kicking
III. Receiving impetus
    A.   Of one's own body in landing from a jump or fall
    B.   Of external objects in catching, trapping, spotting, or intercepting

It may have been noticed that the three major headings in this outline are maintaining erect posture, and giving and receiving impetus. Some may question the reason for treating the maintenance of erect posture as a major category instead of including it under giving impetus to one's own body. The rationale for this decision is that the emphasis here is on *adjustment to the immediate environment* rather than on "making a movement" in the sense that one usually interprets this concept. With one exception, the adjustments are made from a stationary position, the exception being a shift in stance necessitated by standing on a moving base. This does not involve moving from one place to another, but only widening the stance and facing in a different direction for the purpose of maintaining balance.

The initial step in the classification is to determine in which major category the skill belongs, and then in which secondary, and possibly tertiary, category. A forehand drive in tennis, for instance, belongs in the primary category of giving impetus to an external object and in the secondary one of striking. Turning a cartwheel is a form of giving impetus to one's own body, when it is supported by the ground, and is classified further as rotatory locomotion.

In addition to pinpointing the exact categories to which the skill belongs, there are a number of factors that should be considered. Many skills consist of a series of phases that cut across different categories, and these must be considered separately. A tennis serve, like the forehand drive, is a form of striking, but it also involves tossing the ball, a skill that should not be overlooked. Vaults over a gymnasium box or horse consist of the approach, the placement of the hands almost simultaneously with the jump or takeoff, the momentary support by the hands, and the push-off from the box, followed by the projection of the body together with the necessary adjustments of the bodily segments, and finally the landing, which involves movements of the upper extremities and trunk as well as of the lower extremities. In pole vaulting and in hand-over-hand rope climbing using feet as well as hands (the only method that assures continuous movement and avoids the necessity for overcoming inertia at every step), there is a smooth transition from pulling to pushing. In hurdling there is repeated alternation between the run and the hurdle without any break in the rhythm. In many basketball throws for the basket, the throw is accompanied by a jump. All phases of the skill should be included in the analysis.

In many skills, especially those involving either the giving or the receiving of a force of appreciable magnitude, the ability to maintain balance is an important feature. To do so effectively means observing the principles of balance and posture adjustment as well as those relating to the specific form of giving or receiving impetus. Lifting a heavy weight from the floor is a good example of an impetus-giving activity that depends in large part for its effectiveness upon the maintenance of a posture that favors lifting.

The standing long jump shown in Figure 14–1 belongs in the major category of giving impetus to one's own body. The initial phases prior to the takeoff and landing and recovery phases belong in the secondary category of movement on a stationary base, while the "in air" phase is an activity of the unsupported category.

Having classified the skill according to the categories in the outline, and having considered the related factors, the skill may now be analyzed both anatomically and mechanically. In the next two sections the standing long jump in Figure 14–1 is used as an example to show how the analysis might proceed.

Anatomical Analysis

The anatomical analysis of the movement should include an examination of the skeletal-joint action, an account of the muscle participation, and an identification of the neurological mechanisms involved. It should attempt to give specific answers to these questions:

1. Which joints are involved, and what are their exact movements in the motor skill?
2. Are any of the joints used to the limit of their range of motion?
3. Which muscles are responsible for the joint actions, and what is the nature of their contraction?
4. Do any of the muscle groups exert maximal or near maximal effort?
5. Which neuromuscular mechanisms are likely to help or hinder the action, and what is the nature of their involvement?
6. Which anatomical principles contribute to maximal efficiency and accuracy in the performance of the motor skill?
7. Which principles are directly related to the avoidance of injury?

To facilitate answering these questions the technique being analyzed should be divided into units or phases. Each phase is treated as a separate movement and should have a logical beginning and ending in terms of the muscle and joint involvement. The golf drive, for instance, might have four phases: the stance, the preparatory phase, the downswing or force phase ending with the ball contact, and the follow-through. The phases for walking, a repetitive or cyclical movement, are often separated into swing and support phases, with the support phase further subdivided into the restraining and propulsive phases. The standing long jump in Figure 14–1 was divided into the preparatory phase, unsupported phase, and landing and recovery phases.

SKELETAL/JOINT ACTIONS   For each phase of the technique and for each joint participating in the phase, the precise joint action should be identified and recorded as was done for the sample analysis of the force phase of the standing long jump shown in Table 14–2. If it seems desirable to measure the ranges of motion of these joint actions, they can be measured directly using elgons or indirectly on sequential motion pictures of the technique.

MUSCLE PARTICIPATION   The muscular action is identified for each joint movement and recorded next to the joint actions on the chart (Table 14–2). This implies identifying not only the muscles that are contracting, but also their precise function in the movement, the kind of contraction they are undergoing (concentric, eccentric, or static), and an estimate of the force of their contraction (strong, medium, mild). The method of identification of the muscle participation can vary from the relatively simple but least reliable to more complex laboratory procedures. The technique that requires no equipment relies on subjective judgment of the actions of a muscle based on the muscle's attachments, together with its relation to the joint in question. This method must be used with caution, however, as its validity is questionable. To make it worthwhile, assumed muscular actions should be verified whenever possible by referring to related EMG research reports.

Table 14–2   Chart for Anatomical Analysis of a Motor Skill
Skill being analyzed: Standing long jump (see Figure 14–1).
Phase being analyzed: Force phase.

NAME OF JOINT	STARTING POSITION	OBSERVED JOINT ACTION	FORCE FOR MOVEMENT	MAIN MUSCLE GROUPS ACTIVE	KIND OF CONTRACTION	FORCE OF CONTRACTION
Metatarsal phalangeal	Extended	Hyperextension/ flexion	Muscle	Extensors/flexors	Concentric	Strong
Ankle	Dorsiflexed	Plantar flexion	Muscle	Plantar flexors	Concentric	Strong
Knee	Flexed	Extension	Muscle	Extensors	Concentric	Strong
Hip	Flexed	Extension	Muscle	Extensors	Concentric	Strong
Pelvis	Decreased tilt	Increased tilt	Muscle	Spinal extensors	Concentric	Moderate
Lumbar spine	Flexion	Extension	Muscle	Spinal extensors	Concentric	Moderate
Thoracic spine	Slight flexion	Extension	Muscle	Spinal extensors	Concentric	Moderate
Cervical spine	Hyperextended	Flexion	Gravity	Spinal extensors	Eccentric	Mild
Shoulder girdle	Upward tilt	Upward rotation, abduction	Muscle Muscle	Upward rotators Abductors	Concentric Concentric	Moderate Moderate
Shoulder joint	Hyperextension, medial rotation	Flexion	Muscle	Flexors	Concentric	Strong
Elbow	Extended	—	—	Extensors	Static	Mild
Radioulnar	Pronated	—	—	—	—	—
Wrist	Extended	—	—	Extensors	Static	Mild
Phalanges	Extended	—	—	Extensors	Static	Mild

Patterned after format presented in Rasch, P. J., and Burke, R. K.: *Kinesiology and applied anatomy*. 6th ed. Philadelphia: Lea & Febiger, 1978, pp. 339–347. This form for recording an anatomical analysis may be reproduced for class use without specific permission.

There is one experimental technique that is available to everyone. This is palpation and inspection of superficial muscles. In spite of the limitations of this method and its subjective nature, it is recommended for students as it is a valuable learning experience. Students should be cautious, however, about applying their findings to sport skills which, in most cases, are performed under circumstances that differ widely from those under which basic movements are executed.

The most reliable laboratory method of investigating muscular action in present use is electromyography. Evidence of muscle participation and relative quantification of that participation is possible with this methodology.

The recording of isokinetic contraction is another technique for making precise evaluations of muscular and joint performance. It requires the use of an electromechanical device designed specifically for this purpose. This method is discussed in Chapter 21.

NEUROMUSCULAR CONSIDERATIONS   The muscle response patterns of well-learned motor skills involve the integrated action of many reflexes and the inhibition of others. After repeated viewings of the performance "live" or on film, the student should name and discuss the reflexes that could be acting at various points in each phase. The reflexes that should be considered are spindle reflexes (stretch reflex), Golgi tendon organ reflex, joint reflexes, cutaneous responses, labyrinthine reflexes, neck reflexes, and visual righting reflexes. For each reflex, the receptors involved should be identified, the expected action due to the reflex described, and the actual results explained. In the standing long jump in Figure 14–1, the following reflex actions are plausible examples of reflex action:

1. *Reflex:* Labyrinthine head righting reflex is present.
    Time: Preparation for takeoff.
    Evidence: As the trunk leans farther forward, the head and neck become more hyperextended.

2. *Reflex:* Stretch reflexes in extensors of hip, knee, and ankle are present.
    Time: Early preparation for takeoff (crouch).
    Evidence: The stretch reflexes are activated in the extensors as flexion occurs in the hips, knees, and ankles. The result is facilitation of contraction of the extensors.

Mechanical Analysis

The mechanical analysis of an activity involves the identification of laws and principles that help to explain the most appropriate form for the execution of the activity and identify the mechanical reasons for success or failure. In order to assess the mechanical nature of a technique and to make use of this information in helping performers choose movements that will result in skillful motion, the analyzer should attempt to identify those principles and laws which verify the actions as desirable. Once the movement is classified according to an outline such as that on page 415, the analyzer should determine exactly how and when the movements of the performance do or do not satisfy the standards of good performance as explained by the laws and principles of mechanics. Once this process is accomplished, a greater depth of understanding of the skill is achieved, and the basis for making change is founded upon sound knowledge and understanding of the reasons "why."

UNDERLYING MECHANICS OBJECTIVE   The purpose of the standing long jump in performance terms is to jump as far as possible. The focus of this statement is on the desired outcome—i.e., maximum distance. The question now becomes one of determining what must be done in mechanical terms to produce the maximum distance. Since the distance traveled occurs in the air, the body is a projectile, and those factors that cause a projectile to travel the farthest are those which must be considered.

The distance a projectile will travel is governed by the speed and angle of projection and the relation of the landing height to the takeoff height. Maximum horizontal distance occurs when a body is projected into the air with maximum speed and at an angle that will keep it in the air long enough to travel a maximum horizontal distance. An examination of the film record of the jump reveals that the center of gravity is higher at takeoff than it is at landing. Therefore, the optimum angle will be somewhat less than the 45 degrees popularly associated with maximum horizontal distance.

The speed of the projection is related to the total impulse (force × time) exerted during the takeoff, which, in turn, is due to the impulses developed at each joint. The joint impulses in turn are equal to the product of the joint torques (muscle forces) and the time over which they are exerted. Important joint torques in this performance are at the hip, knee, ankle, and shoulder. Thus, in summary, it seems that one appropriate underlying objective for this technique is to maximize the total impulse exerted during the takeoff. A second one is to direct the impulse through the center of gravity at an angle with the horizontal of slightly less than 45 degrees.

NATURE OF MOTION AND FORCES   In this section of the mechanical analysis, the kind(s) of motion and the forces causing or modifying the motion are identified for each phase. In the standing long jump, the type of motion in each phase is as follows:

1. Preparatory force phase—angular movement of the body segments on a stationary base.
2. Unsupported phase—unsupported curvilinear motion of the body as a whole as well as angular movement of the body segments.
3. Landing and recovery phases—angular movement of body segments on a stationary base.

After the jumper leaves the ground the horizontal velocity of the body remains constant, except for the negligible effect of air resistance. The vertical velocity decelerates uniformly owing to the effect of gravity until it reaches zero at the high point. Uniform acceleration then continues until the landing. The rotatory movements of the arms and legs do not contribute to the motion of the body in the air. Their actions are needed solely to get the body segments in the best position for landing.

The forces causing or modifying motion leading up to the takeoff are:

1. *Weight*—applied downward through the center of gravity.
2. *Normal reaction*—applied vertically upward from the contact of the feet with the ground.
3. *Friction*—applied perpendicular to the normal reaction force along the contact surface opposite the direction of the push-off.
4. *Propulsive force*—applied at contact, equal and opposite to reaction and friction forces; generated by the muscles, which in turn produce the velocity of the projection, probably in the ankle, knee, hip, shoulder, and metatarsophalangeal joints.
5. *Drag*—negligible air resistance opposite to the direction of the jump.

MECHANICAL PRINCIPLES   The identification of principles related to the execution of the skill are a first step in establishing the causes of error in the performance of the skill. By focusing on the principles and how they relate to the skill the potential sources of error are suggested.

The following principles are examples of those that should be identified and examined when analyzing jumping techniques, such as in the example of the standing long jump. Only those of importance in preparation for the takeoff (force phase) are considered here.

Projectile Range   The range of a projectile is controlled by three factors: the angle, initial speed, and height at the moment of projection. For maximum horizontal distance, the theoretical angle of projection is 45 degrees. This optimum angle decreases as the initial speed decreases and the distance between takeoff and landing increases.

Impulse   Any change in the body's center of gravity is dependent upon the applied force and the time over which it is applied. The optimum impulse in this instance is one that will give maximum linear velocity to the body for its projectile flight.

Torque   The torque about any point equals the product of the force magnitude and its perpendicular distance from the line of action. The force rotating the body segments depends upon the related joint torques, which are governed by the muscle forces and the location of their attachments. In the broad jump, strength and speed in the lower extremity extensors are necessary for optimal torques in the related joints.

Summation of Moments (Torques)   The resultant moment of a force system equals the sum of the individual moments. Therefore, if a maximum resultant is desired, all body segments that have the capability must contribute to their maximum. Maximum thrust of the body in the jump depends upon maximum resultant torques generated at the individual joints. The sum of these moments applied through the contact point produces the type and speed of motion (rotatory or linear).

Timing of Forces   The timing of individual joint actions affects the resultant force. Poor sequencing and coordination reduce the force of the jump. Because the heavier, more resistant segments of the body take more time to generate maximum speed, they should begin to move first and the lightest levers should move last. In this way the angular velocities of each contributing segment are at maximum velocity at the instant of the thrust. This principle suggests that the thrusting action begin with the hips, followed by the shoulders and knees, ankles, and metatarsophalangeal joints.

Normal Reaction   The thrust of the ground on the feet pushing the body up is equal and opposite to the thrust of the feet on the ground.

VIOLATION OF MECHANICAL PRINCIPLES   Diagnosing the cause of an error is difficult because the cause may be far removed from the observed effect. The purpose in identifying the mechanical principles is to locate potential sources for error. Given the purpose of the skill, which of the principles, if violated, has the greatest potential for limiting performance? How? These are the most troublesome questions to answer. Without quantitative data it is difficult to make any selection with certainty. And, even with the support of such data, which indeed can provide us with much useful information, we still cannot be certain. At this time there is no general method available to identify and establish the order of importance for those factors that limit performance. One must rely primarily upon knowledge of the technique and the principles of mechanics that apply.

Again, using the example of the standing long jump, we know that *speed* and *direction* are the two most important factors in limiting performance. The direction is governed by the direction of impulse of the thrust. It appears, then, that direction might be a good place to start to look for errors. In Figure 14–1A the angle formed by the center of gravity of the jumper, the jumper's toes, and floor at takeoff, when judged by the eyeball method, appears to be less than 45 degrees (measured with a protractor it is actually 52 degrees). What is not known from looking at the picture, however, is the relationship between the lean and the speed due to the coordinated summation of the joint impulses.

The speed of the projection depends upon the ground impulse. The faster the properly timed contributing lower extremities can extend the greater will be the impulse of the ground against the feet. It is important, therefore, to consider the speed and range of extension in the hip, knee, and ankle at takeoff. Although their speeds cannot be judged merely by examining the picture, the range of motion in the joints can be determined. The full extension of those joints at takeoff suggests optimization of the joint impulses through proper sequencing or timing.

Prescription for Improvement of Performance

After the performance has been described in anatomical and mechanical detail and the causes for error have been identified, the analyst must decide on the appropriate strategy for effecting change in the performance so that it conforms to the anatomical and mechanical ideal. Now the analyst becomes an instructor who must decide not only what must be done but how best to communicate that information to the performer in a manner that will make sense. The task is not unlike that of a physician who uses vast medical knowledge to prescribe bed rest as the best cure for an ailment. The cure may be simple but the complexities attached to knowing what to do, and why, and then making that information understandable to the patient, are far from simple. The instructor of motor skills needs to develop ability as a prescriber as well as an analyst. Both talents will improve with practice. As more systematic analyses are performed, the student will become aware of characteristics common to groups of skills. Common errors and their causes will emerge for related skills as well as similar or common prescriptions appropriate for correcting the errors. The important thing to remember is to concentrate on the causes for errors, not on the resultant symptoms. Before the physician can prescribe for a limping gait, the cause must be known and the viable options for treatment identified. Before an instructor of motor skills can prescribe for improvement of a short, standing long jump or any other motor performance, the cause(s) for the error must be known and the valid options for correction determined.

Laboratory Instrumentation for Motion Analysis

The scholarly study of man in motion has interested scientists for centuries, and their contributions have established the foundation for the advances made in kinesiology and biomechanics research in the twentieth century. Methodology has progressed from exclusive dependence upon observations by the naked eye to the use of sophisticated photographic and electronic equipment for analyzing and quantifying the anatomical and mechanical nature of human performance. Although the student in the undergradute course in kinesiology is not expected to have much experience with sophisticated laboratory equipment and methodology, a brief summary of current laboratory approaches to analyses may be of interest.

Photographic Instrumentation

Many types of optical equipment, including the motion picture camera, the still camera, and the sequence camera, have been used to record motion. The most frequently used research instrument is the high-speed motion picture camera coupled with a stop motion film analyzer. Cameras with speeds of up to 500 frames per second and variable shutters provide an ample number of clear data points for analyzing the fastest of human movements. In addition, the camera is a noncontact instrument that does not interfere in any way with the subject's normal movement. When filming is done for research purposes, the camera needs to be centered with respect to the action stationary, level, and perpendicular to the motion plane. Either angular or linear displacement (i.e., motion) may be measured from the films obtained. If velocity, acceleration, or force values are desired, some form of timing device must also be part of the recording process.

The quantitative analysis of movement techniques recorded on processed film requires the use of some type of projector that permits single frame projection so that measurements may be made of the image. This may be done by making tracings of the projected picture frame using a stop action projector and a flat tracing area or a Recordak Film Analyzer (Figure 14–2). Careful marking of body landmarks and segments on sequential frame tracings makes it possible to measure body and segment displacements from which a variety of motion and force values may be obtained.

These approaches to analyzing films are simple but tedious and time-consuming, and subject to error at each step in the process. For these reasons their current uses are primarily for laboratory exercises. They have been replaced in research by more sophisticated analyzers that allow for the direct feeding of data points from the film

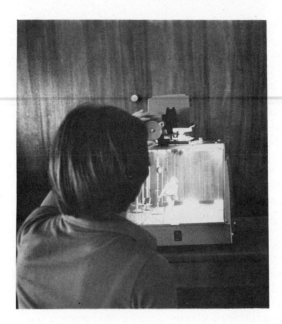

Figure 14–2 The Recordak is used to view single frames of a film and to make tracings of the projected image if desired.

image into an on-line computer using an electronic digital analyzer. Even so, the methodology is still laborious, and it is possible for errors to occur in the methods now used for the numerical treatment of the data obtained from film. This is especially true in the determination of acceleration and, because acceleration values are needed for force estimates, force values obtained through film records may also be suspect. For these reasons experimenters continue to search for alternatives to film analysis.

Forms of instrumentation that are being investigated as suitable alternatives for the motion picture camera involve the use of optoelectronic devices. One of these is polarized light goniometry, or Polgon. The Polgon employs polarized light to measure angles of limb movements. An advantage of this technique is immediate feedback to the subject. Another technique is automatic image analysis, in which a videotape is automatically scanned to detect levels of light intensity. Opaque dots placed on the subject can thus be distinguished, and x, y coordinates identified. The advantage of this technique is also the quick availability of the data; the disadvantage is that television does not as yet have the same resolution and speed rates as motion pictures.

Still cameras are also useful in motion analysis when used with special light sources. The camera shutter is left open during the filming, and the exposure is controlled by the light source. Multiple images on a single picture are the result of a flashing strobe light. Another technique is to attach tiny light bulbs to the joints and extremities. When photographed in a dark room with an open shutter the motion appears as a light streak, and the nature of the movement pattern is revealed. If the electrical supply to the bulbs is interrupted intermittently the streak is similarly interrupted. The length and spacing of the interruptions gives an indication of the speed variations in the motion.

**Electronic
Instrumentation**

There are a number of applications of electronic instrumentation in biomechanical research. The value of this type of instrumentation is that the data may be more accurate because they are obtained directly from the subject rather than indirectly, as is the case with photoinstrumentation. The disadvantage is that the subjects must be in contact with some part of the sensing mechanism of the instrument which, in turn, must be connected by wires or radio waves (telemetry) to the recording device.

Electronic instruments such as the elgon (see Chapter 1) have been developed for measuring displacement data, but the major application has been for the direct measurement of force. Basic to the electronic system for measuring force is a transducer, which serves to sense and convert the quantity of the variable being measured into an electric signal proportional in magnitude to the original signal. After being amplified or conditioned in some other fashion, the output from the transducer is displayed by means of readout equipment that may take the form of pen and ink or light beam paper recorders, magnetic tapes, or cathode ray tubes.

The most common types of electronic transducers used in motion analysis have been the potentiometer and strain gauge. The potentiometer, acting like a light dimmer, converts changes in angular displacement to changes in electrical current—the greater the angle, the greater the current. The strain gauge is a form of force transducer and is used for direct measurement of force. The Elgon (pp. 18–19) is an example. Altered resistance due to strain on the mechanism, which may be made of wire or a semiconductor substance, produces a change in output voltage which may then be recorded.

There have been many applications for recording force over time in sports and basic movement patterns and, with the improved technology in the manufacture of force transducers that has occurred in recent years, it has been possible to measure and evaluate forces more precisely and conveniently than ever before. One instrument that relies on strain gauge transducers to measure reactive force is the force platform. These force-sensing instruments are placed so that forces may be recorded between the feet and the ground in all six modes (vertical and two horizontal directions, and about the three axes) while walking, running, jumping, dancing, or hopping. As the feet or any other body part lands on the platform, linear forces and torques that develop are identified. This instrument's use to measure reactive forces in a variety of activities has increased tremendously over the last decade. So, too, has its value as a research tool increased because of technological improvements in the instrument and in the procedures employed.

The instrumentation used in electromyography is another application of electronics. The action potentials from the muscle are picked up by electrodes (surface or indwelling), amplified, and recorded. The raw EMG record can be modified by the inclusion of an electronic signal conditioner that may rectify or integrate the record. It is also possible to quantify EMG data when appropriate computers and computer programs are tied in to the system.

Probably the form of instrumentation that has most influenced analysis and research procedures in the mechanical analysis of motion is the high-speed computer. Without it the volume of data that can be generated through the use of film and force measuring devices would never be analyzed, because many of the necessary mathematical procedures would be impossible to accomplish. The availability of computers is undoubtedly responsible for the rapid advances in biomechanical research that have occurred in the last two decades. In addition to the facilitation of data treatment, the computer also contributes to the analysis of motion in two other significant ways.

An important application is computer simulation. Complex mathematical equations are used to develop mathematical models that simulate human movement patterns. Once these models are validated against experimental conditions, they may be used to determine the effect of altering selected variables upon the total performance. The third use of computers applied to the analysis of motion is computer graphics—i.e., computer data are displayed graphically. Drawings of the human body have been made by the computer, as have other illustrative charts, graphs, and diagrams. The display of computer simulations is also often "drawn" through the use of computer graphics.

The future of research in the mechanics of human motion will probably be as varied as present and future technologies allow. The use of gamma ray scanners and laser beams are under investigation, as are procedures for automating much of the data gathering that now requires endless hours of attention.

Laboratory Experiences

1. Select three motor skills from different sections of Appendix I and classify them according to the outline of motor skills. Perform a kinesiological analysis for each, following the outline in Table 14–1.
2. Analyze kinesiologically the two performances of the standing long jump portrayed in Figure 14–1. Follow the outline presented in Table 14–1.

References

Berg, K. 1975. A functional approach to undergraduate kinesiology. *J. Phys. Educ. Rec.* 46:43–4.

Cavanagh, P. R. 1976. Recent advances in instrumentation and methodology of biomechanical studies. In *Biomechanics V-A,* ed. P. V. Komi. Baltimore: University Park Press.

Cooper, J., and Glassow, R. 1976. *Kinesiology,* 4th ed. St. Louis: C. V. Mosby.

Gowitzke, B., and Milner, M. 1980. *Understanding the scientific bases of human movement,* 2d ed. Baltimore: Williams & Wilkins.

Grieve, D. W., et al. 1976. *Techniques for the analysis of human movement.* Princeton, N.J.: Princeton Book.

Hay, J. G. 1978. The identification and ordering of the technical factors limiting performance. Paper presented at the XXI World Congress in Sport Medicine, Brasilia, Brazil.

Hoffman, S. J. 1974. Toward taking the fun out of skill analysis. *J. Health Phys. Educ. Rec.* 45:74–6.

Miller, D. I., and Nelson, R. C. 1973. *Biomechanics of sport.* Philadelphia: Lea & Febiger.

Norman, R. Q. 1978. An approach to teaching the mechanics of human motion at the undergraduate level. In *Kinesiology: A National Conference on Teaching,* ed. C. Dillman and R. G. Sears. Urbana-Champaign, Ill.: University of Illinois.

Plagenhoef, S. 1971. *Patterns of human motion—a cinematographic analysis.* Englewood Cliffs, N.J.: Prentice-Hall.

Rasch, P., and Burke, K. 1978. *Kinesiology and applied anatomy,* 6th ed. Philadelphia: Lea & Febiger.

The Standing Posture

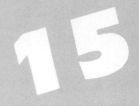

Objectives

At the conclusion of this chapter, the student should be able to:

1. Identify and describe the skeletomuscular and neuromuscular antigravity mechanisms involved in the volitional standing position.
2. Summarize the similarities and differences that occur in the relation of the line of gravity to various body landmarks with good and poor anteroposterior segmental alignment.
3. Discuss the factors that affect the stability and energy cost of the erect posture.
4. Explain the effects that the variables of age, body build, strength, and flexibility have on the alignment of body segments in the standing posture.
5. Name the values, if any, of good posture.

Significance of Posture

There are innumerable concepts of human posture and innumerable interpretations of its significance. Posture may well claim to be "all things to all people." To the physical anthropologist posture may be a racial characteristic, or it may be an indication of phylogenetic development; to the orthopedic surgeon it may be an indication of the soundness of the skeletal framework and muscular system; to an artist it may be an expression of the personality and the emotions; to the actor it serves as a tool for expressing mood or character; to the physician, biologist, fashion model, employer, sculptor, dancer, therapist, psychologist—to each of these, posture has a different significance. Each sees posture within the framework of his or her own profession and interest. This is no less true of kinesiologically oriented therapists and educators. To them, posture is a gauge of mechanical efficiency, kinesthetic sense, muscle balance, and neuromuscular coordination.

For all practical purposes no individual's posture can be described completely. Posture means position, and a multisegmented organism such as the human body cannot be said to have a single posture. It assumes many postures and seldom holds any of them for an appreciable time. Although characteristic patterns become apparent as we observe an individual over an extended period it is difficult, if not well nigh impossible, to measure, or even record, these patterns. It would take a comprehensive series of motion pictures of an individual's varied stance and movement patterns to provide an adequate sample. Perhaps this is the reason why most posture research has been related to the volitional standing position.

Another difficulty in analyzing and evaluating human posture is the varieties of human physique represented, such as those defined by Sheldon (1940). The importance of considering these individual differences of build when evaluating posture has been emphasized by Frost (1938). Hence we see that posture norms are appropriate only for the mythical average figure and apply only to the static standing position, which may or may not be representative of a person's habitual postural patterns.

In view of the fact that activity postures should be of greater concern than static postures to those who specialize in human movement, it may be well to say a word in defense of the practice of examining and photographing the posture of subjects in the erect standing position. It is admitted that the posture in such a position is of little importance in itself. It becomes significant, however, when taken as the point of departure for the many postural patterns assumed by the individual, both at rest and in motion. Since there is an almost endless variety of activity postures and since these are extremely difficult to judge, it is a convenient custom to accept the standing posture as the individual's basic posture from which all other postures stem. Hence, as a reflection of the individual's characteristic postural patterns, the standing posture takes on an importance it would not otherwise have. It should be kept in mind, however, that its importance is in direct proportion *to the extent to which it represents the individual's habitual carriage.*

Support of the Standing Posture

Muscular Activity in Erect Standing

Compared to other mammals humans have very economical antigravity mechanisms, and the muscle energy needed to maintain the erect standing position is not great (Basmajian, 1979). A major reason for the economy of muscle effort required is the major role of the ligaments in supporting and maintaining the integrity of the joints. The muscles that are active are those that aid in keeping the weight-bearing column of bones in relative alignment and that oppose gravity's downward directed force.

According to electromyographic studies reported by Basmajian (1979), the postural muscular activity in the body segments can be expected as follows:

FOOT None of the intrinsic musculature is active during normal standing but becomes active in the push-off for walking or rising on the toes.

LEG The posterior calf muscles are more active than the anterior ones. Any swaying forward or backward produces compensatory muscle action to bring the body back to the vertical balanced position. Rising on the toes or wearing high heels increases the activity of both the anterior and posterior muscles.

THIGH AND HIP   There is very little activity in the thigh muscles during relaxed standing. Swaying produces alternating bursts of activity in the gluteus medius and tensor fasciae latae. The iliopsoas is constantly active, apparently to prevent hyperextension at the hip joint.

SPINE   There is very slight activity in the sacrospinalis or abdominal muscles, depending upon the relation of the line of gravity to the spinal column. Activity is exhibited in *one or the other* of the two sets of muscles. Slight to moderate back muscle activity is at least three times as likely as abdominal muscle activity (Klausen et al., 1978).

UPPER EXTREMITY   The integrity of the joints in the passively hanging extremity is assisted by low-grade activity in a number of muscles. The serratus anterior and the fibers of the trapezius support the shoulder girdle, and the supraspinatus resists downward dislocation of the humerus. There appears to be no activity in the muscles crossing the elbow or wrist joints when the arm hangs passively.

The Neuro-muscular Mechanism for Maintaining Erect Posture

The proprioceptors are responsible for most of the reflex movements necessary for the maintenance of the erect standing position and for the adjustments that must be made to meet changing conditions. They include the receptors of the muscles, joints, and labyrinths, and are accompanied by two exteroceptors, one visual and the other cutaneous. The latter serves as a proprioceptor together with the pressure receptors, especially in connection with the extensor thrust reflex. Volitional postural adjustments are made by the same mechanism that is responsible for all volitional movements (p. 73) and, of necessity, are governed by the structural limitations of the individual.

There are several schools of thought regarding the method of changing habitual postural patterns. Some believe that it can be accomplished by the frequent repetition of carefully selected exercises performed with control and with constant attention to correct form (Goldthwait et al., 1952; Hawley, 1949; Kelly, 1965; Mensendieck, 1937; Rathbone and Hunt, 1965). Others believe that the rebuilding of the necessary neuromuscular pathways can be accomplished only by the indirect method—that is, by influencing the individual's neuromuscular response by means of the thought processes. Mental concepts are utilized for this purpose (Sweigard, 1974; Todd, 1949). Still others seek to establish new postural habits by practicing movements that are believed to develop the natural postural reflexes (Haller and Gurewitsch, 1950). All groups recognize that establishing new postural patterns can take place only within the limits of the individual's structural heritage.

The kinesthetic sense is believed to be a vital factor in the mechanism for establishing and adjusting postural patterns, but this has not yet been demonstrated satisfactorily.

Postural Stability

Hellebrandt (1940) demonstrated that even the erect standing posture is not literally static. "Standing," she concluded, "is, in reality, *movement upon a stationary base.*" Her experiments revealed that the center of gravity did not remain motionless above the base of support no matter how still the subject attempted to stand, but moved forward, backward, and sideward. This motion indicated that the subjects were constantly swaying. When the swaying was prevented by artificial means there was a tendency to faint. Hence the involuntary swaying was seen to serve the purpose of a pump, aiding the venous return, and ensuring the brain of adequate circulation for retaining consciousness.

In the same experiments Hellebrandt found that the oscillations of each individual were balanced so exactly that the average position of the line of gravity, relative to the base of support, was remarkably constant. From this it would seem that we can assume the presence of a controlling factor in our tendency to sway. Apparently the stretch reflex, kinesthetic sense, and vision all operate here to confine the oscillations to a limited area, an area well within the boundaries of the base of support.

Some experimenters have investigated the possibility of a relationship between the position of the line of gravity relative to the base of support and the quality of posture. The findings of the different investigators do not agree, however. It seems obvious that however close the line of gravity is to the center of the base of support, this condition does not necessarily indicate good segmental alignment. One can assume an exaggerated zigzag alignment and still stand in such a way that the line of gravity intersects the center of the base of support, provided the "zags" balance the "zigs," yet the posture may leave much to be desired. In this connection students may find Numbers 3 and 4 of the Laboratory Experiences of particular interest.

In informal class experiments it was found that the relation of the line of gravity to the base of support was not affected significantly or consistently when the subject assumed different positions of the upper extremities or held external objects such as books, a suitcase, or a tray. This would seem to provide evidence of the body's tendency to compensate for deviations of some of its parts from the fundamental standing position. The principle would appear to be established that, under ordinary circumstances, the disalignment of one segment of the body, whether anteroposteriorly or laterally, is accompanied by a compensatory disalignment of another segment or segments. If the disalignment is not exactly balanced, excessive tension in certain muscle groups results. This is particularly apparent when external loads are not adequately compensated. Objective evidence is suggested but is as yet inconclusive.

Alignment of Body Segments

In the literature on posture, statements are frequently seen to the effect that, in the ideal standing posture as viewed from the side, the line of gravity bears a definite relation to certain anatomical landmarks, such as the mastoid process, acromion process, junctions of the anteroposterior curves of the spine, the hip joint (greater trochanter of the femur), knee joint, and lateral malleolus (Figure 15–1). Deviations of the line of gravity away from these landmarks have been viewed as representing "poor" posture in some tests of "perfect" posture. Unfortunately the evaluation of the ideal posture is not that easy, since variations in body build alone result in differences in the anatomical landmarks–line of gravity relationship. Allowances also have to be made for age and body composition. At best the location of the line of gravity should be used as a general indicator of good posture. It might be more realistic to determine a "normal zone" within which the line of gravity might reasonably be expected to lie when the subject is standing in erect posture.

It has been stated that a standing posture in which each weight-bearing segment was balanced vertically upon the segment beneath it made less demand on the muscles than a posture in which the segments formed a zigzag alignment (Kelly, 1965). Good posture, it was said, takes less muscular effort to maintain than poor. The explanation given was that when a segment is not in vertical alignment, the force of gravity is not parallel with its long axis, and hence exerts a rotatory component of force. Although this reasoning may seem logical, it overlooks two facts: first, that one of the most poorly aligned postures is actually a fatigue posture in which the muscles have let go and have left it to the ligaments to prevent complete collapse (Figure 15–2); and second, that even in the most ideal posture some rotatory force is present,

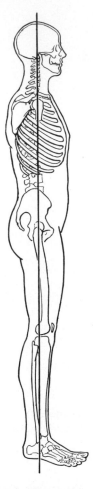

Figure 15–1   Good alignment of weight-bearing segments. Rotatory effect of gravitational force is minimized.

owing to (1) the supporting column of the trunk (i.e., the spine) being situated closer to the posterior surface of the body than to the anterior, (2) the supporting base (the feet) being projected forward from the lower extremities instead of centered beneath them, (3) the spinal column being curved anteroposteriorly, and (4) the chest forming an anterior load upon which gravity is constantly exerting a rotatory force (Figure 15–1). The weight of the breasts in women constitutes an additional anterior weight and thus causes an even greater rotatory component of gravitational force.

There appears to be a definite relationship between the alignment of the body segments and the integrity of the joint structures. It is generally accepted that prolonged postural strain is injurious to these structures. Ligaments that are repeatedly subjected to stretch become permanently stretched, and cartilages that are subjected to uneven pressures and to abnormal friction become damaged. There is adequate clinical evidence to support the contention that prolonged postural strain is a factor in the arthritic changes that take place in the weight-bearing joints. Objective evidence may be lacking, but it might not be difficult to secure if postural records and x-rays of the weight-bearing joints could be obtained for an adequate number of subjects over a

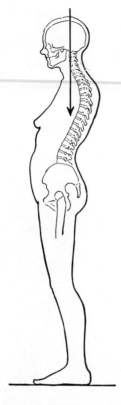

Figure 15–2 Zigzag alignment of weight-bearing segments increases rotatory effect of gravitational force.

10- or 20-year period. Such an investigation might prove or disprove the claim that the human machine functions more efficiently when the weight-bearing segments are in "proper" alignment with a minimum of stress and strain on them.

Factors Related to the Standing Posture

Energy Cost   The question of the energy cost of standing posture has been investigated by both Hellebrandt (1943) and McCormick (1942). Both concluded that when standing, the increase of metabolic rate over the basal rate was so small, compared with the metabolic cost of moving and exercising, as to be negligible. McCormick included both anteroposterior and lateral measurements of body alignment. From these she concluded that the type of posture that involved a minimum of metabolic increase appeared to be one in which the knees are hyperextended as completely as the joints permit, the hips are pushed forward to the limit of extension, the thoracic curve is increased, the head is projected forward, and the upper trunk is inclined slightly backward in a posterior list (Figures 15–3B and 15–4B). As one might expect, this is a typical picture of fatigue posture. A common variation of it is a shift of the weight to one foot with accompanying asymmetrical adjustments in the spine and lower extremities.

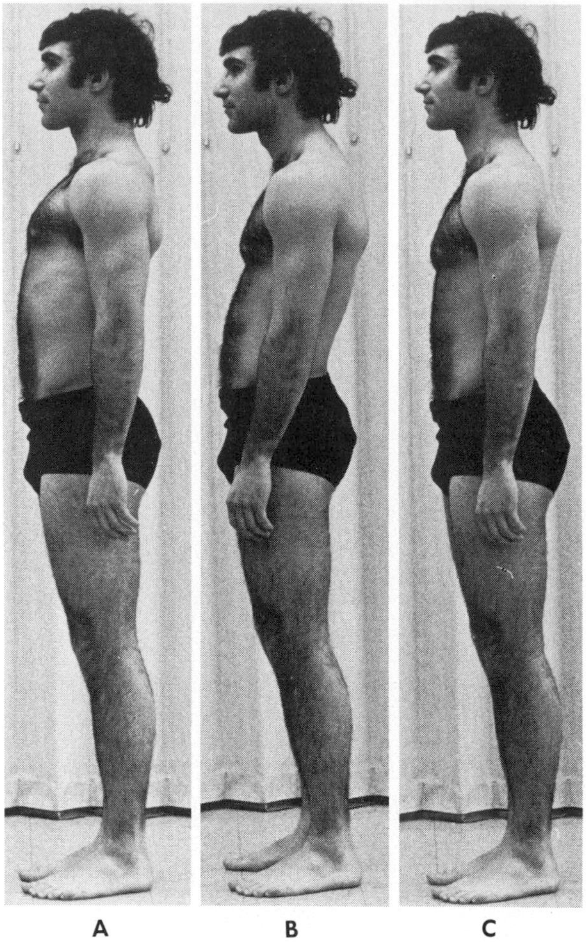

Figure 15–3   *A*, Individual in position of "attention." He is overtense and has exaggerated lumbar curve. *B*, Individual is overrelaxed and has zigzag alignment. *C*. Individual has slightly forward head, round shoulders and slight posterior list of trunk; otherwise there is fairly good alignment.

A   B   C

From these two studies and from the writings of other investigators, such as Basmajian (1979), Evans (1961), Joseph (1960), Steindler (1973), and others, it is seen that there is a lack of agreement concerning the effort required for maintaining upright posture. Doubtless this is partly due to confusion in what is meant by "upright posture." To some, it may mean merely the ability to stay on one's feet and resist the downward pull of gravity. To others, it may mean "good" alignment as opposed to a "zigzag" alignment. The studies based on energy cost appear to indicate that, although it takes little more energy to stand erect than to sit, *minimum* energy expenditure cannot be accepted as a criterion of good posture. Metabolic economy is desirable to a point, as it implies the absence of hypertonicity, but from an overall educator's point of view, well-balanced segmental alignment should not be sacrificed for it.

It would seem that the energy requirement for maintaining erect posture in reasonably good alignment bears a direct relationship to the individual's habitual carriage. It is a matter of common observation that there is a wide range of body alignments seen in "upright posture." Any physical educator who has had the task of

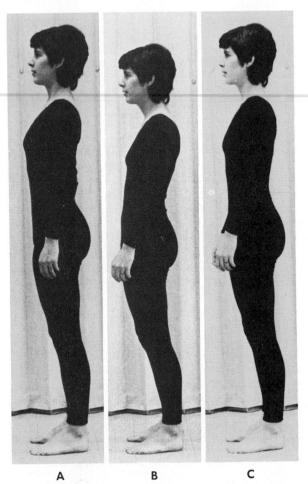

Figure 15–4   *A,* Individual in position of "attention." She has exaggerated lumbar curve but does not show strain. *B,* Individual is overrelaxed and has zigzag alignment. *C,* Individual has a nice easy posture and good alignment except for very slightly forward head.

A   B   C

evaluating the posture of large groups of students and of giving help to those with "poor posture" is impressed with the variation in effort it takes for a student to stand in "good posture." Whereas one individual apparently has no difficulty in assuming this posture because it is the natural one, another cannot assume it even momentarily without the instructor's help and without becoming overtense. It is obvious that the second student is using much more muscular energy than the first. The teacher who is concerned with posture instruction would like to see these individual variations explored more thoroughly. The combination of metabolic determination and electromyography should prove a useful tool for such research. It would be of particular interest to the posture and corrective exercise instructor to learn whether such instruction over a specified period would reveal a relationship between posture improvement and a decrease in the amount of muscular energy required for assuming an "acceptable posture" and maintaining it while participating in selected activities for a specified period of time.

Evolutionary and Hereditary Influences

In tracing the evolution of the human structure and its posture, Morton (1952) has shown the influence that the force of gravity has had on morphological development, first of the terrestrial quadrupeds, then of the arboreal primates, and finally of humans. The evolution from horizontal to vertical posture was achieved, he claimed, by the force of gravity pulling on the suspended body of the arboreal primates when they engaged in brachial locomotion. The changes that developed in human structure, he stated, were the direct result of the shift from a vertically suspended position to a vertically supported one. This shift was responsible not only for the changes in the weight-bearing parts of the musculoskeletal structure, but also for changes in the upper extremities, which were now freed for the development of a great variety of manipulative skills. While no specific principle is derived from this explanation of the role played by the force of gravity in the evolution of human structure, an awareness of it might be of help in the analysis of individual postures.

Attention has already been called to individual variations in posture. In attempting to correct a person's posture one must be realistic and accept the limits imposed by a possible hereditary factor. Improvement can doubtless be made, but one must not expect to effect a radical change in the basic shape of the spine. In addition, certain pathological conditions, such as congenitally dislocated hips, tuberculosis of the spine, cerebral palsy, and poliomyelitis with resultant paralysis of trunk muscles, may cause such changes in an individual's posture that the usual hereditary and environmental influences are obscured.

Organic Function

One frequently mentioned criterion of good posture is the relationship of the alignment of the body to organic function (Goldthwait et al., 1952; Kelly, 1965). Postural patterns are not thought to be good unless they both permit and encourage normal function of the vital physiological processes, particularly those of respiration, circulation, digestion, and elimination. Considerable clinical evidence has been presented to substantiate this belief, but experimental evidence is scarce (Deaver, 1933; Hellebrandt, 1944; Karpovich and Sinning, 1971).

In this regard, Hellebrandt (1944) commented that the concept of the harmful effect of poor posture on visceral function was "based on more or less tenuous evidence without regard for the wide margin of safety under which all organ systems function and the paucity of proof that the anatomical position of a viscus is a valid criterion of the adequacy of its physiologic behavior." There is, however, some evidence of a relationship between menstrual function and posture. Hoffman (1942) studied the findings of the routine orthopedic examination for two groups of college women, one group known as the "dysmenorrhea group," the other as the "no-pain group." The two groups were found to differ significantly with respect to two postural traits, namely anteroposterior pelvic tilt and bilateral hip asymmetry.

Fox (1951) also studied the relation of certain aspects of posture to dysmenorrhea. She investigated the incidence of dysmenorrhea in three groups of young women, one a control group, one a group characterized by sway back (posterior list of the trunk), and one group characterized by faulty pelvic tilt (increased inclination). She found that dysmenorrhea occurred with greater severity among the sway back group than among the control group. Unlike Hoffman, however, she did not find a significant relationship between pelvic tilt and dysmenorrhea.

Strength and Flexibility

That strength and flexibility are factors in posture would seem to be a universally accepted thesis, judging by the preponderance of strength and flexibility exercises included in the majority of corrective programs and also by the strength and flexibility measurements included in posture tests. These exercises relate particularly to the strength of the abdominals, scapular adductors, and thoracic spinal extensors, and in the flexibility of the pectorals and the hamstrings. The results of research in which anteroposterior alignment was correlated with strength or flexibility have been somewhat contradictory. As is often the case, it is difficult to compare results because of significant differences in methodology, especially in the method for measuring the postural alignment and age and sex of the subjects. Although Flint and Diehl (1961) found a significant low correlation between anteroposterior alignment and trunk flexor and extensor strength in elementary school girls, the results of research conducted in Denmark with girls aged 8 to 17 years yielded no correlation between the curves of the spine and the strength of the trunk muscles. However, there was a positive correlation when the same methodology was used with boys aged 6 to 16. The difference between the boys and girls could not be explained, but it was suggested that the differences in muscle strength development between the two sexes could be the cause (Karpovich and Sinning, 1971).

Studies comparing anteroposterior alignment and strength in college-age women have produced results suggesting that there is little or no significant relationship between the strength of the flexors and extensors and postural alignment, but there may be a relationship between alignment and the relative balance between the flexors' and extensors' strength. In addition, poor flexibility of the trunk and hips was found to be more characteristic of college men and women with poor posture than of those with good or average posture (Clark, 1979).

Psychological Aspects

There are several psychological aspects of postural problems with which the instructor should be prepared to deal. For instance, not all posture problems can be explained in terms of physical causes, either musculoskeletal or environmental. Atypical postures may be symptoms of personality problems or emotional disturbances. The hanging head and drooping shoulders of some adolescent girls are often not physical in origin but are symptoms of shyness and poor self-concept. Postural exercises will do little to help such girls unless they are used in conjunction with psychological help. The same is true of the small man whose bantam cock posture is merely an overcompensation for his feelings of inferiority. Proficiency in some sport in which physical size is not important (e.g., swimming or diving) might be much more effective for correcting his lordosis than hours of posture exercises in the corrective gym.

One pernicious psychological cause of undesirable posture among girls is the example set by fashion models. This influence on certain girls is more difficult to combat than almost any other cause of poor posture.

Another type of psychological problem is demonstrated by the emotional reaction of an overly sensitive individual to a conspicuously abnormal posture or body build. As is true of other physical handicaps, it may interfere with the individual's personal and social development unless it can be viewed in its right perspective. The abnormal posture or build may be impossible to correct, in which case the problem is to achieve as much improvement as possible and then to discover ways of standing, sitting, and walking that will minimize the conspicuousness of what cannot be corrected. As in the case of the undersized man, proficiency in some sport can be effective in providing a healthy type of compensation. The instructor's role here is to offer suggestions, to present opportunities, and to be supportive.

In the types of problems described above, the chief principles to follow are (1) to learn as much as possible about the psychology of behavior and adjustment, and (2) when feasible, to work with or at least seek the advice of a psychiatrist or psychologist who is treating the student in question.

An important role of psychology in posture education is that of motivation. No matter how well the teacher or the therapist has selected the exercises, and no matter how conscientiously the student or the patient practices them, they will have little effect in improving the habitual postural patterns unless the student or patient is motivated to *want* to improve them.

And, finally, psychology is used as a technique of treatment by those who like the method of using mental concepts to improve body image, and to change neuromuscular pathways (Sweigard, 1974; Todd, 1949). For success in this method they depend completely upon the cooperation of the individual in mental participation for it is by this means, they believe, that changes in the neuromuscular pathways are effected.

Postural Principles

The following areas appear to be the only ones for which there is objective support:

1. Postural reflex action.
2. Stability of the erect standing position as evidenced by the relationship of the line of gravity to the base of support.
3. The influence of heredity and environment on posture.
4. The relationship between certain postural faults and one type of faulty organic function, namely dysmenorrhea.

Since so much emphasis is placed on posture, it is indeed unfortunate that there is so little objective evidence that our efforts are being made in the right direction. The authors are inclined to be sympathetic toward Miller's (1951) conclusions:

> . . . although orthopedists and physical educators have been working actively for the past fifty years with the problems involved in posture, there is still a seemingly unwarranted lack of agreement among practitioners of both fields. Three basic differences of opinion are implicated in this bewildering lack of unanimity: (1) whether any particular posture is more advantageous physiologically than any other posture; (2) whether prescribed physical activity can actually modify posture; and (3) whether it is possible to agree upon a definition of "good" posture and upon a method of accurately measuring such a concept. Eminent authorities in both physical education and medical circles can be found to support either side of any of these questions.

In view of this lack of evidence and these differences of opinion, what stand shall kinesiologists take in regard to posture education? Shall they ignore it, or shall they formulate tentative principles to guide them in posture education and correction, and shall they adhere to these until they are definitely disproved and indications for other principles have become apparent? The authors believe that, either consciously or unconsciously, the physical educator is bound to be guided by *some* principles of posture, whether they are founded on fact or conjecture. In recognition of the difficulty of devising an accurate measure of habitual posture, the formulation of some guiding principles based on the best knowledge available, incomplete though it may be, would seem to be justifiable, even imperative, if we are to continue to teach "good body mechanics" in our schools and clinics. In full recognition of their limitations and knowing that they may be superseded as new evidence is revealed by further research or by clinical evidence, the following postural principles are suggested:

1. The weight-bearing segments of the body are so aligned in good standing posture* that the line of gravity passes through these segments within certain "normal" limits yet to be defined. Such a definition should either be applicable to all physiques or else indicate to what types of physique it is, or is not, applicable. *It is inappropriate to apply one pattern or formula of good posture to everyone.*

2. Inasmuch as Hellebrandt found that in *every* individual she had observed the average location of the intersection of the line of gravity with the base of support was close to the geometric center of the base, it would seem that the relation of the line of gravity to the base of support is not indicative of body alignment and therefore does not serve as a measure of posture.

3. Good standing posture is a position of extension of the weight-bearing joints. This should be an easy, balanced extension and should not be accompanied by strain or tension (Figures 15–4C and 15–5).

4. From the point of view of energy expenditure, good posture would seem to be a position that requires a minimum expenditure of energy *for the maintenance of good alignment.* Excess energy expenditure indicates hypertonicity or poor neuromuscular coordination, or both. A posture requiring an absolute minimal energy expenditure does not fulfill the requirements of good posture because it is characterized by "hanging on the ligaments"—that is, a dependence upon the ligaments of the weight-bearing joints, rather than upon muscle tonus, for resisting the downward pull of gravity.

5. Good posture, in repose and in activity, permits mechanically efficient function of the joints. In other words, friction in the joints is minimized, tensions of opposing ligaments are balanced, and pressures within the joints are equalized. Hence the skeletal structure is architecturally and mechanically sound and there is a minimum of wear and tear on the joints.

6. Good posture, both static and dynamic, requires normal muscle tonus. This implies adequate development of the antigravity muscles to resist the pull of gravity successfully and to maintain good alignment without excessive effort or tension. It also implies a balance between antagonistic muscle groups. There is no indication, however, that "the stronger the muscles the better the posture."

7. Good posture, both static and dynamic, requires sufficient flexibility in the structures of the weight-bearing joints to permit good alignment without interference or strain. Poor flexibility may be caused by tight ligaments or fasciae, short muscles, or hypertrophied muscles. The flexibility should not be so great, however, that excessive muscular effort is needed to keep the weight-bearing joints in alignment.

8. Good posture requires good coordination. This implies good neuromuscular control and well-developed postural reflexes.

9. Adjustments in posture can be made more readily by individuals who have a good kinesthetic awareness of the postures they assume and of the degree of tension in their muscles.

---

*The term "good standing posture" is used advisedly. Allowances should be made for atypical builds.

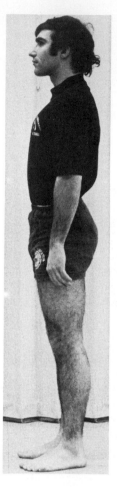

Figure 15-5 Except for a slightly forward head, the subject shows good alignment and extension without strain.

10. Good posture, both static and dynamic, is favorable, or at least not detrimental, to organic function.
11. A relationship exists between habitual posture and personality, and also between habitual posture and extreme emotional states.
12. The characteristics of normal posture change with age. Young children typically have a protruding abdomen and hollow lower back. Loss of muscle strength, inactivity, and balance problems in older persons show up in a wider stance, forward head and rounded upper back, and limited flexibility in the trunk, hips, and knees.
13. An erect body alignment is esthetically pleasing to most people. It would be unusual for anyone to judge a zigzag alignment of forward head, sunken chest and rounded shoulders, protruding abdomen and hollow back, and hyperextended knees as being physically attractive (Clark, 1979).
14. In the last analysis, both the static and dynamic posture of any individual should be judged on the basis of how well it meets the demands made upon it throughout a lifetime.

Postural Adaptation to External Conditions and Special Problems

There are a number of conditions that necessitate postural adjustment if one is to maintain a reasonably balanced standing position. These include standing on either an uphill or a downhill slope, standing on the level but wearing high heels, standing on a moving surface, such as bus, streetcar, subway, or other train, holding a heavy bundle against the front of the body, pregnancy, and standing on one foot. In all of these the body can be relied upon to adjust automatically through the function of proprioceptors and the feedback mechanism. From the point of view of "good body mechanics," however, the nature of the adjustment may not always be desirable. For instance, one can *balance* when standing on an inclined plane by bending at the knees, hips, or spine, but it would be mechanically preferable to maintain vertical segmental alignment, as well as balance. To achieve this position one would need to stand so that the center of gravity of each weight-bearing segment was centered above the base of support. This centering can be achieved only by making the adjustment at the ankles and feet. The same is true for the person wearing high heels and for the pregnant woman, although some women lack the necessary abdominal strength for this action. It is highly desirable for them to strengthen these muscles in order to resist the tendency to lean back from the waist, an adjustment that is almost sure to cause trouble in the lower back. The person carrying a heavy bundle against the front of the body may find that adjustment at the ankles is not enough, especially if the load is excessively heavy. In this case some adjustment at the knees and hips will help, but every effort should be made not to lean back at the waist because of the danger of lower back strain.

When standing in a moving bus, streetcar, or train, there are three adjustments one should be prepared to make: adjustment to acceleration, deceleration, and side-to-side sway. The same principle applies to all three—namely, establishing a comfortably wide stance in the direction of motion (forward-backward for acceleration and deceleration, and sideward for a steady speed, especially if there is a pronounced sway). During sudden acceleration, especially, the person tends to be thrown toward the back of the vehicle, in keeping with Newton's first Law of Motion. The foot toward the rear, therefore, should be well braced, and more weight should be borne by the forward foot in anticipation of the jerk. The reverse is true during deceleration and stopping. In both acceleration and deceleration the body will be less likely to be thrown off balance if the knees are slightly flexed, since this shortens the lever upon which the vehicle's motion acts.

In a crowded vehicle that makes frequent stops it may not be possible to keep adapting the stance, and one may have to rely on a hand grasp to supplement the foot adjustment. A slightly oblique stance, favoring the forward-backward direction, serves as an acceptable compromise.

The adjustment to standing on one foot is a delicate one but is usually managed automatically by the muscle, joint, and labyrinthine proprioceptors, and by the reflex response. The adjustment consists of a shift in the body weight to the single supporting limb and in the support of the pelvis on the side of the free limb. The latter adjustment requires additional effort by the quadratus lumborum and the abductors (gluteus medius and minimus, tensor fasciae latae, and oblique abdominal muscles on the support side). The iliopsoas, which is continuously active during all standing, undoubtedly increases its activity in steadying the lumbar spine (Basmajian, 1979). In addition, there is probably a continuous interplay of the deep muscles of the lumbar spine and possibly of many of the lower extremity muscles. The alternating action of the foot and ankle muscles, especially the tarsal pronators and supinators, is quite pronounced in their effort to keep the center of gravity over the narrow base of support. This problem can be helped somewhat by turning the toes slightly outward (i.e., rotating the thigh slightly outward) before the one-legged stance is assumed. For a more precise muscular analysis of the adjustments made in standing on one foot, an electromyographic investigation is needed.

Laboratory Experiences

1. To demonstrate the alignment of the body segments take from five to seven large wooden blocks, each having a vertical line painted in the center of one side. A layer of thick felt should be glued to the top and bottom of each block and a small hook screwed into each of two opposite sides.
   a. Arrange the blocks in a straight column with the painted lines in front. Connect the hooks on the sides with elastic bands. The elastic "ligaments" will be under equal tension and the felt "cartilages" under equal pressure when the column is in perfect alignment.
   b. Now insert wedges between the blocks in such a way that every other block tips to the left and the alternate blocks tip to the right. The elastic "ligaments" will now be under unequal tension and the felt "cartilages" under unequal pressure. The zigzag alignment of the painted lines illustrates graphically the poor alignment of the segments.

2. To demonstrate good and poor alignment of a single weight-bearing joint, such as the knee, two blocks arranged like those described above may be used in a similar manner.

3. Take two side-view photographs of a subject standing on a reaction board. The first photograph should represent the subject's "best" posture and the second a zig-zag fatigue slump. Have another person read the scale readings at the same time the photographs are taken. Compute the distance of the line of gravity from the scale, using the method described on page 396. The length measurements (total length of board and distance d) are made directly on the photograph instead of on the board itself. Draw the vertical line of gravity from the point at which the line of gravity intersects the board to a point above the head. Compare the postures and the anteroposterior positions of the line of gravity in the two photographs.

4. Take anteroposterior "line of gravity" photographs of several subjects representing various postures. Determine the location of the line of gravity for each photograph using the method described in Number 3. After drawing the line of gravity on each photograph, observe them carefully and note the relation of the line to the head, shoulders, upper trunk, lower trunk, pelvis, knees, and ankles.

5. Take ten anteroposterior "line of gravity" photographs of one subject within a period of 1 week. Compare these.

6. Take anteroposterior "line of gravity" photographs of several subjects representing different physique types. Can you make any generalizations about the relation of physique to posture?

7. Do an original posture study using a small number of subjects.

References

Basmajian, J. V. 1979. *Muscles alive,* 4th ed. Baltimore: Williams & Wilkins.

Brunnstrom, S. 1972. *Clinical kinesiology,* 3d ed. Philadelphia: F. A. Davis.

Clark, H. H. 1979. Posture. *Phys. Fitness Res. Dig.* Series 9, No. 1. Washington, D.C.: President's Council on Physical Fitness and Sports.

Deaver, G. G. 1933. Posture and its relation to mental and physical health. *Res. Q.* 4:221–28.

Evans, F. G., ed. 1961. *Biomechanical studies of the musculo-skeletal system.* Springfield, Ill. Charles C Thomas.

Flint, M., and Diehl, B. 1961. Influence of abdominal strength, back-extensor strength, and trunk strength balance upon antero-posterior alignment of elementary school girls. *Res. Q.* 32:490–98.

Fox, M. G. 1951. The relationship of abdominal strength to selected posture faults. *Res. Q.* 22:141–44.

Frost, L. H. 1938. Individual structural differences in the orthopedic examination. *J. Health Phys. Educ.* 9:90–3, 122.

Goldthwait, J. E., Brown, L. T., Swaim, L. T., and Kuhns, J. G. 1952. *Essentials of body mechanics in health and disease,* 5th ed. Philadelphia: J. B. Lippincott.

Haller, J. S., and Gurewitsch, A. D. 1950. An approach to dynamic posture based on primitive motion patterns. *Arch. Phys. Med.* 31:632–40.

Hawley, G. 1949. *Kinesiology of corrective exercise,* 2d ed. Philadelphia: Lea & Febiger.

Hellebrandt, F. A. 1940. Physiology and the physical educator. *Res. Q.* 11:12–29.

Hellebrandt, F. A. 1944. Postural adjustments in convalescence and rehabilitation. *Fed. Proc.* 3:243–46.

Hellebrandt, F. A., and Franseen, E. B. 1943. Physiological study of the vertical stance of man. *Physiol. Rev.* 23:220–55.

Hellebrandt, F. A., Riddle, K. S., and Fries, E. C. 1942. Influence of postural sway on stance photography. *Physiother. Rev.* 22:88.

Hoffman, E. 1942. *Certain physical and psychological characteristics as related to the incidence of severe dysmenorrhea.* Unpublished M.S. thesis, Wellesley College.

Joseph J. 1960. *Man's posture: Electromyographic studies.* Springfield, Ill.: Charles C Thomas.

Karpovich, P. V., and Sinning, W. E. 1971. *Physiology of muscular activity,* 7th ed. Philadelphia: W. B. Saunders.

Kelly, E. D. 1965. *Adapted and corrective physical education,* 4th ed. New York: Ronald Press.

Kendall, H. O., and Kendall, F. P. 1968. Developing and maintaining good posture. *J. Am. Phys. Ther. Assoc.* 48:319–36.

Klausen, K., Jeppesen, K., and Mogensen, A. 1978. Form and function of the erect spine in young girls. In *Biomechanics VI-B,* ed. E. Asmussen and K. Jorgensen. Baltimore: University Park Press.

McCormick, H. G. 1942. *The metabolic cost of maintaining a standing position, with special reference to body alignment.* New York: King's Crown Press.

Mensendieck, B. 1937. *Mensendieck system of functional exercises.* Portland, Me.: Southworth-Anthoensen Press.

Miller, K. D. 1951. A physical educator looks at posture. *J. Sch. Health* 21:89–94.

Morton, D. J. 1952. *Human locomotion and body form.* Baltimore: Williams & Wilkins.

Rathbone, J. L., and Hunt, V. V. 1965. *Corrective physical education,* 7th ed. Philadelphia: W. B. Saunders.

Sheldon, W. H., Stevens, S. S., and Tucker, W. B. 1940. *The varieties of human physique.* New York: Harper.

Steindler, A. 1973. *Kinesiology of the human body.* Springfield, Ill.: Charles C Thomas.

Sweigard, L. E. 1974. *Human movement potential; its ideokinetic facilitation.* New York: Dodd, Mead.

Todd, M. E. 1949. *The thinking body.* Boston: Charles T. Branford.

Wells, K. F. 1958. What we don't know about posture. *J. Health Phys. Educ. Rec.* 29:31–2.

Moving One's Body on the Ground or Other Resistant Surfaces

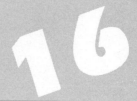

Objectives

At the conclusion of this chapter, the student should be able to:

1. Identify and classify motor skills belonging in the categories that fall under the heading of moving one's body on the ground or other resistant surface.

2. Describe the anatomical and mechanical nature of motor skills representative of the major types of locomotor patterns.

3. Name and state anatomical and mechanical principles that apply to the locomotor patterns of walking, running, and jumping.

4. Evaluate performance of motor skills representative of the major locomotor patterns in terms of application of the related kinesiological principles.

Both nonmanipulative movements performed on a stationary or limited base and all forms of locomotion performed on the ground constitute the category of motor skills of moving one's body on the ground or on other resistant surfaces.

Movements of the Body on a Stationary or Limited Base

This group embraces the majority of calisthenic exercises, such as those for warming-up purposes and for improving muscle tonus, flexibility, agility, and postural alignment. These are segmental movements rather than movements of the body as a whole. The only movement that involves the body as a whole and is performed on a stationary base on the ground is the rotation of the body about its own vertical axis, as when pirouetting on the toes or on ice skates. Rotation about successive points of contact with the ground, such as in a single cartwheel or a single forward roll, might be included, depending upon one's interpretation of "limited base." When performed in a series these activities constitute forms of locomotion.

The following are suggested as the major principles applying to nonmanipulative movements of the body when it is supported by the ground on a stationary or limited base. They are in addition to the principles relating to stability, discussed in Chapter 13.

PRINCIPLE I Law of Inertia: An object that is at rest will remain so unless acted upon by a force. When the "object" is the human body itself, or a segment of it, the force giving impetus to it is usually internal—i.e., muscular contraction. Another force that must not be overlooked is the force of gravity, which is always operative, except in outer space. In many instances a movement is initiated by muscular action and then carried on by gravitational force because of the position in which the segment has been placed. If this is the desired direction of the movement, the muscles that normally perform the opposite movement contract eccentrically in order to control the speed of the segment. These same opposing muscles will check the movement if it is not desired. A common example of this controlling and checking action is seen in slow deep knee bending as the body assumes a squatting position. The movement is started by the momentary contraction of the hip, knee, and ankle flexors and is then carried on by the lengthening contraction of the extensor muscles. If one wishes to stop the movement before a full squat is reached, the same muscles must contract statically with just the right amount of force to balance the gravitational force acting on the lower extremity levers.

PRINCIPLE II Law of Action and Reaction: To every action there is an equal and opposite reaction. In all movements performed in the standing position, the counterpressure of the ground against the feet is essential to the accurate performance of a movement of one or more parts of the body. The performer is usually unaware of this in easy movements, but if attempting vigorous movements standing on soft sand the difference would be noticeable. The principle holds true no matter what part of the body is in contact with the supporting surface.

PRINCIPLE III A long lever has greater velocity at the end than does a short lever moving at the same angular velocity. Hence, in a vigorous arm swing from the shoulder, the hand will have greater velocity if the elbow is kept fully extended. Likewise, in a vigorous movement of the lower extremity, such as a kick, the foot will have greater velocity if the knee is fully extended.

PRINCIPLE IV Centrifugal force is developed in circular movements of bodily segments, as in vigorous arm circling. This should be recognized as a potential source of injury to the shoulder joint, since the centrifugal force creates a dislocating tendency.

PRINCIPLE V The momentum of any part of a supported body can be transferred to the rest of the body. For instance, if one sits on the end of a table with the legs hanging down, then lies down on the back and raises the legs overhead until the feet almost touch the table behind the head, and then vigorously swings both limbs forward-downward, suddenly checking their motion when they touch the table, the trunk will rise to a vertical position. Or, if one stands with one arm extended forward and then flings it horizontally sideward-backward as far as possible, the whole body will tend to follow the arm in horizontal rotation. It is through the application of this same principle that the ballet dancer and the figure skater are able to spin in place. In both cases friction is minimized by the footwear worn and by the smoothness of the supporting surface.

PRINCIPLE VI   Rotational movement of the body as a whole may be decelerated by lengthening the radius, and accelerated by shortening the radius while the spin is in progress. When spinning on the toes (or skates), the dancer and the skater lengthen the radius by extending the arms sideward at shoulder level, and shorten it by bending the arms in close to the body. The spectacular increase in the speed of the spin when the arms are bent gives the impression that an additional force has acted upon the body, whereas the acceleration is merely the result of decreasing the moment of inertia about the vertical axis. The extended arms cause the moment of inertia of the spinning body to increase. Because the angular momentum is conserved the angular velocity decreases and the spinning body slows down.

Locomotion

Locomotion is the act or power of moving from place to place by means of one's own mechanisms or power. Locomotion in humans is the result of the action of the body levers propelling the body. Ordinarily the propulsion is provided by the lower extremities, but it is occasionally provided by all four extremities, as in creeping, or by the upper extremities alone, as in walking on the hands or in suspension. It may involve the use of wheels, blades, skis, or other equipment attached to the feet, or it may involve a vehicle such as a bicycle or wheelchair, or a small craft such as a boat, canoe, or surfboard propelled by means of the arms or legs, with or without the use of a propelling implement such as oars, paddles, or poles. Locomotion may be on the ground or in the water but, at the present writing, not in the air without support. There must be a resistance against which the body part can push if locomotion is to occur. Aside from locomotor activities that are used mostly for utilitarian purposes, there are many skills in which humans indulge for sport and pleasure. For the purpose of systematizing the study of locomotor skills, the following classification is suggested.

On foot
Walking
Running
Climbing (inclined plane, stairs, ladder)
Descending (inclined plane, stairs, ladder)
Jumping, leaping, hurdling
Skipping, hopping, sliding, sidestepping
Progressive dance steps, e.g., polka, mazurka
Snowshoeing
Ski touring (cross-country skiing)
Walking on stilts

On wheels and blades
Bicycling
Roller skating
Ice skating
Propelling self in wheelchair

On hands
Walking on hands
Hand traveling suspended from boom, horizontal ladder, traveling rings

On hands and knees or hands and feet
Creeping
Crutch walking
Stunts (dog running, rabbit hopping)

Rotatory locomotion
Cartwheels
Handsprings
Forward, backward, and sideward rolls

Walking

To the casual observer, the movements involved in walking appear to be relatively simple, yet kinesiological analysis shows them to be exceedingly complex. The dovetailing of muscular action and the synchronization of joint movements beautifully illustrate the teamwork present in all bodily movements. Not even the most complex piece of machinery designed by the most skillful engineers exceeds the movements of the human machine in perfection of detail or in potential smoothness of function.

Research on the gait, such as that conducted at the University of California as part of the Prosthetic Devices Research Project (1953) and that of Dr. Patricia Murray (Murray et al., 1964, 1966, 1967, 1970), Dr. J. V. Basmajian (1979), and many, many others, has served to emphasize the complexity of human locomotion. In the fourth edition of his book, *Muscles Alive,* Basmajian (1979) has written an excellent chapter on this subject and has reported on numerous electromyographic studies.

Description   Walking is accomplished by the alternating action of the two lower extremities (Figure 16–1). It is an example of translatory motion of the body as a whole brought about by means of the angular motion of some of its parts. It is also an example of a periodic or pendulum-like movement in which the moving segment (in this case, the lower extremity) may be said to start at zero, pass through its arc of motion, and fall to zero again at the end of each stroke. In walking, each lower extremity undergoes two phases, the swing or recovery phase and the support phase. The support phase is further divided into a restraining phase (from the moment the foot touches the ground until it is directly under the center of the body) and the propulsion phase (from the moment when the foot is under the center of gravity until it leaves the ground). The beginning of the restraining phase of one leg overlaps the end of the propulsive phase of the other leg. Thus it constitutes a brief phase of double support when both feet are on the ground. This double support phase is characteristic of the walk and serves to

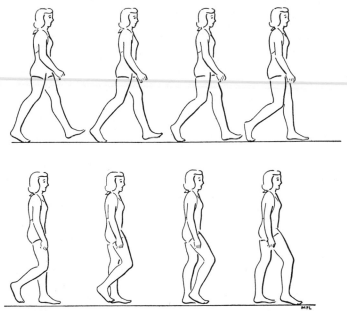

Figure 16–1   Walking is an example of linear motion of the body as a whole resulting from the angular motion of some of its parts.

differentiate it from the run. In the swing phase of the walk, the action of the lower extremity may be likened to that of the pendulum of a clock and, in the support phase, to that of the inverted pendulum of a metronome.

Gravity and momentum are the chief sources of motion for the swing phase; hence, this phase represents a ballistic type of movement (p. 49), particularly when the individual is walking at a natural pace. The source of motion for the support phase is, for the first half, the momentum of the forward-moving trunk (provided by the propulsive action of the other leg) and, for the second half, the contraction of the extensor muscles of the supporting leg. Whether the support phase can also be classed as ballistic movement is open to question. Even the swing phase varies in its ballistic quality according to the speed of the gait and the skill, flexibility, and build of the walker. A tense individual will tend to substitute muscular action for the pendulum swing of the lower extremity, and an individual with tight hamstrings will have to exert additional muscular force to overcome the restraining action of the short hamstrings. An individual who has knock-knees or fat thighs will also have difficulty in achieving a natural, pendulum swing because of friction and interference between the two limbs. In order to avoid this interference the walker would need to increase the lateral distance between the limbs and thus introduce an undesirable lateral component of motion.

Anatomical Analysis

The six major components of walking have been defined as (1) pelvic rotation, (2) pelvic tilt, (3) knee flexion, (4) hip flexion, (5) knee and ankle interaction, and (6) lateral pelvic displacement. Each of these components is essential for efficient walking, and the loss of any one will cause an increase in the energy cost.

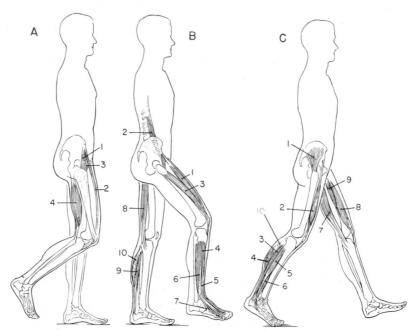

Figure 16–2   The muscles of the lower extremity used in walking. *Key: A: 1*, Tensor fasciae latae; *2*, sartorius; *3*, pectineus; *4*, biceps femoris. *B: 1*, Rectus femoris; *2*, iliopsoas; *3*, vastus lateralis (medius and intermedius are not shown); *4*, tibialis anterior; *5*, extensor hallucis longus; *6*, extensor digitorum longus; *7*, peroneus tertius; *8*, semitendinosus and semimembranosus; *9*, soleus; *10*, gastrocnemius. *C: 1*, Gluteus medius; *2*, rectus femoris; *3*, soleus; *4*, tibialis posterior (underneath); *5*, peroneus longus; *6*, peroneus brevis; *7*, semimembranosus and semitendinosus; *8*, vastus medialis and intermedius (lateralis not shown); *9*, adductor longus; *10*, gastrocnemius.

The action taking place in the joints of the lower extremity consists essentially of flexion and extension. But, in much the same way that the shoulder girdle cooperates with the arm movements of the upper extremity, the pelvic girdle cooperates in movements of the lower extremities. The pelvis has the double task of transmitting the weight of the body alternately first over one limb, then over the other, and of putting each acetabulum in a favorable position for the action of the corresponding femur. The adaptations of the pelvic position are made in the joints of the thoracic and lumbar spine as well as in the hip joints. Thus, as first one foot and then the other is put forward, the flexion and extension movements of the thigh are accompanied by slight rotatory movements and ab- and adduction at the hips, and by slight lateral flexion and rotation of the spine (Figures 16–2 and 16–3).

The muscular analysis presented in the original edition of this text was based on Wells' own investigations (using palpation and inspection), supplemented by information from the literature available prior to 1950. It was later revised to incorporate the findings of two electromyographic investigations, the Prosthetic Devices Research Project at the University of California in Berkeley (1953), and a study by Sheffield et al. (1956). Since then a number of revisions have been made to incorporate findings

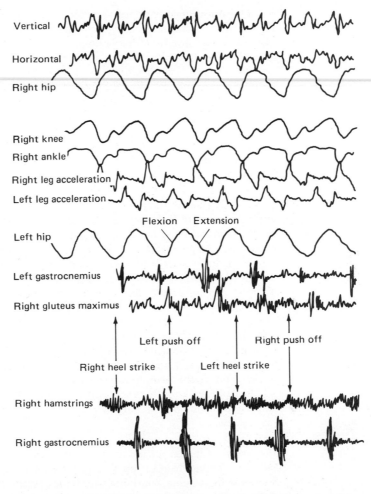

Figure 16–3 Simultaneous tracings recorded during normal walking. From top: vertical and horizontal accelerograms; electrogoniograms of right hip, knee, and ankle; angular accelerograms of right and left legs; electrogoniogram of left hip; electromyograms of left gastrocnemius, right gluteus maximus, right hamstrings, and right gastrocnemius. (After Liberson, W. T.: In *Biomechanics III,* ed. S. Cerquiglini et al. Baltimore: University Park Press, 1973.)

from subsequent EMG investigations. The last word on locomotion has not yet been written, so it behooves all kinesiologists to keep abreast of the research being done in this area.

SWING PHASE   The swing phase begins with toe-off and ends with heel strike.

Spine and Pelvis

1. *Movements:* Rotation of the pelvis toward the support leg and of the spine in the opposite direction; slight lateral rotation of the pelvis toward the unsupported

leg. The simultaneous opposite actions help to prevent excessive motion of the trunk. Pelvic rotation also lengthens the step and decreases the lateral deviation of the center of gravity of the body.

2. *Muscles:* Semispinalis, rotatores, multifidus, and external oblique abdominal muscle on side toward which the pelvis rotates. Erector spinae and internal oblique abdominal muscle on opposite side. (*Note:* Rotation of the pelvis to the right constitutes rotation of the spine to the left. See p. 168.) The psoas and quadratus lumborum help to support the pelvis on the side of the swinging limb.

Hip

1. *Movements:* Flexion; outward rotation (because of pelvic rotation); adduction at beginning and abduction at end of phase, especially if long stride is taken (also because of pelvic rotation, as well as stride length).
2. *Muscles:* The sartorius, tensor fasciae latae, pectineus, *iliopsoas*, rectus femoris, and short head of the biceps femoris contract during the early part of the swing phase, each in its own particular pattern—the sartorius and short head of the biceps, for instance, chiefly at toe-off and the tensor at both toe-off and midswing.

    In the latter part of the swing phase there is no appreciable action of the hip flexors in normal walking on level ground. This is consistent with the ballistic nature of the movement. The hamstrings contract with moderate intensity during the knee extension part of the swing and the gluteus maximus and medius contract slightly at the very end of the swing. The adductors longus and magnus, and presumably brevis, contract slightly after the swinging limb has passed the halfway mark. Just what the function of the adductor magnus is, is not clear. It may help to steady and guide the forward-swinging limb. In any event its action is extremely slight, even in rapid walking.

    In rapid walking there is a noticeable increase in the activity of the sartorius and the rectus femoris and also a slight increase in that of the tensor fasciae latae.

Knee

1. *Movements:* Flexion during the first half; extension during the second half.
2. *Muscles:* As was true in hip flexion (and for the same reason), so also in knee flexion is there remarkably little muscular action in the swing phase of normal walking. The quadriceps extensors contract slightly at the end of this phase. The action of the sartorius, a two-joint muscle, has already been mentioned in connection with the hip. The action of these muscles, as well as that of the medial hamstrings, increases in rapid walking. In an easy gait the movement appears to be initiated by gravitational force and continued by momentum. This force is sufficient to extend the leg at the knee, except perhaps at the very end of the movement. In more vigorous walking the quadriceps femoris provides the force for leg extension.

Ankle and Foot

1. *Movements:* Dorsiflexion; prevention of plantar flexion.
2. *Muscles:* The tibialis anterior, extensor digitorum longus, extensor hallucis longus, and probably the peroneus tertius contract with slight to moderate intensity at the beginning of the swinging phase and taper off during the middle portion of this phase. Basmajian and coworkers (1979) found that the tibialis anterior was actually completely quiescent at midswing. They observed that the foot everted

in the early phase and maintained this eversion during the middle part. This seemed to them to serve the important purpose of providing sufficient clearance between the foot and the ground.

Toward the end of the swing phase this group of muscles contracts again with considerable force in preparation for heel strike. The plantar flexors are completely relaxed throughout the entire swing phase.

SUPPORT PHASE The support phase begins with heel strike and ends with toe-off. The portion between heel strike of the forward foot and toe-off of the other—i.e., the rear foot—constitutes a period of double support that is characteristic of walking but does not occur in running.

Spine and Pelvis

Rotation of pelvis toward same side and spine to opposite side; lateral tilt away from support leg.

Hip

1. *Movements:* Extension; reduction of outward rotation, followed by slight inward rotation; prevention of adduction of thigh and dropping of pelvis to opposite side.
2. *Muscles:* During the first part of the support phase all three gluteal muscles contract with moderate intensity; then the contractions of maximus and medius taper off during the middle part. There is disagreement in the literature as to whether the gluteus maximus participates at all in normal walking but, until the evidence is conclusive, this text is inclined to accept the views of the EMG researchers who found evidence of gluteus maximus activity in the early part of the support phase (Basmajian, 1979). The gluteus minimus continues to contract moderately during the middle portion. The only muscles of the hip that contract appreciably during the last part of the support phase are the adductors magnus, longus, and gracilis, and possibly brevis.

    In rapid walking the gluteus maximus and minimus contract with appreciable intensity during the first part of the support phase, and the adductor longus during the last part. The hamstrings apparently have but a small part in the supporting phase of normal walking. Only the long head of the biceps contracts at all, and it contracts only slightly at the very beginning of this phase. In rapid walking both the long head of the biceps and the semitendinosus contract with moderate intensity during the first half of the support phase.

Knee

1. *Movements:* Slight flexion at moment of contact continuing into midstance; followed by extension until heel-off when flexion for swing phase begins. The flexion during stance flattens the vertical path of the center of gravity of the body, thus increasing the efficiency of the gait.
2. *Muscles:* The quadriceps extensors contract moderately in the early part of the support phase, then gradually relax. They appear to control the slight flexion that occurs in the knee at the moment of heel strike. The vastus intermedius continues to contract throughout the first half of this phase. As the leg reaches the vertical position, the knee apparently locks and makes contraction of the extensors unnecessary. The tension of the stretched hamstrings at the end of the swing phase, especially when a long stride has been taken, may well be the factor that

initiates the slight flexion at heel strike. The hamstrings again show activity at the end of the support phase. In rapid walking all of these muscles contract more strongly and for a longer duration. There is an abrupt increase in their action in the second half of the support phase, which would seem to indicate that the extension of the leg at the knee is much more forceful in rapid walking than in normal walking.

Ankle and Foot

1. *Movements:* Slight plantar flexion, followed by slight dorsiflexion; prevention of further dorsiflexion, which the body weight tends to cause. Plantar flexion of ankle and hyperextension of metatarsophalangeal joints at end of propulsive phase, especially in vigorous walking.

2. *Muscles:* EMG studies reviewed by Basmajian (1979) show that there is considerable action of the tibialis anterior in the early part of the supporting phase, especially at heel strike. It seems likely that this is related to the controlled lowering of the foot by eccentric contraction in order to prevent the foot from slapping down too hard. Contrary to earlier opinions, it does not continue to show activity during the major weight-bearing period, but it becomes active again at toe-off. The extensor digitorum longus and hallucis longus follow a similar pattern. They reach their peak of contraction almost at the moment of transition between the swing and support phases; they relax early in the support phase, commencing to contract slightly at the end of this phase.

Carlin (1963) emphasized the importance of recognizing the influence of the weight-bearing position on the action of the dorsiflexors of the ankle joint. In the stance or support phase of walking the leverage of the leg is reversed because the foot is fixed on the ground. Instead of acting on the foot, the dorsiflexors act on the tibia to pull the upper end forward over the foot. This is an important point and worthy of attention. It is also suggested here, however, that the relative force that these muscles have to exert is probably strongly influenced by individual variations in walking patterns. The tibialis anterior, extensor digitorum longus, and extensor hallucis longus doubtless have to exert more force in a person who habitually walks with a backward list than in a person who tends to keep the weight over the forward foot. It would also seem that the length of stride might be a factor, as it is related to the slant of the forward leg at the moment of contact with the ground, that is, at heel strike.

The tibialis posterior is most active during the middle part of the support phase, one of its functions, according to Basmajian, being to prevent eversion (pronation) of the foot. He points out that the peroneus longus and tibialis posterior apparently cooperate in stabilizing the leg and foot in weightbearing. The gastrocnemius and soleus act to decelerate the lower leg and stabilize the knee at midstance (Winter and Kuryliak, 1978). There is a sharp increase in gastrocnemius and soleus activity beginning after the heel lifts and continuing until the opposite heel contacts the ground. Extension of the knee in the stance phase is always accompanied by calf muscle activity. In *rapid* walking, however, their activity is much more pronounced. The peroneus longus follows a similar pattern but does not seem to contract quite so strongly as the others, except in rapid walking. The peroneus brevis does not start to contract until about the middle of the support phase, but it contracts more strongly than the longus. In rapid walking it starts earlier and contracts with intensity soon after the halfway point has been reached.

The flexor digitorum longus contracts slightly during the middle portion of the support phase and increases abruptly to moderate contraction in the last portion. In rapid walking the contraction becomes strong. The flexor hallucis longus follows the same pattern, except that it does not start to contract until the middle of the phase.

The toe muscles, flexor hallucis longus, flexor digitorum longus, and the short, intrinsic flexors of the toes contract in response to the pressure of the ground against the toes. In the propulsive phase, especially in vigorous walking, this contraction is intensified. In all parts of the support phase the contraction of the toe flexors is greater in barefoot walking than when shoes are worn. This is especially noticeable when walking on turf or sand.

ACTION OF UPPER EXTREMITIES IN WALKING   Unless restrained, the arms tend to swing in opposition to the legs, the left arm swinging forward as the right leg swings forward and vice versa. This is usually accomplished without obvious muscular action and serves to balance the rotation of the pelvis. It is a reflex action. When the arm swing is prevented, the upper trunk tends to rotate in the same direction as the pelvis, causing a tense, awkward gait.

Murray and her coworkers (1967), using the technique of interrupted light photography, investigated the action of the upper extremities in walking. They noted "patterns of sagittal rotation of the shoulder and elbow," or flexion and extension of both joints. They found that, although the amplitudes of the arm swing pattern varied considerably from one subject to another, each individual had a similar pattern in all trials, even at higher speeds. Furthermore, they noted that the increased amplitude accompanying the faster speeds was due mainly to increased shoulder (hyper-) extension in the backward swing and increased elbow flexion in the forward swing. Maximum flexion of both the shoulder and elbow joints occurred at the moment of heel strike of the opposite foot and maximum extension at the moment of heel strike of the foot on the same side.

In an investigation of the muscular action of the arms, Hogue (1969) found that although they appear to swing without muscular effort in walking at a normal pace on level ground, actually their pendular action was caused by a combination of muscular activity and gravity. The mid- and posterior deltoid and the teres major were the muscles that he found to be most concerned, the latter two being active mainly during the backward swing. The posterior deltoid also contracted toward the end of the forward swing, leading one to suspect that it was serving as a brake to check the movement. The middle deltoid was found to be active during both flexion and extension of the arm at the shoulder joint. As this muscle is primarily an abductor, it seems that its function might be to keep the arms from brushing the sides of the body as they swing past it.

INDIVIDUAL VARIATIONS IN THE GAIT   Although the basic anatomical analysis of the gait is valid for all physically normal persons, individual characteristics are present to such a degree that persons are often recognized by their gaits. These variations may be either structural or functional in origin. The structural differences include unusual body proportions as well as differences in the limbs themselves, such as knock-knees and bowlegs. Extreme variations in the angle between the neck and the shaft of the femur and in the obliquity of the femoral shaft are also responsible for atypical gaits.

Variations in the forward-backward distribution of weight and in the length of stride have already been mentioned. Other variations in movement patterns which are not structural in origin are often related to characteristics of the personality. This fact was brought home forcefully to Wells when she attempted to help college students whose gaits were awkward. Almost invariably the students who walked the most awkwardly were those who were extremely shy or lacking in self-confidence. A study investigating the possible relationship between the two might be rewarding.

WALKING UP AND DOWN STAIRS AND RAMPS   In walking up stairs or up a ramp the reactive force resulting from the push of the legs should be directed through the body's center of gravity and in line with the forward-upward slope of the stairs or ramp. The most strain-free way of doing this is to incline the body forward in a straight line from the rear foot. The act of descending stairs or a ramp involves resisting the force of gravity on the body safely. The eccentric contraction of the muscles of the lower extremity enables the body to be lowered at a controlled rate and maintaining the line of gravity toward the back of the base of support prevents forward falls (Figure 16–4). In walking up stairs or up a ramp the swing phase is characterized by an exaggerated knee lift and dorsiflexion of the ankle. According to Joseph and Watson, the hamstrings and tibialis anterior are the chief muscles involved (Basmajian, 1979). In the support phase, when the action is chiefly extension of the knee and hip, with the ankle being either slightly plantar flexed or else maintained in the midposition on the ball of the foot, they found the chief muscular action to come from the gluteus maximus, hamstrings, quadriceps femoris, and soleus, with the gluteus medius helping to maintain stability at the hip joint.

The swing phase of walking down stairs starts with a slight lifting of the rear foot to clear the step. This involves slight knee flexion and dorsiflexion of the ankle. It is followed by slight hip flexion, then hip and knee extension and plantar flexion of the ankle as the foot reaches for the step below the one the supporting foot is on.

The support phase starts with the ankle in plantar flexion and the knee in extension. As the foot assumes the body weight, the ankle, knee, and hip are approximately in their neutral positions with the knee very slightly flexed. As the other foot swings forward, the supporting leg engages in slight hip flexion, increasing knee flexion, and dorsiflexion of the ankle. In the brief period of double support, the knee and ankle flexion reach their maximum. The main muscular action of the supporting limb, according to Joseph and Watson, consists of eccentric contraction of the hamstrings, quadriceps femoris, and soleus, with the gluteus medius contributing to hip stability as it does in ascending (Basmajian, 1979).

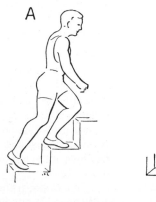
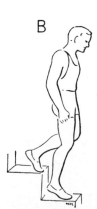

Figure 16–4   Going up and down stairs.

NEUROMUSCULAR CONSIDERATIONS   Walking is a reflex action; no conscious control is necessary. On the contrary, if attention is focused on any part of the gait, tension is likely to develop and the natural rhythm and coordination are disturbed. Reflexes control not only the movements of the limbs but also the extension of both the supporting limb and the trunk in resisting the downward pull of gravity. This extension serves to give stability to the body in the support phases of locomotion, a stability that provides for effective muscular action in producing the necessary movements. Thus, in walking, as in all the motions of the body, smooth, coordinated movement requires properly functioning reflexes, normal flexibility of the joints, and optimum stability of the body as a whole in the weight-bearing phases of the act.

Anatomical Principles Applied to Walking

PRINCIPLE I   Good alignment of the lower extremities reduces friction in the joints and decreases the likelihood of strain and injury.

PRINCIPLE II   Normal flexibility of the joints (i.e., sufficiently long and flexible muscles, ligaments, and fasciae) reduces internal resistance, and hence reduces the amount of force required for walking.

PRINCIPLE III   Speed of walking is increased by increasing both the length of the stride and the tempo of the gait.

PRINCIPLE IV   The longer the stride, the greater the up and down movements of the body, unless the knee is kept slightly flexed during the middle portion of the supporting phase.

PRINCIPLE V   Unnecessary lateral movements result in an ungainly and uneconomical gait.
    a. Failure to keep the gluteus medius contracted when the weight is on the foot results in an exaggerated hip sway caused by the dropping of one side of the pelvis.
    b. Excessive trunk rotation may be caused by an exaggerated arm swing or by restriction of the arm swing. Normally the arm swing exactly counterbalances the hip swing (Murray et al., 1967).
    c. Straight, sagittal plane action of the leg is ensured by keeping the knee and foot pointing straight forward in all phases of the gait.
    d. The rotation of the pelvis should be just enough to enable the leg to move straight forward. Too little or too much rotation tends to cause a weaving gait.
    e. Minimal lateral motions occur when the feet are placed in such a way that their inner borders fall approximately along a single straight line.

PRINCIPLE VI   The tendon action of the two-joint muscles of the lower extremity contributes to economy of muscular action in walking (see page 48).

PRINCIPLE VII   Properly functioning reflexes contribute to a well-coordinated gait.

PRINCIPLE VIII   The stability of the weight-bearing limb and the balance of the trunk over this limb are important factors in the smoothness of the gait.

Mechanical Analysis

Walking is characterized by the translation of the body's center of gravity forward as a result of the alternating pattern of the lower extremity joint movements during the stance and swing phases. The forces that control walking are the external forces of weight, normal reaction, friction, air resistance, and internal muscular forces. The direction and interaction of these forces determine the nature of the gait.

The inertia of the stationary body is overcome by the horizontal component of the propulsive force. Since periodic movement is characterized by an alternating increase and decrease of speed, the inertia must be overcome at every step, and the greater the weight of the body, the greater is the inertia to be overcome. As the center of gravity moves forward, it momentarily passes beyond the anterior margin of the base of support and a temporary loss of balance results. At this point the downward pull of gravity threatens a complete loss of equilibrium. A timely recovery of balance is effected, however, as the foot is placed on the ground. Thus, a new base of support is established and a new support phase is begun. The downward force of the body's weight is counteracted by the vertical reactive force through the feet. If the vertical force exceeds that needed to balance the gravitational force at the time of push-off, an exaggerated lift to the body results, causing a gait characterized by a bounce or unusual spring.

When forward motion has been imparted to the trunk by means of the ground reaction to the backward thrust of the leg and foot, it tends to continue unless restrained by another force. Once the center of gravity passes beyond the base of support, it is essential to restrain the action of the trunk until a new base of support is established. Hence, as the foot is brought to the ground in front of the body at the close of its recovery phase, a restraining phase is constituted. This diminishes as the leg approaches midstance. During the period that the foot is in front of the center of gravity, there is a forward component of force in the thrust of the foot against the ground. This results in a *backward* reactive force of the ground against the foot, which is transmitted to the leg and thence to the trunk.

The degree to which the pressure of the foot actually imparts motion to the body in the propulsive phase and restrains it in the restraining phase is in direct proportion to the counterpressure of normal reactive force of the supporting surface. If the surface lacks solidity, as in the case of mud, soft snow, and sand, it offers too little resistance to give the needed counterpressure. The pressure of the foot results in slipping or sinking, and more pressure must be applied in order to achieve even a slow forward progress. Hence the efficiency of the gait depends upon the right balance between the pressure of the foot and the counterpressure of the supporting surface (Figure 16–5).

Like counterpressure, friction is also an essential factor in the effective application of the forces needed in walking. Because of the diagonal thrust of the leg at the beginning and end of the support phase, friction between the foot and the ground is essential in order that the counterpressure of the ground may be transmitted to the

Figure 16–5 The ground reaction force *R* is equal in action line and magnitude to the downward thrust of the foot during walking, but is opposite in direction. The force is greater at heel-strike than at mid-stance because of the body's momentum, and is greater at push-off because of the plantar flexion thrust of the calf muscles driving the body forward. (From *Williams and Lissner: Biomechanics of human motion*, 2d ed. Philadelphia: W. B. Saunders, 1977.)

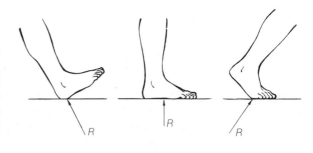

body. For efficient walking, friction must be sufficient to balance the horizontal component of force. If it is insufficient, the thrust of the foot results in a slipping of the foot itself, rather than in the desired propulsion of the body. The greater the horizontal component of force (as when walking with a long stride), the greater the dependence upon friction for efficient locomotion.

The forward-moving trunk meets with air resistance, which tends to push it backward. By inclining the body forward, the pull of gravity is utilized to balance the force of the air resistance. When walking against a strong wind, it is necessary to incline the body farther forward in order to maintain balance. If the air resistance is not balanced by the force of gravity, it must be balanced by the contraction of the abdominal and other anterior muscles of the neck and trunk. If the body is inclined too far forward, however, the force of gravity acts too strongly on it and must be counteracted by tension of the posterior muscles. Thus, the proper degree of forward inclination is a factor in muscular economy.

Mechanical Principles Applied to Walking

PRINCIPLE I   A body at rest will remain at rest unless acted upon by a force. Since walking is produced by a pendulum-like motion of the lower extremities, the inertia of the body must be overcome at every step.

PRINCIPLE II   A body in motion will continue in motion unless acted upon by a force. Since motion is imparted to the trunk by the backward thrust of the leg, the trunk has a tendency to continue moving forward, even beyond the base of support. A brief restraining action of the forward limb serves as a check on the momentum of the trunk.

PRINCIPLE III   Force applied diagonally consists of two components, horizontal and vertical. The vertical component in walking serves to counteract the downward pull of gravity. The horizontal component serves (1) in the restraining phase, to check forward motion, and (2) in the propulsive phase, to produce it. The horizontal component of force in the propulsive phase must exceed that in the restraining phase if the end result is to be progressive forward locomotion.

PRINCIPLE IV   Translatory movement of a lever is achieved by the repeated alternation of two rotatory movements, the lever turning first about one end and then the other end (Steindler, 1973). In walking, the lower extremity alternates between rotating about the foot's point of contact with the ground and the hip joint.

PRINCIPLE V   The speed of the gait is directly related to the magnitude of the pushing force and to the direction of its application. This force is provided by the extensor muscles of the hip, knee, and ankle joints, and the direction of application is determined by the slant of the lower extremity when the force is being applied.

PRINCIPLE VI   The economy of the gait is related to its timing with reference to the length of the limbs. The most economical gait is one which is so timed as to permit pendular motion of the lower extremities.

PRINCIPLE VII   Walking has been described as an alternating loss and recovery of balance (Steindler, 1973). This being so, a new base of support must be established at every step.

PRINCIPLE VIII   As propulsion of the body is brought about by the diagonal push of the foot against the supporting surface, the efficiency of locomotion depends upon the counterpressure and friction provided by this surface.

PRINCIPLE IX   Stability of the body is directly related to the size of the base of support. In walking, the lateral distance between the feet is a factor in maintaining balance.

a. Too narrow a lateral distance between the feet, such as occurs when one foot is placed directly in front of the other, increases the difficulty of maintaining balance as it decreases the width of the base of support.

b. Too wide a lateral distance between the feet increases stability, but tends to cause a weaving gait and to make the body sway from side to side.

c. The optimum position of the feet appears to be one in which the inner borders fall approximately along a single straight line.

Running

Description

Easy running, like walking, is a pendulum type of movement. It is doubtful, however, whether running at top speed can be so classified. The most notable factors differentiating the run from the walk are the period of double support, characteristic of the walk but not present in the run, and the period of no support (a "sailing-through-the-air period"), characteristic of the run but not present in the walk. In the run the foot hits the ground in front of the body's center of gravity as in the walk, but not as far in front. As the speed of the run increases, the distance in front decreases and the foot contact is almost directly under the body's center of gravity. This position reduces the restraining part of the support phase and gives greater emphasis to the propulsive part. At maximum speed, the restraining part disappears completely. The use of the term "driving phase" for the support phase in running indicates its propulsive nature.

There are two major types of running. The first is the kind of running done for its own sake, as in competitive races or jogging. The major concerns here are time and distance in one direction. The second is the type of running that is part of games and sports. Here it is necessary also to consider matters such as change of direction or pace and stability. The technique for a run varies with the purpose, but the basic anatomical and mechanical aspects are the same, regardless of the purpose.

Anatomical Analysis

The difference between the joint actions in walking and running is a matter of degree and coordination. The joint actions are essentially the same but the range of motion in running is generally greater. This is especially apparent in the actions of the swinging leg. The difference in coordination is evident in the period of nonsupport and the absence of the period of double support.

SWING PHASE   The swing phase begins with toe-off and ends with the foot landing (Figure 16–6). It is more muscular than pendular, and is longer than the support phase. In fast running the initial foot contact may be the ball of the foot and, in slow running, the whole foot. The flexed leg in the swing phase brings the mass of the leg close to the hip, reducing the moment of inertia and increasing the angular velocity of the forward swinging thigh, which in turn drives the center of gravity of the body forward.

Spine and Pelvis

1.   *Movements:* Same actions as in walking but through somewhat greater range.
2.   *Muscles:* See walking.

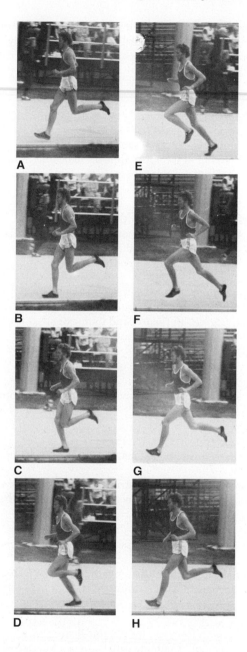

Figure 16–6 Running. *A–E*, Support and drive phase. *F–H*, Non-support phase (*F* shows beginning of swing phase for right leg).

Hip

1. *Movements:* Hyperextension immediately after toe-off; vigorous flexion followed by extension.
2. *Muscles:* The iliopsoas is the major muscle force for hip flexion. During the first half of this action there is decreasing activity in the rectus femoris, biceps

femoris, semimembranosus, and semitendinosus. In the second half, the semitendinosus and semimembranosus sharply increase in activity and are responsible for the slowdown in flexion and the change in direction to extension (Elliott and Blansky, 1979).

Knee

1. *Movements:* Rapid flexion (increases with speed) during the first two-thirds, followed by extension (decreases with speed).
2. *Muscles:* Semimembranosus and semitendinosus during the knee extension phase. The sharp flexion at the knee appears to be due in large measure to reflex action and the transfer of momentum from the forward-moving thigh.

Ankle

1. *Movements:* Dorsiflexion; prevention of plantar flexion.
2. *Muscles:* The tibialis anterior, extensor digitorum longus, and extensor hallucis longus have low-level activity until the last third of the swing when the activity increases in preparation for the foot contact.

SUPPORT PHASE   The support phase begins with the contact of the forward foot and ends at toe-off when the body is driven into the air (Figure 16–6A to E). During this time the knee and ankle "give" in flexion and then extend as the body passes over the foot and is driven into the air. The support time decreases as the speed of the run increases.

Spine and Pelvis

1. *Movements and Muscles:* Same as in walking but more vigorous in reaction to leg movements.

Hip

1. *Movement:* Flexion followed by extension. These actions increase with the speed of the run.
2. *Muscles:* Gluteus maximus at heel strike. The hamstrings and quadriceps contract simultaneously at the time of heel strike to stabilize the hip and pelvis.

Knee

1. *Movement:* Flexion (increases with speed) followed by extension (decreases with speed).
2. *Muscles:* The rectus femoris, vastus medialis, and vastus lateralis are active during knee flexion, reaching maximum activity at heel-off.

Ankle

1. *Movement:* Dorsiflexion followed by plantar flexion.
2. *Muscles:* The soleus and gastrocnemius are active during the whole support phase and show the strongest activity after heel-off as the knee is flexing.

Mechanical Analysis

The speed of running is governed by the length of the stride and the frequency of the stride. Better runners have a greater stride length per given pace than poorer runners. The length of the stride is determined by the length of the leg, the range of motion in the hip, and the power of the leg extensors which drive the entire body forward. Like any projectile, the distance the body will move once it is driven into the air depends upon the angle of takeoff (distance that center of gravity is ahead of takeoff foot), the speed of the body's projection, and the height of the center of gravity at takeoff and landing. The stride rate of the run is affected by the speed of muscle contraction and the skill (technique of the performer).

In running, as in walking, the forces exerted to produce and control the movement are the internal muscular forces and the external forces of gravity, normal reaction, friction, and air resistance. There is no optimal speed in running because the energy needed to run is proportional to the square of the velocity. Therefore, whether the run is an easy jog or a full-speed sprint, economy of effort is a highly desirable objective. To achieve this it is essential that the runner observe the principles that apply to efficient running.

Mechanical Principles Applied to Running

PRINCIPLE I In accordance with the first Law of Motion, a body at rest remains at rest unless acted upon by a force. In running, the problem of overcoming inertia decreases as the level of speed increases. It is greatest at the takeoff and least after acceleration has ceased.

a. The crouching start enables the runner to exert maximum horizontal force at the takeoff by:

(1) Providing a surface against which the foot can push horizontally; moving the rear foot back increases the push-off force but decreases the time to apply the force. The result may be a smaller impulse (Ft).

(2) Putting the legs in a more horizontal position;

(3) Enabling the runner to use maximum hip, knee, and ankle extension in both legs (Figure 16–7).

b. During acceleration the horizontal component of the leg drive gradually diminishes until a level of speed is maintained, during which period it remains uni-

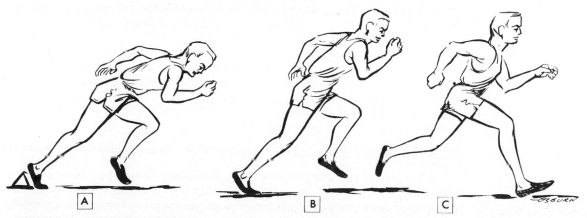

Figure 16–7 The crouch start for a sprint race. The period of acceleration is characterized by a gradual decrease in the forward inclination of the trunk and a lengthening of the stride.

form. The period of acceleration is characterized by a gradual decrease in the forward inclination of the trunk, a lengthening of the stride (made possible by the raising of the center of gravity as the trunk becomes more erect), and a decrease of the knee thrust, resulting from the gradual straightening of the knee at the moment of contact between the foot and the ground.

PRINCIPLE II   Also in accordance with the first Law of Motion, a moving body will move in a straight line unless it is acted upon by a force causing it to change its direction. In order to run in a curved pathway, as when running around a circular or oval track, an additional force is needed to overcome the body's tendency to continue in a straight line. This is achieved by leaning toward the inside, since the slant of the body will introduce a lateral component to the pressure of the foot against the ground. The well-banked curves of indoor tracks do this for the runner.

PRINCIPLE III   In accordance with the second Law of Motion, acceleration is directly proportional to the force producing it. Hence, the greater the power of the leg drive, the greater the acceleration of the runner.

PRINCIPLE IV   In accordance with the third Law of Motion, every action has an equal and opposite reaction.

PRINCIPLE V   Since a long lever develops more speed at the end than does a short lever, the length of the leg during the driving phase of running should be as great as possible when speed is a consideration. This is achieved by full extension at the knee joint at the end of the driving phase.

PRINCIPLE VI   The smaller the vertical component of force, the greater the horizontal or driving component.

   a. In the most efficient run, vertical movements of the center of gravity are reduced to a minimum.

   b. The vertical component of force should be just enough to counteract the downward pull of gravity but not enough to produce an unnecessary bounce in running.

PRINCIPLE VII   The more completely the horizontal component of force is directed straight backward, the greater its contribution to the forward motion of the body. Lateral movements of the arms, legs, and trunk detract unnecessarily from forward propulsion. To ensure forward motion of the body:

   a. The knees should be lifted directly forward-upward with the entire lower extremity kept in the sagittal plane. (Unathletic people sometimes run with a minimal knee lift and with an inward rotation of the thighs, the feet and lower legs being thrown out to the side.)

   b. The arm swing should exactly counterbalance the twist of the pelvis and should not cause additional lateral motion.

PRINCIPLE VIII   Efficiency in running, as in any movement, requires the elimination of all unnecessary force.

   a. The shorter the lever, the less the force required to move it, and the less the reaction to it. By flexing the leg at the knee and carrying the heel high up under the hip in the recovery phase, the leg is moved more rapidly, as well as more economically.

   b. Internal resistance caused by the viscosity of the sarcolemma is reduced by warming up activities.

c. Internal resistance caused by tight muscles, fasciae, and ligaments is reduced by systematic stretching exercises.

d. Unnecessary force in the form of excessively rapid muscular contractions is eliminated by developing as long a stride as can be controlled.

PRINCIPLE IX   The force of air resistance affects performance. More horizontal velocity and forward shift of the center of gravity are needed to counteract a head wind.

Jumping, Hopping, or Leaping

Jumping, hopping or leaping are forms of locomotion familiar from earliest childhood, whether engaged in as a simple expression of joy and exuberance, as a self-testing and competitive activity, or as an integral part of a sport. In each instance the goal is to propel the body into the air with sufficient force to overcome gravity and in the direction to accomplish the desired height or horizontal distance. Like any projectile, the path of the body in the air is determined by the conditions at the instant of projection. The differences between a hop, jump, and leap relate to the landing and takeoff. In the hop, the same foot is used for the takeoff and landing. In the leap, the takeoff is from one foot and the landing on the other. A jumper takes off from one or both feet and lands on both feet. Each of these types of projection may be initiated from a stationary position (vertical jump, standing long jump) or preceded by some locomotor pattern such as running (running long jump, triple jump, high jump, hurdle).

The total horizontal distance covered by the performer of these related patterns is the sum of three distances: (1) the horizontal distance between the takeoff foot and the line of gravity of the performer, (2) the horizontal distance the center of gravity travels in the air, and (3) the horizontal distance the center of gravity is behind the body part that lands closest to the takeoff point. The total height may be considered to be divided into the distance between the ground and the line of gravity at the moment of takeoff and the maximum distance the center of gravity is projected vertically. For some activities, such as the high jump and the pole vault, the vertical distance between the center of gravity and the crossbar may be an additional important unit of distance.

All forms of these activities share the problems of adequate muscle strength to project the body against the force of gravity and the coordination needed for utilizing what might be called secondary motions for achieving maximum height or distance. The force that projects the body is provided by the forceful contraction of the extensors of the hips, knees, and ankles and, to a lesser extent, by the arm flexors in swinging the arms forward and upward.

Principles Applied to Jumping, Hopping, and Leaping

The principles that relate to projectiles—momentum and its transfer, reaction, and impulse—are important to consider when analyzing hopping, jumping, and leaping actions.

PRINCIPLE I   The path of motion of a body's center of gravity in space is determined by the angle at which it is projected, speed of the projection, height of the center of gravity at takeoff, and air resistance.

Applications   *a.* The angle of projection for world-class long jumpers is around 20 degrees. This angle is governed by the speed of the preparatory run and the vertical velocity generated at the takeoff. This angle is lower than the optimum 45 degrees because the time to generate vertical velocity at the takeoff is so small, and the horizontal velocity therefore dominates. A jumper's vertical velocity would have to equal the horizontal velocity in order to have a 45 degrees angle of projection.

b. The speed of a long jumper's projection is a compromise between the runner's ability to run horizontally and the ability to jump vertically. In order to allow time to generate a vertical impulse at takeoff, the runner's speed must be less than maximum and, in order to have a fast takeoff, the runner's vertical impulse cannot be at maximum. Dyson (1970) has suggested that the proportion of horizontal to vertical takeoff velocity should be 2:1.

c. In the high jump the jumper's center of gravity should be projected from as high as possible. At the moment of leaving the ground the jumping leg and trunk should be fully extended, and the free leg and arm raised. Besides technique another important factor in the height of the center of gravity is build. Olympic-class high jumpers are all tall, long-legged individuals.

d. In the standing vertical jump where maximum height is the goal, the center of gravity should be directly over the feet so that the angle of projection will be 90 degrees.

PRINCIPLE II   Jumpers project themselves into the air by exerting a force against the ground that is larger than the force supporting their weight. The *reaction* to this force accelerates them upwards. The faster the leg movements, especially, the more force is produced against the ground.

Applications   *a.* The upward swinging movement of the arms and free leg in the high jump accelerate against the support leg, which in turn causes a reaction thrust from the ground. These are followed by a second reactive thrust due to the extension of the trunk and jumping leg.

b. Long jumpers modify their running strides right before takeoff to lower the center of gravity and to increase the flexion of the hip, knee, and ankle on landing. As the center of gravity moves over and in front of the takeoff leg the free leg and arms flex vigorously, and vigorous extension occurs at the hip, knee, and ankle. The reactive force projects the body into the air.

PRINCIPLE III   The magnitude of the *impulse* that the jumper exerts against the ground is a product of the forces and the time over which they act.

Applications   *a.* The vertical impulses in all jumps are those resulting from the swinging actions of the arms and the extension of the flexed hip, knee, and ankle. The magnitude of the forces depends upon the strength of the muscles, speed of the joint actions, and coordination of the joint movements. The time for generating vertical impulses is greatest in jumps from a stationary start and greater in the high jump than in the long jump.

b. The time for takeoff in the high jump varies with the style of jump and action of the free limbs. The Fosbury flop style generally has shorter times than the straddle style, and jumpers who use a double-arm action and a straight lead leg action have longer takeoff times. Those who use techniques with faster takeoff times appear to have higher jumps, apparently compensating by generating more force for a greater vertical impulse (Hay, 1978).

PRINCIPLE IV   Momentum can be transferred from one part of a body to the whole.

Applications   *a.* The angular momentum built up in the high jumper's free leg at takeoff is transferred to the body for the layout over the crossbar.

b. In the standing long jump the arms swing forcefully forward and up. The momentum of the arm swing is transferred to the body and, if timed properly (summation of forces), will add to the momentum of the jump.

PRINCIPLE V   Angular momentum may be developed by the sudden checking of linear motion or by an eccentric thrust.

Applications   *a.* As the result of planting the pole at the end of the run, the vaulter rotates both around the pole and around the hands.

b. Part of a high jumper's layout in the high jump may be due to eccentric thrust. This will never be great, however, because it diminishes the amount of vertical thrust through the center of gravity.

c. The eccentric thrust of the long jumper at takeoff can produce either forward or backward rotation. The more usual is forward rotation, which jumpers counteract by movements such as the hitch kick or running in air that rotate the body backward. These actions also help to place the legs in the best position for landing (Figure 16–8).

PRINCIPLE VI   For movement to occur, inertia must be overcome. One of the chief problems in jumping from a standing start is overcoming inertia, often with a minimum space in which to do so.

Applications   *a.* If the jump is for the purpose of reaching as high as possible with one hand, as in tipping a basketball, and the player is free to move the feet even slightly, inertia may be overcome by taking a hop or short step before the jump.

b. Two or three preliminary swings forward and back will help to overcome inertia in the standing long jump.

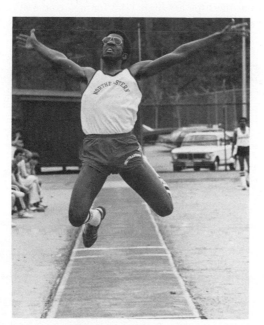

Figure 16–8 The long jump using the hang technique. The extended body position increases the moment of inertia about the horizontal axis, thus decreasing the undesired forward rotation developed at takeoff. (Courtesy of Northeastern University.)

PRINCIPLE VII Muscles can store elastic energy. When concentric contraction is preceded by a phase of active stretching, elastic energy stored in the stretch phase is available for use in the contractile phase. Work done by muscles shortening immediately after stretching is greater than that done by those shortening from a static state.

Applications *a.* There should be no pause between the crouch and thrust phases of the vertical jump.

b. The quick extensions in the long jump and high jump are enhanced by the lengthening contractions in the quick lower extremity flexions that precede.

Additional Forms of Locomotion

**Rotatory Loco-
motion**

In general, the factors responsible for the successful performance of rotatory locomotion are the magnitude, direction, and accurate timing of the forces contributing to the desired movement of the body, including the advantageous use of the force of gravity whenever possible.

The most common activities in this category are forward, backward, and sideward rolls, cartwheels, and handsprings. Each of these is achieved by rotating about the body's successive areas of contact with the supporting surface. In forward rolls, for instance, the body rotates about the hands, shoulders, rounded back, buttocks, and feet (Figure 16–9) and in cartwheels, about each hand followed by each foot with the body rotating laterally in a fully extended position. The impetus for the forward roll is given by the hands and feet, the direction of their thrust being a combination of backward and downward: backward to send the body forward, and downward to resist the downward pull of gravitational force on the head and trunk. When the hands and feet are no longer pushing, the head is tucked forward and the back is rounded with the knees bent close against the body to facilitate the roll. During the foot thrust the hips are high, both for ensuring a stronger backward thrust with the legs and for making greater use of the force of gravity for the roll over the back.

Since a body at rest will remain at rest unless acted upon by a force and a body in motion will continue in motion unless acted upon by a force, it is important to keep the body moving in successive rolls and not to let it come to a momentary halt

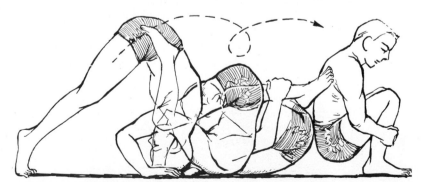

Figure 16–9 The body rotating around its points of contact with the supporting surface. (Redrawn from LaPorte and Renner: *The tumbler's manual*. By courtesy of Prentice-Hall, Inc.)

following each roll. Even the briefest of interruptions necessitates the overcoming of inertia after each revolution. It takes velocity to acquire sufficient momentum to prevent these halts; therefore, each backward thrust of hands and feet against the ground should be as forceful as possible. Rotary movement is accelerated by shortening the radius. In both forward and backward rolls the radius is shortened by tucking the flexed lower extremities close to the body when the back is in contact with the floor.

Locomotion by Specialized Steps and Jumps

Other forms of ground-supported locomotion not involving the use of special equipment include two general categories. One of these consists of acrobatic stunts and athletic events, such as walking on the hands, successive jumping, and hurdling either with or without actual hurdles. The other category consists of activities used both in children's play and in forms of dance. It includes skipping, hopping, galloping, sliding, sidestepping, leaping, and standard dance steps, such as the polka and mazurka.

Off the Ground Locomotion

There are two major categories of locomotion that do not involve support on a solid surface. These are hand-traveling on suspension apparatus and aquatic locomotion, which includes both swimming and boating. These are discussed in the appropriate chapters.

Laboratory Experiences

1. Try this as a class exercise, working in pairs. *A* stands with heels against a wall with the feet otherwise in a comfortable, "natural" position in readiness to walk. *B* holds a ruler across the toes of *A*'s feet and draws a line against the ruler. *A* then stands with feet parallel at right angles to the wall, and again *B* draws a line. Measure the distance between the two lines. This measurement is likely to vary from ¼ inch to 1 inch in a sizable class. *A* and *B* now change places and repeat.

   Assume that you are to engage in a walking race of 1000 yards; also assume that if you toed straight ahead, each step would be 1 yard long. It would therefore take you 1000 steps to cover the distance. But suppose you toed out so that each step was (your measurement) _____ short. How many yards short of the finish line would you be when you had taken 1000 steps? (*Ans:* If the distance between the two lines had been $^3/_{16}$ inch you would be $^3/_{16} \times 1000$ = 187.5 inches or 5.2 yards short.)

   Implication. If you are walking against an opponent who walks at the same rate as you, but who toes straight ahead, you would be 5.2 yards behind when you cross the finish line. Yet, presumably you took the same number of steps.

2. Observe the gait of people on the street or campus, detect individual characteristics, and analyze them in terms of anatomical and mechanical principles.

3. Get a subject to walk in each of the following ways. Observe and note differences in the movements of the head, shoulders, hips, and so forth.
   a. Place one foot directly in front of the other.
   b. Keep a lateral distance of 10 to 12 inches between the feet.
   c. Point the toes out.
   d. Point the toes in.
   e. Point the toes straight ahead.
   f. Take a short stride.
   g. Take a long stride.

4. Select four or five individuals who differ in leg length. Get them to practice walking until each one finds the stride and speed that feel most comfortable. Compare their strides and measure the distance between footprints for each individual.

5. Observe several individuals as they run. Look for the application of the principles listed. Which are "violated" and how?

6. Using the iliac crest as an estimate of the center of gravity, trace the path of the center of gravity on a sequence drawing of some form of jump (see Figure 13–2, page 406). Determine the percentage of the distance jump which can be attributed to each of the following:
   a. Distance center of gravity is in front of takeoff point at the moment of takeoff.
   b. Distance center of gravity travels while body is unsupported.
   c. Distance center of gravity is behind landing point.

7. Compare the segment positions at several points during the execution of a standing long jump or vertical jump as done by several "poor" jumpers and several "good" jumpers. Identify the principles of concern in these jumps. Evaluate the performances in terms of the related principles. Based on this information try to improve the performance of the "poor" jumpers.

8. Choose a locomotor pattern not discussed in this chapter (hurdling, for example). Identify those principles which will help you determine whether or not someone performing this pattern is doing it correctly.

References

Advisory Committee on Artificial Limbs, National Research Council. 1953. *The pattern of muscular activity in the lower extremity during walking.* Berkeley: Prosthetic Devices Research Project, Institute of Engineering Research, University of California.

Basmajian, J. V. 1979. *Muscles alive,* 4th ed. Baltimore: Williams & Wilkins.

Bates, B., et al. 1979. Functional variability of the lower extremity during the support phase of running. *Med. Sci. Sports* 2:328–31.

Brandell, B. R. 1973. An analysis of muscle coordination in walking and running gaits. In *Biomechanics III,* ed. S. Cerquiglini et al. Baltimore: University Park Press.

Broer, M. R., and Zernicke, R. 1979. *Efficiency of human movement,* 4th ed. Philadelphia: W. B. Saunders.

Carlin, E. J. 1963. Human gait. *Am. J. Phys. Med.* 42:181–84.

Cooper, J. M., et al. 1973. Kinesiology of the long-jump. In *Biomechanics III,* ed. S. Cerquiglini et al. Baltimore: University Park Press.

Dyson, G. 1970. *The mechanics of athletics,* 5th ed. London: University of London Press.

Elliott, B., and Blansky, B. 1979. The synchronization of muscle activity and body segment movements during a running cycle. *Med. Sci. Sports* 2:322–27.

Hay, J. 1978. *The biomechanics of sports techniques,* 2d ed. Englewood Cliffs, N.J.: Prentice-Hall.

Hogue, R. E. 1969. Upper-extremity muscular activity at different cadences and inclines during normal gait. *J. Am. Phys. Ther. Assoc.* 49:963–72.

Liberson, W. T. 1973. Discussion of the paper of Dr. Brandell. In *Biomechanics III,* ed. S. Cerquiglini et al. Baltimore: University Park Press.

Murray, M. P., Drought, A. B., and Kory, R. C. 1964. Walking patterns of normal men. *J. Bone Joint Surg.* 46A:335–60.

Murray, M. P., Kory, R. C., Clarkson, B. H., and Sepic, S. B. 1966. Comparison of free and fast speed walking patterns of normal men. *Am. J. Phys. Med.* 45:8–24.

Murray, M. P., Kory, R. C., and Sepic, S. B. 1970. Walking patterns of normal women. *Arch. Phys. Med. Rehab.* 51:637–50.

Murray, M. P., Sepic, S. B., and Barnard, E. J. 1967. Patterns of sagittal rotation of the upper limbs in walking. *J. Am. Phys. Ther. Assoc.* 47:272–84.

Saunders, J. B. deC. M., Inman, V. T., and Eberhart, H. D. 1953. The major determinants in normal and pathological gait. *J. Bone Joint Surg.* 34A:543–58.

Sheffield, F. J., Gersten, J. W., and Mastellone, A. F. 1956. Electromyographic study of the muscles of the foot in normal walking. *Am. J. Phys. Med.* 35:223–36.

Sinning, W., and Forsyth, H. 1970. Lower limb action while running at different velocities. *Med. Sci. Sports* 2:28–34.

Steindler, A. 1973. *Kinesiology of the human body.* Springfield, Ill.: Charles C Thomas, Lectures 37 and 38.

Winter, D., and Kuryliak, W. 1978. Dynamic stabilization in human gait: The biomechanical relationships between the triceps surae and the metatarsophalangeal joint. In *Biomechanics VI-A,* ed. E. Asmussen and K. Jorgensen. Baltimore: University Park Press.

Moving One's Body When Suspended and When Free of Support

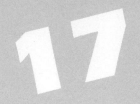

Objectives

At the conclusion of this chapter, the student should be able to:

1. Explain how each of the following influences the action of swinging bodies: weight of the body, length of the pendulum, angular momentum, potential-kinetic energy, centrifugal-centripetal force, friction.
2. Describe how to initiate pendular action, increase the height of a swing, alter the period, change grips, and dismount safely.
3. Explain how each of the following influences the flight path of unsupported bodies: angle of projection, vertical velocity, gravity, angular momentum.
4. Describe how to initiate and control rotation of unsupported bodies.
5. Analyze the performance of a suspension and a nonsupport movement. For each, identify the basic anatomical and mechanical considerations, as well as those factors that appear to limit performance.

Suspension Activities

Climbing, hanging, swinging, and other suspension activities were more commonly engaged in by our early ancestors than by members of more recent generations. The modern version of these brachial activities is seen in the trapeze activities of the aerial artist at the circus, in gymnastics events on the high bar, parallel bars, uneven bars, and rings, and in various forms of hanging on ladders and ropes in the gymnasium and on the playground. Success in suspension activities depends upon considerable strength and endurance, particularly of the hand, arm, and shoulder musculature, and the ability to adjust body positions to counteract or take advantage of the forces acting on the body (Figure 17–1). Ladder or rope climbing and brachial locomotion are modifications of locomotion. Where swinging movements of a suspended body are involved the principles of a pendulum, angular momentum, and centripetal-centrifugal forces are major considerations.

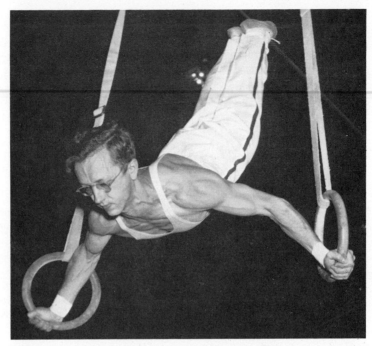

Figure 17–1 Movement of the body in suspension. This maneuver on the still rings illustrates the need for good muscular development in the arms and shoulders. (Courtesy of Springfield College.)

Principles Related to Swinging Movements

Principle I

The movement of a pendulum is produced by the force of gravity. This presupposes a starting position in which potential energy is present. In other words, the pendulum must be moved from its resting position before the force of gravity can make it swing downward.

APPLICATIONS

 a. The initial problem of the child on the swing and of the gymnast on the flying rings is that of being given potential energy. Without the help of an assistant, the swinger must find a way of being put into a position with potential energy. This is usually done in one of three ways. The performer may move the apparatus to some position other than its normal position of rest before being suspended (i.e., the rings or swing are pulled as far back and up as can be reached); the performer may initiate the swing with a push of the feet against the floor or with small running steps; or a pumping action may be used to get started. For the gymnast swinging on the rings, the last alternative involves bending the legs up in front of the body and then extending them as high as possible. The range of the arc of motion may be increased by the repetition of this procedure on the forward-upward phase of the swing. The child in the swing accomplishes the same result by inclining the trunk backward and raising the feet forward, while at the same time pulling the ropes toward the body and pressing forward against the seat.

b. Initiating a pendulum swing on the traveling rings is achieved by flexing each arm alternately. Because of the wide distance between the traveling rings, this procedure moves the body a considerable distance from its resting position and thus puts it in favorable position for the force of gravity to act on it.

Principle II

As the pendulum swings downward, gravity causes its speed to increase; as it swings upward, gravity counteracts its speed, diminishing it until the zero point is reached. Hence the pendulum's speed is greatest at the bottom of the arc and least (zero) at each end of the arc.

APPLICATION   Caution must be exercised to maintain a firm grip on the supporting surface (rings, bar, or ropes), particularly at the bottom of the swing where the tendency to fly off is the greatest.

Principle III

The upward movement of a pendulum is brought about by the momentum developed in the downward movement. The swinging body moves through an arc, first in one direction, then in the reverse direction (one-half the arc's distance is called the amplitude). Thus it undergoes partial rotation about a center of motion. Since this rotation takes place in a vertical plane, the influence of gravitational pull must be taken into consideration. Whereas the force of gravity *produces* the downward swing, it *opposes* the upward swing. Nevertheless it is indirectly responsible for the latter, inasmuch as the upward swing is caused by the momentum which was built up in the preceding downward swing.

APPLICATION   This relationship is especially important in skills performed on the uneven bars when long, swinging actions are involved. The higher the position from which the downswing is initiated, the higher will be the upswing. The range of a swing depends upon the height from which the movement is initiated.

Principle IV

The potential energy of the pendulum is greatest at the height of the swing and zero at the bottom. Conversely, kinetic energy is greatest at the bottom and zero at the top. In a perfect mechanical system a pendulum would continue to swing with a constant amplitude with the required energy supplied by the perpetual conversion from potential to kinetic energy. Most of the potential energy is converted to kinetic energy in the downswing and reconverted on the upswing. Some is lost, however, due to friction and air resistance, and a pendulum left to its own devices will gradually decrease in amplitude and stop.

APPLICATION   In order to make up for the lost mechanical energy, supplemental energy in the form of properly timed muscular action of the swinger must be used. Maximum repetitions of a pendulum left to its own devices will occur if the initial height is maximum and friction is minimized.

Principle V

The height of a swing may be increased by lengthening the radius of rotation on the downswing and decreasing it on the upswing (Figure 17–2). Shortening the radius on the upswing decreases the moment of inertia and therefore increases the angular velocity. This occurs because the angular momentum is conserved and, since angular momentum = $I\omega$, a decrease in I requires an increase in ω. The increased angular velocity is accompanied by an increase in kinetic energy and consequently more height results. The increased height for the start of the downswing and the length-

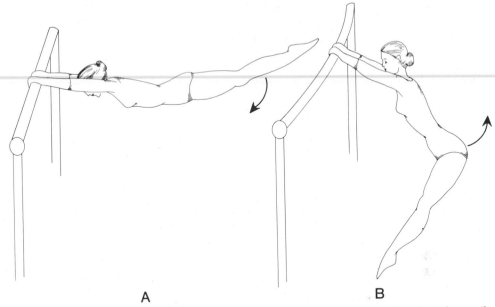

Figure 17–2 The height of a swing may be increased by lengthening the radius of rotation on the downswing and decreasing it on the upswing.

ened radius of rotation produce a gain in angular momentum on the downswing because gravity has a longer time to act on the body before it reaches the bottom of the swing. When the shortening of the radius occurs for the next upswing, the increased momentum is conserved and, once again, there is an increase in angular velocity. The equation for angular momentum, $I\omega$, also shows that the greater the angular velocity on the downswing the less the body has to be shortened to decrease I in order to reach its desired height on the upswing.

APPLICATION   A swinging performer may shorten the radius of rotation by moving body parts toward the axis of rotation. This may be done by flexing at the hips, hunching the shoulders by depressing the shoulder girdle, or arching the back. A performer in the giant swing depresses the shoulder girdle and flexes at the hips on the upswing, and may also arch the back slightly. In a circle from a front uprise, the head is thrown back to shorten the radius on the upswing.

Principle VI   *To increase height, the decrease in radius should be initiated at the moment that the center of gravity of the body is directly under the axis of rotation. In the movement of a pendulum, speed is greatest at the bottom of the arc. Shortening the radius at this point accelerates its angular velocity more than at any other position.*

APPLICATION   In the backward hip circle on the uneven parallel bars the movement is started with the body extended so that there is a long radius of rotation on the downswing. At the moment the legs pass under the hands, the hips are flexed to shorten the radius on the upswing and increase the angular velocity.

Principle VII   *The time taken by the pendulum to make a single round-trip excursion (known as its period) is related to the length of the pendulum.* The longer the pendulum, the more slowly it swings. Specifically, the period of the pendulum is proportional to the square root of its length.

APPLICATIONS

    a. When the hands are the axis of rotation, such as in the preparatory movements for the giant swing, the period is longer than in swings about a hip axis or a knee axis.

    b. When swinging on ropes, the supporting ropes should be lengthened for a slow swing and shortened for a fast swing.

Principle VIII   *The period of the pendulum is not influenced by its weight.* A heavy body will swing no faster than a lighter one, or vice versa. This is consistent with the behavior of freely falling bodies.

APPLICATION   Trapeze artists take advantage of this principle. A performer swinging from one trapeze knows that an empty trapeze of the same length, swung from an opposite platform of the same height and at the same time as the trapeze artist's, will have the same period. Consequently the performer also knows that it is safe to let go of the original bar at the height of its swing and turn around in midair, because the empty bar will be right there to be grasped, also at the height of its swing.

Principle IX   *When a pendulum reaches the end of its arc, just before it reverses its direction, it reaches a zero point in velocity.* At this precise moment the force of gravity is momentarily neutralized by the upward momentum.

APPLICATION   The performer can take advantage of this situation by using this moment to perform position changes such as changing grips, reversing direction, and performing dismounts and cutaways. The underswing half-turn on the unevens is executed best and is most easily controlled when the twist and grip change are both completed during the height of the underswing.

Principle X   *When a body consisting of two segments reaches the vertical, with the proximal segment leading on the downswing, the distal segment will accelerate relative to the other segment and precede it into the upswing. If, on the other hand, the distal segment reaches the vertical first, the reverse will occur. The distal segment will decelerate and the proximal segment will lead into the upswing* (Figure 17–3).

APPLICATION   Action at the bottom of a swing, which forces the hips through in front of the feet, increases the acceleration on the upswing owing to hip flexion in shortening the radius. Such swings are called "beat" swings. "Beat" swings are used to set up hechts and flyaways on the high or uneven bars and stutzes and somersaults on the parallel bars.

Principle XI   *The rotation of a gymnast's hands about a bar is opposed by frictional forces.* This accounts for some loss in swinging energy as it is converted to heat energy. Evidence of this is the appearance of friction blisters and skin irritations on the gymnast's hands. These friction forces tend to strengthen the gymnast's grip when the swing is in the direction the palms are facing and weakens it when the swing is in the reverse direction.

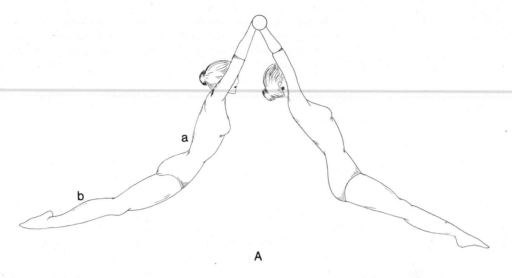

A

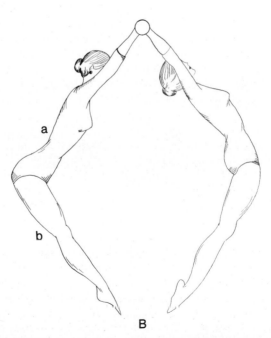

B

Figure 17–3 *A,* Double pendulum swing. If segment **a** precedes segment **b** to the vertical, segment **b** accelerates and precedes **a** in the upswing. *B,* When segment **b** precedes **a** to the vertical, **a** will lead into the upswing, but the whole pendulum decelerates.

APPLICATION   Gymnasts reverse their grasps when the swing is reversed. This is usually done at the peak of the swing at the point of "weightlessness" when the pressure on the hands is at a minimum. Gymnasts also sand the bar before each performance to assure its smoothness and to minimize the friction on the hands.

Principle XII   *In all mounting exercises involving swinging, the center of gravity must be brought as near as possible to the center of rotation.* This is usually done when the center of gravity is directly under the bar on the downswing.

APPLICATION   In the glide kip on the unevens the performer swings the body forward and back, alternately flexing and extending to gain momentum. At the end of the glide the gymnast flexes fully at the hips so that the feet are near the bar. This sharp flexion increases the angular velocity by decreasing the moment of inertia. As the center of gravity passes under the bar on the downswing, the hips are extended vigorously. This movement raises the body and places the center of gravity close to the bar, thus further decreasing the moment of inertia and enabling the body to rotate until it is in a front support position with the center of gravity located at the fixed point of the grip.

Principle XIII   *The centripetal-centrifugal force in pendular movements increases as the mass or velocity increases and decreases as the radius increases* $(C_F = \dfrac{mv^2}{r})$. The centripetal force is greatest at the bottom of the swing where the velocity is the greatest, and decreases to zero at the height of the swing. However, bodies develop proportionately more centripetal force and need more strength to maintain a grasp and counteract the opposing centrifugal force than do those of less weight. When centripetal force ceases to act on a swinging performer, the body will obey Newton's first law and will fly off tangent to the arc of the swing at that instant.

APPLICATIONS

   a. Great care should be taken with beginners and children. The hands should be watched for indications of slippage, particularly at the bottom of the swing where the centripetal force needed is maximal. Probably the safest way for children and novices to dismount is for them to stop swinging, come to a "dead stop," and then drop down.

   b. Stunts requiring the release and resumption of the grasp should be executed at the peak of the swing where velocity, and hence centripetal and centrifugal forces, is zero. Dismounts and cutaways are timed to occur at that point where the tangent of the arc at the instant of release coincides with the desired line of flight.

   c. The centripetal force has been calculated to be four to five times the body weight as the body swings under the bar in a giant swing. To resist the equal and opposite outward-pulling centrifugal force, strong hands and arms are essential. The heavier the gymnast, the greater must be the hand and arm strength.

Principle XIV   *In support swings the center of gravity should be at the point of support.*

APPLICATION   Hip circles forward or backward require the center of gravity of the body to be close to the hand supports. In this position it takes less effort to keep the body against the bar while turning because the torque between the center of gravity of the body and the axis of rotation is kept at a minimum.

Principles Related to Hand Traveling and Hanging Activities

Principle I

In hanging activities the muscles of the arm and shoulder girdle must contract to protect the joints. The pull of the body's weight puts stress on the joints by tending to separate them.

Principle II

Hand traveling is a locomotor pattern. It is governed by the principle of action and reaction. As in walking, force applied against a supporting surface in one direction causes the body to move in the opposite direction.

APPLICATION   Hand traveling sidewards on a boom or along the side of a horizontal ladder without swinging is achieved by alternately moving one hand away from the other hand, and then moving the second hand toward the first. As the first hand moves, the second hand pushes laterally against the apparatus. Both hands share the weight equally for a moment, then the second hand is released and brought toward the first hand, while at the same time the first hand is pulling laterally on the apparatus.

Principle III

The action used in hand climbing activities is essentially a chinning action.

APPLICATIONS
   a. In rope climbing with or without the use of the legs, the body is raised through a forceful chinning action of the arms.
   b. In the back kip to support on the still rings, the performer chins forcefully from a piked inverted hang. As the performer rises upward, the body is extended upward and the chinning action is converted to a push-up, ending in a straight-arm support position.

Principle IV

In accord with Newton's Law of Inertia, sequential hand support movements should be continuous. The momentum of one action contributes to the next action.

APPLICATIONS
   a. In the kip-up on the still rings there should be no pause between the pulling phase and the pushing phase of the hands and arms.
   b. Hand traveling on a horizontal bar or ladder should be a continuous hand-over-hand action.

Nonsupport Activities

The unsupported body moves through the air along a pathway determined prior to the beginning of flight. The flight path of the body may be primarily horizontal, as in a long jump, mostly vertical, as in springboard diving or high jumping, or somewhere in between, as in vaulting and tumbling events. Principles governing the flight path of the body relate to those of the projectile. Additional principles explaining the effect of the body's lean at the moment of takeoff and the twisting movements in the air are derived from Newton's third Law of Action-Reaction and the conservation of angular momentum.

Principles Related to Nonsupport Activities

Principle I

The path of motion of the body's center of gravity in space is determined by the angle at which it is projected into space, the force of the projection, and the force of gravity.

APPLICATIONS

a. Nothing a diver can do will alter the pathway of the center of gravity, once the feet have left the diving board. Divers who, by pulling the head down, attempt to "correct" dives they believe to be too far away from the board merely cause additional rotation about the transverse axis. The horizontal velocity of the diver remains constant and the path of the center of gravity is not altered.

b. A trampolinist must direct the body's projection in a totally vertical direction in order to ensure landing back in the middle of the bed. A diver must leave the board with some degree of lean to ensure *not* hitting the board after takeoff.

Principle II

The time a body remains unsupported depends upon the height of its projection, which is governed by the vertical velocity of the projection (Figure 17–4).

APPLICATION The more complicated or lengthy the stunt a diver or trampolinist wishes to perform, the higher the peak of projection must be. A diver must emphasize vertical rather than horizontal distance.

Principle III

The angular momentum (Iω) of an unsupported body is conserved. It cannot be increased or decreased.

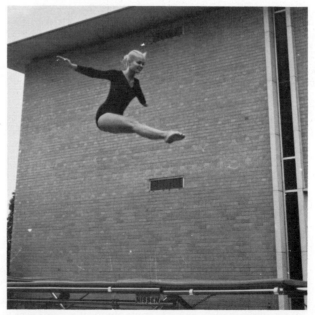

Figure 17–4 Movement of the body in the air, free of support. The height of projection is dependent upon its vertical velocity. (Judi Ford, Miss America, 1969; Junior Women's National A. A. U. Trampoline Champion, 1968. Courtesy of Mrs. Virgil Ford.)

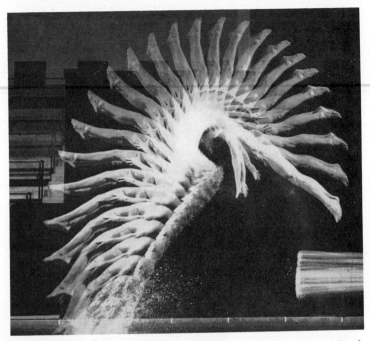

Figure 17–5 Front somersault dive in layout position. An example of rotatory movement of the body about its center of gravity while undergoing unsupported parabolic motion. (Courtesy of H. E. Edgerton.)

APPLICATIONS

a. A performer executing a forward tuck somersault may decrease the angular velocity by increasing the moment of inertia. This is done by increasing the radius of rotation—i.e., decreasing the amount of tuck. A tuck somersault has less angular inertia than a pike somersault and a pike somersault has less than a layout.

b. If a somersault starts with a twist from the board or trampoline bed, the twist can be increased by decreasing the arch or pike of the spin and by moving the arms close to the body. Each of these moves decreases the moment of inertia and increases the angular velocity of the twist.

Principle IV   *Most rotatory movements are initiated before the performer leaves the supporting surface.*

APPLICATIONS

a. In the front somersault dive (Figure 17–5), the diver's center of gravity must be in front of the feet at the moment of takeoff for a rotatory or torque force to exist and for the dive to be possible.

b. In a back somersault with a twist (Figure 17–6), the diver pushes the feet sideways as well as diagonally backward against the board as the upper body leads the twist in the opposite direction. In keeping with Newton's third law, the direction of the twist is opposite to the direction in which the feet push against the supporting surface.

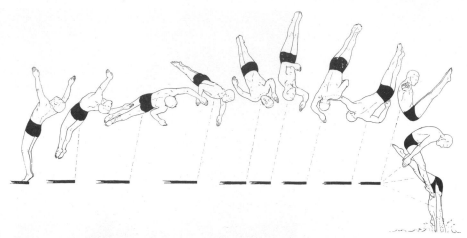

Figure 17–6 Back one-and-one-half somersault, one-and-one-half twist, free. (From Armbruster, D. A., et al.: *Swimming and diving*. 5th ed. St. Louis: C. V. Mosby, 1968.)

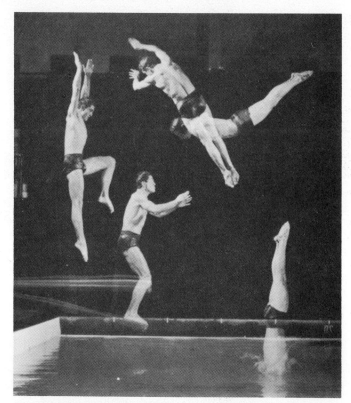

Figure 17–7 The reverse dive layout with one-half twist. (From Batterman, C.: *The techniques of springboard diving*. Cambridge: MIT Press, 1968.)

Principle V

When a body is free in space, movement of a part in one direction results in movement of the rest of the body in the opposite direction.

APPLICATIONS

a. In a back dive in the pike position, the diver should wait until the legs have rotated past the vertical before the pike is opened. As the trunk and arms move back, the legs will react in the opposite direction and therefore move back to the vertical position.

b. A reverse dive layout with a one-half twist (Figure 17–7) may be performed by initiating the twist in the air rather than from the board. The diver will cause the body to twist to the opposite direction by moving one arm across the chest after the body is in a layout position in the air. The arm must then be moved overhead, keeping it close to the body so that another equal and opposite reaction does not occur. This method for initiating a twist is slow and is not usually used for more than a half-twist.

Principle VI

A performer who is rotating about a horizontal axis in the air may initiate a twist about a vertical axis by tilting the body to one side.

APPLICATION   In any twisting somersault, a diver can tilt to the side by moving one arm from the side horizontal to a position over the head and the other arm sideward downward across the body. This happens because of action-reaction. As the arms move in one direction in the frontal plane, the body moves in the other direction. The twist will occur in the direction of the raised arm and be directly proportional to the spin. That is, the faster the performer is rotating forward or backward, the faster will be the twist (Figures 17–6 and 17–8).

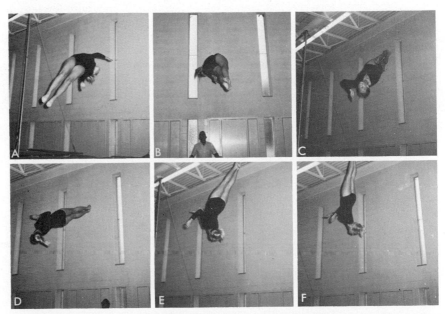

Figure 17–8.   Double twisting back somersault. (Judi Ford, Miss America, 1969; Junior Women's National A. A. U. Trampoline Champion, 1968. Courtesy of Mrs. Virgil Ford.)

Analysis of Suspension and Nonsupport Movements

Movements from both categories are so numerous, particularly in gymnastics or diving, that it would be impossible to analyze them all. The movements selected for analysis here are chosen as examples to illustrate the further application of principles related either to the body suspended or to the body free of support.

Nonsupport Example

THE REVERSE DIVE LAYOUT WITH ONE-HALF TWIST   A twisting dive is one in which the body makes at least one-half turn about the vertical axis. Twisting dives may be combined with somersaults in the tuck, pike, or layout positions. Divers may face forward and leave the board with a forward spinning action or a backward spinning action (reverse spinning dives). They may also initiate dives from a backward stance and spin backward or forward (inward spinning dives). In the reverse dive layout with a one-half twist pictured in Figure 17–7 the diver starts the dive facing the end of the board. He performs a reverse spinning somersault about a transverse axis in a layout position completing a one-half revolution. At the same time he twists one-half of a revolution about the vertical axis.

Mechanical Essentials   In starting a reverse dive the diver must end the forward approach by pushing backward toward the back end of the board with the feet. The rebounding board will push back with an equal and opposite reaction, causing the legs to move forward. This action of the board causes the reverse spin to develop in the body as the feet and legs move forward and the head and upper trunk rotate backward. It also causes the entire body to move forward away from the board. Because the feet push back against the board in reverse dives and force the body forward, less lean is needed on takeoff than with forward dives, where the feet push forward toward the tip of the board. The amount of rotation (spin) about the transverse axis must be determined in large measure at takeoff in this dive because usual methods of controlling the rate of spin by decreasing the moment of inertia through tucking or piking are not permitted. The angular momentum of the dive is determined and conserved at takeoff and cannot be altered, although some control may be exercised by varying the arch in the back in the initial layout. An increase in the arch will increase the rate of rotation.

The twist in this dive is accomplished through the use of two methods of initiating twists. As the diver leaves the board, he not only pushes back to create the reversed spin, but he also pushes slightly to the right to initiate a twist to the left. Once the diver is in the air the principle of action-reaction is used to complete the twist. As the diver twists to the left the left arm is brought across the chest, causing his body to move in the opposite direction (left) in reaction. He continues to aid the twist by circling the arm down next to the body, close to the axis of rotation. Keeping the head in line with the body and the right arm overhead during the twist decreases the moment of inertia of the rotating body and increases the speed of the twist. Turning the head left toward the water helps in the turn and in the diver's orientation. The diver's twist is completed so that he enters the water with the back to the board and at the point where the center of gravity was predetermined to land the instant the feet left the board. In spite of the spin of the body about both a vertical and a horizontal axis, the body's center of gravity follows a perfect parabolic curve controlled only by the velocity and angle of projection and the downward acceleration of gravity.

The entry of the dive must take into account the fact that the forward rotation of the dive will continue because of the Law of Conservation of Momentum. The stretched position of the body with the arms overhead creates the greatest moment of inertia possible and therefore the slowest rotation, but there is still some rotation. For this reason the diver should continue to turn underwater in the same direction. The angle of entry of the dive should be a natural continuation of the parabolic path of the center of gravity of the body. For reverse dives the entry would be almost vertical.

Anatomical Essentials As with all dives from a diving board, this dive requires good strength, flexibility, and control, particularly in the trunk and legs. Good range of motion in the ankle joint is essential since the feet contact the end of the board, dorsiflex as the board is depressed, and then ride it upward and extend until the toes leave the board. Strength in the extensors of the hip and knee are also important in lifting the body from the board and maintaining the extended position in the air. Strength of the abdominals and back extensors is of prime importance to divers. Vertical alignment in the air relies on control by these muscles, as does the entry position. The abdominals also are important in the initiation and control of rotations, and in the prevention of overarching the back. Contrary to popular belief, extreme extension mobility of the back is not desirable in dives and should be avoided. In the dive described here, overarching would decrease the height of the dive and slow the twist, as it causes an increase in the moment of inertia about the vertical axis. Flexibility of the back and hips for full flexion in tuck and pike positions is desirable, however.

Suspension Example

HALF-TURN FLYING HIP CIRCLE WITH HECHT DISMOUNT—UNEVEN PARALLEL BARS Gymnasts who perform on the uneven parallel bars have numerous combinations of movements from which to choose. Each routine starts with a mount and concludes with a dismount. In between the gymnast selects from a series of movements, including those characterized as circling, swinging, or kipping movements. Grip release and regrasps must also be incorporated. Movements are classified as being of medium or superior difficulty, and each performance should contain four medium and two superior moves in its 12 to 14 moves. The moves shown in Figure 17–9 and described here are of medium difficulty. The gymnast starts in a handstand position on the high bar (A). As she begins to swing downward she performs a half-twist so that she faces in the direction of the swing (B, C). At the bottom of the swing she begins to flex at the hips in preparation for continuing in a back hip circle around the low bar (D, E). Toward the end of the hip circle she extends at the hip joint and dismounts forward over the low bar in a move called a *hecht* (F, G). She lands with the back to the bars (H).

Mechanical Essentials In starting the downward swing from the handstand position the gymnast pushes against the bar. Because of action-reaction the bar pushes back in the opposite direction. The give of the bar adds to the reactive force and thus increases the total energy of the system. The push of the gymnast backward and the accompanying stretch increase the distance between the center of gravity and the axis of rotation and thus increase the torque on the downward swing. The time for gravity to act on the downward swinging body is also increased. The half-twist is performed at the beginning of the downswing when the forces acting on the hands are minimal and the grip change can be accomplished with ease (B). At the bottom of the swing the gymnast flexes at the hips, thus shortening the radius of rotation and increasing her angular velocity on the upswing. This piked position also enables her

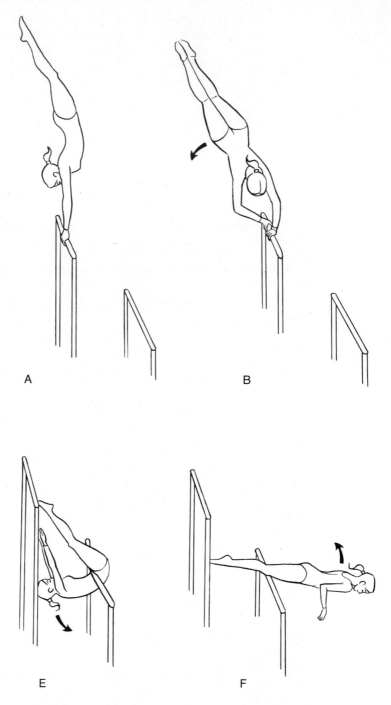

Figure 17–9   Half-turn flying hip circle with hecht dismount. (Drawn from motion picture film tracings.)

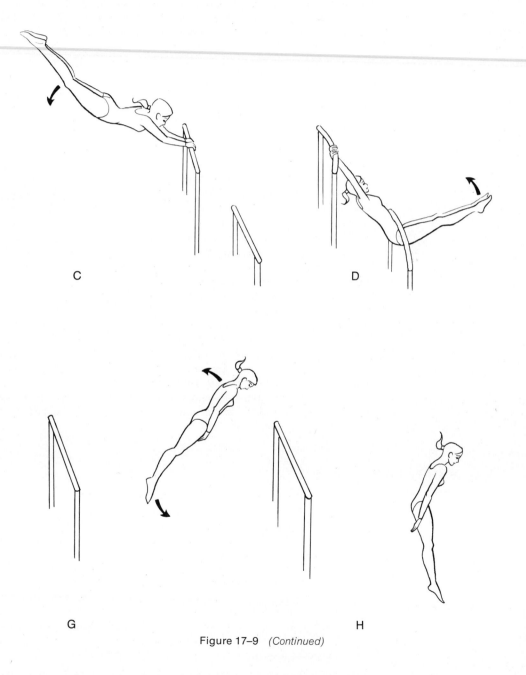

C

D

G

H

Figure 17–9   *(Continued)*

to "wrap" around the low bar as she moves into the backward hip circle (D). There should be no pause between one movement and the next. Any slowing down would require more energy to pick up again (law of inertia) and fluidity would be lost. As the gymnast's hands leave the high bar, she pushes up and forward, causing the reactive force to add to the downward trunk rotation (E).

The hip circle should be accomplished with the hips close to the bar so that the center of gravity is near the axis of rotation. Otherwise, centrifugal force would tend to pull the body away from the bar. Toward the completion of the hip circle the gymnast forcefully extends by lifting the upper trunk and arms foward and upward (F). This action causes several things to happen. In reaction, the legs also extend so that the whole body is straight. The moment of inertia about the transverse axis is increased, and the rate of rotation decreases. The body pushes down and back against the bar causing the bar to push the body forward and up. All of this results in the body rotating up and away from the bar for the dismount. Once the body has left the bar the back should be arched to again decrease the radius slightly and aid in the rotation of the body, allowing the feet to move slightly ahead of the center of gravity at the moment of landing (H). The success of the hecht dismount depends upon sufficient angular momentum being developed in the downswing and hip circle and a forceful, properly timed extension of the body at the end of the hip circle.

Anatomical Essentials   The anatomical essentials for successful performance in this movement series are strength and flexibility. Strength of the shoulders, arms, and hands is especially important for swinging movements. Grip strength is essential, and until one is sure of such strength certain swinging movements should not be attempted without the assistance of a spotter. Arm and shoulder strength can be checked by testing onself with push-ups and pull-ups. According to Frederick (1969) beginning gymnasts should be capable of doing at least one of each. Strong abdominal and back extensor muscles are also important. These muscle groups play a significant role in maintaining and changing the trunk position in the downward swing, the hip circle, and the hecht dismount as shown here. Range of motion is also needed for these movements, particularly in the shoulder during the swing, and in the hip and lower back during the pike of the hip circle.

Laboratory Experiences

1. Observe a partner perform the following moves on a trampoline. In each instance identify the underlying principles which explain the resulting action.
   a. Jump straight up and down a few times. At the peak of a jump, try to move forward so that upon landing you are 6 inches in front of your previous landing spot. Do *not* initiate your forward move until you are in the air.
   b. At the peak of a vertical jump, move one arm sharply across the front of the body. Observe the effect on the rest of the body.
   c. Perform a swivel hips. Observe the action of the head, arms, hips, and feet. Explain how and why these actions contribute to the successful completion of the swivel hips.
   d. Initate a 90-degree turn from the trampoline bed. Next, perform a 6-inch jump forward, backward, and sideward. Note the direction in which the feet push against the bed of the trampoline in each move.

2. Hang motionless from a rope or a pair of rings. Now start swinging without the help of anyone else. How was the swing accomplished? Explain.

3. Swing on a pair of rings without attempting to get much height. Perform the following movements. Explain the results in terms of the underlying principles. Be sure to have mats placed under the swinging area.
    a. Reverse the grasp of one hand. At what point in the swing is this accomplished most easily?
    b. Dismount at various positions along the arc of the swing. Note the effect on the body.

4. Perform the following movements in the water and explain the actions in terms of underlying principles. (Except for the factor of increased resistance, the actions simulate those of an unsupported body.)
    a. Lie on the side and swing both legs forward vigorously, keeping the knees straight. Note the effect on the trunk.
    b. Lie on the back with the arms in a side horizontal position. Keeping the elbows straight, swing both arms in a clockwise direction across the surface of the water in a 90-degree arc as you roll to the right into a prone float. Note the direction in which the feet now point compared to the starting position.

References

Batterman, C. 1968. *The techniques of springboard diving*. Cambridge: MIT Press.

Borms, J., et al. 1976. Biomechanical study of forward and backward giant swings. In *Biomechanics V-B,* ed. P. V. Komi, Baltimore: University Park Press, pp 309–13.

Bowers, C. O., Fie, J. U., Kjeldsen, K., and Schmid, A. B. 1972. *Judging and coaching women's gymnastics*. Palo Alto: National Press.

Bunn, J. W. 1972. *Scientific principles of coaching,* 2d ed. Englewood Cliffs, N.J.: Prentice-Hall.

Cooper, J. M., and Glassow, R. B. 1972. *Kinesiology,* 3d ed. St. Louis: C. V. Mosby.

Dyson, G. 1970. *The mechanics of athletics,* 5th ed. London: University of London Press.

Fairbanks, A. R. 1963. *Teaching springboard diving*. Englewood Cliffs, N.J.: Prentice-Hall.

Frederick, A. B. 1966. *Women's gymnastics*. Dubuque, Iowa: William C. Brown.

Frederick, A. B. 1969. *Gymnastics for men*. Dubuque, Iowa: William C. Brown.

Hay, J. G. 1978. *The biomechanics of sports techniques,* 2d ed. Englewood Cliffs, N.J.: Prentice-Hall.

Jensen, C. R., and Schultz, G. W. 1970. *Applied kinesiology*. New York: McGraw-Hill.

Zinkovsky, A., et al. 1978. Biomechanical analysis of the formation of gymnastic skill. In *Biomechanics V-B,* ed. P. V. Komi, pp. 322–25. Baltimore: University Park Press.

Moving One's Body When It Is Supported by Water

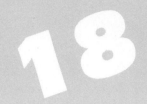

Objectives

At the conclusion of this chapter, the student should be able to:

1. Name those factors that contribute to the propulsion of a swimmer.
2. Name those factors that impede the progress of a swimmer.
3. Explain how the propulsive and resistive factors named affect the length or frequency of a swimming stroke.
4. Analyze the performance of a swimmer in a racing stroke by identifying the anatomical and mechanical factors important to success in the selected stroke, as well as those factors that appear to limit the particular performance.

Aquatic Locomotion: Swimming

The problem of moving the body through the water is fundamentally not so different from that of moving it on land. As in walking, it is necessary to push against something in order to move the body from one place to another. The chief differences between locomotion in the water and locomotion on land are that (1) in the water the body is concerned with buoyancy rather than with the force of gravity, (2) the substance against which it pushes affords less resistance to the push, (3) the medium through which it moves affords more resistance to the body, and (4) as a means of getting the greatest benefit from the buoyancy and of reducing the resistance afforded by the water, it is customary to maintain a horizontal, rather than a vertical, position. (Review the discussion of buoyancy on pages 334 to 336). The practical problem in swimming is not to keep from sinking, as novices are inclined to believe, but to get the mouth out of the water at rhythmic intervals in order to permit regular breathing. This is a matter of coordination, not buoyancy.

In swimming, as in all motion, the initial mechanical problem is to overcome the inertia of the body. Once the body is in motion, the problem is to overcome the forces that tend to hinder it. In terrestrial locomotion the body exerts its force against the supporting surface—the ground—in order to overcome inertia. The forces resisting the progress of the body are the force of gravity and air resistance. In aquatic locomotion the water is both the supporting medium and the source of resistance. In swimming, the hands and feet depend upon the counterpressure of the water in order that the force may be transmitted to the body. Yet, at the same time, the body must overcome the resistance afforded by the water.

The speed obtained in swimming any stroke depends upon the stroke length and stroke frequency. The *length* of the stroke is the result of the forces that move the swimmer forward in reaction to the movements of the arms and legs, and of the resistance of the water in the opposite direction. In the front crawl the arms are the primary source of power, while in the breast stroke the legs dominate. Regardless of the stroke the actions of the arms and legs appear to result in a combination of lift and drag forces that then propel the body forward.

There are four different types of water resistance that act to decrease the stroke length. *Frontal* or *head-on drag* is the resistance due to the surface area of the front of the body as it meets the oncoming water. This type of resistance has the greatest effect on retarding the swimmer. Streamlining the body by changing its position in the water decreases frontal resistance. *Surface drag* is caused by the resistance of the water next to the body. Although it has little effect on the forward progress of swimmers, they have been known to shave the hair from their bodies as a means of decreasing skin friction. A third form of drag is that which occurs at the surface as the body moves along, partially in water and partially in air. The *waves* caused form an additional resistance to forward progress. The amount of this resistance depends upon both the speed and movements of the body as it progresses through the water. A fourth but minor resistance is *suction* or *eddy* resistance that forms behind the body, causing it to pull some water along with it.

The *frequency* of the stroke depends upon the amount of time spent per stroke cycle. This in turn is related to the nature of the stroke pattern and the muscle torques of the arms and legs. Thus, the major problem in the mechanics of swimming is the minimization of the resistance due to the water, which is either pushed out of the way or dragged along, and the advantageous application of the force of the arms and legs. The swimmer reduces resistance by streamlining the body position through relaxing in the recovery phase of the stroke and by eliminating useless motion and tensions. The propulsive force is increased with improvements in technique and conditioning.

Principles Applied to Swimming

Principle I

Less force is needed to keep an object moving than to overcome its inertia.

APPLICATION   Force in swimming should be applied so that the progress through the water is even rather than consisting of cycles of speeding up and slowing down. In the front crawl, the beginning of one arm pull should start before the other arm finishes its pull. In strokes such as the breast stroke and side stroke, too long a glide will result in a reduction in momentum and the need to expend extra energy to overcome inertia in starting up again.

Principle II

The body will move in the opposite direction from that in which the force is applied. For instance, a backward thrust will send the body forward, downward pressure will lift it, and pressure to the right will send it to the left.

APPLICATION   In the crawl stroke, too much force at the beginning of the arc will have too great a downward component, thereby tending to lift the body. This increases resistance and is a needless expenditure of energy. In a similar manner, a wide recovery of the arm in the front crawl or back crawl will result in an opposite lateral reaction in the legs, and thus cause additional resistance. In the breast stroke, the two arms balance each other; hence, too great an outward force at the beginning of the stroke or inward force at the end of the stroke does not produce lateral motion but results in a waste of energy.

Principle III

Maximum force is attained by presenting as broad a surface as possible in the propulsive movements of the limbs and by exerting a backward pressure through as great a distance as possible, provided undesirable forces are not inadvertently introduced.

APPLICATIONS
  a. The full surface of the hand should be used.
  b. The use of fins increases the force of the leg stroke.
  c. The hand should not enter the water so soon that it shortens the stroke unduly. In the crawl stroke care must be taken not to reach too far, however, as this involves lifting the shoulder and is likely to introduce a lateral force acting on the trunk.

Principle IV

Momentum may be transferred from one body or part to another body or part as momentum is conserved.

APPLICATION   If the breast stroker or backstroker checks the momentum of the arms at the end of the recovery, the momentum will be transferred to the body, forcing the head and body downward and thus setting up a bobbing stroke and additional resistance.

Principle V

The height of the body position in the water depends upon the swimmer's buoyancy and speed of moving through the water.

APPLICATION   Even though a "high" position in the water will have less drag resistance, the swimmer can do nothing about achieving it. The buoyancy of a swimmer is determined by body composition and cannot be changed. Swimmers should not try to ride high in the water by raising the head or pushing down, because each action will be followed by an opposite reaction and additional wave resistance due to the bobbing.

Principle VI

A rapidly moving body in the water leaves a low pressure area immediately behind it. This creates a suction effect and tends to pull the body back.

APPLICATION   Although this backward pull cannot be entirely eliminated, it can be reduced in the crawl stroke by keeping the feet close together.

Principle VII

When a body is free in a fluid, movement of a part in one direction results in movement of the rest of the body in the opposite direction.

APPLICATION   Swimming with the head out of water, as in water polo, lifesaving, or synchronized swimming causes the feet to drop. This position produces more frontal drag than the flat horizontal position and therefore requires more energy on the swimmer's part to overcome the additional resistance.

Principle VIII

The sudden or quick movement of a swimmer's body, or one of its parts, at the surface of the water tends to cause whirls and eddies. These create low pressure areas that have a retarding effect on the swimmer.

APPLICATION   The low pressure areas can be reduced by slicing the hand into the water and by eliminating movements which do not contribute to forward progression. In the flutter kick, movements of the feet in the air do not contribute to the propulsion of the body; hence, the feet and legs should be kept just below the surface of the water.

Principle IX

The more streamlined the body, the less the resistance to progress through the water.

APPLICATIONS
The streamlining of the body in the crawl stroke is accomplished by five actions.
  a. Carrying the head so that the water level is somewhere near the hairline, depending upon the buoyancy and speed of the swimmer.
  b. Carrying the body parallel with the surface of the water.
  c. Carrying the buttocks just below the surface of the water.
  d. Keeping the legs, ankles, and feet close together.
  e. Wearing a smooth, tight-fitting suit.

Principle X

The resistance of a body in any fluid increases approximately with the square of the velocity.

APPLICATIONS
  a. The underwater recovery phase of the arms in the breast stroke or elementary backstroke should not be rushed. Too rapid a movement will add unnecessarily to the resistance to forward movement.
  b. The entry of the recovery arm in the front or back crawl should not be rushed. Because it is moving in a direction opposite the forward progress of the swimmer, the rapid entry serves to increase the resistance. The speed of the recovery should be close to that of the pull.

The Sprint Crawl

As an example of aquatic locomotion, the sprint crawl (Figure 18–1) has been chosen for analysis. The position of the head and trunk and the movement of the head in breathing are described briefly. The arm and leg strokes are described in somewhat greater detail, and their propulsive phases are analyzed anatomically.

The Head and Trunk

The head and trunk have three important functions in swimming, particularly in speed swimming. These are minimizing resistance, enabling the swimmer to breathe, and providing a stable anchorage for the arm and leg muscles to effect a maximum propulsive force. The position of the body is the key to reducing resistance. The body is as horizontal as possible, with the feet below the surface and the head breaking the water at hairline level. The flatter the body the less drag there will be to decrease the swimmer's speed. The exact position of the body varies with the anatomical build and buoyancy of the individual, as well as with the speed of the stroke. The greater the buoyancy and speed, the higher the body will ride in the water. A common mistake is to lift the head too much. If the head is held too high or tipped back too far, it makes

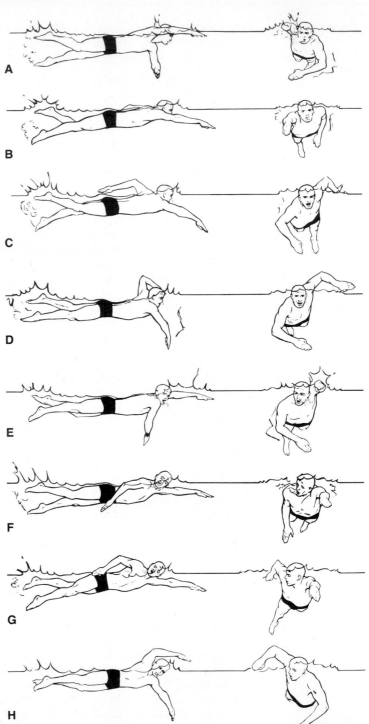

Figure 18–1   The crawl stroke. (From James E. Counsilman: *The Science of Swimming*, © 1968, pp. 61–65. Reprinted by permission of Prentice-Hall, Inc., Englewood Cliffs, N.J.)

the swimmer's legs drop, causing a broader frontal surface and therefore more resistance. Armbruster et al. (1968) emphasize the importance of keeping the chin and nose in the midplane of the body in order to keep the body on a even keel. By static contraction of the rectus abdominis the spine is held in a position of slight flexion—or at least of incomplete extension—and the pelvis in a position of slightly decreased inclination.

Lateral movements of the trunk will also increase the resistance to forward movements and should be minimized. Any circular movement of the arms or legs causes a countermovement in the rest of the body. A wide swing of the arms on recovery produces a lateral, opposite fishtail action of the legs. Lateral flexion of the head and neck also results in a counteraction. The turning of the head for inhaling must be accomplished with the least possible interference with the rhythm of the arm and leg action and with the progress of the body through the water. It is essential not to lift the head for breathing but rather to rotate it on its longitudinal axis while at the same time tucking the chin in close to the side of the neck. In this position the face appears to be resting on the bow wave, and the mouth is just above the surface of the water. After a quick inhalation the face is again turned forward with the eyes in the horizontal plane and the nose and chin in the midsagittal plane of the body. Although breathing with every arm cycle is preferable in distance events, sprints are better swum with fewer breathing cycles since the turning of the head, even when done properly, causes additional resistance.

In order to provide a firm base of attachment for the muscles of the arms and thighs the trunk must be held steady. By the alternating action of the left and right oblique abdominals and spinal extensors, the spine and pelvis are stabilized against the pull of the shoulder and hip muscles. Thus, they permit the latter to exert all their force on the limbs for the propulsive movements.

The Arm Stroke

ENTRY AND SUPPORT Since the arm stroke provides approximately 85 percent of the total power, it is most important that the entry of the arm into the water should place it in the most advantageous position for exerting force that will be effective in driving the body forward. Its position on entry is with the forearm high and the elbow pointing to the side. The hand passes in front of the shoulder in preparation for the entry and then, reaching forward, it is driven forward and downward into the water directly in front of the shoulder. The elbow is slightly flexed at the beginning of the hand entry but extends during the entry. The brief moment between entry and the beginning of the chief propulsive action is known as the *support phase*, and its purpose is to keep the head and shoulders above the surface. The pressure of the forearm and hand is mostly downward and then backward, thus producing an upward and forward reactive force (Figure 18–1A, B).

CATCH, PULL, AND PUSH The moment at which the chief propulsive action changes from downward to backward constitutes the catch. This occurs when the hand is 5 to 10 inches below the surface and involves a quick inward movement of the hand and arm that serves to bring the hand to a position in front of the axis of the body in such a way that the body weight is balanced above the arm. The upper arm is approximately vertical, a position that favors the large muscles (sternal portion of the pectoralis major and latissimus dorsi) for their task of pulling the arm downward and backward. Since the purpose of the stroke is to drive the body forward, it is essential to apply maximum force over the longest possible distance. This is best done by keeping the elbow high during the first part of the pull and by bending the elbow as the arm is pulled under the body (Figure 18–1C, D). The maximum bend occurs halfway through the pull, when the hand begins to push the water backward. Armbruster et al. (1968) give the following three reasons for flexing the elbow during the pull:

1.   It permits the hand and forearm to assume a position in which they can exert their force more nearly in line with the body's long axis.
2.   It shortens the lever arm and thus permits greater speed with less energy expenditure.
3.   It favors the transition from pull to push.

The transition from pull to push occurs as the arm passes under the shoulder. The upper arm remains nearly vertical as the forearm gradually extends until it is in front of the hip, at which time the upper arm extends and the hand gives a quick push backward (Figure 18–1E, F).

It would seem that the ideal direction of the swimmer's force should be directly backward for maximum forward horizontal movement. In actuality the path of the hand of most good swimmers is more like an inverted question mark. Counsilman (1968) suggests that one reason for the lateral part of the pull is to counteract opposing lateral forces in another part of the stroke. Another reason may be to get the hand in position to push the water in a line parallel to the longitudinal axis of the body throughout the entire pull phase. There is also increasing evidence that lift plays an important part in propulsion in all four basic strokes (Hay, 1978; Lundholm and Ruttieri, 1976). For lift to occur the hand would have to be at an angle to the direction of water flow (see Bernouilli's principle, p. 337), and the hand would have to be moving laterally with respect to the path of the body. In studying the butterfly stroke, Barthels and Adrian (1975) concluded that both lift and drag contributed to the propulsion: lift during the insweep and drag during the push. They also observed that some angle of attack in the hands was maintained throughout the stroke.

BRIEF ANATOMICAL ANALYSIS OF PROPULSIVE PHASE OF ARM STROKE

Shoulder Joint   Strong extension, inward rotation, slight "horizontal" flexion-adduction in oblique plane, followed by continued extension and possibly slight hyperextension. Muscles: Latissimus dorsi, teres major, sternal portion of pectoralis major, posterior deltoid.

Shoulder Girdle   Downward rotation, adduction, slight upward tilt. Muscles: Rhomboids and pectoralis minor.

Elbow and Radioulnar Joints   Flexion, slight pronation; partial extension toward end. Muscles: (flexors) brachialis, brachioradialis, probably biceps brachii because of resistance; (pronators) pronator teres, pronator quadratus; (extensors) triceps, anconeus.

Wrist   Held in midposition, possibly slight flexion toward end of propulsion. Muscles: Palmaris longus, flexor carpi radialis (longus and brevis), flexor carpi ulnaris.

Fingers   Held in extension and adduction. Muscles: Probably flexors and adductors in static contraction.

RELEASE AND RECOVERY   The elbow is now near the surface with the hand slightly lower and posterior to it and the palm facing mostly upward. The pressure of the forearm and hand now being relaxed, the elbow and shoulder are raised until the hand is out of the water. As this occurs, the palm turns toward the body. The elbow leaves the water first and swings forward and upward with the hand trailing behind it, moving from a position near the hip to a position in front of the shoulder, preparatory to a new entry (Figure 18–1G, H). The movement of the arm from release to the completion of recovery is continuous. It is important that no break occur, since this would mean a loss of momentum and would necessitate an additional force for overcoming inertia, or at least for regaining the lost velocity.

As the elbow is brought forward it remains above the level of the hand throughout the recovery and entry, the forearm being virtually horizontal as the arm moves forward past the shoulder and the hand staying in line with the forearm. Finally, as the hand passes the head, the arm reaches forward in preparation for the entry, the shoulder girdle remains high, the tip of the elbow is above shoulder level pointing to the side, and the forearm then points downward from the elbow with the wrist slightly flexed, the palm facing the water, and the fingers aiming forward and downward into the water.

Armbruster et al. (1968) mention that there are various other styles of arm recovery in the crawl stroke, the chief differences being in the position of the elbow. Counsilman (1968) also discusses various forms of arm recovery and attributes the variety to variations in shoulder flexibility. He even goes so far as to express the opinion that if all swimmers had equal degrees of flexibility they might all use similar recoveries.

BRIEF ANATOMICAL ANALYSIS OF RECOVERY PHASE OF ARM STROKE

Shoulder Joint   Hyperextension followed by horizontal flexion. Muscles: posterior deltoid, teres major, and latissimus dorsi, followed by pectoralis major, anterior deltoid, coracobrachialis, and biceps. After the initial contraction, the momentum of the action continues it in a modified ballistic manner.

Shoulder Girdle   Slight elevation, upward rotation, and abduction. Muscles: trapezius, serratus anterior, and pectoralis minor.

Elbow   Extension. Muscles: triceps.

Wrist and Fingers   Relaxed flexion until end of phase, when there is slight extension. Muscles: Extensor carpi radialis brevis, extensor carpi ulnaris, extensors digitorum indices and digiti minimi, the pollicis longus, and the intrinsic hand muscles.

The Leg Stroke

NATURE OF MOVEMENT   The leg stroke most often used in the sprint crawl is the flutter kick. Whether or not it contributes to the propulsive force has been questioned. Counsilman (1968) believes that the primary role for the kick is that of a stabilizer and neutralizer, and that therefore its timing with respect to the arms' action is critical. In this stroke the legs are relatively close together as they alternate in an up and down movement, with the feet attaining a maximum stride of about 1 to 2 feet. The width of the kick depends upon such factors as the swimmer's build and strength and the speed of the stroke. In both the upstroke and downstroke the movement, described as whiplike or lashing, starts at the hip joint and progresses through the knees to the ankle and feet. Unlike the arms, whose movements alternate between propulsion and recovery, both phases of the leg stroke are propulsive, if anything. Flexibility in the ankles is important in the kick, and those with a greater range of plantar flexion have an advantage. In the downstroke the thrust is downward and backward and, in the upstroke, upward and backward.

DOWNSTROKE   The downstroke begins with a downward drive of the thigh. The thigh flexes only slightly and the knee, which was in a position of flexion at the completion of the upstroke, extends completely by the end of the downward movement. The ankle and foot remain in plantar flexion, probably being held in this position by the pressure of the water against the dorsal surface of the foot (Figure 18–1 A, B). It seems likely that the dorsiflexors contract statically to stabilize the foot against this pressure. Throughout the downstroke the foot remains in a slight toeing-in position. Armbruster et al. (1968) warn that the heels should not be allowed to drift apart in an attempt to facilitate the in-toeing, since this would involve rotation of the thigh and would cut down on the driving power of the limb.

BRIEF ANATOMICAL ANALYSIS OF DOWNSTROKE

Hip Joint   Partial flexion. Muscles: Iliopsoas, tensor fasciae latae, pectineus, sartorius, and gracilis.

Knee Joint   Strong extension. Muscles: Quadriceps femoris.

Ankle Joint   Incomplete plantar flexion probably caused by pressure of water. Muscles: Tibialis anterior, peroneus tertius, extensor digitorum longus, and extensor hallucis longus may contract statically to stabilize foot against pressure of water.

Tarsal Joints   Adduction and inversion. Muscles: Tibialis posterior and anterior, flexor digitorum longus, and flexor hallucis longus.

UPSTROKE   At the completion of the downstroke the thigh is in a position of slight flexion, the knee is completely extended, the ankle is incompletely plantar-flexed. The upstroke begins with thigh extension. Slight knee flexion develops near the end of the stroke at the same time the opposite leg is finishing the downstroke. The movements of the three major segments of the lower extremity are forceful in the upstroke but are under such good control that the foot stops just below the surface of the water. To break through the surface constitutes a major error as it causes an immediate reduction in propulsive force (Figure 18–1 D–F).

BRIEF ANATOMICAL ANALYSIS OF UPSTROKE

Hip Joint   Strong extension. Muscles: Hamstrings and gluteus maximus.

Knee Joint   Slight flexion against resistance. Muscles: Hamstrings, sartorius, gracilis, popliteus, and gastrocnemius.

Ankle Joint   Plantar flexion. Muscles: Gastrocnemius, soleus, peroneus longus and brevis, tibialis posterior, flexor digitorum longus, and flexor hallucis longus.

Tarsal Joints   Plantar flexion, especially in final part of stroke. Muscles: Peroneus longus and brevis, tibialis posterior, flexor digitorum longus, and flexor hallucis longus.

Additional Factors

Other factors of importance to the crawl-stroke swimmer and to the coach are the timing and coordination of the arm and leg strokes and of the breathing, the rhythm of the stroke as a whole, the relaxation of the body, and the flexibility of the joints, particularly of the shoulders and ankles. Of these, possibly the last named is of greatest interest to the kinesiologist. The serious swimmer will want to know how to increase the range of motion in the shoulder joints and ankles—that is, how to stretch the pectorals and anterior ligaments of the shoulders and how to gain greater plantar flexion of the feet. Armbruster et al. (1968) and Counsilman (1968) have both suggested a few exercises for these purposes. The kinesiology student should be able to originate several others.

Sample Analysis of a Common Fault in the Crawl Stroke

A *rigid flutter kick* is a common fault of beginners learning the standard crawl stroke. This was analyzed by Vollmer (1951) as part of a graduate project at Wellesley College.* It is included in this text as an example of how the kinesiologist can analyze a common fault and use the analysis as a basis for making constructive suggestions in teaching.

DESCRIPTION   In the rigid flutter kick the movement is one of alternate flexion and extension of the entire lower extremity, with the movement confined to the hip joint instead of being transmitted successively through the thigh to the knee joint and thence through the leg to the ankle and foot. The knee joints are fully extended throughout the kick, and the feet and ankles are held in an unchanging position of plantar flexion, the exact degree of this flexion varying with individuals. This results in a narrower kick. A rigid flutter kick is obviously less efficient than the correct kick. In brief, the rigid flutter kick deviates from the correct form in that there is an absence of knee and ankle flexion, an absence of relaxation at the end of the downkick or beginning of the upkick, and an absence of fishtail action of the sole of the foot against the water.

ANATOMICAL ANALYSIS   In the correct downkick the upward pressure of the water against the lower leg causes flexion at the knee. In the rigid kick, however, this is prevented by the tension of the quadriceps extensors. Normally, the slight flexion at the knee is followed by extension during the course of the downstroke but, when the knee is already rigidly extended, this extension cannot take place. Similarly, the reduction of plantar flexion which should take place at the end of the downstroke fails to occur because of the continuous contraction of the plantar flexor muscles (soleus, peroneus longus and brevis, tibialis posterior, flexor digitorum longus, and flexor hallucis longus).

In the upstroke the tension of the quadriceps extensors again prevents the slight knee flexion which occurs when the kick is correctly performed (see Figure 18–1). Throughout the stroke the extensors of the lower back and the abdominal muscles contract to stabilize the pelvis against the pull of the hip flexors and extensors. Normally they relax momentarily just before the legs reverse their direction. The tension in the muscles of the lower extremities spreads to these, however, and the excess tension of these muscles causes interference with the action of the diaphragm. This, in turn, results in less efficient breathing and is an additional factor in causing fatigue.

MECHANICAL ANALYSIS   The propulsive component of force that drives the body forward is that which pushes the water directly backward. In the downstroke this is provided most effectively by the instep of the foot, and in the upstroke, by the sole. The amount of propulsive force developed depends upon the angle at which the instep and the sole of the foot are held with respect to the surface of the water. In the upstroke the best angle for the sole of the foot is possible only when the knee is flexed. In the rigid kick the knee is straight, and the sole of the foot is therefore not in the best position for providing propulsive force.

In the correct form each limb acts as a series of levers—thigh, lower leg, and foot—but in the rigid kick each limb acts as one long lever with the force arm extending from the distal attachments of the hip flexors and extensors to the axis of

---

*Used by permission of Mrs. Lola Vollmer Shepherd.

the hip joint. The resistance arm consists of the entire length of the lever from the instep or from the sole of the foot to the hip joint. The force acting on this lever comes solely from the muscles of the hip joints. The muscles of the knee and ankle do not contribute to the motion of this lever, but when the limb is used as a series of levers, they provide additional force.

Inertia must be overcome with each reversal of direction in the kick. Since, in the rigid flutter kick, the stroke is shorter and faster than it should be, the muscles of the hip joint, which have the double task of overcoming both the inertia of the limb and the resistance of the water, are overburdened. They must work harder and faster to meet the demands made on them by the frequent changes of direction and the increased resistance of the water due to the speed of movement. Ordinarily the upstroke has an advantage over the downstroke because, when the stroke is performed correctly, the sole of the foot is in a better position to push back against the water than is the instep on the downstroke. In the rigid kick this advantage is lost.

TEACHING SUGGESTIONS   The rigid crawl flutter kick is associated with undue tension of the quadriceps extensors at the knee joint, and of the plantar flexors at the ankle joint, during the changes of direction in both the downkick and the upkick. There may also be unnecessary tension of the abdominal muscles and the spinal extensors. As the kick is inefficient, it is carried on at a faster rate and through a narrower arc than would be the correct kick for the individual swimmer. Conversely, a rapid, narrow kick tends to be a rigid kick. These factors aid in its recognition. In the teaching of the kick, it would seem the best procedure to insist on a slow, deep kick in the student's first attempts, and to increase the rhythm gradually to the desired rate. Motivation should not be directed toward speed in the performance of the "kick glide" in the teaching progression. Neither is it desirable to emphasize that the legs be held straight at the knees. The emphasis should be put on the increased action at the hips and at the ankles. Furthermore, land drills to increase ankle flexibility seem to be advisable (Spears, 1966).

Aquatic Locomotion: Boating and Canoeing*

On the whole, the principles which apply to swimming apply also to boating and canoeing. This is particularly obvious in canoeing, for the paddle is used in much the same way as are the arms in swimming. The use of the oars in rowing is more limited, since they must be kept in the oarlocks at all times. In paddling, as in the arm movement of the crawl stroke, too much force at the beginning of the stroke has too great a downward component, and hence too great a lifting effect. Conversely, too much force at the end of the stroke has too great an upward component, and hence a depressing effect on the canoe. In order to make the canoe move smoothly in a horizontal direction without unnecessary bobbing up and down, it is essential to

---

*Although it might seem that these activities should be classified with those of giving impetus to an external object, like bicycling, they are forms of locomotion by self-propulsion. The primary purpose of boating and canoeing is locomotion of the self on the water, and the locomotion of the craft is of secondary importance. An additional reason for including the discussion of rowing and paddling in this chapter is that the principles of locomotion in the water are the same, regardless of whether the locomotion is caused by movement of the hands and feet or of oars and paddles.

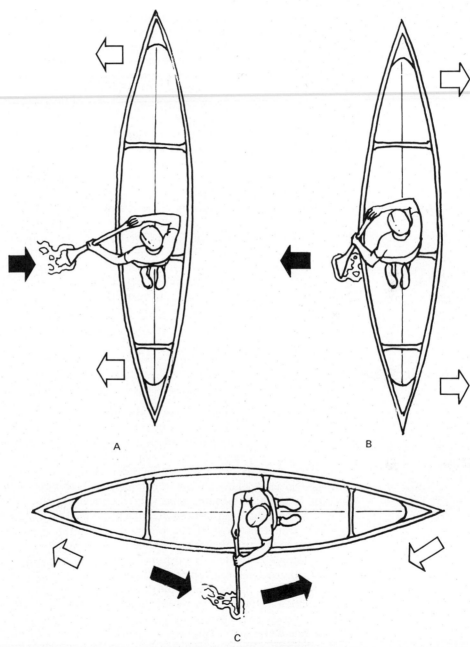

Figure 18-2 Movement in a canoe occurs in the direction opposite to that in which the force is applied. *A,* Movement toward the paddling side occurs when the paddle is *drawn toward* the center of the canoe. *B,* The canoe moves away from the paddling side when the paddle is *pushed away* from the canoe. *C,* The sweep stroke pushes the bow away from the paddling side and draws the stern toward it, causing the canoe to move forward in a sweeping turn away from the paddling side. (Black arrows indicate the path of the paddle, and white arrows indicate the path of the canoe.)

reduce these two components to a minimum and to emphasize the backward movement of the blade.

The techniques of steering the canoe are based on this same principle (Figure 18–2). Assuming that there is only one paddler who is paddling from the center of the canoe, if he wishes to move the canoe broadside to the paddling side, he would put the paddle in the water, blade parallel to the keel, directly opposite the center of the canoe, as far out as he can conveniently and safely reach, and then draw the blade squarely toward him at right angles to the keel of the canoe. If he wishes to move broadside away from the paddling side, he would slice the blade into the water opposite the center of the canoe and close to it, with the blade parallel to the keel, and then push it directly away from him at right angles to the keel. In order to turn the canoe, he would have to reach either forward or backward and press the blade toward or away from the canoe at a point as far from the canoe's center of buoyancy as he can conveniently reach. A drawing stroke nearer the bow would make the canoe turn toward the paddling side; a drawing stroke nearer the stern would make the canoe turn away from the paddling side. (The direction taken by the canoe as a whole is stated in terms of the bow. As the stern of the canoe moves toward the paddling side, the bow moves away from it.) Steering a canoe is logical and simple when one remembers the principle that movement occurs in the direction opposite to that in which the force is applied and, at the same time, remembers that a canoe tends to rotate about its center of buoyancy when force is applied at any point other than one in line with this center.

Aquatic Stunts

Aquatic stunts are an integral part of synchronized swimming or aquatic art. Together, with various aquatic locomotor patterns, they are used to help the swimmer express a theme or idea. Individually, they are used as a measure of the performer's competence in the same manner in which school figures are used in figure skating.

Aquatic stunts are executed in different directions on or below the water's surface. No matter how simple or complex the technique, most of the principles of aquatic locomotion pertain. Especially significant is the principle of reaction. All stunts are brought about by observing the principle that the body moves in a direction opposite from that in which the force is applied to it. A swimmer lying on the back will move in the direction of the head by using the hands to push the water toward the feet, sideways to the left by pushing the water to the right, and toward the feet by pushing the water toward the head (Figure 18–3). Pushing toward the feet with one hand and toward the head with the other causes the swimmer to rotate. To submerge, the direction of the push is toward the surface and, to move toward the surface, the push is downward. The downward action is often used to keep the entire body on the surface while some action such as ballet legs is performed. With the leg out of the water the body's buoyancy is decreased, and the downward body weight must also be opposed with an upward force. The vigorous downward sculling action of the hands causes the equal and opposite force that helps to keep the body on the surface (Figure 18–4).

In the process of performing a stunt, the body may be rotated about the vertical, frontal-horizontal, or sagittal-horizontal axes, and those principles relating to rotating

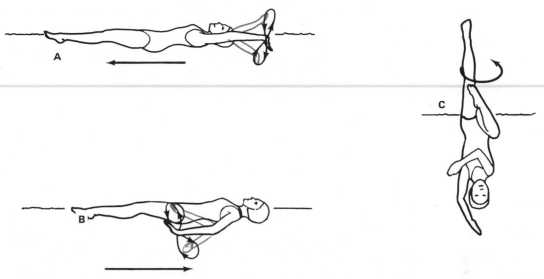

Figure 18–3   The body moves in the direction opposite that in which the force is applied. *A,* The figure-eight sculling action of the arms with the palms facing away from the feet moves the body in the direction of the feet. *B,* The hands face the feet to scull head first. *C,* The swimmer spins to the right by pressing the right forearm across the body toward the left. (Adapted from Lundholm, J., and Ruttieri, M.: *Introduction to synchronized swimming.* Minneapolis: Burgess Publishing, 1976.)

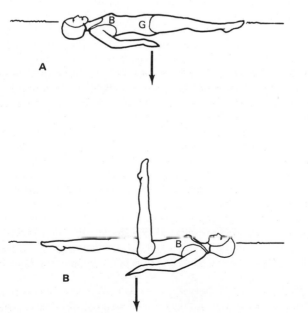

Figure 18–4 Keeping the body on the surface of the water. *A,* A body will rotate around its center of buoyancy (B) unless opposed. The action of the hands against the water provides an upward force that prevents the hips and legs from rotating downward. *B,* The sculling action must increase in intensity when the ballet leg is performed, because additional downward forces of the heavy unsupported leg must be opposed. (Adapted from Lundholm, J., and Ruttieri, M.: *Introduction to synchronized swimming.* Minneapolis: Burgess Publishing, 1976.)

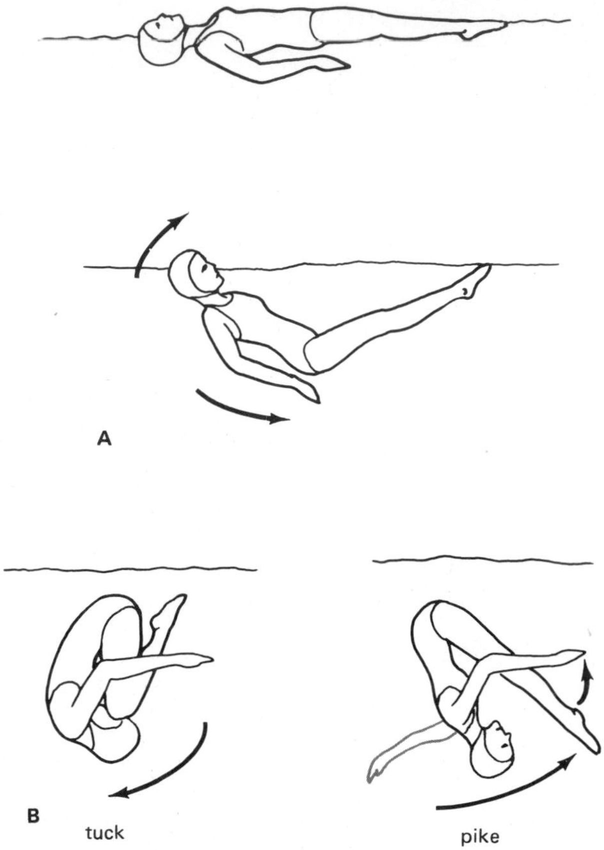

Figure 18–5 Rotating in an aquatic medium. *A*, Action of an unsupported body causes an equal and opposite action of another part. (Lifting of head causes feet to rise and hips to drop.) *B*, Rotating in a tuck position is faster and takes less effort than in a pike position. (Adapted from Lundholm, J., and Ruttieri, M.: *Introduction to synchronized swimming.* Minneapolis: Burgess Publishing, 1976.)

bodies apply. It is important to remember that the body is twisting or rotating in a fluid medium and will therefore behave as a nonsupported rotating body. Movement in one part of the body in one direction results in movement of the rest of the body in the opposite direction (Figure 18–5A). The reaction will also be more evident and slower than in air because water is a denser fluid.

Like all rotating bodies, momentum is conserved in rotating aquatic stunts. The speed of angular rotation of a tuck somersault, for instance, will decrease if it is turned into a pike somersault because the moment of inertia has increased (angular momentum $= I\omega$). It will also take less time to rotate with a short radius than with a long one. Shortening the radius increases the angular velocity and lengthening the radius decreases it (Figure 18–5B).

As the swimmer engages in twists and rotations below the surface of the water disorientation may occur, especially in the inverted position. The usual feeling of weight is absent, and visual cues may be confusing. In addition, the various righting reflexes that rely on gravity to act may be of little use. The stunt performer has to learn to be particularly sensitive to proprioceptive feedback, such as joint position and muscle effort, which will help with the body awareness needed to control the position of the body segments and perform the technique properly.

Laboratory Experiences

1. Do the arm movement of the crawl stroke and deliberately press hard with the hand as soon as it enters the water and, at the end of the stroke, instead of taking the hand out of the water at the proper time, continue the movement of the arm until the hand has pressed upward against the water. What is the effect of these two errors on the body?

2. Observe or perform the following swimming stunts and analyze them in terms of the direction in which the body is moved and the direction of the application of force:
   a. Dolphin.
   b. Side sculling.
   c. Foot foremost surface dive.
   d. Tub.

3. Analyze any of the standard strokes—e.g., breast, side, elementary back, back crawl. Either observe or practice the stroke before analyzing it.

4. Analyze other forms of aquatic locomotion—e.g., paddling and rowing. Either observe or practice each before analyzing it.

5. Analyze the following common faults kinesiologically and suggest coaching points for avoiding or correcting each fault: too wide a pull with the arms in the breast stroke; a short, choppy stroke in paddling; "catching a crab" in rowing (crew style).

References

Armbruster, D. A., Allen, R. H., and Billingsley, H. S. 1968. *Swimming and diving,* 5th ed. St. Louis: C. V. Mosby.

Barthels, K., and Adrian, M. 1975. Three-dimensional spatial hand patterns of skilled butterfly swimmers. In *Swimming II,* ed. L. Lewillie and J. Clarys, pp. 154–60. Baltimore: University Park Press.

Counsilman, J. E. 1968. *The science of swimming.* Englewood Cliffs, N.J.: Prentice-Hall.

Dyson, G. H. G. 1970. *The mechanics of athletics,* 5th ed. London: University of London Press.

Hay, J. 1978. *The biomechanics of sport techniques,* 2d ed. Englewood Cliffs, N.J.: Prentice-Hall.

Lewillie, L. 1971. Graphic and electromyographic analysis of various styles of swimming. In *Biomechanics II,* ed. J. Vredenbregt and J. Wartenweiler, pp. 253–57. Baltimore: University Park Press.

Lundholm, J., and Ruttieri, M. 1976. *Introduction to synchronized swimming.* Minneapolis: Burgess Publishing.

Miller, D. 1975. Biomechanics of swimming. In *Exercise and sport science reviews,* Vol. 3. ed. J. Wilmore and J. Keogh. New York: Academic Press.

Spears, B. 1966. *Fundamentals of synchronized swimming.* Minneapolis: Burgess Publishing.

Vollmer, L. T. 1951. Kinesiological analysis of common faults in selected activities. Unpublished M.A. thesis, Wellesley College.

Welch, J. H.: A kinematic analysis of world-class crawl stroke swimmers. In *Biomechanics IV,* ed. R. Nelson and C. Morehouse, pp. 217–22. Baltimore: University Park Press.

Giving Motion to External Objects

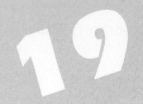

19

Objectives

At the conclusion of this chapter, the student should be able to:

1. Classify activities involving imparting motion to external objects according to the nature of the force application and joint action patterns.
2. Identify the anatomical and mechanical principles that apply to imparting force to external objects.
3. Analyze the performance of someone imparting force to an external object under each of these force application conditions: momentary contact; projection; continuous application.
4. Identify the anatomical and mechanical factors important to optimum performance for each analysis, as well as those factors that appear to limit the particular performance.

Classification of Patterns for Moving Objects

A baseball pitcher throws a baseball across the plate and the batter hits it to center field, a man pushes a lawnmower over the lawn, a school teacher opens the window, a traveler lifts a suitcase and places it on an overhead rack, an archer shoots an arrow from a bow, a boy pitches horseshoes, and a girl practices serving tennis balls against a backboard. As widely diverse as these activities seem, they all have a common denominator. Each involves moving an external object, either directly by some part of the body or by means of an implement held in the hand or hands.

There is an almost endless variety of ways in which an individual may move an object, and there are many factors to consider. For instance, what is the objective in moving it? Is it speed or distance, or perhaps accuracy in reaching a specified target? Is the purpose to project it into the air, to roll or slide it along the ground, or something other than either of these? What part of the body or what kind of implement is used for transmitting motion to the object? Is it the hand, the foot, the head, or some other part of the anatomy, or is it some kind of racket or stick, or perhaps scoop or basketlike structure on the end of a stick? What kind of movement is used and, within this type, what anatomical adjustments are required to meet the needs or limitations of the situation and to achieve the objective? In spite of the numerous ways in which an object can be put into motion, these conveniently fall into only three or four categories. This simplifies the kinesiologist's task of judging them on the bases of their effectiveness and the effect that they have on the body itself.

As an aid to analysis, activities involving imparting force to external objects should be classified according to both the *nature of the force application* and the *joint action patterns*.

Nature of Force Application

MOMENTARY CONTACT   Movements such as striking, hitting, and kicking are characterized by a momentary contact made with an object by a moving part of the body or by an implement held by or attached to a moving segment of the body. The object itself may be either stationary or moving. This category includes all forms of striking, such as hitting with the hand (as in handball or volleyball), striking with a club or racket (as in baseball, golf, and tennis), and kicking and heading (as in soccer) (Figure 19–1).

PROJECTION   This type of force application is characterized by the development of kinetic energy in a movable object that is usually held in the hand or hands or in an implement such as a lacrosse stick, followed by the release of the object at the moment of desired speed and direction (Figure 19–2).

CONTINUOUS APPLICATION   Movements in this category are characterized by the continuous application of force, usually by the hand or hands, but the legs may also be included. These movements are usually of the push-pull type of joint action (Figure 19–3).

A push, pull, or lift may be applied either directly or indirectly to the object. In the latter instance the push or pull pattern is used for the purpose of developing potential energy in an elastic structure, such as a bow or slingshot. When the elastic structure is released, it imparts its force to the movable object, causing the arrow or shot to be projected into the air.

Joint Action Patterns

Broer was perhaps the first to call attention to the similarity of movement patterns used in seemingly dissimilar activities, such as a softball pitch, bowling, and a badminton serve (Broer and Zernicke, 1979). Objective evidence of such similarities between throwing and striking activities within each of the three major upper extremity patterns (overhand, underhand, and sidearm) was revealed by the Broer and Houtz EMG investigations (1907). The investigators also noted that representative activities from these categories showed a greater similarity in the muscular action of the lower extremities than they expected. Similarly, push-pull activities share the same pattern of joint activities. The volleyball pass and the basketball chest pass are examples of two-handed push patterns, while the one-handed set shot, boxing jab, and shot-put are examples of one-handed patterns.

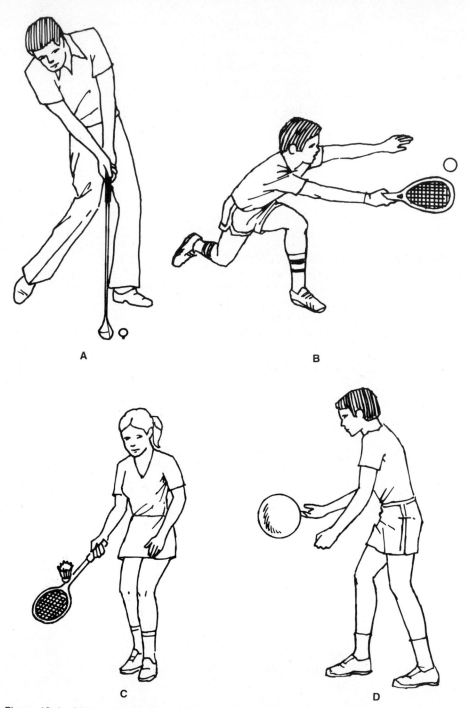

Figure 19–1   Different methods of giving motion to an external object by striking. *A*, Golf drive. *B*, Racketball stroke. *C*, Badminton serve. *D*, Volleyball serve.

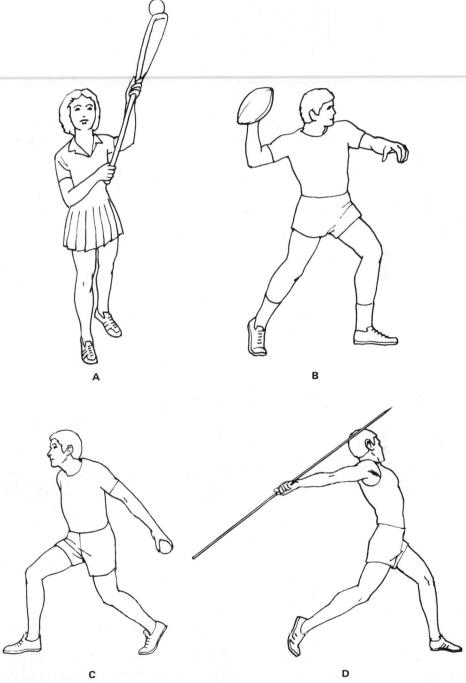

Figure 19–2   Different forms for giving motion to an external object by projection. *A*, Lacrosse throw. *B*, Football pass. *C*, Softball pitch. *D*, Javelin throw.

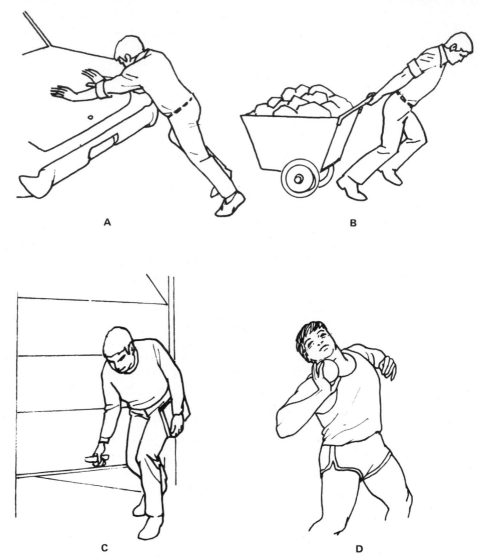

Figure 19–3   Different applications for giving motion to external objects by pushing, pulling, or lifting.

OVERHAND PATTERN   This kind of throw or strike is characterized by rotation at the shoulder joint. In the backswing or preparatory phase the abducted arm rotates laterally, and in the forward or force phase the arm rotates medially. Some elbow extension, wrist flexion, and spinal rotation occur in the force phase. These movements are accompanied by rotation of the pelvis at the hip joint of the opposite limb, resulting in medial rotation of the thigh (Figures 19–4 and 19–5).

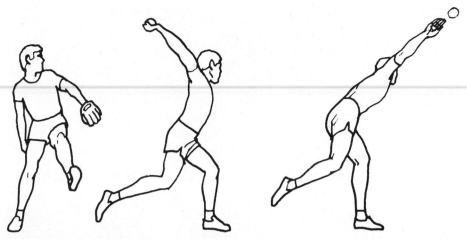

Figure 19–4   Overhand pattern applied in baseball pitch. The forward force phase is character-ized by medial rotation of the arm, elbow extension, spinal rotation, and medial rotation of the pelvis at the contralateral hip joint.

+ wrist flexion

UNDERHAND PATTERN   This pattern consists of a forward movement of the extended arm in the sagittal plane, usually starting from a position of hyperextension and ending in a forward reach. The basic joint action of the arm is flexion. The actions of the wrist, spine, and pelvis are the same as those observed in the overhand pattern.

SIDEARM PATTERN   In this pattern the basic movement is medial rotation of the pelvis on the opposite hip with the arm usually in an abducted position. The arm is moved forward in a horizontal plane due to the pelvic action and spinal rotation. The range of the upper extremity movement may also be enlarged by the addition of horizontal flexion at the shoulder, and by a forward step. The elbow is maintained in

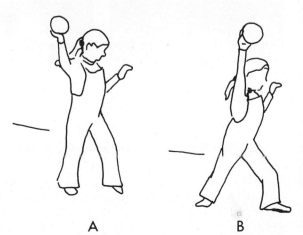

A   B

Figure 19–5   Overhand throw by a girl aged 3 years 10 months who had not been given any di-rections regarding how to throw. Note elbow extension, pelvic ro-tation, step and weight shift. (Drawn from motion picture film tracing.)

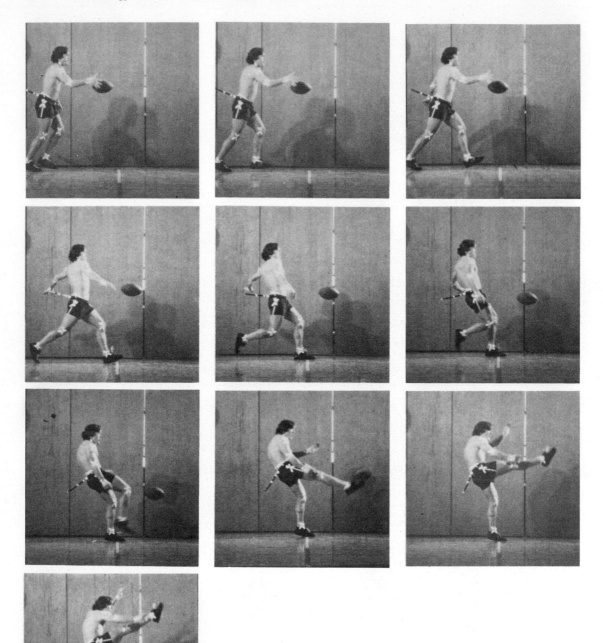

Figure 19–6   The kicking pattern as used in the football punt.

extension or is extended from a slightly flexed position, depending upon the nature of the skill in question (e.g., basketball throw for distance, tennis forehand drive, or batting). Wrist flexion may also be part of the action in some techniques. Indeed, in the badminton drive, it is extremely important.

PUSH-PULL PATTERNS   In this pattern the basic joint actions are flexion and extension in one or more of the extremities. The joint actions in the upper extremities are characterized by flexion and extension in the elbow while the opposite movement is occurring in the shoulder. In the lower extremities extension occurs simultaneously in the hip, knee, and ankle. Movements of this pattern are used for hitting or striking (basketball dribbling), projecting (throwing darts), or continuous force application (weight lifting).

KICKING   The kicking pattern (Figure 19–6) is a modification of a locomotor pattern in which the force imparted to the external object is accomplished during the forward swing of the non-weight-bearing limb. The basic actions are flexion or diagonal adduction at the hip and rotation of the pelvis toward the support leg, followed by vigorous extension at the flexed knee. Movements in this pattern are used primarily in the sports activities of soccer and football.

Table 19–1 summarizes the classification, and presents examples of the patterns used to give motion to external objects.

TABLE 19–1   Classification of Sample Activities According to the Nature of Joint Action Patterns and Force Application

FORCE APPLICATION	JOINT PATTERNS				
	Overhand	Sidearm	Underhand	Push-Pull	Kicking

Momentary contact	Badminton clear
	Volleyball serve
	Tennis serve
	Tennis smash
		Tennis forehand
		  or backhand
		Baseball batting
		Golf drive*
		Racketball
			Polo
			Badminton serve
			Volleyball serve
			Handball
				Boxing jab
				Volleyball pass
				Billiards
				Dribbling
					Football punt
					Football place
					  kick
					Soccer kick

Projection	Football forward
	  pass
	Javelin throw
	Baseball pitch
	Lacrosse throw
		Discus throw
		Shot-put
		Basketball throw
		  for distance
		Jai alai
			Bowling
			Curling
			Horseshoes
			Softball pitch
				Chest pass
				Lay up shot
				Shot-put
				Darts	

Continuous				Weight lifting Rowing and paddling Tackling Archery	

* Although this movement is in a plane similar to that of the underhand pattern, it appears to be more similar to the sidearm patterns in joint action and coordination.

Principles and Applications of Giving Motion

However motion is given, whether by hand, foot, head, or implement, it involves the imparting of force. And force, or effort, is described in terms of its magnitude, direction, and point of application. These three aspects of force provide the basis for the principles that apply to giving motion to external objects, the latter on occasion being other human bodies. Supplementing these aspects are the factors that relate to the stability of the body at the moment of giving motion; those that relate to the interaction between the body and the surface that supports it (for unless the body is stable when it is giving impetus, much of the force is wasted); and those that relate specifically to struck objects. The underlying mechanical principles have been presented in Part Two. Stated briefly in descriptive terms, they are as follows.

Principles Relating to the Magnitude of Force

Principle I

The object will move only if the force is of sufficient magnitude to overcome the object's inertia. The force must be great enough to overcome not only the mass of the object but also all restraining forces. These include (1) friction between the object and the supporting surface, (2) resistance of the surrounding medium (e.g., wind or water), and (3) internal resistance. Warming up helps to prevent injury as well as to decrease resistance. Increasing range of motion through training is also important and effective.

Principle II

The pattern and range of joint movements depends upon the purpose of the movement. If maximum force magnitude is not needed, the optimum movement pattern should be changed with respect to the range, speed, and number of joint actions until it is the most efficient for the task. Throwing a ball to a small child 10 feet away does not require the same pattern as that of pitching a baseball.

Principle III

Force exerted by the body will be transferred to an external object in proportion to the effectiveness of the counterforce of the feet (or other parts of the body) against the ground (or other supporting surface). This effectiveness depends upon the counterpressure and friction presented by the supporting surface. The force applied to a ball thrown while in midair or while treading water is less than that applied to it while pushing against the ground.

Principle IV

Linear velocity is imparted to external objects as a result of the angular velocity of the body segments. The linear velocity at the end of any segment is the product of the angular velocity and the length of the segment. Thus, for a given angular speed, the linear speed imparted to a tennis ball with a tennis racket is much greater than that of a ball hit with the hand. On the other hand, more force is needed to move the longer of the two levers.

Principle V

Optimum summation of internal force is needed if maximum force is to be applied to move an object. For maximum velocity of each contributing body segment to occur at release of, or impact with, the external object, the slower or heavier segments must start to move first and the lightest and quickest ones last. The optimum sequence for a forceful overarm pattern is pelvic rotation, spinal rotation, shoulder motion, elbow extension, wrist flexion, and finger extension. It is quite possible in any of the arm patterns for the slower joints to begin their forward movements while the faster joints are still completing the backswing.

Principle VI   For a change in momentum to occur, force must be applied over time (impulse). If maximum force is desired in projection-type activities maximum muscle torques should be applied over as long a time as possible.

Principles Relating to the Direction of Force

Principle VII   The direction in which the object moves is determined by the direction of the force *applied* to it. If the force consists of two or more components, the object will move in the direction of the resultant of those components. After being projected or struck the direction will be modified by gravity and air resistance.

Principle VIII   If an object is free to move only along a predetermined pathway (as in the case of a window or sliding door), any component of force not in the direction of this pathway is wasted and serves to increase friction.

Principles Relating to the Point at Which the Force is Applied

Principle IX   Force applied in line with an object's center of gravity will result in linear motion of the object, provided the latter is freely movable.

Principle X   If the force applied to a freely movable object is not in line with the latter's center of gravity, it will result in rotatory motion of the object.

Principle XI   If the free motion of an object is interfered with by friction or by the presence of an obstacle, rotatory motion may result, even though the force is applied in line with the object's center of gravity.

Principles Relating to the Impact of a Struck Ball

Principle XII   Momentum is conserved in all collisions. The momentum before impact must equal the momentum after impact, provided that none is lost through friction or other forces.

Principle XIII   Any change in the momentum of colliding objects is related to the force and duration of the collision. The greater the impulse *(Ft)*, the greater will be the change in momentum. This is the reason for the importance of the follow-through. The longer the missile can be carried along by the striking implement at its greatest velocity, the greater will be the change in velocity of the missile.

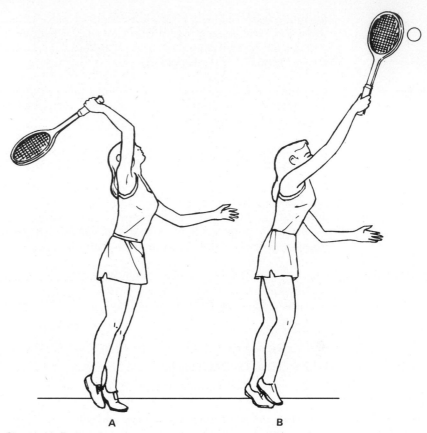

Figure 19–7 Tennis serve, an overhead pattern of striking. Note how the entire body acts as a lever to impart maximum force to the ball.

Principle XIV   The greater the velocity of the approaching ball, the greater the velocity of the ball in the opposite direction after it is struck, other things being equal.

Principle XV   The greater the velocity of the striking implement at the moment of contact, the greater the velocity of the struck ball, other things being equal. Obviously, a full-powered swing will send the ball farther and faster than will a bunt. Increasing the length of the lever (Figure 19–7) and striking with a good follow-through (Figure 19–8) both help to increase the velocity of the striking implement and therefore to increase the force of impact.

Principle XVI   The greater the mass of the ball, *up to a point*, the greater its velocity after being struck, other things being equal. A hard baseball will travel farther and faster than a softball. Nevertheless an iron ball would offer too much resistance for the average batter using an average bat.

Principle XVII   The greater the mass of the striking implement, *up to a point*, the greater the striking force, and hence the greater the speed of the struck ball, other things being equal. A

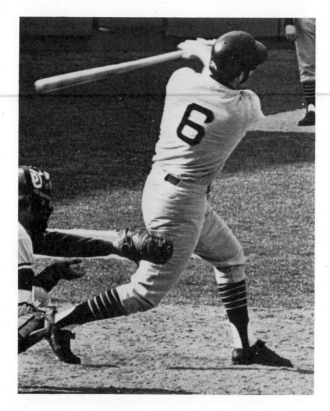

Figure 19–8 Batting: At end of follow-through. (Courtesy of Northeastern University.)

good baseball player usually selects a heavy bat. Too heavy a bat, however, is inadvisable because of the difficulty of swinging it with sufficient speed and control.

Principle XVIII

The higher the coefficient of restitution (the elasticity) of the ball and of the striking implement, the greater the speed of the struck ball, other things being equal.

Principle XIX

The direction taken by the struck ball is determined by four factors: (1) the direction of the striking implement at the moment of contact; (2) the relation of the striking force to the ball's center of gravity (an off-center application of force causes spin, and spin affects direction); (3) degree of firmness of grip and wrist at moment of impact; and (4) the laws governing rebound (see pages 330–334).

Applications

Throwing

The efficiency of imparting force to a ball is judged in terms of the speed, distance, and direction of the ball after its release. The purpose of the throw determines which of these is given the greater emphasis. Both the speed and distance of the thrown ball are directly related to the magnitude of the force used in throwing it and to the speed of the hand at the moment of release. The speed the hand is able to achieve depends upon the distance through which it moves in the preparatory part of the act and the summed angular velocities of the contributing body segments. Hence, the longer the preparatory backswing and the greater the distance that can be added by means of rotating the body, shifting the weight, and perhaps even taking a step, the greater the opportunity for accelerating. Approximately 50 percent of the ball speed is obtained from the forward step and body rotation. The remaining speed is contributed by the joint actions in the shoulder, elbow, wrist, and fingers. This is why the technique of a baseball pitcher is designed to allow maximum time and distance over which to accelerate the ball before its release. In addition, if the ground reaction force is to be maximal, the surface against which the thrower pushes must be firm and there must be no sliding between the ground surface and the foot. The more the direction of the body thrust is backward, the more important the friction becomes and the value of cleated shoes appreciated. If distance is a major objective of the throw, the angle of projection and the effects of gravitational force and air resistance must also be taken into consideration.

The accuracy with which a ball is thrown depends upon accurate judgment of the distance and direction of the throw's target. The ball will leave the hand in the direction it is moving at the instant of release and continue in that direction except for modifications due to gravity and air resistance. Therefore the effect of gravity, wind, and spin must be considered, as well as the release direction. If the hand is traveling in an arc at release, the ball will follow a path tangent to the arc, and timing of the release is highly critical. Flattening the arc of the ball's path prior to release increases the margin of error by allowing more time over which the ball can be released in the desired direction. This may be done by taking a step and shifting the weight forward while flexing at the forward knee. The rotation of the pelvis and spine also help.

When the object being thrown is other than a small ball, such as a javelin, discus, bowling ball, or horseshoe, the general principles are the same but must be modified according to the nature of the object and the regulations of the sport.

Striking, Hitting, Kicking

As in the case of throwing, the effectiveness of striking, hitting, and kicking is judged in terms of the speed, distance, and direction of the struck ball. All the factors that apply to these aspects of a thrown ball apply similarly to a struck ball. There appear to be five major factors that apply to the speed of a struck ball. These are:

1. The speed of the oncoming ball and the striking implement.
2. The mass of the ball and the striking implement.
3. The coefficient of restitution (elasticity) between the ball and the striking implement.
4. The direction the ball and the implement are moving at the time of impact.
5. The point of impact between the ball and the implement.

The speed of the approaching ball and the speed of the striking implement may be further analyzed into secondary factors. For instance, the speed of the striking implement is determined by the magnitude of the force exerted, and the magnitude of the force is dependent upon the distance of the preparatory backswing and the speed of muscular contraction. The distance of the preparatory backswing is further dependent upon the range of motion in the joints and the timing of the swing. Furthermore, the effectiveness of the force exerted by the body is completely dependent upon a strong grip and a firm wrist for transmission of the force from the body to the striking implement, and a firm ground support for transmission of the normal reactive force to the body.

**TABLE 19–2   Ball and Striker Velocities Before
and After Impact and Time of Impact***

	BALL VELOCITY (ft/sec)		STRIKER VELOCITY (ft/sec)		TIME OF IMPACT (sec)
	Before	*After*	*Before*	*After*	
Baseball	hit from tee	128	103	90	1/800
Badminton	30 ft/sec	112	97.2	95	1/800
Football punt	0	92	60	39	1/125
Football kickoff	0	85	60	47	1/125
Golf, 7 iron	0	177	155	133	1/800
Golf drive	0	225	166	114	1/1000
Handball serve	0	76	63	47	1/80
Paddleball	0	115	90	70	1/200
Soccer kick	0	85	58	42	1/125
Soccer, head	25	42	11	8.6	1/44
Squash, hard serve	0	160	145	111	1/333
Softball	hit from tee	100	105	71	1/285
Tennis serve	0	167	123	107	1/250
Tennis forehand	0	93	71	41	1/200
Volleyball serve	0	72	65	45	1/100

*From Plagenhoef, S. 1971. *Patterns of human motion.* Englewood Cliffs, N.J.: Prentice-Hall.

Objects that have been hit through their centers of gravity will have linear motion, whereas those that have been hit off center may curve due to a resultant spin. The more the striking force is eccentric in its application, the less is the linear speed imparted to the ball. Furthermore, balls that hit a striking surface at an angle to the surface will rebound at an angle approximately equal and opposite to the rebound angle.

Some examples of ball and striker velocities before and after impact are presented in Table 19–2.

Pushing, Pulling, Lifting

There are relatively few sports that involve the continuous pushing or pulling of external objects. Archery is a notable example, since it consists of pulling with one hand while pushing with the other. The same is true of using a forked stick slingshot. Pushing is also used in football and both pushing and pulling are used in wrestling. Weight lifting is the prime example of a sport activity involving lifting.

Rowing and paddling, while classified as forms of aquatic locomotion, may also be considered activities that involve external objects. Oars and paddles are both moved by continual pushing and pulling movements. Pole vaulting, rope climbing (previously classified as locomotor), and all suspension activities might also be included in the pushing and pulling category, provided one accepts activities that involve the moving of the body by means of pushing or pulling an external object, the object in such cases also serving as the means of body support. The great majority of pushing, pulling, and lifting activities undoubtedly occur in everyday tasks.

The magnitude of the force used in pushing, pulling, and lifting can be increased in two ways. The immediate way is by using the lower extremities and, in some instances, the body weight to supplement the force provided by the upper extremities.

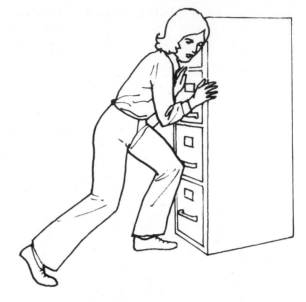

Figure 19–9 Using the lower extremities and body weight to supplement the upper extremities in a pushing task.

In many, if not most, of the activities the direction and point of application of force are interrelated. They both have an important bearing on the effectiveness of the force exerted, and also on the economy of effort and avoidance of strain. Economy of effort is ensured when the force is applied in line with the object's center of gravity and in the desired direction of motion. When this application of force is not feasible, the undesirable component of force should be as small as possible. For instance, if one desires to push a low trunk across the floor, it would be difficult to stoop low enough to push with the arms or even the forearms in a horizontal position. One should stoop as low as conveniently possible, however, in order to reduce the downward component of force that would tend to increase friction. If it were necessary to move the trunk down a long corridor, it would be more efficient to tie a rope to the handle at one end and pull it. By using a long rope, the horizontal component of force would be relatively great and the vertical or lifting component relatively small. Some lifting component would be desirable, however, as it would serve to reduce friction.

When friction is a major obstacle, as when pushing a tall object such as a filing cabinet across a carpeted floor, the horizontal push should be applied close to the cabinet's center of gravity at a point found by experimentation (Figure 19–9). When this point is found, it will be possible to push the cabinet without tipping it. When it does not seem practical to slide a heavy object along the floor, one may try "walking" it on opposite corners. This involves tipping the object until it is resting on one edge of its base and then, by a series of partial rotations, alternately pivoting it first on one corner and then on the other. This is the method often used for moving a wardrobe trunk. The arms alternate in a lever action, one hand holding the upper corner that corresponds to the lower one that is serving as the pivot, and the other hand pushing the diagonally opposite upper corner forward.

When attempting to pull an object, the same general directions apply but with this exception. As in the case of pulling the low trunk by a rope, it may be advantageous to pull in a slightly upward direction since the lifting effect would help to reduce friction. Nevertheless, unless one wishes to rotate the object, the pull should be applied in line with the object's line of gravity.

When applying a pull or a push to an object that must move on a track, such as a window or a sliding garage door, it is essential to apply the force in the direction that the track or runway permits. Force in any other direction is wasted and friction is increased. Trying to open a heavy window or one that sticks can be done by standing with the right side next to it, the arm close to the body, elbow fully flexed, and the heel of the hand placed beneath a crosspiece of the frame, and then pushing vertically upward. If more force is needed, the knees and hips should be flexed and the hands placed against a lower crosspiece. The extension of the lower extremities then supplements the force exerted by the arm. If this action is inadequate, both hands can be used by twisting the trunk to face the window. In pulling the window down one should face it, stand as close as possible, and use both hands, being careful to apply the force vertically downward.

Lifting is a form of pulling; it is pulling a movable object vertically or obliquely upward. The more nearly vertical the pull and the more in line with the object's center of gravity, the more efficient is the lift. The principle involved here is that of minimizing the resistance arm of a lever in order to reduce the amount of effort needed to lift a given weight. For instance, to give an extreme example, it takes less effort to lift and hold a heavy package close to the body than it does to lift and hold it at arm's length. Likewise it takes less effort to lift a suitcase by bending the knees than by bending from the waist with the knees kept straight (Figure 19–10). In bending, the weight arm of the lever is the horizontal distance from the center of the knee joint to the body's line of gravity; in bending from the waist the weight arm of the lever is the horizontal distance from the center of the hip joint to the body's line of gravity. There are other factors involved here too, but the relative length of the resistance arm is an important one. Also, because of the shorter resistance arm, it takes less effort to lift by bending with the trunk inclined slightly forward than with the trunk held in, or close to, a vertical position. That this is a mechanically more efficient method of stooping (and rising from a stoop) may easily be demonstrated by the use of line-of-gravity photographs (Figure 19–11).

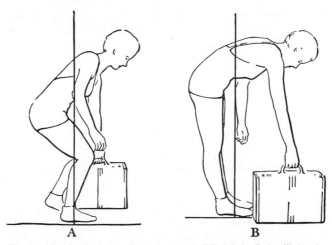

Figure 19–10   Picking up a suitcase. *A*, Efficiently. *B*, Inefficiently.

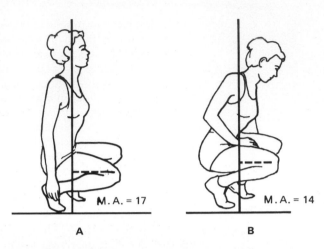

Figure 19–11 Stooping. *A,* Attempting to keep the trunk vertical. *B,* Inclining the body slightly forward. (M.A. = the moment arm of the thigh lever.)

M.A. = 17

A

M.A. = 14

B

In stooping the thigh serves as the lever, the knee joint as the fulcrum, and the point at which the line of gravity intersects the thigh as the resistance point. The weight or resistance moment arm is the horizontal distance from the fulcrum to the line of gravity. Figure 19–11 is based on two line-of-gravity photographs taken by Wells of one subject with the first (A) attempting to keep the trunk as nearly vertical as possible, and the other (B) inclining the trunk slightly forward from the hips in what felt to the subject like a comfortable position. In the original photographs the moment arm of the lever in Figure 19–11A measured 17 mm and in B, 14 mm. The actual (life-sized) difference in the two moment arms was approximately 4.5 cm. Although it is true that more effort is required to lift the weight of the torso itself from a full stoop than from a bend at the waist, the latter method endangers the joints and muscles of the lower back (Figure 19–10B). It requires strong action of the hip and spine extensors, and the latter muscles are forced to work in a stretched condition.

If the body is used in this manner for lifting heavy objects, an additional burden is put upon the muscles of the back, one that they can ill afford to take. Strait et al. (1947) have made the interesting observation that bending from the waist to touch the floor, without flexing the knees, creates a tensile force of 450 pounds in the erector spinae muscle and a compression force of nearly 500 pounds on the fifth lumbar vertebra (Figure 19–12). If a 50-pound weight is held in the hands, the tensile force is

Figure 19–12 Bending from the waist to reach the floor not only puts a strain on the back muscles but also subjects the fifth lumbar vertebra to a compression force of nearly 500 pounds.

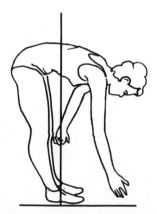

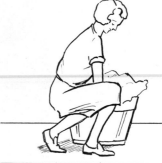

Figure 19–13 Lifting a load with both hands at one side of the body. Note that the foot that is farther from the load is placed forward. This gives better balance.

increased to 750 pounds and the compressional force to 850 pounds. The spinal extensors are not powerful muscles and are easily strained. It is unwise to expose them to the danger of strain when this can be avoided by observing the principles of good mechanics (Figures 19–13 and 19–14).

Common Examples of Giving Motion to External Objects in Sports and Everyday Tasks

The Forehand Drive

Description

The forehand drive (Figure 19–15) is one of the fundamental strokes of tennis. Its objective is to send the ball over the net and deep into the opponent's court close to the base line.

STARTING POSITION The player faces the net with the feet about shoulder width apart and the weight on the balls of the feet. The racket is held with an eastern or shake hands grip.

Backswing The player pivots the entire body so that the shoulder and hips of the nonracket side are toward the net. At the same time the racket is taken back at shoulder level in either a straight or circular manner, with the head of the racket above the wrist and its face turned slightly down. The weight of the body is over the rear foot (racket side).

Figure 19–14 A safe and efficient method of lifting a heavy object.

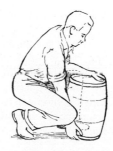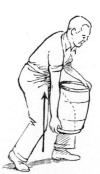

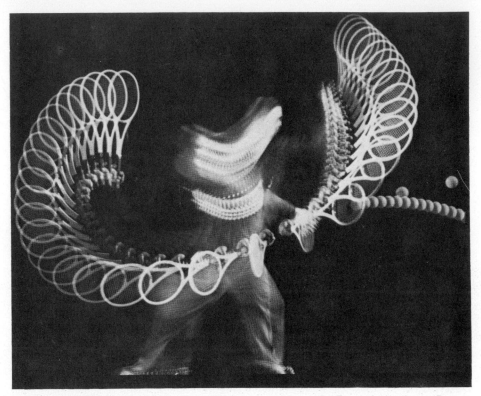

Figure 19–15   The forehand drive. (From Braden, V., and Bruns, B.: *Tennis for the future.* Boston: Little, Brown, 1977.)

Forward Swing and Follow-through   The player bends the knees to drop the racket and racket arm below the intended contact point (still keeping the racket head above the wrist with its face turned down) and steps toward the ball with the nonracket foot. The pelvis and spine rotate so the trunk faces forward, and the weight is shifted to the forward foot as the racket is swung forward and up. The racket face is perpendicular to the court at ball impact, thus imparting top spin to the ball as it swings through and up. The follow-through continues toward the intended target, with the racket arm swinging across the body and up toward the chin.

Mechanical and Anatomical Factors

The movement involved in the forehand drive is classified as "giving motion to an object," in this instance, striking a ball with a racket using a sidearm pattern. (See page 512 for the principles of giving motion to an external object and page 516 for specific principles that apply to striking.) The action is ballistic in nature and, as such, is initiated by muscular force, continued by momentum, and finally terminated by the contraction of antagonistic muscles. The chief lever participating in the movement consists of the arm, trunk, and racket together with the fulcrum located in the opposite hip joint (see Figure 12–18), the point of force application at a point on the pelvis that represents the combined forces of the muscles producing the movement (mainly the gluteus medius and minimis and the adductor magnus), and the resistance point at the center of gravity of the trunk-arm-racket lever. At the moment of impact, however, the resistance point may be considered to be the point of contact of the ball with the racket face. The additional lever actions due to the rotation of the spine, the horizontal flexion at the shoulder, and flexion at the wrist, if present, should also be recognized.

In considering the force involved in the forehand drive, it is important to distinguish between the force applied to the lever and the force applied by the lever to the ball. Whereas the force applied to the lever is muscular force, the force applied to the ball is the force of momentum. It is determined by both the mass and velocity of the implement that makes contact with the ball. These, in turn, are related to the distance of the point of contact from the fulcrum—in other words, the length of the temporary resistance arm of the lever ("temporary" because the distance from the fulcrum to the point of contact with the ball constitutes the resistance arm of the lever only for the brief moment of impact). In addition to the rotatory movement of the trunk-arm-racket lever, the linear motion produced by the forward movement of the body (due to weight shift) adds to the force which meets the ball.

The purpose of the forehand drive is to return the ball so that it will not only land within the opponent's court, but will land in such a place and manner that it will be difficult to return. For the player to achieve this requires both high speed and expert placement of the ball. Hence, imparting maximum speed to the ball and, at the same time, placing it with accuracy are the two major skills that the player seeks to develop.

The force of impact is determined by the speed of the racket at the moment of contact with the ball, and maximum velocity can be obtained only when maximum distance is used for accelerating. The function of the backswing is to provide this distance. There are two types of backswing, the straight and the circular. The straight backswing has the advantage of greater ease in controlling the direction of the racket and in timing the movement, but the disadvantage of necessitating the overcoming of inertia in order to reverse the direction from the back to the forward swing. On the other hand, the circular backswing permits the arm to move in one continuous motion over a longer path, thereby providing more than twice the distance for building up momentum. For the more skillful player who is able to control both the direction of the racket and the timing of the entire movement, it is the more efficient method.

Whichever backswing is used, an important anatomical factor is the strength of the muscles responsible for keeping the arm abducted and for assistance in the forward swing as the arm is carried along by the rotating spine and pelvis. Those whose muscles lack the strength to swing the outstretched arm with speed are likely to flex the arm at the elbow or adduct the arm, bringing the racket closer to the trunk and thus shortening the resistance moment arm. Among the muscles that were tested by Broer and Houtz (1967) and found active in the forward swing of the forehand drive were the anterior deltoid and, to a lesser degree, the middle deltoid, trapezius (especially the middle and upper parts), pectoralis muscles, especially the clavicular portion of the major at the end of the swing, biceps, brachioradialis, and triceps, the latter in two short bursts, the first at the beginning of the forward swing, and the second at the moment of impact. One might wonder why the trapezius, an adductor of the scapula, should be active in this action of the upper arm. It seems reasonable to assume that it stabilizes the scapula against the pull of the deltoid in order to permit the latter to exert all of its force on the humerus.

Starting with the pelvic rotation and weight shift and working out toward the racket, each movement in turn gets under way before the next one commences. If the timing is correct, the cumulative effect of these movements is to produce maximum velocity. If any of the movements is added to the preceding one either too early or too late, the potential velocity will not be realized.

Other important factors that contribute to the force applied to the ball, and therefore to the speed of the ball on its return flight, include the following:

1. The use of the arm in an almost fully extended position increases the length of the lever, thereby giving greater velocity to the racket head than would be the case if the upper arm were close to the body. This is only true, however, if the racket can be moved with the same angular velocity in both positions.
2. The effort needed to resist the force of the ball hitting the racket is less when the racket lever arm is shortened.
3. It takes less time to swing a shortened racket lever into the striking position than it does a fully extended one. (These first three related factors help to explain why beginners and children bend the forehand elbow or choke up on the racket handle.)
4. The concentration of mass at the level of the shoulders moving forward at the moment of impact ensures maximum speed for striking.
5. A skillful player tends to use a relatively heavy racket because, other things being equal, the greater the mass of the striking implement, the greater the striking force, and hence the greater the speed of the struck ball.
6. A new ball and a well strung racket ensure a good coefficient of restitution (elasticity), thereby increasing the speed of the struck ball.
7. The bending of the knees at the beginning of the forward swing followed by the extension of the legs and shift of weight as the racket is swung forward and up increases the ground reactive force imparted to the body and thus to the ball.
8. It has been generally accepted that a firm wrist and grip are essential for maximum impulse to be applied by the racket to the ball. Recent research results appear to contradict this belief, however, and further investigation seems warranted (Watanabe, 1979).
9. Placement of the ball is a matter of direction. It will be recalled that the direction taken by a struck ball is determined by four factors:
   a. The direction of the striking implement at the moment of impact.
   b. The relation of the striking force to the ball's center of gravity—in other words, the control of spin.
   c. Firmness of grip and wrist at the moment of impact.
   d. Angle of incidence.

   The first of these is obvious. The beginner may be less aware of the importance of the other three factors. For successful placing of the ball, an understanding of the effect of spin and the skill of imparting the desired spin to the ball are essential. Firmness of grip is dependent upon wrist and finger strength and is closely related to the angle at which the racket face makes contact with the ball. Since the angle of rebound equals the angle of incidence (actually slightly less than this in the case of tennis balls because of their compressibility), it will be seen that firmness of grip is therefore an important factor in the direction taken by the struck ball.

Archery

Archery requires a strong pulling action, not on the object to be moved but on an elastic structure—a string stretched between the ends of a flexible bow—and a simultaneous strong pushing action on the bow. A notched arrow is fitted against the string and its shaft rests lightly on the index finger knuckle of the hand holding the bow. As the string is drawn back the arrow moves with it, and when it is suddenly released the string springs back, pushing the arrow forward and, in so doing, projecting it into flight. Meanwhile, the hand holding the bow is engaged in what might be called a static pushing action to maintain it in correct position.

As in other motion-giving activities, magnitude of force and direction of application are all important. All the fine points of technique relative to stance, head and trunk alignment, and bow arm and string arm action are related to these factors. The speed of the arrow depends upon the weight, design, and flexibility of the bow, length of the draw, and technique in the release. The direction is governed by the accuracy of the arm, the release technique, air resistance, and the "trueness" of the arrow. In archery, perhaps more than in other activities, the attempt to impart adequate force is the main cause of the difficulty in controlling direction.

The chief anatomical action of the drawing arm consists in horizontal extension of the humerus combined with adduction of the shoulder girdle. Flexion of the distal phalanges of the second, third, and fourth fingers is required for exerting a steady pull on the string. In the bow arm the push consists of abduction at the shoulder and extension at the elbow. The deltoid and supraspinatus are active at the shoulder and the triceps muscle is responsible for exerting a steady push at the elbow. The latter is maintained in *incomplete* extension, as complete extension, especially hyperextension, would increase the difficulty of holding the hand and wrist properly and would almost certainly cause the rebounding string to hit against the elbow region, resulting in a painful bruise.

A common fault in archery, due to insufficient force, is creeping on the release. An analysis of this is presented below.*

Description

The fault known as creeping may be caused by either arm. It may be due to a forward movement of the right hand prior to or at the moment of the release or it may be due to the relaxation of the left arm at both the shoulder and elbow joints. If the creeping is due to the right arm, the normal follow-through is omitted entirely; if it is due to the left arm, the follow-through is reduced because of the loss of tension between the bow and the string preceding the release.

Anatomical Analysis

The arms are maintained at shoulder level by the deltoid and supraspinatus muscles and are drawn back in horizontal extension chiefly by the posterior deltoid, infraspinatus, and teres minor, assisted by the latissimus dorsi. The scapulae are strongly adducted by the rhomboids and middle trapezius. Both the horizontal extension of the arm and the adduction of the scapula are stronger on the side of the drawing arm than of the bow arm. The muscles of both arms are first in phasic contraction and then in

*Used by permission of Mrs. Lola Vollmer Shepherd.

static contraction. The elbow extensors and the ulnar flexors of the wrist are in strong static contraction to resist the pressure of the bow.

When creeping is the fault of the drawing arm, it is caused by premature relaxation or by lengthening contraction of the scapular adductors and the horizontal extensors of the shoulder joint. This results in insufficient resistance to the pull of the string. When creeping is the fault of the bow arm, it is caused by tiring and consequent relaxation of the muscles that must resist the pressure of the bow, particularly the triceps muscle.

Mechanical Analysis

Creeping before or during the release reduces the tension between the string and the bow, and thereby reduces the potential energy which the string has acquired. Thus the amount of force imparted to the arrow by the string is decreased. Furthermore, this fault introduces a variable factor, as the amount of creeping will tend to vary with each shot.

> A study has been made on the effect of creeping when the archer holds the anchor and aims correctly [see Hickman, 1947]. A reduced draw, or a creep, of one-half inch resulted in hits 5.9 inches below the target center at forty yards, and 9.4 inches below the center at fifty yards. A creep of three-quarters inch resulted in hits 8.8 inches below the center of the target at forty yards and 13.8 inches below at fifty yards.

Teaching Suggestions

The student should be instructed to keep drawing actively with the right arm and to be constantly aware of the pull between the shoulder blades until after the release. Absence of a follow-through is usually an indication of creeping. Since creeping may be caused by using too heavy a bow, the teacher should check to see that the bow is the right weight for the student. In addition, a check should be made to ensure that the student has a correct anchor and that the draw position is not held too long.

Working with Long-Handled Implements

Working with implements such as a hoe, rake, mop, or vacuum cleaner involves a combination of pushing, pulling and, in some instances, lifting. The last is usually only for short distances, but it may occur with considerable frequency. One characteristic of working with implements such as these is that the body must maintain a more or less fixed posture for relatively long periods of time causing tension and fatigue. Hence the chief problem is that of using the body in such a way that tension will be minimized and fatigue postponed for as long as possible. If the implement is used back and forth in front of the body, the tendency of the worker is to lean forward. This necessitates static contraction of the extensors of the spine in order to support the trunk against the downward pull of gravity. Because implements such as the rake and hoe are lifted at the end of each stroke and carried to position for the next stroke, the force of gravity acts on the implement as well as on the worker's body. Although the implement may not weigh much in itself, its forward position means that the lever has a long weight arm, the effect of which must be balanced by the muscles. This gives an added burden to the back muscles and not infrequently causes a backache. A better method is to stand with the side turned toward the work site and the feet separated in a fairly wide stride, and work the implement from side to side. The reach can then be obtained by bending the knee of the leg on the same side as the implement and by inclining the body slightly to the same side. Those who are familiar with gymnastics will recognize this as a side lunge position. On the recovery, the knee and the trunk are both straightened. Thus there is an alternating contraction and relaxation of muscles and there is no necessity for any of the trunk muscles to remain in static contraction. Temporary relief can also be obtained by changing sides.

The use of a spade or snow shovel involves primarily the act of lifting. Because the load is taken on the end of a mechanical lever held in a more or less horizontal position, it is inevitable that the weight arm of the lever be relatively long. It can be shortened somewhat, however, by sliding one hand as far down the shaft as possible, using this hand as a fulcrum, and providing the force with the other hand by pushing down on the outer end of the handle. As a variation of this technique, when getting a particularly heavy load on a shovel, it is possible to bend one knee and brace the shaft against the thigh, thus using the thigh as a fulcrum. This is only for the initial lift, however; the hands must then be shifted to the position previously described in order to carry or throw the load.

Aside from taking and lifting the load on the spade, there is the factor of lowering the body to reach the load and of assuming the erect position for moving it. As in the case of stooping to lift a heavy object from the floor, the chief problems are economy of effort, maintenance of stability, and avoidance of strain. These problems are intensified by the additional factor of taking the load on a long-handled implement instead of directly in the hand. As before, separating the feet to widen the base of support, bending at the knees instead of bending from the waist to lower the body, and inclining the trunk forward only slightly will, respectively, increase stability, shorten the anatomical levers involved in the stooping and divide the muscular work among the knee, hip, and back extensors instead of making the back muscles assume too large a share of the work. Since the lower back is easily strained by heavy shoveling, it is of great importance to protect it by observing the principles of good body mechanics.

Laboratory Experiences

1. Raise a window from the bottom:
   a. Standing at arm's length.
   b. Standing close, facing the window, and using both hands.
   c. Standing close, side to the window, and pushing it up with one hand with the elbow bent and the forearm in a vertical position.
   Which is the best method for a heavy window or a window that sticks? Explain in terms of components of force and the direct application of force.

2. Open (or close) a sliding door.
   a. Standing at arm's length.
   b. Standing close, facing the door.
   c. Standing close, facing in the direction that the door is to move, using a pushing motion with the forearm parallel with the door.
   Which is the best method? Explain in terms of direction of application of force and of components of force.

3. Push a heavy piece of furniture. Experiment to find the most efficient method.
   a. At what part of the object did you apply the force? Explain the underlying principles.

      b. What was the position of your arms? Explain the advantage.

      c. What was the position of your body? Explain the advantage.

4. Throw a tennis ball or baseball for distance.

      a. Standing still, facing in the direction of the throw.

      b. Standing with the left side toward the direction of the throw, with the feet apart and the weight evenly distributed, using a full arm swing and body twist with the throw.

      c. Same as in *b,* except with the weight on the right foot to begin with, shifting to the left as the ball is thrown.

    Compare the three methods for distance. Explain in terms of length of backswing, speed at moment of release, and total distance used in applying force to ball before releasing it.

5. If possible, observe a small child or an untrained youth and then a trained boy or girl throw a small ball as forcefully as possible at a target 20 or 30 feet away. Analyze the motions of each with reference to the pathway of the hand immediately preceding, at the moment of, and following the release. Explain the factors differentiating the good throws from the poor.

6. Observe slow motion films of throwing, striking, and other forms of giving motion. Look for the application of the principles stated in this unit or for the lack of such application.

References

Braden, V., and Bruns, B. 1977. *Tennis for the future.* Boston: Little, Brown.

Broer, M. R., and Houtz, S. J. 1967. *Patterns of muscular activity in selected sport skills.* Springfield, Ill.: Charles C Thomas.

Broer, M. R., and Zernicke, R. 1979. *Efficiency of human movement,* 4th ed. Philadelphia: W. B. Saunders.

Cooper, J., and Glassow, R. 1976. *Kinesiology,* 4th ed. St. Louis: C. V. Mosby.

Dyson, G. 1970. *The mechanics of athletics,* 5th ed. London: University of London Press.

Hatze, H. 1976. Forces and duration of impact and grip tightness during the tennis stroke. *Med. Sci. Sports,* 8:88–95.

Hickman, C. N., et al. 1947. *Archery, the technical side.* Milwaukee: North American Press.

Strait, L. A., Inman, V. T., and Ralston, H. J. 1947. Sample illustrations of physical principles selected from physiology and medicine. *Am. J. Physics,* 15:375–82.

Toyoshima, S., et al. 1973. Contribution of the body parts to throwing performance. In *Biomechanics IV,* ed. R. Nelson and S. Morehouse, pp. 169–74. Baltimore: University Park Press.

Vollmer, L. T. 1951. Kinesiological analysis of common faults in selected activities. Unpublished M.A. thesis, Wellesley College.

Watanabe, T., et al. 1979. Tennis: The effects of grip firmness on ball velocity after impact. *Med. Sci. Sports,* 11:359–61.

Receiving and Intercepting Impetus

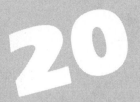

Objectives

At the conclusion of this chapter, the student should be able to:

1. Name the common problems associated with the diverse forms of giving impetus.
2. Explain how the work-energy, impulse-momentum, and pressure-area relationships apply to receiving the impetus either of one's own body or of external objects.
3. State the principles related to avoiding injury while receiving impetus, and furnish an application for each.
4. State the principles related to maintaining and regaining equilibrium while receiving impetus, and furnish an application for each.
5. State the principles related to accuracy and control while receiving impetus, and furnish an application for each.

The Meaning of Impetus and its Reception

The word impetus is derived from a Latin word (*impetere*, to attack) and, interestingly, shares its derivation with the word "impetuous." Both words are used to convey the sense of motion and force, and both of their dictionary definitions include reference to impulse. Receiving or intercepting of impetus is opposing or resisting in some manner the force with which a moving body tends to maintain its speed and direction. The impetus opposed may be that of one's own body, as in landing from a jump or fall, or that of external objects, as in catching or spotting.

Impetus of one's own body is experienced by anyone who falls through space. Such motion, which occurs subsequent to a downward jump, a dive, or an accidental

529

fall, has a rapidly increasing velocity due to the uniform acceleration effect of gravitational force. When the body lands on a supporting surface, its impetus is said to have been received. Likewise, the impetus of a horizontally moving body is received when its motion is stopped as the result of contact with a resisting surface, such as a wall or other obstacle.

Examples of receiving the impetus of external objects are commonly seen in sports. Baseballs are caught or fielded with the hands, hockey balls and pucks are received with a stick, soccer balls are trapped with the feet, and blows from an opponent's fists are received by various parts of the body. Examples of receiving the impetus of external objects are also seen in industry and in daily life. Cartons and tools are tossed from one person to another, red-hot rivets are tossed and caught with tongs, and victims from a fire are caught in nets.

Problems and Concepts

What are the particular problems involved in these diverse forms of receiving impetus, and what are the principles that enable us to solve these problems satisfactorily? In the reception of the body's own impetus, the chief problems would seem to be those of *avoiding injury* and *regaining equilibrium promptly*. There appear to be three problems involved in receiving the impetus of external objects: *avoiding injury, maintaining equilibrium,* and *receiving the object with accuracy and control.*

Whether the moving object is one's own body or an external one, the basic concepts enabling us to understand and solve these problems are the same. The first concept is the **kinetic energy-work relationship.** *When a body or object is "received" it has work done on it equal in amount to the change in kinetic energy of the moving body* (see p. 344). If, for example, the velocity of an object is reduced to zero, all its kinetic energy would be used to do work on the receiver. Since work equals the product of force and distance, the work done in "receiving" may consist of any combination of force and distance as long as the product is equivalent to the kinetic energy lost by the moving object.

The second applicable concept is the **momentum-impulse relationship** (see p. 321). *Any change in momentum requires a force applied over a period of time (impulse) and is equal to the product of that force and the time.* Again, the reduction in momentum of any object can be accomplished by any equivalent product combination of force and time. Both impulse and kinetic energy are proportional to the mass and velocity (momentum) of any object, and will change if the momentum does.

The third concept involves **pressure,** and is especially important with respect to avoiding injury. *The pressure that any part of the body must absorb is inversely proportional to the area over which the force is applied.*

Reception of the Body's Own Impetus

It is the abrupt loss of motion resulting from collision with an unyielding surface that is likely to cause an injury. In order to avoid injury it is necessary to find some means of losing the body's kinetic energy more gradually. This is achieved by increasing the distance and time over which the kinetic energy and momentum are lost. Landing on "giving" surfaces, such as mats or sawdust, controlled flexion at the joints of the landing extremities through eccentric contraction of the antagonist muscles, and rolling are important contributors to the gradual decrease in momentum without injury.

Another factor in injury that should not be overlooked is the *relation of the force of impact to the size of the area that bears the brunt of the impact.* A force of 100 pounds concentrated on 1 square inch of body surface, for instance, is likely to cause more serious injury than the same amount of force spread over an area of 36 square inches. Hence, the problem is to increase the size of the area which receives the force of impact. This is especially important when there is limited opportunity for increasing the distance over which the kinetic energy is lost.

The problem of regaining equilibrium is largely a problem in *controlling the placement of the limbs in preparation for landing,* for equilibrium is regained when an adequate base of support is established. This requires sufficient control to place the feet, or perhaps both the hands and the feet, in a position that will provide a favorable base. The problem of regaining equilibrium is closely related to that of avoiding injury, since establishing an adequate base is dependent upon the integrity of the bones and joints that receive the force of impact.

Various methods of falling are taught in classes in tumbling and modern dance. Perhaps one of the most effective measures for the prevention of injury in accidental falls is this kind of instruction, followed by the practice of a variety of falls until the techniques have been mastered. This helps to establish the right patterns, patterns that will be followed automatically when accidental falls occur.

Receiving Impetus of External Objects

As in the case of receiving the impetus of one's own body, avoidance of injury in catching or receiving external forces is achieved by increasing the distance over which the object's kinetic energy is lost. When catching a swift baseball, the experienced player will not hold his hands rigidly in front of him but will "give" with the ball. By moving his hands toward his body through a distance of 10 to 20 inches as he receives the ball, he is making it possible for the ball's kinetic energy to be lost gradually. This same principle is likewise true for the player who is reaching for a high ball with one hand. The extended arm acts as a lever, the force being applied by the impact of the ball on the palm. The moment of force is therefore the product of the force of impact and the perpendicular distance from the shoulder joint to the ball's line of flight at the instant it is caught. If this line of flight is perpendicular to the outstretched arm, the moment of force is the product of the force of impact and the length of the arm. Catching a fast ball with the arm extended can put a tremendous strain on the shoulder joint, as well as endanger the bones of the hands. To avoid injury the player should "give" by reaching somewhat forward for the ball and drawing his arm back at the moment of impact, and by rotating his body and by stepping back if the force is sufficiently great. If he lets the elbow flex slightly, he will shorten the lever of his arm and thus reduce the moment of force.

Another factor in avoiding injury when catching swift balls is the position of the hands. Beginners often reach with outstretched arms and point their fingers toward the approaching ball. This leads to many a "baseball finger." The fingers should be pointed either down or up, according to whether the ball is below or above waist level. Balls approaching at approximately waist level can be caught above the waist if the player bends the knees.

The second problem in receiving the impetus of external objects, that of *maintaining equilibrium,* is often neglected. The receiver should prepare for it in advance, for a swift ball or a sudden blow can easily cause anyone caught "off balance" to lose equilibrium. The stance is of great importance here. The base needs to be widened in the direction of the ball's flight, thus making it possible for the catcher to shift the weight of the body from the forward to the rear foot at the moment of impact. This action not only increases the chances of maintaining equilibrium but also contributes to the gradual reduction of the ball's motion. Widening the stance in a direction at right angles to the flight of the approaching ball does little to increase the catcher's stability.

The third problem—that is, receiving the ball or other object with accuracy and control—is perhaps the one given the most emphasis in a game situation. As in the attempt to avoid injury, one of the key factors is the gradual loss of the object's kinetic energy. This reduces the danger of the ball's bouncing off the hands. Accurate vision, judgment, and positioning of the body are of vital importance. "Keeping the eye on the ball" is essential to judging its speed and direction, and hence to adjusting the position of the body. Thus, accurate judgment depends upon accurate vision, and accurate adjustment of the body depends upon both of these, as well as upon agility and smoothness of neuromuscular response. Together, these factors make up what is known as "hand-eye and foot-eye coordination." To a certain extent this is innate, but it is also developed and improved by practice.

Intercepting a ball or puck is another illustration of receiving impetus. Ice hockey, field hockey, basketball, and football are all games in which a player tries to intercept a pass. The same principles that apply to catching apply to intercepting, but with this difference. Whereas in catching there is usually time to place oneself in a favorable position and to use one's arms and hands advantageously, in intercepting one must take advantage of the opportunity when it comes. There is no time for preparation. The important principle to observe is to "give" with the hands or stick the moment that contact is made with the ball or puck in order to keep control of it; otherwise it is likely to bounce off.

In receiving both the impetus of one's body and that of external objects, an important factor to be considered is the subsequent movement one expects to make. It may be the determining factor in deciding on the stance to assume. For instance, if a run is anticipated, a forward-backward stance will be more favorable than a lateral one. Furthermore, it will be desirable to have the weight over the forward foot. If a catch is to be followed immediately by a throw, the movements used for "giving" may be blended into the preparatory movements of the throw. These are fine points that have much to do with the degree of one's skill in an activity.

A summary of the principles to observe in receiving impetus, both that of one's own body and that of external objects, is presented below, together with some representative applications of these principles.

Principles of Receiving Impetus

Related to Avoiding Injury

Principle I

The more gradually the momentum (or kinetic energy) of a moving body is lost, the less likely is the loss to cause injury.

APPLICATIONS TO RECEIVING THE IMPETUS OF ONE'S OWN BODY

a. For landing from jumps wear rubber-soled shoes and use landing pit or gymnasium mat.

b. When landing from a fall, attempt to land on the more heavily padded parts of the body.

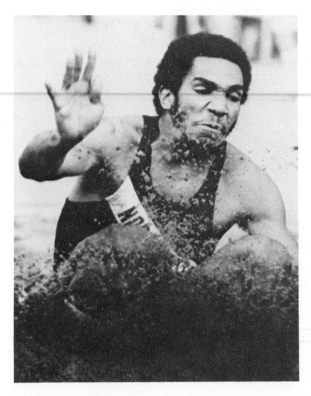

Figure 20–1 Landing from the running long jump. The momentum of the moving body is decreased through the controlled flexion at the ankles, knees, and hips and the "give" of the landing surface. (Courtesy of Northeastern University.)

c. When landing from a jump, attempt to land on the balls of the feet, and immediately let the ankles, knees, and hips flex, controlling the action by means of eccentric contraction of the extensor muscles of these joints (Figure 20–1).

d. When horizontal motion is terminated by a fall or jump, as in the case of falling off a horse, tripping and falling when running, jumping off a moving vehicle, and so on, attempt to diminish the horizontal motion gradually by rolling, somersaulting, taking a few running steps or doing a series of "frog jumps" (Figure 20–2).

e. When landing from a jump, if the suggestions in *c* are not adequate, attempt to transfer the downward motion of the body to horizontal motion by rolling or somersaulting.

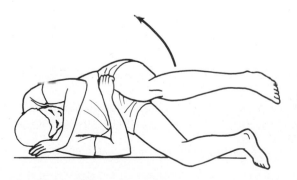

Figure 20–2 To avoid injury when landing from a jump or fall, the horizontal motion should be decreased gradually. An effective technique is the shoulder roll. The action is controlled by landing and rolling on the more heavily padded parts of the body.

f. When landing from a fall following horizontal motion, if the suggestions in *d* are not feasible, attempt to take some of the weight on the hands, letting the arms "give" at the wrists, elbows, and shoulders. When falling forward in an extended position, attempt to arch the back as the hands take the weight, turn the face to the side, and rock down on the front of the body. This method is especially applicable to tripping and falling when running. It takes a high degree of skill, however.

APPLICATIONS TO RECEIVING THE IMPETUS OF EXTERNAL OBJECTS

a. Wear a thickly padded glove when catching fast balls. This reduces the shock of impact for the hand in the same manner as wearing thick rubber-soled shoes does for the feet when landing from a jump. The greater the mass of the ball, the thicker the padding needed.

b. When catching a ball with both hands, "give" with the arms by pulling them in toward the body at the moment of impact and, if necessary, shift the weight backward and take a backward step or two. The speed of flexion in the joints due to the momentum imparted by the fast ball will be controlled by the antagonist muscles in eccentric contraction.

c. When catching a high ball with one hand, allow the arm to move horizontally backward and rotate the body in the same direction. By bending at the elbow the likelihood of straining the shoulder will be reduced. By placing oneself in a favorable position in the first place, the need for overreaching will be prevented.

d. The method of reducing kinetic energy gradually when catching a ball may be adapted in such a way that it will serve as the preparatory movement for throwing. In catching a basketball, for instance, swinging the arms down to one side and rotating the body not only ensure a gradual loss of the ball's velocity but also serve to put the hands and ball in a favorable position for throwing. The transition from catching to throwing is thus made with one continuous motion.

e. The principle of "giving" when catching balls applies also to "spotting" and to receiving in apparatus work in the gymnasium. In receiving the weight of another person the "giving" is effected by a lowering and bending of the arms and bending of the knees or by taking several steps, according to whether the motion is chiefly vertical or horizontal.

Principle II   The larger the area receiving the force of impact, the less will be the force per unit of surface area.

APPLICATIONS

a. When falling forward, rocking onto the front of the body serves to increase the area which receives the force of impact, as well as to effect a gradual loss of kinetic energy.

b. When one seems to be in danger of falling on the elbow, a slight twist may make it possible to roll onto the upper arm and shoulder and thus increase the area receiving the force of impact.

c. When one seems to be in danger of falling on one knee, it may be possible to twist onto the side of the leg and rock onto the side of the thigh, perhaps using one arm to help absorb the shock.

d. Wear a thickly padded glove when catching fast balls. The glove reduces the shock of impact by distributing the force of the ball over a broader area than that of the bare hand (Figure 20–3).

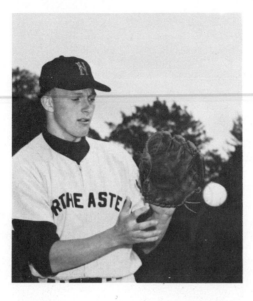

Figure 20-3 Catching a baseball with the aid of a glove. The shock of impact is reduced because of the broad area of the glove and its thick padding. (Courtesy of Northeastern University.)

Related to Maintaining and Regaining Equilibrium

Principle III

Other things being equal, the larger the base of support in the direction of the impetus, the greater will be the body's equilibrium.

APPLICATIONS TO RECEIVING THE IMPETUS OF ONE'S OWN BODY

a. In any jump or fall the body's equilibrium is temporarily lost. In order to gain prompt control of the body upon landing, a favorable base of support can be established by adjusting the position of the feet *before landing* in such a way that they will provide a base of adequate width when the landing is made.[*]

b. In connection with the above, the position assumed by the feet should be such that it will facilitate the equal distribution of body weight over them.

c. External aids to making a controlled landing include a smooth landing surface and appropriate footwear. These help to prevent turned ankles and stubbed toes, which might spoil an otherwise good landing.

d. When one lands with so much force that it is difficult to establish an adequate base of support with the feet alone, one or both hands should be used to establish a temporary base large enough to assure a quick recovery of equilibrium.

e. In order to provide an adequate base of support for the recovery of balance following forceful horizontal movements, the larger dimension of the base should be parallel with the direction of the horizontal movement. This will necessitate a for-

---

[*]The practice of teaching landing with the feet together when vaulting over gymnastic apparatus is not in keeping with this principle. This method of landing is not to be condemned for that reason, but it should be recognized as a test of skill. The skillful gymnast can regain balance in spite of a narrow base of support. Beginners should be permitted to land with their feet separated.

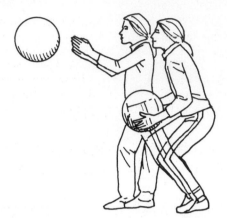

Figure 20–4   Catching a medicine ball. The principles of stopping a heavy object are demonstrated. The feet are separated in the direction of the oncoming ball; the line of gravity is forward in preparation for catching the heavy ball; there is a gradual "give" in the joints of the arms and legs and a backward weight shift so that the momentum of the ball may be reduced gradually; the stability of the receiver is improved by lowering the center of gravity.

ward-backward stance if one is facing in the direction of the horizontal motion. It will necessitate a sideward stance if one lands facing sideward with reference to the direction of motion. This adjustment of stance is particularly applicable to vaulting and tumbling activities. When one trips while running, the body automatically uses this method in its attempt to prevent a fall.

APPLICATIONS TO RECEIVING THE IMPETUS OF EXTERNAL OBJECTS AND FORCES

a. In preparation for catching a swift ball, especially a heavy one such as a medicine ball, assuming a moderately wide stance with the feet separated in the direction of the approaching ball will enable the catcher to maintain balance. It also enables increasing the distance for stopping the ball's velocity (Figure 20–4).

b. When standing in a moving train or bus, balance is maintained more readily as the vehicle accelerates and decelerates if one takes a moderately wide stance parallel with the long axis of the vehicle—in other words, with the direction of movement.

c. If the body is subjected to pushes, pulls, or blows, it can maintain and regain balance more readily if the feet are separated in a stance which is parallel with the direction of the force.

Principle IV   At the moment of impact, the line of gravity should intersect the base of support at a point allowing the greatest range of movement within the area of the base with respect to the direction of the motion.

APPLICATIONS

a. In any *vertical* landing from a jump or fall, the center of gravity should be centered above the base. This position will provide maximum distance in any direction should it be necessary to adjust for any horizontal forces upon landing.

b. In order to provide for maximum distance for the establishment of balance after landing from a forceful *horizontal* movement, the line of gravity should be located close to the near edge of the base of support at the moment of landing.

c. The line of gravity should be near the front edge of the base of support and the knees bent in preparation for receiving an object with large *horizontal* momentum. In this way the horizontal distance over which the center of gravity can move and still stay over the base during the act of catching is maximal.

Related to Accuracy and Control in Receiving External Objects

Principle V

The more gradually the velocity of an external object is reduced, the less likely is the object to rebound when its impetus is received.

All the methods suggested for avoiding injury and maintaining equilibrium when receiving the impetus of external objects also apply to preventing rebound.

Principle VI

"Keep the eye on the ball." Whether the object whose impetus is about to be received is a ball, carton, or fist, keeping the eyes on it will enable one to judge its speed and direction and to respond accordingly. The tendency of some novices to shut the eyes should be corrected at the outset.

Principle VII

Catching an external object with accuracy and control is dependent largely upon the position of the catcher relative to the direction of the approaching object. Putting oneself in the most favorable position possible is an essential objective for accurate

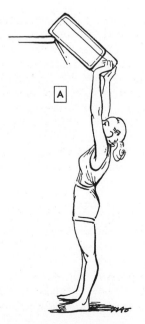
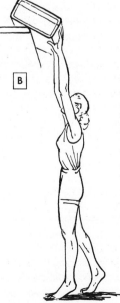

Figure 20–5 Lifting a suitcase down from a high shelf. *A*, Inefficiently. *B*, Efficiently. In *B* the woman is prepared to take a step backward if necessary and to bring the suitcase down close in front of her body. The base of support is widened in the direction of the force being received, and the center of gravity is located over the front edge of the base of support.

catching. This applies to such everyday tasks as lifting a heavy suitcase or carton down from a high shelf, as well as to catching objects that are approaching more or less horizontally (Figure 20–5). This is basic to the prevention of injury and the maintenance of equilibrium.

Classification of Activities for Receiving Impetus in Sports and Dance

Of ball or similar object
> *With hand or hands*
>> Baseball
>> Basketball
>> Field hockey (occasionally)
>> Football
> *With implement held in hand or hands*
>> Hockey (field and ice)
>> Jai alai
>> Lacrosse
> *With feet or legs*
>> Field hockey
>> Soccer

Of another human body
> Boxing (other than striking)
> Dance
> Spotting in gymnastics
> Wrestling

Of own body, landing from a jump or fall
> Baseball (sliding)
> Dance (acrobatic, ballet, and modern)
> Football
> Gymnastics (vaults and tumbling)
> Ski jumping
> Track and field (high jump; long jump; triple jump; pole vault)
> Trampolining

Laboratory Experiences

1. Jump from a low bench to the floor, landing on both feet.
   a. Landing with minimum "give," that is, with as little flexion at the ankles, knees, and hips as possible.
   b. Landing with maximum "give," that is, allowing the ankles, knees, and hips to flex to a full squat position. The head should be kept erect.
   c. Landing as in *b,* but looking down at the feet.
   Which method is preferable? Why?

2. Trip on the edge of a mat and fall forward, landing first on the knees, then on the hands.

    a. Keeping the arms rigid, elbows straight.

    b. Letting the elbows flex, arching the back, rocking down onto the abdomen and chest, with the head turned sideways.

3. Jump down from a table or gymnasium box, using the parachute landing technique, that is, landing on the toes with the feet together, bending the knees slightly and turning sideward, rolling onto the side of the leg, thigh, and hip, then onto the back of the shoulder, keeping the arms close in front of the chest and the head flexed forward.

4. Catch a medicine ball thrown straight toward your chest.

    a. With your arms rigidly outstretched.

    b. With your hands held close in front of your chest.

    c. With your arms outstretched at first, but brought in toward your chest at the moment of impact.

    Which method is preferable? Why?

5. Receive a hard drive in field hockey, *a* with and *b* without "giving" with the stick. Compare the results both as to control of the ball and sensation in the hands.

Exercises for Special Purposes

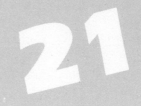
Objectives

At the conclusion of this chapter, the student should be able to:

1. Define flexibility, muscular strength, and endurance, and state how each can be developed.
2. State the principles that should be followed when prescribing or engaging in exercises for flexibility.
3. Develop an appropriate exercise for improving range of motion in any joint.
4. Name and describe the four types of exercise programs used for muscle strength and development.
5. Identify the advantages and disadvantages of each type of muscle strength and endurance program.
6. Develop a graded exercise series for strengthening each of three muscle groups, and justify the selection and order of the exercises.
7. Analyze a postural fault and design an exercise program that will encourage appropriate postural adaptations.

Kinesiology and Exercise Programs

The objectives of exercise programs are to effect musculoskeletal, circulatory, and respiratory adaptations that will make possible increases in strength, flexibility, and work capacity. Indeed, the objectives are well explained by the somewhat old-fashioned term for such exercises: calisthenics. According to Webster's *New Collegiate Dictionary,* calisthenics means "the science of bodily exercise without apparatus, or with light hand apparatus, to promote strength and gracefulness." The Greek origins of the word are indeed apropos—*kallos,* meaning beauty, and *sthenos,* meaning strength. A balance between the two is an appropriate expression of the objectives of an exercise program.

The realm of exercise is one where the interests of the exercise physiologist and the kinesiologist overlap. Both are concerned with the energy, work, and power aspects and the musculoskeletal and neuromuscular dimensions of exercise. They diverge in their concerns with the physiologist's focus on energy sources and demands and the kinesiologist's focus on forces causing the motion and analysis of technique. Knowing what to select for an appropriate conditioning or therapeutic exercise or program requires knowledge of both exercise physiology and kinesiology. As might be expected, the discussion in this chapter is limited primarily to the kinesiology of selected exercises.

A knowledge of kinesiology is important when exercises are required for three special purposes: flexibility or increased range of joint motion, development of muscle strength or endurance, and improvement of postural alignment.

Exercises for Flexibility

Flexibility is the ability of the tissues surrounding a joint to yield to stretching and then to relax. The tissues to be stretched include not only the ligaments, fasciae, and other connective tissue related to the joints but, in many instances, the antagonistic muscles as well—that is, the muscles that oppose the movement in which the joint action is limited. For instance, the restriction in a person who is unable to bend over and touch the floor without bending the knees is even more likely due to tight tendons of the hamstring muscles than to tight knee ligaments. And the person who lacks the shoulder flexibility needed for raising the arms forward-upward and past the head is hampered at least as much, if not more, by tight pectoral muscles as by tight anterior shoulder ligaments.

Developing Flexibility

Joint flexibility is an important element of general health and physical fitness. Adequate flexibility is desirable for all individuals, and is considered to be a possible preventer of low back pain and some of the aches and pains that accompany aging. In addition, improved performance in many sports activities, as well as prevention of injury and soreness, can result from an appropriate program of flexibility development. Using stretching exercises as part of warm-up and cool-down for other types of exercises is especially helpful in reducing injuries and soreness.

SPECIFICITY OF FLEXIBILITY Flexibility is joint- and activity-specific. The range of motion about a joint depends upon the structure of the joint and the pattern of movement to which it has been subjected. The range of motion of the shoulder is far greater than most other joints for all sports participants, but swimmers and baseball players have greater shoulder flexibility than do basketball players or weight lifters. Moreover, a large degree of flexibility in one joint does not mean that there will be a large degree of flexibility in another joint. For example, weight lifters have below average flexibility in the shoulder and above average flexibility in the trunk, whereas swimmers have above average wrist flexibility and average trunk flexibility. Individuals participating in specific activities should know the joint range of motion de-

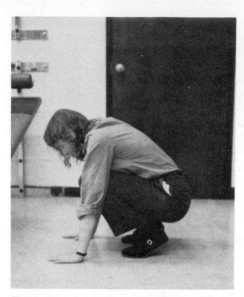
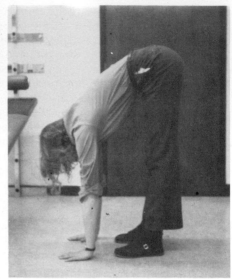

Figure 21–1   An example of active static stretching. The muscles of the lower back and posterior leg are stretched as a result of the contraction of the contralateral muscles of the legs.

mands necessary for optimum performance in the activity and select appropriate flexibility exercises for each involved joint.

A general program of flexibility exercises should include those that stretch the tissues crossing the lower back, hip, shoulder, knee, and ankle. Exercises for other joints should be added as appropriate for the demands of a given activity.

BALLISTIC AND STATIC STRETCHING   The development of range of motion in a joint may be accomplished using either the *ballistic* or *static* method. The ballistic method consists of an active bobbing or bouncing action that makes use of the momentum of the moving body part to force the involved tissues to stretch. In the static method the tissues are gradually stretched up to the point of discomfort and the resulting position is held for a minimum of 30 seconds. Both methods have been shown to be equally effective in developing flexibility but the static stretch has become the preferred method because there is less danger of tissue damage through sudden overstretching, the energy requirement is less, and there is not only less postexercise muscle soreness but this method also helps to alleviate it. Another advantage is that a slow static stretch will not invoke the stretch reflex contraction of the muscle being stretched.

Regardless of whether they are ballistic or static, stretching exercises may be classified as active or passive according to the source of the stretching force.

ACTIVE STRETCHING   In active stretching the antagonists of joint actions are stretched by the concentric contraction of the contralateral muscles. In the cat stretch shown in Figure 21–1 the muscles in the lower back and posterior leg are stretched due to the contraction of the extensors of the knee and ankle. In Figure 4–4 of Appendix I the pectoral muscles and anterior shoulder structures are stretched due to the contraction of the antagonists, posterior shoulder muscles, and scapular adductors.

Another exercise in the active category is bending the spine sideward when sitting astride a gymnasium bench. In an attempt to localize the bend high in the spine the subject brings one hand up under the armpit and pushes either the fist (with wrist straight) or the heel of the hand high against the side of the ribs. The other arm is curved above the head but not touching it, and in this position the subject pushes it vigorously toward the opposite side while bending the spine (not the waist) to that side. This position of the two arms is called the "S" position. The arm reach provides some stretch force but the trunk muscles should make as much effort as they can (see Figure 4–6, Appendix I).

Active stretching has the advantage of the use of reciprocal innervation. When motor neurons transmit impulses to muscles, causing them to contract, the motor neurons that supply the antagonists are simultaneously inhibited (see p. 76).

PASSIVE STRETCHING   The passive exercise requires the help of another person or gravity unless the part of the body is one on which the subject can use another body part, such as the hands, to apply the stretch. *Except for conditions where the individual is unable to provide adequate force (as in paralysis), the assistance of another person is not a preferred method because of the danger of overstretching and injury.*

There are numerous exercises that use the force of gravity as the stretching agent. A strong pectoral stretching exercise in which gravity does the stretching is passive hanging from a horizontal bar, trapeze, or pair of rings. For a somewhat greater stretch, swinging on a trapeze or pair of flying rings is usually enjoyable as well as effective. A still different kind of pectoral stretching exercise using gravity calls for the individual to stand in an open doorway with the arms extended diagonally sideward and upward with the hands braced against the door frame. Keeping them in that position, the subject leans forward from the ankles. The weight of the body in the slanting position puts the pectoral muscles and the anterior joint tissues on a stretch (see Exercise 3–1 in Appendix I).

Gravity also provides a stretch for the ankles in two exercises. In one, the subject stands on the bottom or next to the bottom rung of the stallbars and holds the body close to the bars by grasping a bar at about shoulder or chin level. With the feet kept parallel, the heels are lowered as far as possible in a position of dorsiflexion. This stretches the Achilles tendon as well as the posterior ligaments of the ankle (see Exercise 3–3 in Appendix I). In the second exercise, as the subject leans toward the wall with the feet flat on the floor, the calf muscles crossing the posterior ankle are stretched by the downward torque of the body weight applied at its center of gravity. The weight of the body also forces the heel stretch in Exercise 3–2 (Appendix I).

The quadriceps stretching exercise shown in Figure 21–2 is a good example of a passive exercise in which the subject uses the hands to apply the force for the stretch. With the knee flexed, the ankle is grasped behind the body and the anterior hip and thigh are stretched by pulling up on the leg. Another good example is a hamstring stretching exercise used in the Niels Bukh School of Gymnastics in Denmark. While lying on the back with one knee bent to the chest, the subject grasps the instep with the opposite hand. Maintaining this hold without twisting the foot, the subject pushes against the front of the knee with the other hand attempting to straighten the leg in a vertical and upward direction. A third example applied to the hip is used for stretching in the direction of abduction and outward rotation. The subject assumes the position shown in Figure 3–8 in Appendix I and presses down on the knees.

Whatever the method of stretching used, the instructor needs to be thoroughly

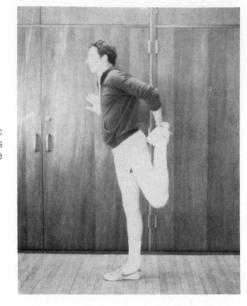

Figure 21–2 An example of passive static stretching. The anterior hip and thigh muscles are stretched by pulling up on the foot with the hand.

familiar with the structure and function of the joint in question. Not only must the degree of limitation of motion be known, but it must also be known which tissues are responsible for the limitation. The effect that the various reflexes may have and the conditions under which they are likely to be active must also be considered.

Measuring the Range of Motion

In instances of unusual restriction, especially if the exercises have been prescribed by a physician, it is desirable to measure the range of motion at the beginning and at regular intervals during the term of instruction. The reader is referred to Chapter One for the method of performing this technique. This activity is also desirable for a student who may want to increase the flexibility of a joint in order to perform better in a specific motor skill. Serious swimmers, for instance, often want to increase the plantar flexion of their ankles, and they would be interested in keeping a progress record.

Exercises for Muscle Strength and Endurance

The one who selects exercises for muscular strength and muscular endurance must be aware of the meaning of each of these elements of physical conditioning and understand the relationship that exists between them. **Muscle strength** is the force a muscle or muscle group can exert against a resistance in one maximum effort. **Muscle endurance** is the ability to perform repeated contractions of the muscle(s) or to sustain a contraction against a submaximal resistance for an extended period of time. These elements are related so that training with an emphasis on strength will have an effect on endurance. However, different adaptations occur within the muscle, with different training emphases. For this reason conditioning programs should be selected to be specific to the needs of a particular activity, and should be patterned after the demands placed on the muscle in the activity. The most important factor in maximum strength development is the *amount of resistance* employed to overload the muscle. In endurance development the emphasis is placed on the *number of repetitions* of the movement.

Principles Relating to Muscle Strength and Endurance

**Principle I:
Overload**

This principle has long been recognized as the essential physiological requirement for strength development. A muscle must be exercised at or near maximal strength and endurance capacity for a specified period of time if strength and endurance are to develop. It has been suggested that, although this process is commonly called overloading, a more accurate term might be "loading to full capacity" (Hislop and Perrine, 1967). The strength of a muscle exercised against normally encountered resistances will not increase.

**Principle II:
Specificity**

Strength or endurance training activities must be specific to the demands of the particular activity for which strength or endurance is being developed. The full range of joint action, the speed, and the resistance demands of the movement pattern should be duplicated in the training activity.

**Principle III:
Progressive
Resistance**

The resistance against which a muscle group is exercised must be increased periodically. Since the overload program increases strength, the original overload eventually becomes inadequate and must be supplemented with progressive increases in resistance.

**Principle IV:
Frequency**

A regular program of exercises should be established and followed at least three to five times per week. The exact number of repetitions for strength development has not yet been established, but sufficient resistance to enable the performance of six to ten repetitions performed in three sets in each workout period is a generally accepted guideline. For muscular endurance the maximum number of repetitions used depends upon the specific demands of the activity.

**Principle V:
Exercise Order**

The order in which different muscle groups are exercised should be arranged so that each muscle group has a rest period between two exercises that both stress that muscle group. The exercise order should also be planned so that the more easily fatigued muscles (the weaker ones) are exercised last.

**Principle VI:
Warm-Up**

All muscle strengthening and endurance workouts should be preceded by warm-up and followed by cool-down exercises. The warm-up prepares the muscles and joint tissues by increasing their temperature and makes them less susceptible to strains and tissue tears. The cool-down helps to speed recovery by removing accumulated lactic acid and, if slow static stretching is used, it also helps to alleviate muscle soreness.

**Principle VII:
Maintenance**

Once muscular strength and endurance are developed they may be maintained with less frequent workout sessions. The loss of strength and endurance progresses at a slower rate than its gain. Therefore, much will be retained for an extended time after training stops. Fox and Mathews (1981) suggest that once the difficult development phase has been accomplished, retention of strength and endurance is possible with exercise sessions once every 1 or 2 weeks, provided maximum contractions are used.

Strength and Endurance Exercise Programs

There are four types of strength and endurance exercise programs, each using a different type of muscular contraction: isometric, concentric, eccentric, and isokinetic. It is not unusual to find exercises that utilize either or both concentric and eccentric contraction referred to as isotonic exercises. The word isotonic means *equal* tension, a condition that does not exist throughout these types of exercises. Therefore, its use to describe them is erroneous and should be discouraged.

Concentric Exercise

As generally practiced, this involves the lifting of free weights—e.g., dumbbells, disk weights, or stack weights, such as used on the Universal Gym, through a specified range of motion. The resistance to the contracting muscles is not only the actual magnitude of the weight lifted but is the product of the weight and length of the resistance arm of the anatomical lever involved. Hence, the maximum resistance occurs only when the gravitational force is acting at right angles to the lever. The clinical value of such exercise, therefore, has been said to be "limited by its inability to impose maximum tension and work demands on a muscle throughout its range of action." Another way of expressing this is that "resistance is constant and greatest at the extremes of the range of motion" (Rosentswieg and Hinson, 1972).

During the late 1940s DeLorme and Watkins (1951) increased our awareness of the overload principle by their emphasis on "progressive resistance exercise" (PRE), and by the concept of the "repetition maximum" (RM). A repetition maximum is the maximum resistance a muscle group can lift a given number of times before fatiguing. Their principles for using sets of repetition maximum to develop concentric muscle strength gains are followed in most such programs today. They were in full agreement with Brouha and Radford (1973), who said that "the strength of the muscles can be developed only by exercising them against gradually increasing resistance such as pulling or pushing springs, lifting weights, or moving the body at increasing speed."

Eccentric Exercise

The return movement of concentric type exercises, when done in a slow, controlled manner, uses eccentric contraction of the antagonist muscles. Because a muscle can sustain more tension in eccentric contraction than it can develop in concentric contraction, exercise physiologists had thought that eccentric contraction exercises should be more effective in strength development than concentric exercises. The results of research to date do not support this theory. Eccentric exercises have been shown to be as effective as concentric exercises, but no more effective. Moreover, there is evidence that eccentric exercises can produce more muscle soreness than concentric exercises. Based on information currently available, it would seem that eccentric exercise programs should not be used exclusively but that they may have a value if the activity to which the training is related contains eccentric contraction movement patterns.

Isometric Exercise

Whereas "isotonic exercise involves muscular contractions against a mechanical system providing a constant load, . . . isometric exercise denotes muscular contractions against a load which is fixed or immovable or is simply too much to overcome" (Hislop and Perrine, 1967).

In the same decade when progressive resistance exercise was so widely publicized, the use of isometric exercise for rapid strengthening of muscles was introduced by two German physiologists, who claimed that one 6-second isometric contraction at two-thirds maximum performed once each day for 5 days was sufficient for 5 percent per week strength gain (Muller and Hettinger, 1954). Subsequent studies have failed to support the claim of such dramatic strength gain, but they do provide evidence that strength gains can occur from this type of program. Most current isometric programs use five to ten maximum contractions held for 5 seconds and repeated 3 days per week.

Because of the misleading publicity received by Hettinger and Muller's claims in newspapers and popular magazines, the public tends to have a distorted interpretation of the value of isometric exercise programs as well as a total lack of appreciation of their potential harmfulness. One common misconception of the value of isometric exercise is that it is an effective method for building total physical fitness, whereas its only function is increasing muscular strength. It does not increase cardiovascular endurance or joint flexibility, nor does it contribute to any objectives of physical fitness other than those related to strength. Moreover, strength development is greatest at the specific angle of the static contraction. If isometric contraction is desired over the full range of a joint action, then isometric exercises must be done at many angles spread over the entire range.

Inasmuch as the extreme effort exerted in isometric exercises causes considerable internal pressure, especially if the breath is held, it is not wise for persons out of condition, such as the middle-aged or the elderly, to engage in them. The strain might be injurious to anyone with a cardiovascular impairment or with a weakness in the abdominal wall. For those in good health and good cardiovascular condition isometric exercises, when given under proper supervision, have proved to be an effective and relatively quick method of increasing muscular strength. They appear to be particularly useful for strengthening muscle groups that have been weakened as the result of injuries to joints.

Isokinetic Exercise

This form of exercise stands out in contrast to the other forms in that it permits maximum muscle contraction throughout the full range of joint movement. It is referred to as "accommodating resistance exercise" (Hislop and Perrine, 1967). The resistance varies in proportion to the changing muscular capability at every point in the range of motion, the variation being controlled so that at all times it equals the product of the muscular strength and the perpendicular distance from the application of effort to the axis of motion ($E \times EMA = R \times RMA$).

Performance of isokinetic exercise requires the use of specialized equipment. Currently there are two major types, with one type involved in controlling the speed of the exercise. Awareness of the importance of the speed factor in muscle strengthening exercises is not new. What is new is the means of controlling it while applying maximum force throughout the range of the motion. No matter how much force the individual applies, the speed will not change, thus allowing maximal resistance throughout the range of the exercise. This was made possible in the 1960s by the development of an electromechanical device (Figure 21–3) that can be preset to run at any speed between 0 and 25 revolutions per minute, while keeping the motion of a body segment at a constant, predetermined velocity. It has been determined by the use of this device for isokinetic exercise that the muscle's capacity for work increases more rapidly than it does in either isotonic or isometric exercise. (Moffroid and Whipple, 1970; Moffroid et al., 1969).

The use of such devices (the Cybex is an example) grew markedly during the

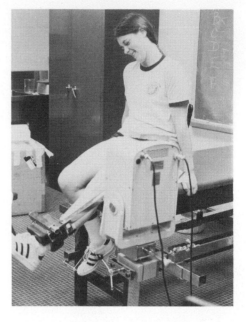

Figure 21–3   Isokinetic exercise for knee extensors using a Cybex machine.

1970s, with the two predominant areas of use being in research and rehabilitation. Attention is called to two articles representing these two areas, namely, "Comparison of isometric, isotonic and isokinetic exercises by electromyography" by Rosentswieg and Hinson (1972) and "Isokinetic exercise: Clinical usage" by Coplin (1971).

The other type of equipment for isokinetic exercise utilizes a cam to change the moment arm of the selected resistance to coincide both with the change in moment arm of the muscle effort and the change in tension due to muscle length change. The

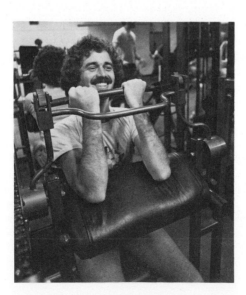

Figure 21–4   One of the machines of the Nautilus system. Isokinetic exercise is possible with a different machine for each muscle group and joint action.

resistance thus accommodates the continuous changes in muscle force that occur throughout the range of motion; it is greatest when the muscle forces are maximal and least when they are minimal. The changes in the resistance arm on the machine are determined and preset to coincide with *average* strength curves for the various joint actions. Equipment of this type designed to provide this very specific type of resistance requires a separate machine for each muscle group and joint action. The Nautilus system, which is most popular with sports and fitness enthusiasts, is an example (Figure 21–4).

Modification of Common Exercises to Fit the PRE Concept

Although isokinetic exercise is admittedly the superior technique for building muscular strength, it requires expensive equipment and is not feasible for class use. A practical procedure is to modify familiar exercises in such a way that the resistance to be overcome can be progressively increased. This can be done by either or both of two ways: (1) by increasing the length of the resistance arm of the involved lever and (2) by increasing the magnitude of the resistance. Among some common exercises that lend themselves well to such modifications are the sit-up, push-up, and pull-up.

The Sit-Up

The sit-up is a popular exercise for the development of abdominal strength and endurance. Consequently much has been written about it, and considerable research has been done on muscle and joint participation during its execution. There are many forms of the sit-up, some more rigorous than others and some more hazardous. Because of the many possible modifications, the exercise is easily adapted to form a series of safe, graded exercises once the related anatomical and mechanical factors are identified.

STARTING POSITION   Supine lying position with hands resting lightly on thighs, feet flat on the floor, and knees bent to approximately 90 degrees.

MOVEMENT   The subject pulls in the chin and curls up to a sitting position. The action is then reversed and the subject curls back down to the starting position.

ESSENTIAL JOINT AND MUSCLE ANALYSIS
Head and cervical spine
Curl-up: flexion followed by extension (concentric contraction of neck flexor muscles followed by concentric contraction of the many neck extensors).
Curl-down: flexion followed by extension (eccentric contraction of neck extensors followed by eccentric contraction of neck flexors).
Thoracic and lumbar spine
Curl-up: flexion followed by extension (rectus abdominis and oblique abdominals followed by thoracic and lumbar portions of spinal extensors).
Curl-down: flexion followed by extension (abdominals, especially the rectus abdominis, in eccentric contraction).
Hip joints
Curl-up: flexion (iliopsoas and rectus femoris in concentric contraction).
Curl-down: extension (iliopsoas and rectus femoris in eccentric contraction).

In the initial stage of the sit-up the rectus abdominis and external oblique muscles are acting as movers to flex the spine; the iliopsoas and other hip flexors act

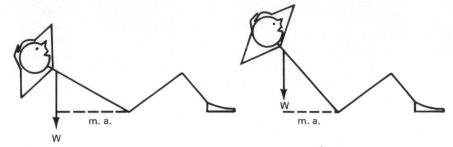

Figure 21–5   During the course of a sit-up the length of the resistance moment arm (m.a.) changes, decreasing as the trunk moves toward the vertical and increasing as the trunk moves toward the horizontal.

as stabilizers to fix the pelvis against the pull of the abdominal muscles. In the last half or two-thirds of a full sit-up or curl-up the hip flexors are acting as movers to flex the trunk as a whole on the thighs. If no further spinal flexion occurs, the abdominal muscles serve as stabilizers to fix the pelvis against the pull of the hip flexors. The major abdominal muscle in a straight sit-up is the rectus abdominis. If strengthening of the oblique abdominals is an objective, the sit-up action should include rotation of the spine.

GRADED EXERCISE SERIES   A set of abdominal exercises that can be performed either as a partial curl-up or a full curl-up series and that are graded from easy to more difficult according to muscular effort necessary might be as follows. All exercises are performed with the feet unsupported and the knees bent.
1. Reverse curl. Slowly curl down from sitting position with hands on thighs. Push back up to sitting position using hands. Repeat.
2. Sit-up, hands under thigh to help pull up.
3. Sit-up, hands resting lightly on thighs.
4. Sit-up, fingertips on shoulders and elbows reaching forward.
5. Sit-up, hands clasped behind head.
6. Sit up holding weight on top of head. Increase difficulty with increased weight.
7. Sit-up on inclined board. (Why does the incline increase the difficulty?)

DISCUSSION   The sit-up provides a clearcut example of the effect that lengthening the resistance moment arm has on the effort needed (Figure 21–5). As the trunk is flexed at the hip by the hip flexors, the action is resisted by the weight of the trunk applied at the center of gravity of the trunk. The downward torque to be overcome is greatest when the trunk is nearest the horizontal because the resistance moment arm is greatest at this point. Thus, the muscular effort needed to move the trunk is also greatest at this part of the sit-up.

Muscular effort may be increased throughout the range of the action if the resistance moment arm is increased in length by moving the center of gravity of the trunk closer to the head, either by moving the arms up or by adding weights (Figure 21–6). If the arms are moved and the magnitude of the weight increased, the demand made on the muscles will be increased markedly (Figure 21–7).

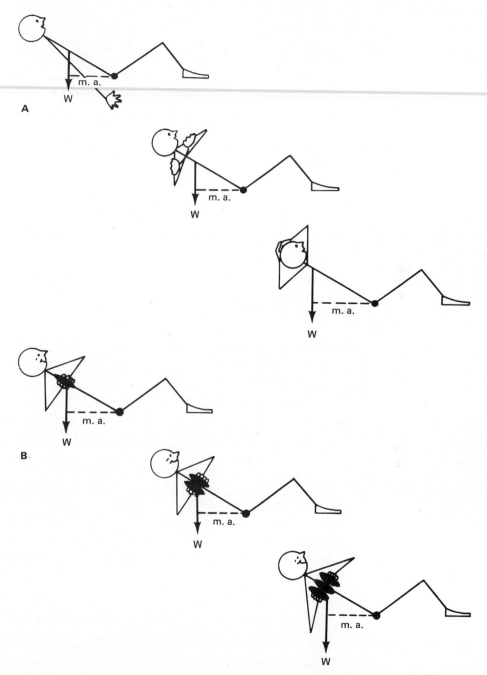

Figure 21–6   The sit-up. *A,* Increasing the effort requirement by lengthening the moment arm of the trunk (m.a.). By moving the arms higher, the weight line, W, is moved higher, thus making m.a. longer. *B,* Increasing the effort requirement by increasing the magnitude of the weight W.

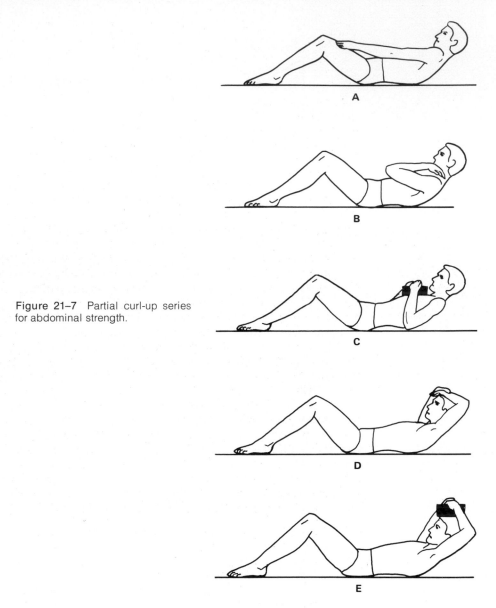

Figure 21–7 Partial curl-up series for abdominal strength.

There has been a good deal of controversy over whether the sit-up should be done in the straight leg or bent knee position, feet anchored or unanchored. Present thinking favors the bent knee, unanchored position because it is safer and requires more abdominal and less hip muscle participation than the straight leg or anchored types. In the straight-leg sit-up the hip flexors are on more of a stretch than in the bent knee position, and the extended legs provide a greater force moment to resist the pull of the trunk. As might be expected, the action potentials of the hip flexors are greater in the straight-leg position than in the bent knee, while the action potentials of the

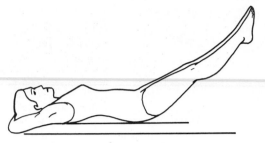

Figure 21–8 Slow leg lowering. Note the increased curve of the lumbar spine.

rectus abdominis are greater in the bent knee than in the straight-leg sit-up. Moreover, the results of x-ray studies suggest that there are possible dangers in the straight-leg sit-up because it causes the lordosis angle of the spine to increase, forward displacement of the fifth lumbar vertebra, and increased disc compression. It is for these same reasons that double leg raising and slow leg lowering from the supine position (Figure 21–8) are not recommended as abdominal strengthening exercises.

Anchoring the feet during the sit-up facilitates action of the hip flexors because it gives those muscles a firm anchor against which to pull. The action does result, however, in diminished electrical activity in the abdominals.

The strongest action of the abdominals is during the first half of the sit-up and the last half of the sit-back. Lifting just the head and shoulders from the floor in a partial curl-up is an exercise that is often employed as an alternative or a lead-up to the full curl-up (Figure 21–9). Its primary difference in form is the elimination of the hip flexion. There is also less electrical activity of the abdominals as compared to the full sit-up (Noble, 1979).

A common fault in the sit-up is coming up or at least starting too quickly, using momentum rather than gradual muscle contraction. This nullifies the value of the exercise. Beginners are sometimes tempted to push off with the elbows, but this can be prevented if care is taken to see that the arms are in the correct position.

In addition to the partial curl-up and sit-up the following exercises have been suggested by various investigators as effective for strengthening abdominal muscles. Their conclusions were reached as a result of EMG studies of the abdominal muscles (Flint, 1965a and b; Flint and Gudgell, 1965; Noble, 1979).

1. Basket hang (double knee bending to chest from hanging position).
2. Side lying with legs supported, trunk lifting sideward (Figure 21–10).
3. Kneeling with hips and spine extended—i.e., with trunk and thighs vertical, leaning backward to a 60- to 45-degree angle.
4. The "V" sit-up (from hook-lying, trunk raising, and double leg extending upward at the same time).

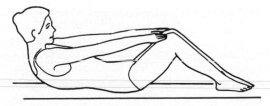

Figure 21–9 The partial curl-up. The head and shoulders are raised until the scapulae are clear of the floor.

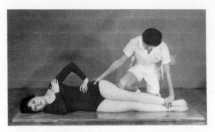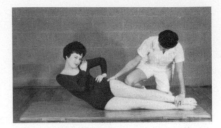

Figure 21–10   Lying on side with legs supported, trunk lifting sideward; a strong exercise for abdominal and spinal muscles. (From Wells, K. F.: *Posture exercise handbook—a progressive sequence approach.* Copyright © 1963, The Ronald Press Company, New York.)

PRINCIPLES FOR SELECTING ABDOMINAL EXERCISES

1.   The criterion for an abdominal exercise performed in the supine position is the performer's ability to prevent the tilting of the pelvis and the hyperextension of the lumbar spine. If the pelvic tilt and lumbar curve increase, it would seem to indicate the failure of the abdominal muscles to stabilize the pelvis and spine against the pull of the iliopsoas. Since the task is too great for these muscles, there is danger of straining them and stressing lumbar vertebrae and discs.

2.   An objective in building a strong abdominal wall is to strengthen all four of the abdominal muscles: rectus abdominis, external oblique, internal oblique, and transversus abdominis. To do this successfully requires a knowledge of the exercises in which these muscles participate and of the relative intensity of their action.

3.   It seems reasonable to assume that a protruding abdomen indicates that the abdominal muscles have been stretched. It would seem to be a function of abdominal exercises, therefore, to shorten as well as to strengthen these muscles. This suggests that exercises such as back bends that put the abdominal wall in a stretched position are not desirable for strengthening.

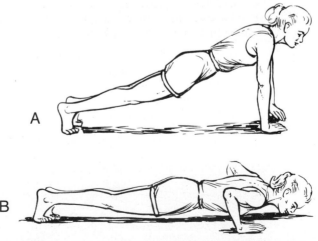

A

B

Figure 21–11   The push-up. *A,* The starting and ending position. *B,* The dip.

The Push-Up   The push-up is an exercise for strengthening the elbow extensors and the anterior shoulder and chest muscles. The basic exercise is described and analyzed first, and then a graded series of variations of this activity is suggested.

STARTING POSITION   The front-leaning-rest position—i.e., semiprone with the body extended, the arms extended vertically toward the floor, and the weight supported by the hands and toes. The body is in a straight line from head to heels; there is no sag at the spine nor hump at the hips. The hands are approximately shoulder width apart with the palms flat on the floor.

MOVEMENT   With the body kept straight the elbows are allowed to bend, and the body is lowered until the chest almost touches the floor. By pushing the hands vigorously against the floor, the body is raised until it regains the starting position.

ESSENTIAL JOINT AND MUSCLE ANALYSIS

   The Dip   Flexion at the elbow joint accompanied by a lowering of the body until it almost touches the floor (Figure 21–11B).
      Shoulder joints
         Horizontal extension: pectoralis major, anterior deltoid, coracobrachialis, and subscapularis in eccentric contraction
      Shoulder girdle
         Adduction: pectoralis minor and serratus anterior in eccentric contraction
      Elbows
         Flexion: triceps and anconeus in eccentric contraction
      Wrists
         Reduction of hyperextension: extensor carpi radialis longus and brevis and extensor carpi ulnaris in eccentric contraction
Maintenance of straight alignment from head to heels against the pull of gravity
      Head and neck: cervical extensors in static contraction
      Lumbar spine: rectus abdominis and external and internal obliques in static contraction
      Hips: flexors in static contraction
   The Push-Up   Extension at the elbow joints until the body is again in the position shown in Figure 21–11A.
      Shoulder joints
         Horizontal flexion: pectoralis major, anterior deltoid, coracobrachialis, and subscapularis
      Shoulder girdle
         Abduction: serratus anterior and pectoralis minor
      Elbows
         Extension: triceps and anconeus
      Wrists
         Hyperextension: extensor carpi radialis longus and brevis and extensor carpi ulnaris
Maintenance of straight alignment from head to heels: Same as above

GRADED EXERCISE SERIES   In the push-up, the familiar form of the exercise represents the most difficult level in the series. Starting at what might be considered the lowest level and working up, the following push-up exercises are suggested.

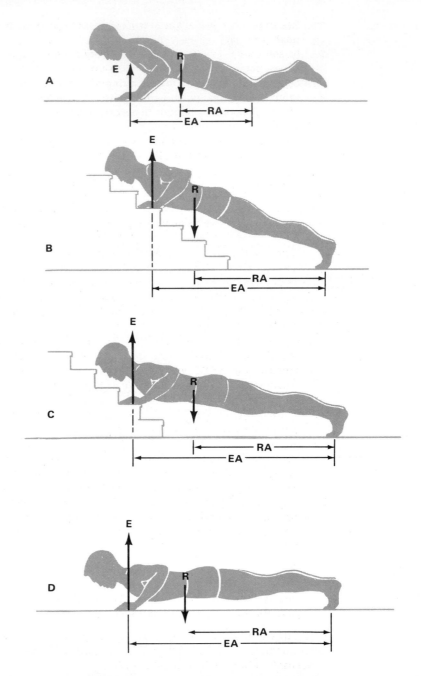

Figure 21–12   Push-up series for arm strength. As the ratio of the resistance moment arm *(RA)* to the effort moment arm *(EA)* increases in magnitude, the effort must also increase so that $E \times EA$ is greater than $R \times RA$. Only then will the push-up occur. The order of increasing difficulty in this series is A, B, C, D.

1. Resting on hands and knees with hip and knee joints bent at right angles, dip and push up.
2. In semiprone position with hips straight and weight supported by hands and knees, perform a half-dip and push-up (Figure 21–12A).
3. Same position as for 2, but complete the full dip and push-up.
4. Front-leaning-rest position, facing stairs with feet on floor and hands on fourth or fifth step, body in a straight line from head to heels, dip and push up (Figure 21–12B).
5. Continue, placing hands on lower step until able to perform regulation push-up from floor (Figure 21–12D).

DISCUSSION A student may have to work up to a full push-up in any of the positions by first performing only the let-down or a half push-up, i.e.—a push-up from a half dip position. Whatever type of push-up is practiced, the student should be able to repeat it several times in good form before being permitted to try a more advanced type.

There are two common faults that must be guarded against in the push-up. These are (1) a sagging back and (2) humped up hips. The latter fault is usually caused by an "overcorrection" of the first one—namely, maintaining a flexed position at the hips in order to prevent the back from sagging. The correction of both of these faults lies in strengthening the abdominal muscles and training them to prevent hyperextension of the lumbar spine when the body is in the extended position. Until the subject is kinesthetically aware of this position, the use of a mirror may be helpful.

The differences in difficulty among the forms of push-up shown in Figure 21–12 are primarily due to the length of the resistance moment arm in proportion to the effort moment arm. As the proportion of RMA to EMA increases in size, the effort in relation to the resistance also must increase ($E \times EMA = R \times RMA$). This can be demonstrated by placing a bathroom scale under each hand. An additional reason for the ease of the push-up from the knees (Figure 21–12A) is the fact that less body weight (lower legs subtracted) is being pushed up.

The push-up from a half-dip is easier than the push-up from a full dip in any given position because the weight of the body is lifted through a shorter distance and because the joint positions permit the muscles of the elbows and shoulders to work to better advantage. The reverse dip is easier to execute than the push-up from any given level because the muscles are performing negative rather than positive work—that is, they are engaging in eccentric (lengthening) rather than concentric (shortening) contraction.

The Pull-Up

The pull-up is an exercise for strengthening the elbow flexors, shoulder joint extensors, scapular adductors, and downward rotators.

STARTING POSITION Straight arm hanging from a horizontal bar with the hands approximately shoulder width apart, the palms facing the body, and the thumb in opposition to the fingers (Figure 21–13C).

MOVEMENT From a "dead hang" and with a minimum of movement of the trunk and lower extremities, the subject pulls steadily upward until the chin is level with the bar.

JOINT AND MUSCLE ANALYSIS

Shoulder joints

Extension: pectoralis major (sternal portion), latissimus dorsi, teres major, posterior deltoid

Shoulder girdle

Downward rotation combined with some adduction toward end: Rhomboids, trapezius 3 and 4, probably pectoralis minor

Elbows

Flexion: biceps, brachialis, brachioradialis

Radioulnar

Maintained in supination by fixed position of hands

Wrists

Possibly slight flexion; muscles probably stabilize wrist for action of finger and thumb muscles

Fingers and thumb

Flexion: static contraction of all flexors

Thumb adduction of carpometacarpal joint: static contraction of adductor pollicis

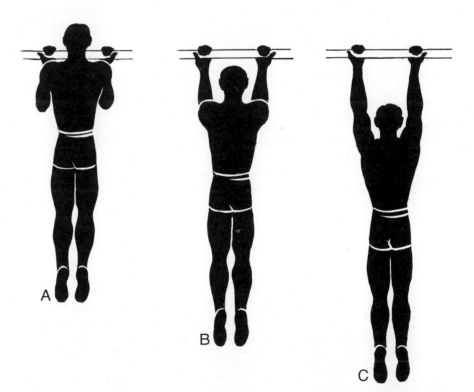

Figure 21–13   Pull-up series for arm strength. *A*, bent arm hanging: *B*, half way position; *C*, straight arm hanging. (For pull-up, start with *C* and end with *A*.)

RETURN MOVEMENT   Reverse joint action of shoulder joints and girdle and elbows; same muscles but contracting eccentrically instead of concentrically; finger and thumb muscles remain in static contraction

GRADED EXERCISE SERIES
Easier pull-ups
1. Bent arm hang, with chin above bar and with legs straight and feet off the ground (Figure 21–13A).
2. Reverse pull-up—that is, slow let-down from bent arm hanging position that can be reached by stepping onto a stool or by jumping.
3. Modified pull-up from low boom or bar with body in semisupine hanging position, arms straight, heels on floor, and body straight from heels to head.
4. Standing on bench high enough to permit subject to grasp bar (or rings) with elbows partially flexed, pull up the rest of the way.

More difficult pull-up   Basic pull-up with weights attached to waist or ankles.

DISCUSSION   The pull-up is a popular exercise for testing upper arm and shoulder girdle strength, and some form of the exercise is commonly included in most fitness test batteries. There is no general agreement, however, about the forearm position to be taught for this exercise. Some tests specify a pronated forearm grasp and others a supinated grasp. Still others suggest the semipronated position as a compromise. Research evidence (functional tests as well as EMG studies) appears to support the supinated forearm grasp as the one most subjects find easiest. The main reason for this may be that the biceps brachii has a mechanical advantage in this position because of its straight line of pull. In the pronated position the line of pull is oblique due to the twisting of the radius to which the biceps tendon attaches.

Advocates of the supine grasp position cite its mechanical efficiency and the fact that those with low strength capabilities will have greater success with this form. Those who favor the prone position identify its use in tasks such as scaling walls or in gymnastics events on the uneven or high bars. From a kinesiological point of view it appears that the supinated grasp should be used because of its performance superiority whenever a choice is appropriate, but that both forms of pull-up should be mastered in anticipation of those situations where choice is not an option.

Exercises for Improving the Posture

The problem of posture improvement and correction is so individualized that exercises for this purpose should be selected on an individual basis if at all possible. This presupposes a postural examination or inspection for analyzing the student's present posture and identifying his or her particular needs.

The following section represents one small sample from the field of posture improvement. Its purpose is to demonstrate how kinesiology may be applied to the corrective uses of exercises. No attempt is made to demonstrate its application to all the problems associated with the corrective aspects of postural education. These are far too extensive and complex to be covered in a general kinesiology text. The appropriate sources for such information are textbooks in corrective and adapted physical education. Furthermore, in addition to kinesiological principles of posture correction, there are equally important physiological, psychological, and pedagogical principles not ordinarily discussed in kinesiology texts.

Round Shoulders

In order to illustrate the application of kinesiology to posture problems and their treatment, one common fault and an exercise for its correction have been selected for analysis (Figure 21–14). The postural fault is the condition commonly referred to as "round shoulders," a misnomer, as the entire body is involved. The *most directly* involved aspects are protracted shoulders, forward head, and rounded back. The exercise selected is specific for this condition.

Anatomical Analysis

HEAD AND NECK   Hyperextended. The head is tipped back with the chin lifted.

THORACIC SPINE   Convexity increased. The increased thoracic curve causes a forward head. Owing to the forward head the sternocleidomastoid and scaleni muscles, which have their upper attachments on the head and neck, no longer exert their normal lifting tension on the sternum and upper ribs. The thoracic portions of the erector spinae and other extensors are elongated because of the increased convexity.

SHOULDER GIRDLE   Abducted and tilted laterally. The rhomboids and middle trapezius are elongated, and the pectoralis minor and serratus anterior are shortened. The pectoralis minor fails to exert its usual lifting tension on the third, fourth, and fifth ribs. The pectoral fascia is likely to be tight.

SHOULDER JOINTS   Inward rotation. The abduction of the scapulae causes the arms to hang farther forward than usual and to turn slightly inward so that the palms face to the rear. Since the pectoralis major attaches to the upper part of the arm, it no longer exerts its usual lifting tension on the ribs.

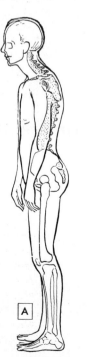 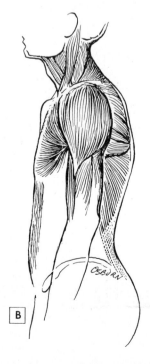

Figure 21–14 Anatomical views of forward head and round shoulders. *A*, Skeletal alignment. *B*, Chief muscles affected.

CHEST   Depressed. The failure of the sternocleidomastoid, scaleni, and pectoral muscles to exert their usual lifting effect on the sternum and ribs results in a lowered position of the chest. This in turn lowers the diaphragm, making it impossible for it to travel through as large an excursion as usual during respiration.

This description here is not complete because compensatory adjustments take place through the entire body. The joints mentioned, however, are those most directly concerned in the posture defect of round shoulders.

A Corrective Exercise

A typical corrective exercise—front lying, head raising with palms turning outward—has been selected for analysis. Its purpose is to strengthen and shorten the muscles that have become unduly stretched.

DESCRIPTION   The subject lies face downward with the arms at the sides, palms down (Figure 21–15). She raises the head from 3 to 6 inches, looking at the floor directly beneath the nose. She should attempt to stretch the top of the head forward, making the body feel as long as possible. As she raises her head, she lifts the hands from the floor, turning the thumbs up and the palms outward. At the same time that she is raising and turning her arms she should pull her shoulder blades together vigorously. After holding the position for at least 5 seconds she returns to the starting position and relaxes. The exercise should be repeated 10 to 20 times.

A more effective but more difficult form of this exercise is to precede the head and arm movement with contraction of the abdominal and gluteal muscles, and to hold this contraction throughout the movement of the head and arms.

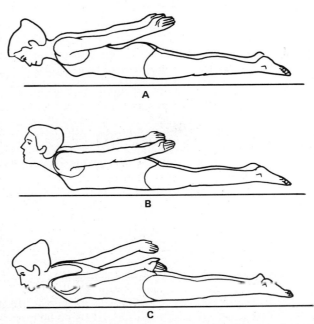

Figure 21–15   Front lying, head raising with palms turning outward. *A,* Correct form. *B,* Incorrect; the head and neck are hyperextended. *C,* Incorrect; the arms are rotating inward instead of outward.

PURPOSE To correct a forward head and round shoulders by strengthening the extensors of the thoracic spine, the adductors of the scapulae, and the outward rotators of the arms.

JOINT AND MUSCLE ANALYSIS

Head and Neck

Holding in extension (but not hyperextension) against the pull of gravity: splenius cervicis and capitis, upper portions of erector spinae, semispinalis, and so on (static contraction).

Thoracic and Lumbar Spine

Extension and slight hyperextension; maintaining position against the pull of gravity: erector spinae, semispinalis, multifidus, rotatores (concentric, followed by static contraction).

Shoulder Joints

Outward rotation and hyperextension: infraspinatus, teres minor, posterior deltoid, latissimus dorsi, teres major.

Shoulder Girdle

Adduction and reduction of lateral tilt: rhomboids, middle trapezius.

Elbows and Forearms

Extension and supination: triceps, anconeus, supinator.

Stabilization of Pelvis

Gluteus maximus, hamstrings.

COMMON FAULTS AND THEIR CORRECTION

Hyperextending the Head and Neck This can be prevented by insisting that the subject look at a spot beneath the nose.

Lifting the Body Too High Because of this the lumbar spine is hyperextended. This can be prevented by telling the subject to lift the head not more than 3 inches off the floor. (Although the subject will probably lift the head more than this, it is not likely that the 6-inch limit will be exceeded.)

Rotating the Arms Inward Instead of Outward This is more likely to occur if the subject is not told to start with the palms down. If the problem continues after the movement of the hands has been carefully explained, the subject should try turning the arms both ways several times and learn to recognize the kinesthetic "feel" of the movements of the shoulder joints and shoulder girdle. Once these movements can be distinguished, the subject will know when the arms have been turned the wrong way and should aim at "pinching the shoulder blades together."

EVALUATION This is one of the best exercises for correcting a forward head and round shoulders when it is done correctly. Unless the subject can be carefully supervised, however, it might be wise not to give it to anyone who has a tendency toward lordosis (hollow back). In such cases the exercise should be done with abdominal and gluteal contraction and the amount of lifting should be carefully regulated. Placing a small pillow beneath the abdomen is helpful.

The exercise is more strenuous than those involving the same movements in a sitting or standing position because in the horizontal position the movements are performed against the resistance of gravitational force.

The total program is likely to include approximately 8 to 15 exercises, and these are changed periodically as improvement in range of motion and strength are apparent. Although the problems in this area appear to be mostly anatomical—limited range of motion and muscular inadequacy being predominant—there are mechanical aspects that need to be considered.

Evaluating Exercises

If the discussions and applications of exercises that have been presented in this chapter have helped give the student a sound basis for developing an effective exercise program, the chapter will have served its purpose. Exercise instructors who have a good kinesiological background should be able to analyze and evaluate exercises, not only those with which they are already familiar but also those that are brought to their attention by their students or are seen on television or in popular magazines. They should be able to tell whether exercises are suitable for the inexperienced performer, a performer of moderate experience and ability, or an advanced performer. They should know whether the exercises have undesirable features such as the danger of straining ligaments, encouraging posture faults, or causing excessive tension. They should also recognize the mechanical problems that may be involved such as problems of balance, leverage, or momentum. In brief, evaluation of exercises should be based on the answers to the following questions:

1. What is the purpose of the exercise?
2. How effectively does it accomplish its purpose?
3. Does it violate any principles of good body mechanics?
4. What are the chief joint and muscular actions involved in it?
5. What are its intensity and difficulty? (Is it suitable for a beginner, a moderately experienced performer, or an advanced performer?)
6. Are there any elements of danger, injury, or strain against whch precautions should be taken?
7. Is it likely to call forth any undesirable or harmful responses against which the performer should be on his guard?
8. If the exercise is a difficult one, what preliminary exercise would serve to prepare the performer for it?

When the exercise instructor has acquired skill in answering such questions as these and in analyzing the individual needs of students, he or she will have become what Huelster (1939) has so aptly called a "practical kinesiologist." To assist in the achievement of this goal the student should find it profitable to analyze as many exercises as possible. Appendices E and I should prove helpful in this connection.

Laboratory Experiences

1. Turn to Appendix I. State the purpose and give the essential joint and muscle analysis for as many of the exercises as possible in Series 1 through 4.
2. Find a subject who has an increased lumbar curve and increased pelvic tilt. Analyze the posture, select two or three appropriate exercises, and suggest a sport that might be beneficial and also one that might be harmful to the subject's posture.

3. Do the same for a subject who has weak lower back muscles.

4. Do the same for a subject who has severely pronated feet.

5. Select from three to ten exercises seen in popular magazines, newspapers, or on television. Using the examples in this chapter as guides, analyze and evaluate these exercises and answer the eight questions in the section above.

6. Observe someone doing a conditioning exercise. Analyze the exercise, using the examples in this chapter as guides.

7. Originate an exercise for stretching the hamstring muscles that will not tend to accentuate a round upper back.

8. In the straight leg lowering exercise from supine lying, identify the resistance moment arm of the lever and also the rotatory component of the resistance (see page 553).

9. Devise an exercise for a swimmer who wants to increase ankle flexibility, especially plantar flexion. (*Note:* Merely plantar-flexing the feet volitionally is not forceful enough to increase the range of motion.)

10. Devise an exercise for a person who is unable to get out of the deep end of a pool onto the deck without using the stairs.

References

Clarke, H. H. (ed.). 1976. Exercise and the abdominal muscles. In *Physical fitness research digest.* Washington, D.C.: President's Council on Physical Fitness and Sport, Series 6, No. 3.

Clarke, H. H. (ed.). 1978. Endurance of arm and shoulder girdle muscles. In *Physical fitness research digest.* Washington, D.C.: President's Council on Physical Fitness and Sport, Series 8, No. 4.

Coplin, T. H. 1971. Isokinetic exercise: Clinical usage. *J. Natl. Athletic Trainers Assoc.,* 6:222–25.

DeLorme, T. L., and Watkins, A. L. 1951. *Progressive resistance exercise.* New York: Appleton-Century-Crofts.

Falls, H. B., et al. 1980. *Essentials of fitness.* Philadelphia: Saunders College.

Flint, M. M. 1965a. Abdominal muscle involvement during the performance of various forms of sit-up exercises. *Am. J. Phys. Med.,* 44:224–34.

Flint, M. M. 1965b. An electromyographic comparison of the function of the iliacus and the rectus abdominis muscles. *J. Am. Phys. Ther. Assoc.,* 45:248–53.

Flint, M. M., and Gudgell, J. 1965. Electromyographic study of abdominal muscular activity during exercise. *Res. Q.* 36:29–37.

Fox, E. L., and Mathews, D. K. 1981. *The physiological basis of physical education and athletics,* 3d ed. Philadelphia: Saunders College.

Hinson, M. M. 1969. An electromyographic study of the push-up for women. *Res. Q.* 40:305–11.

Hislop, H. J., and Perrine, J. J. 1967. The isokinetic concept of exercise. *J. Am. Phys. Ther. Assoc.,* 47:114–17.

Holland, G. J. 1968. The physiology of flexibility; a review of the literature. In *Kinesiology review 1968.* Washington, D.C.: Am. Assoc. Health, Phys. Educ. Rec., pp. 49–62.

Huelster, L. J. 1939. Learning to analyze performance. *J. Health Phys. Educ.,* 10:84, 120–21.

Kendall, F. P. 1965. A criticism of current tests and exercises for physical fitness. *J. Am. Phys. Ther. Assoc.,* 45:187–97.

LaBan, M. M., Raptou, A. D., and Johnson, E. W. 1965. Electromyographic study of function of iliopsoas muscle, *Arch. Phys. Med. Rehab.,* 46:676–79.

Moffroid, M. T., and Whipple, R. H. 1970. Specificity of speed exercise. *J. Am. Phys. Ther. Assoc.,* 50:1699–1704.

Moffroid, M., Whipple, R., Hofkosh, J., Lowman, E., and Thistle, H. 1969. A study of isokinetic exercise. *J. Am. Phys. Ther. Assoc.,* 49:735–46.

Muller, E. A., and Hettinger, T. W. 1954. Die Bedeutung des Trainingerlaufes für die Trainingsfestigkeit von Muskeln. *Arbeitsphysiol.,* 15:452.

Noble, L. 1979. Integrated muscle action potentials of the abdominal musculature during performance of various types of sit-ups. A paper presented at the AAPHER National Convention, New Orleans.

Partridge, M. J., and Walters, C. E. 1959. Participation of the abdominal muscles in various movements of the trunk in man; an electromyographic study. *Phys. Ther. Rev.,* 39:791–800.

Piscopo, J. 1974. Assessment of forearm positions upon upper arm and shoulder girdle strength performance. In *Kinesiology IV.* Washington, D.C.: American Association of Health, Physical Education, and Recreation.

Rosentswieg, J., and Hinson, M. M. 1972. Comparison of isometric, isotonic and isokinetic exercises by electromyography. *Arch. Phys. Med. Rehab.,* 53:249–60.

Ward, J., and Fisk, G. H. 1964. The difference in response of the quadriceps and the biceps brachii muscles to isometric and isotonic exercise. *Arch. Phys. Med. Rehab.,* 45:614–20.

Implications for Teaching

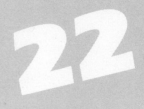

Objectives

At the conclusion of this chapter, the student should be able to:

1. Identify the characteristics of skillful performance.
2. Name the anatomical and neuromuscular principles that contribute to skillful performance.
3. Explain the conditions under which a knowledge of kinesiology is most likely to be effective in motor skill instruction and learning.

Characteristics of Skillful Performance

Now that we have this fund of knowledge about human motion, what are we going to do with it? What use are we going to make of it in our teaching careers? There can be no one single answer. Much depends upon the abilities, experience, and attitudes of the students we are teaching; much also depends upon the nature of the material to be taught and upon us, ourselves—our experience, our convictions, our philosophy, even our own personalities. The purpose of this concluding chapter is to direct the reader's attention to ways in which the study of kinesiology can contribute meaningfully to effective teaching of physical education.

Looking back on the course that we are now completing, we realize that we have learned something about the mechanism of human movement. We see the body as a living machine functioning in accordance with the universal laws of motion and mechanical principles. We see it as an intricate structure of bones, joints, ligaments, and muscles capable of amazing versatility in the movements it can perform. Yet the muscles themselves are only able to pull. Nevertheless, by means of the coordinated action of related segments, each being pulled by the muscles acting upon it, the body as a whole has an almost limitless repertoire of movement patterns. Not only can it pull; it can also push, lift, strike, throw, kick, walk, run, jump, and swim, to name but a few of its amazing capabilities. Note the ways in which these diverse movement patterns can be organized into sports and games, such as tennis, football, or obstacle relay races; gymnastic activities, such as the face vault, the cartwheel, or rope climbing; and the dance—e.g., modern, folk, or tap. These movement patterns are performed with many gradations of skill, according to the experience and ability of the performer.

Teachers of human motion must be prepared to teach a great variety of motor skills. Furthermore, they must teach the ways in which these skills are modified and combined in order to adapt to the requirements of a particular sport, dance, or gymnastic activity. They hope that their teaching will be such that their students will become proficient both in the individual motor skills and in each total activity of which they form a part. They are vitally concerned, therefore, with knowing the characteristics of skillful performance.

Efficient motion is one of the most important of these characteristics. Efficiency refers to the relationship between the amount of work accomplished and the force or energy expended. In mechanics we have seen that efficiency is expressed as the ratio of output to input. In human motion it is the ratio of the external work accomplished to the muscular energy expended. Whereas one of the greatest hindrances to mechanical efficiency is friction, in human motion it is unproductive muscular effort. The poorly coordinated person and the novice tend to make superfluous movements or to tense the muscles unnecessarily. The characteristic of efficient bodily motion is the absence of wasted movements, the use of the correct muscles with no more than the needed amount of force, and the relaxation of all muscles that do not contribute either directly or indirectly to the task. It results in smoothness and grace, in what is commonly called well-coordinated movement. In relaxation terminology the same quality is known as "differential relaxation." This means simply the ability to relax the unneeded muscles while performing a motor skill. It is an important characteristic of skillful performance, since wasted movements and unnecessary tensions not only make for awkward performance but also hasten the onset of fatigue and increase its intensity. As Steindler (1973) has said, ". . . skillful or perfect motion always involves the least expenditure of effort . . ." for the work accomplished. In rapid movements efficiency is characterized by a ballistic type of motion.

Another characteristic of skillful performance is **accuracy.** One may shoot at a basket with a beautifully coordinated and efficient movement but, unless the ball goes into the basket, the player is not considered skillful. Accuracy is based on a combination of factors, namely good judgment of direction, distance, and force, proper timing, and good muscular control. It is needed in simple acts such as lifting a forkful of food to the mouth as well as in more complicated skills such as pole vaulting and pitching a baseball.

Closely related to the characteristics already mentioned are those of **adequate strength, speed,** and **power.** Power implies the speed with which force is exerted. It is an important characteristic of skillful performance in such activities as high jumping, broad jumping, throwing, striking, and kicking, and in speed events such as sprinting and swimming.

Judgment has already been mentioned as a factor in accuracy. It is more than that, however. In dual and team games and in boxing and wrestling, good judgment is one of the most important characteristics of skillful performance. It implies a sizing up of the situation and choosing wisely among several possible responses. It marks the difference between using one's head and acting blindly, between intelligent and unintelligent participation.

The general characteristics of skillful performance may therefore be summed up as *efficiency, accuracy, good judgment,* and *adequate speed, strength,* and *power* for the task. Of course motivation is an all-important factor, and there are also the various individual factors of *special aptitudes* that make one person a potential sprinter and another a potential high jumper. These are related to build, constitution, and temperament. It is a matter of common observation that greater skillfulness is achieved by individuals who happen to be endowed with greater aptitudes or innate capacities for certain kinds of accomplishments. Great individual differences are seen with respect to the various factors of motor ability such as hand-eye coordination, agility, reaction time, and finger dexterity. To be sure, all these can be developed by practice, but not everyone can develop them to the same degree, for there is a wide range in native capacity.

The truly skillful performer is one who habitually obeys the principles of both the anatomical and the mechanical aspects of human motion. Neuromuscular coordination is at a peak performance; muscular function is highly efficient; kinesthetic sense is well developed; flexor and extensor reflexes are dependable; the movements of joints are commensurate with individual structure; and techniques of motion are in accord with the laws of the physical environment. In short, he or she has learned how and has made it a practice to observe the principles of skillful motion.

Anatomical Principles Applied to Motor Skills

The mechanical principles that apply to specific motor skills have already been emphasized. The anatomical principles are more general in nature. Most of them have been mentioned elsewhere in the text, but it may be helpful to bring them together here.

Relating to the Structure and Function of Joints

Principle I   Since the range of motion may be limited by tight muscles, fasciae, or ligaments, it may be increased by the stretching of these tissues.

Principle II   The stretching of tight muscles, fasciae, or ligaments should be done gradually and should be preceded by warm-up activities. The danger of rupturing soft tissues is minimized when they have been adequately "warmed-up."

Principle III   Increase gained in the range of motion will be lost unless it is deliberately retained by means of continued exercise.

Principle IV   Flexibility of weight-bearing joints should not exceed the ability of the muscles to maintain the body segments in good alignment.

Relating to the Muscular System and Neuromuscular Function

Principle I

Muscles contract more forcefully if they are first put on a stretch, provided they are not overstretched. This principle suggests the function of the "wind-up" in pitching and of the preliminary movements in other sport skills.

Principle II

Increase in muscular strength is brought about by increasing the demands made on muscles. This is known as the overload principle. It means that a muscle must be loaded beyond its customary load if strength is to be increased. This principle forms the basis for conditioning exercises and is the principle upon which the system of "progressive resistance exercise" is based. *Strength will not be progressively developed by the mere repetition of exercises of the same intensity.*

Principle III

Unnecessary movements and tensions in the performance of a motor skill mean both awkwardness and unnecessary fatigue; hence they should be eliminated. This is achieved by first developing kinesthetic awareness of muscular tension and then by learning how to relax unneeded muscles.

Principle IV

Skillful and efficient performance in a particular technique can be developed only by practice of that technique. Only in this way can the necessary adjustments in the neuromuscular mechanism be made to ensure a well-coordinated movement.

Principle V

Fatigue from overpractice diminishes skillful performance. It can be avoided by introducing properly spaced rest periods in the practice period.

Principle VI

The most efficient type of movement in throwing and striking skills is ballistic movement. Skills that are primarily ballistic should be practiced ballistically, even in the earliest learning stages. This means that from the beginning the emphasis should be placed on form rather than on aim. Accuracy of aim will develop with practice. If the emphasis is placed on accuracy in the learning stages, the beginner tends to perform the skill as a "moving fixation" or as a slow, tense movement. Once this pattern of movement is established, it is extremely difficult to change it later to a ballistic movement.

Principle VII

An important factor in the learning and perfecting of a motor skill is kinesthetic perception. There is no evidence of a general kinesthetic sense, however. Kinesthetic perception appears to be specific for the skill in question.

Principle VIII

Reflex responses of the neuromuscular system should be recognized and should be utilized when such utilization is clearly indicated (This statement is intentionally general, because much more needs to be learned about some of the physiological reflexes before specific principles can be derived from them.) Of the more familiar reflexes, the extensor reflex is closely related to postural adjustments, and reciprocal innervation is closely related to ballistic motion.

Principle IX   When there is a choice of anatomical leverage, the lever appropriate for the task should be used—i.e., a lever with a long resistance arm for movements requiring range or speed, and a lever with a long effort arm for movements requiring strength. For example, kicking is an effective way of imparting force to a football because the leg provides a lever with a long resistance arm but, for the same reason, it is a poor way of moving a heavy suitcase along the floor.

Utilization of Knowledge of Mechanical and Anatomical Principles

Value in Teaching   In the introduction to the study of kinesiology it was stated that such study had a dual purpose for the teacher of human motion—namely, perfecting of performance in motor skills as well as perfecting the performer (see p. xiv). This brings us to a more specific consideration of ways and means. As we look back over the two kinds of basic information that have been represented in the study of kinesiology, we realize that we have received two sets of tools. One has to do with the mechanical aspects of motor skills, and the other is involved with the anatomical and neurophysiological aspects. Both are related to the human structure and its movements, but their uses differ as widely as do those of woodworking tools and metalworking tools. They serve two totally different purposes. The purpose previously referred to as "perfecting performance" includes presenting the skill and its purpose with such clarity that the students will learn it with a minimum of difficulty. This is what Lawther (1968) means when he advocates giving the student a "gross frame-work idea" of the skill. It also includes analyzing the student's performance, diagnosing difficulties, and making effective suggestions for correcting them.

A student's difficulty may be due to the violation of a mechanical principle, in which case the teacher should make the appropriate suggestion, or it may be due to some physical inadequacy such as lack of strength in a particular group of muscles or limited flexibility in some joint. In these cases it might be desirable to give the student a series of strengthening or flexibility exercises. This would be an example of "perfecting the performer." The entire exercise program—physical fitness, conditioning, and posture correction—belongs in this category. It involves the ability to identify the needs of the individual, to evaluate the exercises from the point of view of their effect on the human structure, and to judge their appropriateness for the age, ability, and specific requirements of the individual.

The usefulness of a kinesiology course depends upon how well the student can put theory into practice. The more knowledgeable and perceptive the instructor is concerning the role of mechanics in performance, the better equipped he or she should be to become an effective teacher of motor skills. Likewise, the better the understanding of the proper functioning of muscles and joints and of the effects of specific exercises, the more skillful should be the prescribing and teaching of physical fitness, conditioning, and postural exercises.

Whether or not this great store of knowledge is useful to the teacher of motor skills in perfecting the performer or the performance depends in large measure upon the instructor's observations, diagnoses, and communication skills. What the instructor, coach, or therapist knows about the kinesiology of motion will have little effect unless specific errors in performance can be detected and properly diagnosed, and the necessary treatment imparted to the performer in unambiguous, specific, and comprehensible instructions that result in appropriate change. The ability to see errors and interpret them correctly is not easy, but it has been established that this facility can be improved with training. It is important for students preparing to be instructors of motor skill to engage in this type of practice so that their study of kinesiology will have optimum practical value and not be restricted to academic interest only.

Value in Learning

KNOWLEDGE OF MECHANICAL PRINCIPLES Whether the learning of motor skills is facilitated by understanding the mechanical principles that apply to them is a question of prime interest to physical education teachers, athletic coaches, and therapists. Of four studies with which the authors are familiar, two indicated that a knowledge of mechanical principles was beneficial to performance. Daugherty (1945) found that the junior high school boys who were taught certain principles demonstrated greater accuracy and force in selected skills than did the boys who were unfamiliar with the principles. Mohr and Barrett (1962) had similar results with college women who were taught the mechanical principles of certain swimming strokes in conjunction with the usual swimming instruction. On the other hand, Good et al. (1979) found that an introduction of mechanical principles and how they apply to tennis strokes had no significant effect upon the skill test scores of college students. The introductions to mechanical principles did, however, have a significant effect upon the level of knowledge of techniques, velocity, mechanics, and transfer techniques and mechanics from forehand to backhand.

The approach of the fourth investigator, Colville (1957), was somewhat different. She selected three mechanical principles and devised experiments that involved their application. The principles investigated and the skills used were as follows:

First Principle: The angle of incidence is approximately equal to the angle of reflection.
Skill: Rolling a ball against a surface or surfaces from which it would rebound.

Second Principle: In stopping a moving object, the force opposing the momentum must be equal to the force of the momentum and, if the object is to be caught, this momentum must be dissipated by reducing the resistance of the catching surface.
Skill: Catching a tennis ball in a lacrosse stick and catching a badminton bird on a tennis racket.

Third Principle: An object set in forward motion through the air by an external force is acted upon by gravitational acceleration.
Skill: Archery.

(For the details of each test the reader should consult the article.)

For all three tests the results gave no indication of a significant difference in performance level between the experimental and control groups. Both methods (instruction with and without using part of the time for learning the principles) resulted in a significant amount of learning which was similar in pattern as well as in amount.

Without having full information about the study one cannot help but have certain questions and comments. For instance,

1. Was instruction given regarding the application of the principles?
2. Might not the first and second tests, because of their artificial nature, have been comparable to nonsense syllables in verbal tests and therefore lacking in motivation for the subjects?

3. It would seem that a better choice of principles might have been made, for instance, principles that were more directly related to the quality of performance.

Lawther (1968) has reported several additional studies listed below:

1. Hendrickson and Schroeder: "Transfer of training in learning to hit a submerged target." This has to do with the principle of light refraction as it affects success in hitting underwater targets.
2. Frey: "A study of teaching procedures in selected physical education activities for college women of low motor ability." This investigates the effect of giving detailed reasons for specific forms used in teaching tennis, volleyball, and rhythmic activities.
3. Cobane: "A comparison of two methods of teaching selected motor skills." This is somewhat similar to Colville's study but is applied to the teaching of tennis.
4. Nessler: "An experimental study of methods adapted to teaching low skilled freshman women in physical education." There was no report of the methods used, but the implication seemed to be that a knowledge of mechanical principles was one of the factors included.
5. Broer: "Effectiveness of general basic skills curriculum for junior high school girls." This included the factor of instruction in simplified mechanics prior to the teaching of volleyball, basketball, and softball.
6. Halverson: "A comparison of three methods of teaching motor skills." Knowledge of mechanical principles constituted one factor in this study. The skill was one-handed shooting in basketball.

Of the ten studies, six reported either negative or negligible results, and four reported positive results. The latter were the studies by Daugherty (1945), Mohr and Barrett (1962), Hendrickson and Schroeder, and Broer. Lawther (1968) observed that most of the studies used beginners as subjects. He suggested that a knowledge of the appropriate mechanical principles might be of greater value at the higher skill levels than at the early stages of learning.

The lack of agreement shown by the results of the studies concerning the value to the learner of a knowledge of mechanical principles is also evident in the opinions of physical education instructors. Those who take the negative side may do so for a number of reasons. They may have had poor results in their own teaching experience and assumed that the procedure itself was ineffective without considering the fact that their own presentation may have been at fault. They may have talked too much in their explanation of the mechanical principles (a fault guaranteed to bore the class if not actually cause resentment); they may have failed to make their explanations clear; they may not have been convinced of the value of such explanations in the first place, and consequently they may have lacked enthusiasm in their presentation; they may have been influenced by some of the research studies which reported negative results.

It is significant that instructors who teach kinesiology tend to use this teaching technique in their sports classes and their coaching. McCloy (1960) asserted that one of the best ways to be sure that the students would attain the correct objectives was to teach the activities in such a way that the mechanics of each type of skill would be clear to the student. He advocated using simplified vocabulary and explanations so that the student would understand how the skill was to be performed and why the method taught was effective. Furthermore, based on his own experience, he claimed that this technique of teaching could be used successfully with children as young as 10 or 12 years of age.

Broer and Zernicke (1979), Bunn (1972), Dyson (1970), and Rasch and Burke (1978) are also among those who advocate giving instruction in mechanical principles when teaching or coaching athletic skills.

KNOWLEDGE OF ANATOMY AND ANATOMICAL PRINCIPLES   Wells knows of no research in this area and therefore offers her own opinion based upon her teaching experience in the field of corrective physical education. This has included all grades from first grade through college. As a result of this experience, she is convinced of the value of giving brief, simple anatomical explanations accompanied by the use of such visual aids as muscle charts, a human skeleton, various anatomical models, and drawings on the blackboard. These explanations and demonstrations have been found to arouse the intelligent interest of pupils from about the fourth or fifth grade on. Obviously they must be geared to the age. Whether the students actually perform the exercises with greater energy and zest may be open to question, but there is no question that they tend to perform them with a greater degree of accuracy and precision.

Teaching for Understanding

Any teachers of human movement who have good knowledge of motor skills can probably teach them. If, in addition, they have a good understanding of kinesiology they will be better able to select effective techniques and methods and to diagnose and remedy individual difficulties. They will thus be improving methods of teaching students how to learn new skills and how to improve their performance. This is desirable but it does not go far enough. Some students may be satisfied with it but the more intelligent students will want to know the *why* of the directions given by the instructor or coach. They want to understand the reasons for what they do and why one approach is more effective than another.

For the majority of students, greater understanding leads to greater interest, and greater interest leads not only to greater effort but also to more productive effort. This constitutes genuine motivation, and finding effective motivation for students has always been one of the major challenges faced by the instructor.

It is the conviction of the authors that the solution to the quest for motivation is to *teach for understanding*, and that an effective way of doing this is to instruct the students in regard to mechanical and anatomical principles and to supplement this with simple demonstrations. If the explanations and the demonstrations are to be meaningful to the student, they must be geared to an appropriate intellectual and educational level. They should drive home essential points vividly and succinctly if they are to make a lasting impression. An example of a simple and meaningful demonstration may be found in Exercise 1 on page 467. Often such a demonstration will be more effective than a meticulously accurate scientific explanation.

As an aid to the beginning teacher who is interested in explaining the appropriate mechanical and anatomical principles, the following guidelines are suggested.

1. Only those instructors who are convinced of the value of this technique or who are at least open-minded about it should use it.
2. The explanations should be kept brief. Preferably, they should not take over 5 minutes, or possibly 10 at the most, out of a 45- to 50-minute period. It is well to remember Lockhart's (1966) warning about keeping oral instructions at a minimum. As she says, most teachers of motor skills talk too much. This has the unfortunate effect of defeating their purpose. Making oneself understood is desirable, but overexplaining to the point of boring or antagonizing one's listeners may be disastrous.

3. Whenever feasible, visual aids and demonstrations should be used in conjunction with explanations.
4. The explanatory talks on mechanical principles and anatomy should be given only occasionally, not as a part of every lesson.
5. Explain only those aspects of a subject that you consider of vital importance to learning the skill in question and that you believe cannot be taught effectively during the activity practice.
6. Avoid any but the simplest mechanical principles unless you know that your students are familiar with physics.
7. In general, save the finer points of instruction in mechanical principles for intermediate and advanced classes.
8. Do not be surprised to discover that adequate preparation for a brief effective explanation may take as long as preparation for an hour's lecture. It takes time to select, condense, and simplify.

Finally, the whole purpose of kinesiology can be summed up in three phrases. It is (1) to provide the motor skill instructor with the tools needed in order to *teach for understanding*, (2) to guide students in acquiring proficiency in motor skills, and (3) to aid students in improving their own physiques when such a need is indicated.

References

Broer, M. R., and Zernicke, R. F. 1979. *Efficiency of human movement,* 4th ed. Philadelphia: W. B. Saunders.

Bunn, J. W. 1972. *Scientific principles of coaching,* 2d ed. Englewood Cliffs, N.J.: Prentice-Hall.

Colville, F. M. 1957. The learning of motor skills as influenced by knowledge of mechanical principles. *J. Educ. Psychol.,* 48:321–27.

Daugherty, G. 1945. The effects of kinesiological teaching on the performance of junior high school boys. *Res. Q.* 16:26–33.

Dyson, G. H. G. 1970. *The mechanics of athletics,* 5th ed. London: University of London Press.

Good, L., et al. 1979. The learning of tennis skills as influenced by a knowledge of mechanical principles. A paper presented at the AAHPER Convention, New Orleans.

Hoffman, S. 1977. Toward a pedagogical kinesiology. *Quest,* 28:38–48.

Lawther, J. D. 1968. *The learning of physical skills.* Englewood Cliffs, N.J.: Prentice-Hall.

Lockhart, A. 1966. Communicating with the learner. *Quest,* VI:57–67.

McCloy, C. H. 1960. The mechanical analysis of motor skills. In *Science and medicine of exercise and sports,* ed. W. R. Johnson. New York: Harper & Row, Chapter 4.

Mohr, D. R., and Barrett, M. E. 1962. Effect of knowledge of mechanical principles in learning to perform intermediate swimming skills. *Res. Q.* 33:574–80.

Rasch, P. J., and Burke, R. K. 1978. *Kinesiology and applied anatomy,* 6th ed. Philadelphia: Lea & Febiger.

Steindler, A. 1973. *Mechanics of normal and pathological locomotion in man.* Springfield, Ill.: Charles C Thomas.

Appendix A*

Outline for Studying the Joints and Their Movements

Name of joint _____ Bones involved _____

Type of joint, movement, and number of axes of motion (check below).

Type of joint:

_____ Diarthrodial
    _____ Irregular   Type of movement:
    _____ Hinge
    _____ Pivot   _____ Gliding
    _____ Condyloid (ovoid)   _____ Axial or rotatory
    _____ Saddle
    _____ Ball-and-socket

_____ Synarthrodial   Axis of motion:
    _____ Cartilaginous
    _____ Ligamentous   _____ Nonaxial
    _____ Fibrous   _____ Uniaxial
                       _____ Biaxial
                       _____ Triaxial

Name or describe briefly:

Articulating processes and surfaces _____

_____

_____

_____

Ligaments and cartilages _____

_____

_____

_____

_____

_____

_____

*The checklists in Appendices A and E may be reproduced for class use without specific permission.

Movements (check)   Comments

___Flexion and extension   _____

___Hyperextension   _____

___Abduction and adduction
   or lateral flexion   _____

___Rotation   _____

   ___Outward (lat.)
   ___Inward (med.)   _____

Movements (check)

   ___Upward and downward   _____

   ___Right and left   _____

   ___Supination and pronation _____

Other: _____

   _____   _____

   _____   _____

   _____   _____

   _____   _____

Appendix B

Classification of Joints and Their Movements

TYPE	ARTICULATION	MOVEMENT
	Diarthrodial: Nonaxial	
	Shoulder Girdle	
	Sternoclavicular	Limited motion of outer end of clavicle in all three planes
		Elevation-depression
		Forward-backward
		Rotation: forward-downward; backward-upward
	Acromioclavicular	Movements of scapula (including motion in both joints)
Irregular;		Elevation-depression
Arthrodial;		Rotation: upward-downward
Plane		Abduction-adduction
		Upward tilt–reduction of same
	Intercarpal	Slight gliding movements in cooperation with movements of wrist and metacarpals
	Intertarsal	Slight gliding movements in cooperation with movements of talonavicular and ankle joints
	Diarthrodial: Uniaxial	
	Elbow	
	Humeroulnar	Flexion-extension-hyperextension (slight)
	Knee	
	Tibiofemoral	Flexion-extension-hyperextension (slight)
Hinge;	Ankle	
Ginglymus	Talotibial and talofibular	Dorsiflexion–plantar flexion (extension)
	Fingers and thumb	
	Interphalangeal	Flexion-extension
	Toes	
	Interphalangeal	Flexion-extension
	Forearm	
Pivot;	Proximal and distal radioulnar	Supination-pronation
Screw;	Neck	
Trochoid	Atlantoaxial (first and second cervical)	Rotation: right-left

TYPE	ARTICULATION	MOVEMENT
	Diarthrodial: Biaxial	
	Wrist	
	Radiocarpal	Flexion-extension-hyperextension Abduction-adduction
	Fingers	
Condyloid; Ovoid; Ellipsoidal	Metacarpophalangeal	Flexion-extension Abduction-adduction
	Toes	
	Metatarsophalangeal	Flexion-extension-hyperextension
	Head	
	Occipitoatlantal	Flexion-extension-hyperextension Lateral flexion: right-left

Saddle;
Seller;
Reciprocal
  reception
	Thumb
	  Carpometacarpal
		Flexion-extension-hyperextension
		Abduction-adduction
		Opposition (combination of abduction, hyperflexion, and possibly slight inward rotation)*

	Diarthrodial: Triaxial	
	Shoulder	
	Glenohumeral	Flexion-extension-hyperextension Abduction-adduction Rotation: outward-inward Horizontal flexion (from abduction) Horizontal extension (from flexion)
Ball-and-socket; Enarthrodial	Hip	
	Femoro-acetabular	Flexion-extension-hyperextension Abduction-adduction Rotation: outward-inward Horizontal flexion (from abduction) Horizontal extension (from flexion)

Shallow ball-
  and-socket
	Foot
	  Talonavicular
		Dorsiflexion–plantar flexion (very slight)
		Abduction-adduction (slight)
		Inversion-eversion (very slight)

Combination Diarthrodial Nonaxial and Fibrocartilaginous Synarthrodial

Triaxial simulated ball-and-socket	Vertebral bodies Intervertebral cartilages	⎧Flexion ⎪Extension ⎨Hyperextension
Nonaxial irregular	Vertebral arches	⎪Lateral flexion: right-left ⎩Rotation: right-left

*Opinions differ with respect to inward rotation.

Appendix C

Joint Range of Motion*

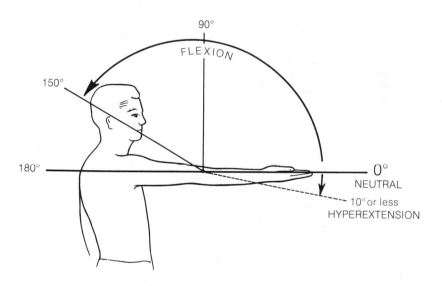

Figure C–1 Range of elbow joint motion: flexion-extension and hyperextension.

---

*The material in Appendix C is adapted from the booklet *Joint motion: Method of measuring and recording,* published by the American Academy of Orthopaedic Surgeons, 430 North Michigan Avenue, Chicago, Illinois 60611.

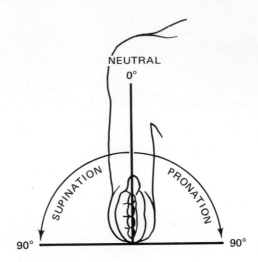

Figure C–2   Range of forearm motion: pronation and supination.

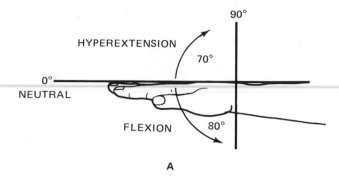

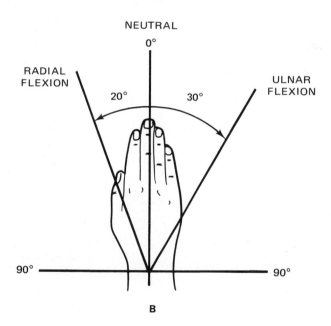

Figure C–3   Range of wrist joint movement. *A*, Flexion-extension and hyperextension. *B*, Radial and ulnar flexion.

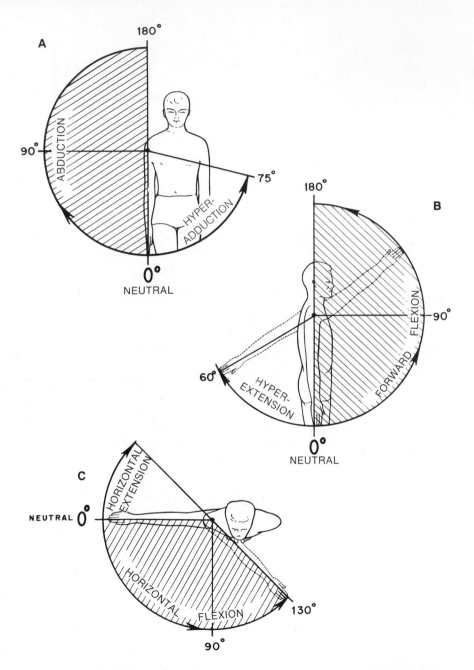

Figure C–4   Range of arm movement on trunk (involving both shoulder joint and shoulder girdle). *A,* Sideward-upward elevation. *B,* Forward-upward elevation and backward elevation. *C,* Horizontal flexion and extension.

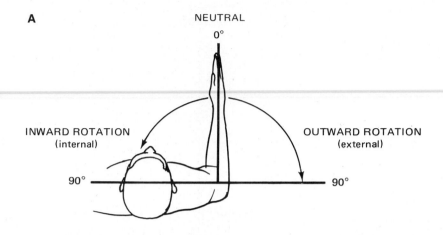

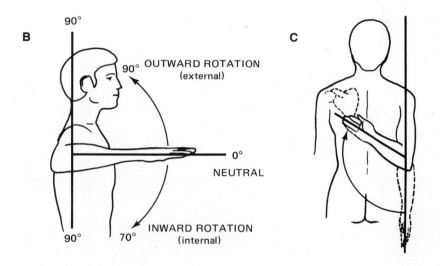

Figure C–5   Range of arm movement on trunk (involving both shoulder joint and shoulder girdle). *A,* Rotation with arm at side, *B,* Rotation with arm in abduction. *C,* Internal rotation posteriorly.

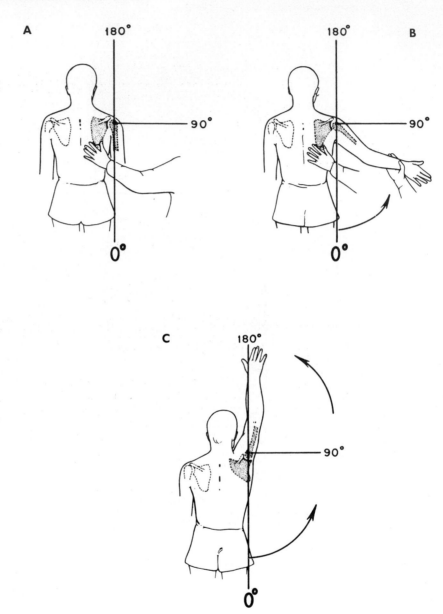

Figure C–6 Range of shoulder joint (glenohumeral) motion. *A,* Starting position. *B,* Abduction. *C,* Sideward-upward elevation of arm (combining abduction of arm and upward rotation of scapula).

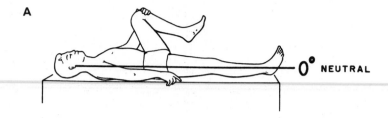

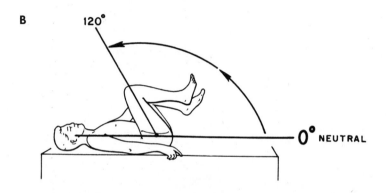

Figure C–7   Range of hip joint flexion. *A*, Starting position. *B*, Maximal flexion without rotating pelvis.

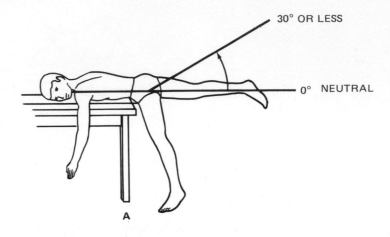

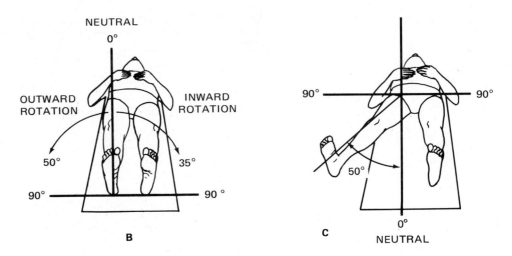

Figure C–8   Range of hip joint movement. *A,* Hyperextension. *B,* Inward and outward rotation. *C,* Abduction.

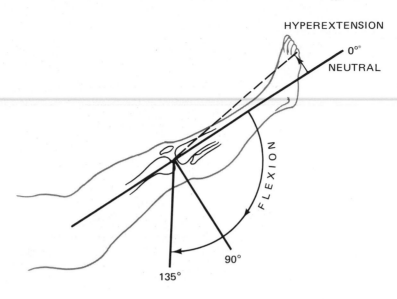

Figure C–9   Range of knee joint motion: flexion-extension and hyperextension.

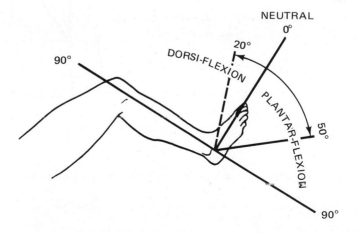

Figure C–10   Range of ankle joint dorsiflexion and plantar flexion with knee in flexed position.

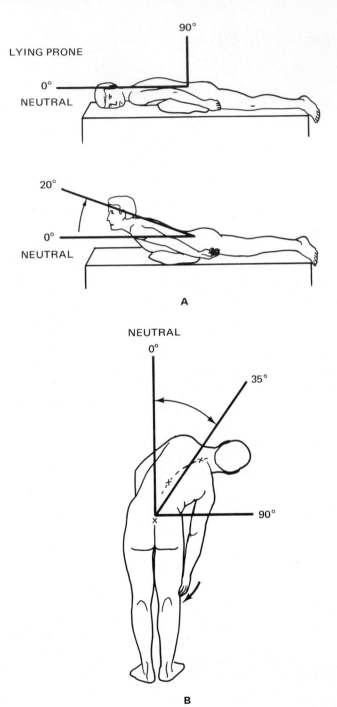

Figure C–11   Range of motion in the thoracic and lumbar spine. *A*, Hyperextension, *B*, Lateral flexion.

Appendix D

Muscular Attachments and Nerve Supply

THE UPPER EXTREMITY*

MUSCLE	PROXIMAL ATTACHMENTS	DISTAL ATTACHMENTS	NERVE SUPPLY
Shoulder Joint			
Coracobrachialis	Coracoid process of scapula	Inner surface of humerus opposite deltoid attachment	Musculocutaneous nerve
Deltoid	Anterior: anterior border of outer third of clavicle Middle: acromion process and outer end of clavicle Posterior: lower margin of spine of scapula	Lateral aspect of humerus, near midpoint	Axillary (circumflex) nerve
Infraspinatus and teres minor	Axillary border and posterior surface of scapula below scapular spine	Posterior aspect of greater tuberosity of humerus	Suprascapular and axillary nerves
Latissimus dorsi	Spinous processes of lower six thoracic and all lumbar vertebrae; posterior surface of sacrum; crest of ilium; lower three ribs	Anterior surface of humerus below head by flat tendon just anterior to, and parallel with, tendon of pectoralis major	Thoracodorsal (middle subscapular) nerve
Pectoralis major	Medial two thirds of clavicle; anterior surface of sternum; cartilages of first six ribs; slip from aponeurosis of external oblique abdominal muscle	Lateral surface of humerus just below head by flat tendon 2 to 3 inches wide	Medial and lateral anterior thoracic nerves
Subscapularis	Entire anterior surface of scapula	Lesser tuberosity of humerus	Subscapular nerve
Supraspinatus	Medial two-thirds of supraspinatus fossa above scapular spine	Top of greater tuberosity of humerus	Suprascapular nerve
Teres major	Posterior surface of inferior angle of scapula	Anterior surface of humerus below head, just medial to latissimus dorsi tendon	Lower subscapular nerve
Shoulder Girdle			
Levator scapulae	Transverse processes of first four cervical vertebrae	Vertebral border of scapula between medial angle and scapular spine	Dorsal scapular and branches from third and fourth cervical nerves
Pectoralis minor	Anterior surface of third, fourth, and fifth ribs near cartilages	Tip of coracoid processes of scapula	Medial anterior thoracic nerve

*See Chapters 4 and 5.

589

THE UPPER EXTREMITY (Continued)

MUSCLE	PROXIMAL ATTACHMENTS	DISTAL ATTACHMENTS	NERVE SUPPLY
Rhomboids: major and minor	Spinous processes of seventh cervical and first five thoracic vertebrae	Vertebral border of scapula from spine to inferior angle	Dorsal scapular nerve
Serratus anterior	Outer surface of upper nine ribs at side of chest	Anterior surface of vertebral border and inferior angle of scapula	Long thoracic nerve
Trapezius	Occipital bone; ligamentum nuchae; spinous processes of seventh cervical and all thoracic vertebrae	Part I: posterior border of lateral third of clavicle Part II: top of acromium process Part III: upper border of scapular spine Part IV: root of scapular spine	Spinal accessory and branches from third and fourth cervical nerves

Elbow and Forearm

MUSCLE	PROXIMAL ATTACHMENTS	DISTAL ATTACHMENTS	NERVE SUPPLY
Anconeus	Posterior surface of lateral epicondyle of humerus	Lateral side of olecranon process and posterior surface of upper part of ulna	Branch from radial nerve
Biceps brachii	Long head: upper margin of glenoid fossa Short head: apex of coracoid process of scapula	Bicipital tuberosity of radius	Musculocutaneous nerve
Brachialis	Anterior surface of lower half of humerus	Anterior surface of coronoid process of ulna	Musculocutaneous and branch from radial nerves
Brachioradialis	Upper two-thirds of lateral supracondylar ridge of humerus	Lateral side of base of styloid process of radius	Radial nerve
Pronator teres	Medial epicondyle of humerus and medial side of coronoid process of ulna	Lateral surface of radius near middle	Medial nerve
Pronator quadratus	Anterior surface of lower one-fourth of ulna	Anterior surface of lower one-fourth of radius	Branch from median nerve
Supinator	Lateral condyle of humerus; adjacent portion of ulna; radial collateral and annular ligaments	Lateral surface of upper third of radius	Branch from deep radial nerve
Triceps brachii	Long head: infraglenoid tuberosity Lateral head: posterior surface of upper half of humerus Medial head: posterior surface of lower two-thirds of humerus	Olecranon process of ulna	Radial nerve

Wrist

MUSCLE	PROXIMAL ATTACHMENTS	DISTAL ATTACHMENTS	NERVE SUPPLY
Extensor carpi radialis brevis	Lateral condyle of humerus	Posterior surface of base of third metacarpal	Radial nerve
Extensor carpi radialis longus	Lateral epicondyle of humerus and supracondylar ridge above	Posterior surface of base of second metacarpal	Radial nerve
Extensor carpi ulnaris	By two heads from lateral epicondyle of humerus and middle third of posterior ridge of ulna	Posterior surface of base of fifth metacarpal	Deep radial nerve

THE UPPER EXTREMITY (*Continued*)

MUSCLE	PROXIMAL ATTACHMENTS	DISTAL ATTACHMENTS	NERVE SUPPLY
Flexor carpi radialis	Medial epicondyle of humerus	Anterior surface of base of second metacarpal	Median nerve
Flexor carpi ulnaris	By two heads from medial condyle of humerus and medial border of olecranon process of ulna	Palmar surface of pisiform and hamate carpal bones, and base of fifth metacarpal	Ulnar nerve
Palmaris longus	Medial epicondyle of humerus	Transverse carpal ligament and palmar aponeurosis	Median nerve

Thumb and Fingers

MUSCLE	PROXIMAL ATTACHMENTS	DISTAL ATTACHMENTS	NERVE SUPPLY
Abductor pollicis longus	Dorsolateral surface of ulna below anconeus, dorsal surface of radius near center, and intervening interosseous membrane	Lateral surface of base of first metacarpal	Deep radial nerve
Extensor digiti minimi	Proximal tendon of extensor digitorum	Fifth finger's extensor digitorum tendon	Deep radial nerve
Extensor digitorum	Lateral epicondyle of humerus	By four tendons, one to each finger, each tendon dividing into three slips, the middle one attaching to dorsal surface of second phalanx and the other two uniting to attach to dorsal surface of base of distal phalanx	Deep radial nerve
Extensor indicis	Dorsal surface of lower half of ulna	Index finger's extensor digitorum tendon	Deep radial nerve
Extensor pollicis brevis	Dorsal surface of radius below abductor pollicis longus	Dorsal surface of base of first phalanx	Deep radial nerve
Extensor pollicis longus	Dorsal surface of middle third of ulna	Dorsal surface of base of distal phalanx	Deep radial nerve
Flexor digitorum profundus	Upper two-thirds of anterior and medial surfaces of ulna	By four tendons (one to each finger) to base of distal phalanx, after passing through tendon of flexor digitorum superficialis	Interosseous branch of median nerve
Flexor digitorum superficialis	Humeroulnar head: medial epicondyle of humerus, ulnar collateral ligament, medial margin of coronoid process / Radial head: oblique line on anterior surface of radial shaft	By four tendons to the four fingers, each tendon splitting to attach to either side of base of middle phalanx	Median nerve
Flexor pollicis longus	Anterior surface of middle half of radius	Anterior surface of base of distal phalanx of thumb	Volar interosseous branch of median nerve
Abductor digiti minimi	Pisiform bone and tendon of flexor carpi ulnaris	Ulnar side of base of first phalanx of fifth finger and ulnar border of aponeurosis of extensor digiti minimi	Ulnar nerve
Abductor pollicis brevis	Anterior surface of transverse carpal ligament, greater multangular and navicular bones	Radial side of base of first phalanx of thumb	Median nerve

THE UPPER EXTREMITY (*Continued*)

MUSCLE	PROXIMAL ATTACHMENTS	DISTAL ATTACHMENTS	NERVE SUPPLY
Adductor pollicis	Carpal (oblique) head: deep carpal ligaments, capitate bone, and bases of second and third metacarpals Metacarpal (transverse) head: lower two-thirds of anterior surface of third metacarpal	Ulnar side of base of proximal phalanx of thumb	Deep palmar branch of ulnar nerve
Flexor digiti minimi brevis	Hook of hamate bone and adjacent parts of transverse carpal ligament	Ulnar side of base of first phalanx of fifth finger	Palmar division of ulnar nerve
Flexor pollicis brevis	Superficial head: greater multangular bone and adjacent part of transverse carpal ligament Deep head: ulnar side of first metacarpal	Superficial head: radial side of base of first phalanx of thumb Deep head: ulnar side of base of first phalanx of thumb	Median nerve
Interossei dorsales	By two heads from adjacent sides of metacarpals in each interspace	Base of proximal phalanx and aponeurosis of extensor muscles on each side of middle finger, on thumb side of index finger, and on ulnar side of fourth finger	Palmar branch of ulnar nerve
Interossei palmares	First: ulnar side of second metacarpal	First: ulnar side of base of first phalanx of index finger and expansion of extensor digitorum tendon	Ulnar nerve
	Second: radial side of fourth metacarpal	Second: radial side of base of first phalanx of fourth finger and expansion of extensor digitorum tendon	
	Third: radial side of fifth metacarpal	Third: radial side of base of first phalanx of fifth finger and expansion of extensor digitorum tendon	
Lumbricales	Tendons of flexor digitorum profundus in center of palm	Extensor aponeuroses on radial side of proximal phalanges	First and second: median nerve; third and fourth: ulnar nerve
Opponens digiti minimi	Hook of hamate bone and adjacent parts of transverse carpal ligament	Entire length of ulnar border of fifth metacarpal	Deep palmar branch of ulnar nerve
Opponens pollicis	Anterior surface of greater multangular bone and transverse carpal ligament	Entire radial border of anterior surface of first metacarpal	Median nerve

THE LOWER EXTREMITY*

MUSCLE	PROXIMAL ATTACHMENTS	DISTAL ATTACHMENTS	NERVE SUPPLY

Hip Joint

Adductor brevis	Outer surface of body and inferior ramus of pubis	Line from lesser trochanter to linea aspera and upper fourth of linea aspera	Obdurator and accessory obdurator nerves

*See Chapters 6 and 7.

THE LOWER EXTREMITY *(Continued)*

MUSCLE	PROXIMAL ATTACHMENTS	DISTAL ATTACHMENTS	NERVE SUPPLY
Adductor longus	Anterior surface of pubis	Medial lip of middle half of linea aspera	Obdurator nerve
Adductor magnus	Inferior rami of pubis and ischium and lateral border of inferior surface of ischial tuberosity	Linea aspera, medial supracondylar line, and adductor tubercle on medial condyle of femur	Obdurator nerve
Biceps femoris, long head	Lower and medial impression on tuberosity of ischium	Lateral side of head of fibula and lateral condyle of tibia	Sciatic nerve
Gluteus maximus	Posterior gluteal line of ilium and adjacent portion of crest; posterior surface of lower part of sacrum and side of coccyx	Posterior surface of femur on ridge below greater trochanter; iliotibial tract of fascia lata	Inferior gluteal nerve
Gluteus medius	Posterior surface of ilium between crest, posterior gluteal line, and anterior gluteal line	Oblique ridge on lateral surface of greater trochanter	Superior gluteal nerve
Gluteus minimus	Posterior surface of ilium between anterior and inferior gluteal lines	Anterior border to greater trochanter	Superior gluteal nerve
Gracilis	Anterior aspect of lower half of symphysis pubis and upper half of pubic arch	Medial surface of tibia just below condyle	Obturator
Iliopsoas	Psoas major: sides of bodies and intervertebral cartilages of last thoracic and all lumbar vertebrae; front and lower borders of transverse processes of lumbar vertebrae / Iliacus: anterior surface of ilium and base of sacrum	Both: lesser trochanter of femur and for a short distance below along medial border of shaft	Femoral nerve
Pectineus	Pectineal line between iliopectineal eminence and tubercle of pubis	Pectineal line of femur, between lesser trochanter and linea aspera	Femoral nerve
Rectus femoris	Anterior inferior iliac spine and groove above brim of acetabulum	Base of patella, as part of quadriceps femoris tendon; by means of patellar ligament it attaches to the tibial tuberosity	Femoral nerve
Sartorius	Anterior superior iliac spine and upper half of notch below it	Anterior and medial surface of tibia just below condyle	Femoral nerve
Semimembranosus	Upper and lateral impression on tuberosity of ischium	Horizontal groove on posterior surface of medial condyle of tibia	Sciatic nerve
Semitendinosus	Lower and medial impression on tuberosity of ischium with biceps femoris	Upper part of medial surface of shaft of tibia	Sciatic nerve
Six deep outward rotators	Outer and inner surfaces of sacrum and of pelvis in region of obturator foramen	Posterior and medial aspects of greater trochanter	Third, fourth, and fifth lumbar and first and second sacral nerves
Tensor fasciae latae	Anterior part of outer lip of iliac crest and outer surface of anterior superior iliac spine	Iliotibial tract of fascia lata on lateroanterior aspect of thigh, about one-third of the way down	Superior gluteal nerve

THE LOWER EXTREMITY (Continued)

MUSCLE	PROXIMAL ATTACHMENTS	DISTAL ATTACHMENTS	NERVE SUPPLY
Knee Joint			
Biceps femoris	Long head: lower and medial impression on tuberosity of ischium Short head: lateral lip of linea aspera	Lateral side of head of fibula and lateral condyle of tibia	Sciatic nerve
Gracilis	See hip joint		
Popliteus	Lateral surface of lateral condyle of femur	Posterior surface of tibia, above popliteal line	Tibial nerve
Rectus femoris sartorius, semimembranosus, semitendinosus	See hip joint		
The three vasti	V. lateralis: upper part of intertrochanteric line; anterior and lower borders of greater trochanter; lateral lip of gluteal tuberosity; upper half of linea aspera V. intermedius: anterior and lateral surface of upper two-thirds of shaft of femur V. medialis: lower half of intertrochanteric line; medial lip of linea aspera; upper part of medial supracondylar line	The tendons of the three vasti muscles unite with that of rectus femoris to form the quadriceps femoris tendon; this attaches to the base of the patella and, indirectly, by means of the patellar ligament, to the tuberosity of the tibia	Femoral nerve
Ankle Joint, Foot, and Toes			
Extensor digitorum longus	Lateral condyle of tibia and upper three-fourths of anterior surface of fibula	Dorsal surface of second and third phalanges of four lesser toes	Deep peroneal nerve
Extensor hallucis longus	Middle half of anterior surface of fibula	Dorsal surface of base of distal phalanx of hallux (great toe)	Deep peroneal nerve
Flexor digitorum longus	Posterior surface of middle three-fifths of tibia	Plantar surface of base of distal phalanx of each of the four lesser toes	Tibial nerve
Flexor hallucis longus	Posterior surface of lower two-thirds of fibula	Plantar surface of base of distal phalanx of hallux (great toe)	Tibial nerve
Gastrocnemius	Posterior surface of each femoral condyle and adjacent parts by two separate heads	Posterior surface of calcaneus by means of calcaneal tendon (tendon of Achilles)	Tibial nerve
Peroneus brevis	Lateral surface of lateral two-thirds of fibula	Tuberosity on lateral side of base of fifth metatarsal	Superficial peroneal nerve
Peroneus longus	Lateral condyle of tibia; lateral surface of head and upper two-thirds of fibula	Lateral margin of plantar surface of first cuneiform and base of first metatarsal	Superficial peroneal nerve
Peroneus tertius	Anterior surface of lower third of fibula	Dorsal surface of base of fifth metatarsal	Deep peroneal nerve

THE LOWER EXTREMITY *(Continued)*

MUSCLE	PROXIMAL ATTACHMENTS	DISTAL ATTACHMENTS	NERVE SUPPLY
Soleus	Posterior surface of head of fibula and upper two-thirds of shaft; popliteal line and medial border of middle third of tibia	Posterior surface of calcaneus by means of calcaneal tendon (tendon of Achilles)	Tibial nerve
Tibialis anterior	Lateral condyle and upper two-thirds of lateral surface of tibia	Plantar surface of base of first metatarsal and medial surface of first cuneiform	Deep peroneal nerve
Tibialis posterior	Posterior surface of upper two-thirds of tibia beginning at popliteal line; medial surface of upper two-thirds of fibula	Tuberosity of navicular bone with branches to sustentaculum tali of calcaneus, to three cuneiforms, to cuboid, and to bases of three middle metatarsal bones	Tibial nerve

THE SPINAL COLUMN*

MUSCLE	LOWER ATTACHMENTS	UPPER ATTACHMENTS	NERVE SUPPLY
Deep posterior spinal muscles	Posterior surface of sacrum and posterior processes of all the vertebrae	Spinous and transverse processes and laminae of vertebrae slightly higher than lower attachments	Branches of spinal nerves for all but levator costorum, which is innervated by intercostal and eighth cervical nerves
Erector spinae	Thoracolumbar fascia; posterior portions of lumbar, thoracic and lower cervical vertebrae; angles of ribs	Angles of ribs; posterior portions of cervical and thoracic vertebrae; mastoid process of temporal bone	Posterior branches of spinal nerves
Hyoid muscles	Suprahyoid: hyoid bone; Infrahyoid: sternum, clavicle, and scapula	Temporal bone and mandible; Hyoid bone	Facial, inferior alveolar, hypoglossi, and ansa hyperglossi
Levator scapula	See shoulder girdle		
Obliquus externus abdominis	Anterior half of crest of ilium; aponeurosis from ribs to crest of pubis	Lower border of lower eight ribs by tendinous slips that interdigitate with those of serratus anterior	Lower seven intercostal nerves and iliohypogastric nerves
Obliquus internus abdominis	Inguinal ligament; crest of ilium; thoracolumbar fascia	Anterior and middle fibers into crest of pubis, linea alba, and aponeurosis on front of body; posterior fibers, by three separate slips, into cartilages of lower three ribs	Lower three intercostal nerves, the iliohypogastric and the ilioinguinal nerves
Prevertebral muscles	Anterior surfaces of various parts of cervical vertebrae and of upper three thoracic vertebrae	Anterior portions of occipital bone and of cervical vertebrae	Cervical nerves
Psoas	See hip joint		
Quadratus lumborum	Crest of ilium and iliolumbar ligament	Lower border of twelfth rib and tips of transverse processes of upper four lumbar vertebrae	Branches from the upper three or four lumbar nerves
Rectus abdominis	Crest of pubis	Cartilages of fifth, sixth, and seventh ribs	Anterior branches of lower six intercostal nerves
Scalenes (three)	First two ribs	Transverse processes of cervical vertebrae	Branches from second to seventh cervical nerves inclusive

*See Chapter 8.

THE SPINAL COLUMN (Continued)

MUSCLE	LOWER ATTACHMENTS	UPPER ATTACHMENTS	NERVE SUPPLY
Semispinalis thoracis, cervicis, and capitis	Transverse processes of all thoracic and seventh cervical vertebrae; articular processes of lower four cervical vertebrae	Spinous process of upper four thoracic and lower five cervical vertebrae; occipital bone	Posterior branches of cervical and upper six thoracic nerves
Splenius capitis and cervicis	Lower half of ligamentum nuchae; spinous processes of seventh cervical and upper six thoracic vertebrae	Mastoid process of temporal bone and adjacent part of occipital bone; transverse processes of upper three cervical vertebrae	Branches from second, third, and fourth cervical nerves
Sternocleidomastoid	By two heads from top of sternum and medial third of clavicle	Mastoid process of temporal bone and adjacent portion of occipital bone	Accessory and branches from the second and third cervical nerves
Suboccipitals	Posterior portions of atlas and axis	Occipital bone and transverse process of atlas	Branches from the first two cervical nerves

MAJOR RESPIRATORY MUSCLES*

MUSCLE	PERIPHERAL ATTACHMENT	CENTRAL ATTACHMENT	NERVE SUPPLY
Diaphragm	Circumference of thoracic outlet	Central tendon, a cloverleaf-shaped aponeurosis	Phrenic nerve

MUSCLE	UPPER ATTACHMENTS	LOWER ATTACHMENTS	NERVE SUPPLY
Intercostales externi	Lower border of each rib but last	Upper border of rib immediately below	Branches from corresponding intercostal nerves
Intercostales interni	Inner surface and costal cartilage of each rib but last	Upper border of rib immediately below	Branches from corresponding intercostal nerves
Levatores costarum	Transverse processes of seventh cervical and upper eleven thoracic vertebrae	Upper eight: each to rib immediately below, between tubercle and angle Lower four: by two bands each, one to rib immediately below and other to second rib below	Branches from corresponding intercostal nerves
Serratus posterior inferior	Lower borders of lower four ribs	Spinous processes and ligaments of lower two thoracic and upper two or three lumbar vertebrae	Branches from ninth, tenth, and eleventh intercostal nerves
Serratus posterior superior	Spinous processes and ligaments of lower two or three cervical and upper two thoracic vertebrae	Upper borders of second, third, fourth, and fifth ribs	Branches from the first four intercostal nerves

*See Chapter 8.

MAJOR RESPIRATORY MUSCLES *(Continued)*

MUSCLE	UPPER ATTACHMENTS	LOWER ATTACHMENTS	NERVE SUPPLY
Transversus abdominis	Inguinal ligament, crest of ilium, thoracolumbar fascia, and cartilages of lower six ribs	Linea alba and crest of pubis	Branches of lower six intercostal nerves, iliohypogastric, and ilioinguinal nerves
Transversus thoracis	Lower borders and inner surfaces of costal cartilages of second, third, fourth, fifth, and sixth ribs	Lower half of inner surface of sternum and adjoining costal cartilages	Branches from upper six thoracic intercostal nerves

ADDITIONAL MUSCLES THAT PARTICIPATE IN RESPIRATION

Muscles of shoulder joint or shoulder girdle
    Pectoralis major
    Pectoralis minor
    Trapezius I and II
Muscles of the spinal column
    Quadratus lumborum
    Scalenes: anterior, posterior, medialis
    Sternocleidomastoid

Appendix E

Checklists for the Muscular Analysis of Movements of the Major Body Segments

These checklists were originally devised for the recording of the muscular actions identified in the palpation experiments described in the section headed Laboratory Experiences at the ends of Chapters 4 through 8. For the most part only the basic movements of individual body segments were used in these exercises. Although it is recognized that the palpation method is not as accurate as the electromyographic method for ascertaining muscular actions, the palpation method is invaluable as a method for studying muscular activity and for supplementing book study.

In addition to their use in identifying the actions of muscles in basic movements, the checklists are useful for the recording of the muscular analyses of postural and conditioning exercises and of the typical motor skills of familiar sports, gymnastic and tumbling events, dance techniques, and so on. For this purpose an ample number of duplicate copies of the lists should be available inasmuch as a complete set may be needed *for each phase* of a movement that involves the entire body. It would be helpful if spaces were provided on these for the student's name and the name of the motor skill being analyzed.

For developing skill in analyzing movements anatomically, much practice is needed. It is therefore suggested that the student start as soon as feasible to make such analyses, progressing from the basic movements to more complex motor skills as rapidly as possible. The following suggestions may prove helpful.

Procedure for Making an Anatomical Analysis of a Movement*

1. Have someone demonstrate the movement to be analyzed both before and at frequent intervals throughout the analysis. In lieu of this, motion pictures (preferably slow motion films shown on a projector which can be stopped at will) are an excellent substitute. If these are not available, a series of still shots or even a single photograph or sketch is helpful.

2. Divide the movement into logical phases, such as

   a. Essential act or propulsive phase and return movement or recovery phase. (Appropriate for calisthenic exercises, swimming strokes, and other two-part movements.)

   b. Preparatory movement, essential act, and follow-through or recovery. (Appropriate for throwing, striking, and kicking activities.)

3. Consider the starting position of the body (vertical, horizontal—prone, supine, side, or other) and the means of its support (ground, water, suspension apparatus, none). In this connection consider the effect of gravity on the muscular action.

4. Consider the nature of the movement, whether fast or slow, ballistic or nonballistic, against or not against resistance, and so on. Consider the effect of this on the muscular action.

5. Identify the movement of each body segment and analyze the joint actions. These may be recorded on the checklists by placing a check in the appropriate spaces across the top of the checklist.

6. Considering all the essential factors, analyze the muscular action and record on the checklist.

   a. Elementary method. Place a check mark in the appropriate space for each muscle that contributes positively to the movement.

---

*See Appendix I for illustrations of conditioning and postural exercises, sports movements, and gymnastic techniques that serve as material for practice in making kinesiological analyses.

b. *Advanced method*
    (1) To differentiate between principal and assistant muscles use P and A.
    (2) To differentiate between concentric (shortening), eccentric (lengthening), and static contraction, use different colored pencils.

7. After completing the muscular analysis consider the following questions:
    a. Are there any clearcut examples of the neutralizing or of the mutually neutralizing action of muscles? If so, identify and explain.
    b. Are there any clearcut examples of stabilization of a segment of the body by muscular action? If so, identify and explain.
    c. Are there any pertinent mechanical aspects or principles which should be taken into consideration in this exercise? If so, identify and explain.

Checklists follow

CHECKLIST FOR MUSCULAR ANALYSIS OF MOVEMENTS OF THE ARM ON THE BODY*

	SIDE-WARD ELEV. OF ARM	SIDE-WARD DEPR. OF ARM	FWD. ELEV. OF ARM	FWD. DEPR. OF ARM	BKWD. ELEV. OF ARM	HOR. BKWD. SWING OF ARM	HOR. SIDE-WARD FWD. SWING	OUT-WARD ROT'N OF ARM	IN-WARD ROT'N OF ARM	ELEV. OF SHOUL. GIRD.	DEPR. OF SHOUL. GIRD.	ABD. OF SCAP.	ADD. OF SCAP.
Shoulder Girdle													
Subclavius													
Pectoralis minor													
Serratus anterior													
Levator scapulae													
Trapezius I													
Trapezius II													
Trapezius III													
Trapezius IV													
Rhomboids													

*The checklists in Appendices A and E may be reproduced for class use without specific permission.

CHECKLIST FOR MUSCULAR ANALYSIS OF MOVEMENTS OF THE ARM ON THE BODY (Continued)

	SIDE-WARD ELEV. OF ARM	SIDE-WARD DEPR. OF ARM	FWD. ELEV. OF ARM	FWD. DEPR. OF ARM	BKWD. ELEV. OF ARM	HOR. BKWD. SWING OF ARM	HOR. SIDE-WARD FWD. SWING	OUT-WARD ROT'N OF ARM	IN-WARD ROT'N OF ARM	ELEV. OF SHOUL. GIRD.	DEPR. OF SHOUL. GIRD.	ABD. OF SCAP.	ADD. OF SCAP.
Shoulder Joint													
Deltoid: middle													
Deltoid: anterior													
Deltoid: posterior													
Supraspinatus													
Pect. major: clavicular													
Pect. major: sternal													
Coracobrachialis													
Subscapularis													
Latissimus dorsi													
Teres major													
Infrasp. and teres minor													

CHECKLIST FOR MUSCULAR ANALYSIS OF MOVEMENTS OF THE FOREARM AT THE ELBOW AND RADIOULNAR JOINTS

	FLEXION	EXTENSION	SUPINA-TION	PRONA-TION
Muscles of Elbow and Forearm				
Biceps				
Brachialis				
Brachioradialis				
Pronator teres				
Pronator quadratus				
Supinator				
Triceps				
Anconeus				
Muscles of Wrist				
Flexor carpi radialis				
Flexor carpi ulnaris				
Palmaris longus				
Extensor carpi radialis longus				
Extensor carpi radialis brevis				
Extensor carpi ulnaris				

CHECKLIST FOR MUSCULAR ANALYSIS OF MOVEMENTS
OF THE HAND AT THE WRIST

	FLEXION	EXTENSION	ULNAR FLEXION	RADIAL FLEXION
Muscles of Wrist				
Flexor carpi radialis				
Flexor carpi ulnaris				
Palmaris longus				
Extensor carpi radialis longus				
Extensor carpi radialis brevis				
Extensor carpi ulnaris				
Muscles of Thumb and Fingers				
Flexor digitorum superficialis				
Flexor digitorum profundus				
Extensor digitorum				
Extensor indicis				
Extensor digiti minimi				
Flexor pollicis longus				
Extensor pollicis longus				
Extensor pollicis brevis				
Abductor pollicis longus				

**CHECKLIST FOR MUSCULAR ANALYSIS OF
MOVEMENTS OF THE FINGERS**

	METACARPOPHALANGEAL				INTERPHALANGEAL	
	FLEX.	EXT.	ABD.	ADD.	FLEX.	EXT.
On Forearm						
Flexor digitorum superficialis						
Flexor digitorum profundus						
Extensor digitorum						
Extensor indicis						
Extensor digiti minimi						
In Hand						
Lumbricales						
Palmar interossei						
Dorsal interossei						
Abductor digiti minimi						
Flexor digiti minimi brevi						
Opponens digiti minimi						

CHECKLIST FOR MUSCULAR ANALYSIS OF
MOVEMENTS OF THE THUMB

	CARPOMETACARPAL					METACARPO-PHALANGEAL		INTERPHA-LANGEAL	
	FLEX.	EXT. & HYP. EX.	ABD.	ADD. & HYP. ADD.	OPP.	FLEX.	EXT.	FLEX.	EXT.
On Forearm									
Flexor pollicis longus									
Extensor pollicis longus									
Extensor pollicis brevis									
Abductor pollicis longus									
In Hand									
Flexor pollicis brevis									
Abductor pollicis brevis									
Opponens pollicis									
Adductor pollicis									

CHECKLIST FOR MUSCULAR ANALYSIS OF
MOVEMENTS OF THE PELVIC GIRDLE

	INCREASED INCLINATION	DECREASED INCLINATION	LATERAL TILT*	ROTATION*
Rectus abdominis				
External oblique				
Internal oblique				
Erector spinae				
Quadratus lumborum				
Psoas				
Gluteus maximus				
Gluteus medius and minimus				
Tensor fasciae latae				
Others:				

Note: Because of the numerous two-joint muscles found in the lower extremity, the checklist for the muscular analysis of movements of the hip is combined with that for the knee. See following page.

*Indicate left (L) or right (R).

**CHECKLIST FOR MUSCULAR ANALYSIS OF
MOVEMENTS OF THE THIGH AND LEG**

	HIP						KNEE			
	FLEX.	EXT.	ABD.	ADD.	OUT. ROT.	INWD. ROT.	FLEX.	EXT.	OUT. ROT.	INWD. ROT.
Iliopsoas										
Sartorius										
Pectineus										
Tensor fasciae latae										
Gluteus maximus										
Gluteus medius										
Gluteus minimus										
Six deep rotators										
Adductor magnus										
Adductor longus										
Adductor brevis										
Gracilis										
Biceps femoris										
Semitendinosus										
Semimembranosus										
Rectus femoris										
Vastus intermedius										
Vastus lateralis										
Vastus medialis										
Popliteus										
Gastrocnemius										

CHECKLIST FOR MUSCULAR ANALYSIS OF
MOVEMENTS OF THE ANKLE, FOOT, AND TOES

	ANKLE		FOOT				TOES	
	DORSI-FLEX.	PLANT. FLEX.	DORSI-FLEX.	PLANT. FLEX.	INV. & ADDUC.	EVERS. & ABD.	FLEX.	EXT.
Tibialis anterior								
Extensor hallucis longus								
Extensor digitorum longus								
Peroneus tertius								
Peroneus longus								
Peroneus brevis								
Tibialis posterior								
Gastrocnemius								
Soleus								
Flexor hallucis longus								
Flexor digitorum longus								

CHECKLIST FOR MUSCULAR ANALYSIS OF MOVEMENTS
OF THE HEAD AND NECK

	FLEXION	EXTENSION	LATERAL FLEXION	ROTATION SAME SIDE*	ROTATION OPPOSITE SIDE*
Anterior					
Prevertebral muscles					
Hyoid muscles					
Lateral					
Three scalenes					
Sternocleidomastoid					
Levator scapulae					
Posterior					
Splenius					
Suboccipitals					
Erector spinae					
Semispinalis					
Deep posterior muscles					
Other					

*Indicate left (L) or right (R).

CHECKLIST FOR MUSCULAR ANALYSIS OF MOVEMENTS
OF THE THORACIC AND LUMBAR SPINE

	FLEXION	EXTENSION	LATERAL FLEXION	ROTATION SAME SIDE*	ROTATION OPPOSITE SIDE*
Anterior					
Rectus abdominis					
External oblique abdominis					
Internal oblique abdominis					
Lateral					
Quadratus lumborum					
Posterior					
Erector spinae					
Semispinalis thoracis					
Deep posterior muscles					
Other					

*Indicate left (L) or right (R).

CHECKLIST FOR MUSCULAR ANALYSIS OF MOVEMENTS
INVOLVED IN RESPIRATION

	NORMAL INHALATION	VIGOROUS INHALATION	VIGOROUS EXHALATION
Muscles of Respiration			
Diaphragm			
External intercostals			
Internal intercostals, anterior			
Internal intercostals, posterior and lateral			
Levatores costarum			
Serratus posterior superior			
Serratus posterior inferior			
Transversus thoracis			
Transversus abdominis			
Muscles of the Spine			
Sternocleidomastoid			
Three scalenes			
Thoracic extensors			
Rectus abdominis			
External oblique			
Internal oblique			
Muscles of the Shoulder Girdle and Joint			
Pectoralis minor			
Trapezius I			
Levator scapulae			
Others			

Appendix F

Mathematics Review

1. Order of Arithmetic Operations:

Certain arithmetic operations take precedence over others. In completing problems with a series of operations the following guidelines apply:

    a.   Addition or subtraction may occur in any order.

        Example: $4 + 8 - 7 + 3 = 8$ or $8 + 3 + 4 - 7 = 8$

    b.   Multiplication or division must be completed before addition or subtraction.

        Example: $48 \div 6 + 2 = 10$ *Example:* $4 + (2/3)(1/2) = 4\,1/3$

    c.   Any quantity above a division line, under a division line or a radical sign ($\sqrt{}$), or within parentheses or brackets must be treated as one number.

        Example: $\sqrt{36 - 25} = \sqrt{11}$ *Example:* $2(5 + 3 - 4) = 8$

        Example: $\dfrac{9 + 2}{3} = \dfrac{11}{3}$

2. Fractions, Decimals, and Percents:

    a.   To add (or subtract) fractions, the denominator in each term must be the same. (Choose the lowest common denominator for each term. Multiply each term by the common denominator and then add [or subtract].)

        Example: $\dfrac{3}{4} + \dfrac{5}{3} = \dfrac{29}{12} = 2\dfrac{5}{12}$ (lowest common denominator $= 12$)

        Solution:

$$\left(\frac{\frac{3}{4} \times 12}{12}\right) + \left(\frac{\frac{5}{3} \times 12}{12}\right) = \frac{9}{12} + \frac{20}{12} = \frac{29}{12} = 2\frac{5}{12}$$

        Example: $\dfrac{cd}{x} + \dfrac{x}{c} = \dfrac{c^2 d + x^2}{xc}$ (lowest common denominator $= xc$)

        Solution:

$$\left(\frac{\frac{cd}{x} \cdot xc}{xc}\right) + \left(\frac{\frac{x}{c} \cdot xc}{xc}\right) = \frac{c^2 d}{xc} + \frac{x^2}{xc} = \frac{c^2 d + x^2}{xc}$$

    b.   To multiply fractions, multiply the numerators by each other and the denominators by each other.

Example: $\dfrac{3}{8} \cdot \dfrac{2}{3} = \dfrac{6}{24} = \dfrac{1}{4}$

Example: $pq\left(\dfrac{p}{q}\right) = \dfrac{p^2q}{q} = p^2$

c.   To divide fractions, invert the divisor and multiply.

Example: $\dfrac{3}{8} \div \dfrac{9}{2} = \dfrac{3}{8} \times \dfrac{2}{9} = \dfrac{6}{72} = \dfrac{1}{12}$

Example: $\dfrac{n}{r} \div \dfrac{s}{t} = \dfrac{n}{r} \times \dfrac{t}{s} = \dfrac{nt}{rs}$

Example: $\left(\dfrac{1}{a} + \dfrac{1}{b}\right) \div \left(\dfrac{1}{a} - \dfrac{1}{b}\right) = \dfrac{b+a}{ab} \cdot \dfrac{ab}{b-a} = \dfrac{b+a}{b-a}$

d.   To convert a fraction to a percent, divide the numerator by the denominator and multiply by 100.

Example: $\dfrac{3}{8} = .375 \times 100 = 37.5\%$

Note: To convert a percent to a decimal move the decimal point two places to the left.

e.   When *dividing* by a decimal divide by the integer and add sufficient zeros to move the decimal point the appropriate number of digits to the *right*.

Example: $36 \div .04 = 900$ or $36 \div 4 = 9$ plus 00. = 900

(appropriate number of digits to right = 2)

When *multiplying* by a decimal multiply the integer and add enough zeros to move the decimal point the appropriate number of digits to the *left*.

Example: $6 \times .012 = .072$ or $6 \times 12 = 72$ plus 0 to left = .072

(appropriate number of digits to left = 3)

f.   Decimals may be expressed as positive or negative powers of 10:

$10^0 = 1$	$10^{-1} = 0.1$
$10^1 = 10$	$10^{-2} = 0.01$
$10^2 = 100$	$10^{-3} = 0.001$
$10^3 = 1000$	$10^{-4} = 0.0001$

Example: $5624 = 56.24 \times 10^2$
$= 5.624 \times 10^3$
$= .5624 \times 10^4$

Example: $.0379 = 3.79 \times 10^{-2}$
$= 37.9 \times 10^{-3}$
$= 379 \times 10^{-4}$

3.   Proportions, Formulas, and Equations

The location of values in proportions, equations, or formulas may be shifted provided that whatever addition, subtraction, multiplication, or division is performed on one side of the equation is also performed on the other side.

Example: $\dfrac{a}{b} = \dfrac{c}{d}$

Solve for d: $d \cdot \dfrac{a}{b} = \dfrac{c}{d} \cdot d$

$$d \cdot \dfrac{a}{b} \cdot \dfrac{b}{a} = c \cdot \dfrac{b}{a}$$

$$d = c \cdot \dfrac{b}{a}$$

Example: $v^2 = u^2 + 2as$

Solve for s: $2as = v^2 - u^2$

$$s = \dfrac{v^2 - u^2}{2a}$$

4. **Right Triangles and Trigonometric Equations:**

   a.   In a right triangle one angle always equals 90°. The other two angles will always be acute angles and the sum of these two angles will be 90° since the sum of the angles in any triangle is 180°.

   b.   In a right triangle the *sides* are related to each other so that the square of the longest side or *hypotenuse (c)* is equal to the sum of the squares of the other two sides: $c^2 = a^2 + b^2$. This is the Pythagorean Theorem.

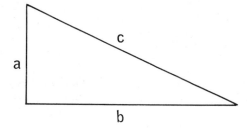

   c.   In triangle *ABC*, side *a* is called the side opposite angle *A*, side *b* is opposite angle *B*, and the hypotenuse, *c*, is opposite the right angle. Side *b* is named the side *adjacent* to angle *A* and side *a* is the side adjacent to angle *B*.

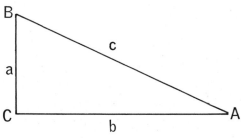

   d.   *Trigonometric functions* are ratios between the sides of a right triangle and are determined by the value of one of the acute angles. There are six trigonometric functions, the sine, cosine, tangent, cotangent, secant, and cosecant, but it will be necessary to consider only the first four here.

   In $\triangle ABC$ the ratio between the side opposite one of the acute angles and the hypotenuse is called the **sine** of the angle. For angle *A* it would be written as

   the sine $\angle A = \dfrac{a}{c}$, or $\sin A = \dfrac{a}{c}$;

   the sine $\angle B = \dfrac{b}{c}$, or $\sin B = \dfrac{b}{c}$.

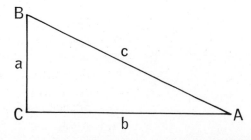

The **cosine** expresses the ratio between the side adjacent and the hypotenuse. For angle A, $\cos A = \dfrac{b}{c}$; for angle B, $\cos B = \dfrac{a}{c}$.

The **tangent** and **cotangent** represent ratios between the two sides of the triangle. For angle A, $\tan A = \dfrac{a}{b}$ and $\cot A = \dfrac{b}{a}$; for angle B, $\tan B = \dfrac{b}{a}$ and $\cot B = \dfrac{a}{b}$. A glance at these values shows that $\sin A = \cos B$, and that $\tan A = \cot B$.

As can be seen from studying these ratios, two functions may have the same ratio. For instance, the $\sin A = \cos B$ and the $\tan A = \cot B$.

In general terms these trigonometric functions are expressed as follows:

$$\sin \theta^* = \frac{\text{side opposite}}{\text{hypotenuse}} \quad or \quad \sin \theta = \frac{\text{opp}}{\text{hyp}}$$

$$\cos \theta = \frac{\text{side adjacent}}{\text{hypotenuse}} \quad or \quad \cos \theta = \frac{\text{adj}}{\text{hyp}}$$

$$\tan \theta = \frac{\text{side opposite}}{\text{side adjacent}} \quad or \quad \tan \theta = \frac{\text{opp}}{\text{adj}}$$

$$\cot \theta = \frac{\text{side adjacent}}{\text{side opposite}} \quad or \quad \cot \theta = \frac{\text{adj}}{\text{opp}}$$

e.   Values of trigonometric functions may be obtained from tables of trigonometric functions (see Appendix F) or from hand-held calculators with trigonometric function capability.

Example: $\sin 60° = .8660$
$\cos 30° = .8660$
$\tan 22° = .4040$
$\cot 68° = .4040$

Tables of trigonometric functions usually go up to 90°. Angles greater than 90° may be handled as follows:

(1) Functions of angles greater than 90° but less than 180° are the same as functions of an angle equal to 180° minus the angle in question. All functions of angles in this range are negative except the sine.

Example: $\sin 120° = \sin 60°$
$\tan 150° = -\tan 30°$

(2) Functions of angles greater than 180° but less than 270° are the same as functions of an angle equal to 270° minus the angle in question. Functions of angles in this range are negative except for the tan and cot.

Example: $\cos 220° = -\cos 50°$
$\tan 195° = \tan 75°$

(3) Functions of angles greater than 270° but less than 360° are the same as functions of an angle equal to 360° minus the angle in question. All functions of angles in this range are negative except the cosine.

*θ (Greek letter, *theta*) is the symbol for angle.

Example: cot 300° = −cot 60°
   sin 330° = −sin 30°

f. Through the use of trigonometric functions, it is possible to determine the values of all components of a triangle when the values of *one side and one angle* or the values of *two sides* are known.

Example 1: In triangle ABC, angle $A = 25°$ and the length of the hypotenuse is 15 ft. Find the length of the other two sides.

Solution:

(1) $\sin 25° = \dfrac{a}{c} = \dfrac{a}{15}$

   $a = 15 \sin 25°$

   $a = (15)(.4226)$

   $\boxed{a = 6.34 \text{ ft}}$

(2) $\cos 25° = \dfrac{b}{c} = \dfrac{b}{15}$

   $b = 15 \cos 25°$

   $b = (15)(.9063)$

   $\boxed{b = 13.59 \text{ ft}}$

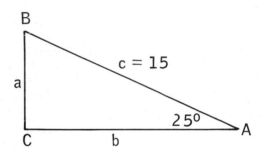

Example 2: In triangle ABC the lengths of the sides are 3 in and 5 in. What is the length of the hypotenuse and the size of both acute angles?

Solution:

(1) $\tan A = \dfrac{a}{b} = \dfrac{3}{5}$

   $A = \arctan .600$

   (i.e., A = angle whose tan is .600)

   $\boxed{A = 31°}$

(2) $B = 90 − A;$ $\boxed{B = 59°}$

(3) $\sin A = \dfrac{a}{c} = \dfrac{3}{c}$

   $C = \dfrac{3}{\sin A} = \dfrac{3}{\sin 31°}$

   $C = \dfrac{3}{.5150} = \boxed{5.83 \text{ in}}$

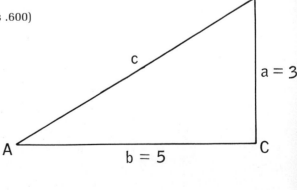

Note: C may also be found using the Pythagorean Theorem: $C^2 = a^2 + b^2$

5. **Geometry of Circles**

a. The circumference of a circle is calculated using the formula $C = 2\pi r$, where C is the circumference, r is the radius, and π (pi) is a constant value of 3.1416. Pi is the ratio that exists between the diameter of a circle and its circumference.

b. In making one complete turn about a circle the radius goes through one revolution, 360° or 2π radians. A radian is the angle subtended by an arc of a circle equal in length to the radius. One radian equals $\dfrac{360°}{2\pi}$ or 57.3°. Some equivalents for these angular units of measure are as follows:

Revolutions	Radians	Degrees
1	2π or 6.28	360°
0.5	1π or 3.14	180°
0.25	0.5π or 1.57	90°
2	4π or 12.56	720°

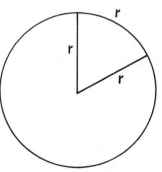

(1) To convert degrees to revolutions divide by 360.

   Example: 1260° = 3.50 rev

(2) To convert radians to revolutions divide by 6.28.

   Example: 15.75 radians = 2.51 rev

(3) To convert degrees to radians divide by 57.3.

   Example: 360° = 6.28 radians

(4) To convert revolutions to radians multiply by 6.28.

   Example: 2.3 rev = 14.44 radians

(5) To convert revolutions to degrees multiply by 360.

   Example: 2.3 rev = 828°

(6) To convert radians to degrees multiply by 57.3.

   Example: 7.6 radians = 435.5°

Appendix G

Table of Trigonometric Functions*

DEGREES	SINES	COSINES	TANGENTS	COTANGENTS	
0	.0000	1.0000	.0000		90
1	.0175	.9998	.0175	57.290	89
2	.0349	.9994	.0349	28.636	88
3	.0523	.9986	.0524	19.081	87
4	.0698	.9976	.0699	14.301	86
5	.0872	.9962	.0875	11.430	85
6	.1045	.9945	.1051	9.5144	84
7	.1219	.9925	.1228	8.1443	83
8	.1392	.9903	.1405	7.1154	82
9	.1564	.9877	.1584	6.3138	81
10	.1736	.9848	.1763	5.6713	80
11	.1908	.9816	.1944	5.1446	79
12	.2079	.9781	.2126	4.7046	78
13	.2250	.9744	.2309	4.3315	77
14	.2419	.9703	.2493	4.0108	76
15	.2588	.9659	.2679	3.7321	75
16	.2756	.9613	.2867	3.4874	74
17	.2924	.9563	.3057	3.2709	73
18	.3090	.9511	.3249	3.0777	72
19	.3256	.9455	.3443	2.9042	71
20	.3420	.9397	.3640	2.7475	70
21	.3584	.9336	.3839	2.6051	69
22	.3746	.9272	.4040	2.4751	68
23	.3907	.9205	.4245	2.3559	67
24	.4067	.9135	.4452	2.2460	66
25	.4226	.9063	.4663	2.1445	65
26	.4384	.8988	.4877	2.0503	64
27	.4540	.8910	.5095	1.9626	63
28	.4695	.8829	.5317	1.8807	62
29	.4848	.8746	.5543	1.8040	61
30	.5000	.8660	.5774	1.7321	60
31	.5150	.8572	.6009	1.6643	59
32	.5299	.8480	.6249	1.6003	58
33	.5446	.8387	.6494	1.5399	57
34	.5592	.8290	.6745	1.4826	56
35	.5736	.8192	.7002	1.4281	55
36	.5878	.8090	.7265	1.3765	54
37	.6018	.7986	.7536	1.3270	53
38	.6157	.7880	.7813	1.2799	52
39	.6293	.7771	.8098	1.2349	51
40	.6428	.7660	.8391	1.1918	50
41	.6561	.7547	.8693	1.1504	49
42	.6691	.7431	.9004	1.1106	48
43	.6820	.7314	.9325	1.0724	47
44	.6947	.7193	.9657	1.0355	46
45	.7071	.7071	1.0000	1.0000	45
	COSINES	SINES	COTANGENTS	TANGENTS	DEGREES

*Note: With angles above 45° be sure to use the headings that appear at the *bottom* of the columns.

Appendix H

English-Metric Equivalents

TO CONVERT FROM	TO	MULTIPLY BY
Inches	Centimeters	2.54
Centimeters	Inches	0.39
Feet	Meters	0.305
Meters	Feet	3.28
Yards	Meters	0.91
Meters	Yards	1.09
Miles	Kilometers	1.61
Kilometers	Miles	0.62
Pounds	Kilograms	0.45
Kilograms	Pounds	2.21
Pounds	Newtons	4.45
Newtons	Pounds	0.225
Slugs	Kilograms	14.59
Kilograms	Slugs	0.068
Ft-lb	Joules	1.36
Joules	Ft-lb	0.735
Ft-lb/sec (power)	Watts	1.36
Watts	Ft-lb/sec	0.735

Appendix I

Exercises for Kinesiological Analysis

These exercises and techniques, intended as laboratory material for the student, are presented for analysis (major joint and muscle action) of movements. Many are commonly used to develop strength, increase flexibility, and improve posture. In most instances they are organized according to the major body segments (the upper and lower extremities and the trunk-head-neck). Many of the exercises are illustrated by three views: (1) the starting position, (2) the movement, and (3) the return to the starting position. The various exercises were selected on the basis of their use in (1) physical fitness and posture programs, (2) conditioning programs for improving athletic performance, and (3) tests for assessing strength and muscular endurance. The sports and gymnastics techniques are representative of movements involving the imparting of motion to one's own body and to external objects. The exercises are organized in the following series:

Series 1   Weight Training Exercises (barbells and weighted pulleys)
Series 2   Isometric Tension Exercises (singly and with partners)
Series 3   Flexibility Exercises
Series 4   Posture Exercises
Series 5   Selected Sports and Gymnastics Techniques

The exercises within each series are numbered consecutively in the following manner: The first exercise in Series 1 is numbered 1–1, the second, 1–2. The first exercise in Series 2 is numbered 2–1, followed by 2–2, and so on in similar fashion.

SERIES 1. WEIGHT TRAINING EXERCISES
THE UPPER EXTREMITY

STARTING POSITION

MOVEMENT

RETURN TO STARTING POSITION

Exercise 1–1.

Exercise 1–2.

Exercise 1–3.

SERIES 1. WEIGHT TRAINING EXERCISES
THE UPPER EXTREMITY

STARTING POSITION   **MOVEMENT**   **RETURN TO STARTING POSITION**

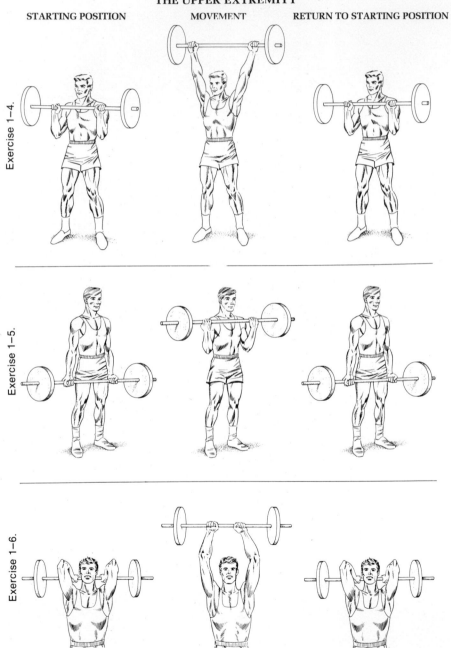

Exercise 1–4.

Exercise 1–5.

Exercise 1–6.

SERIES 1. WEIGHT TRAINING EXERCISES
THE UPPER EXTREMITY

STARTING POSITION   MOVEMENT   RETURN TO STARTING POSITION

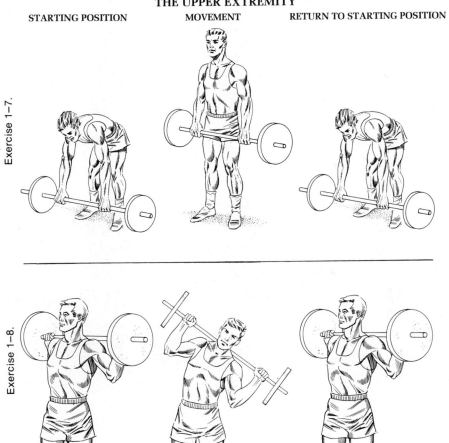

Exercise 1–7.

Exercise 1–8.

SERIES 1. WEIGHT TRAINING EXERCISES
THE LOWER EXTREMITY

STARTING POSITION   **MOVEMENT**   **RETURN TO STARTING POSITION**

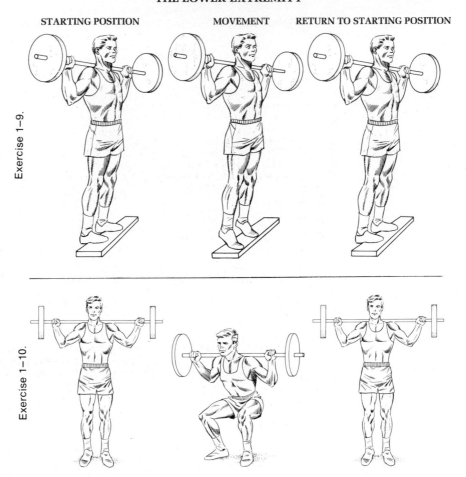

Exercise 1–9.

Exercise 1–10.

SERIES 1. WEIGHT TRAINING EXERCISES
THE LOWER EXTREMITY

STARTING POSITION   MOVEMENT   RETURN TO STARTING POSITION

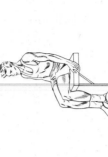 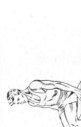 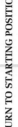

Exercise 1–11.

THE UPPER EXTREMITY

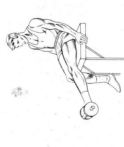 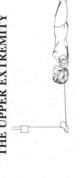 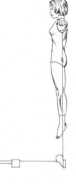

Exercise 1–12.

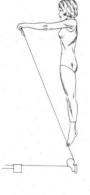 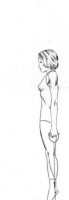

Exercise 1–13.

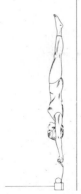 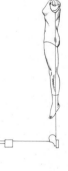

Exercise 1–14.

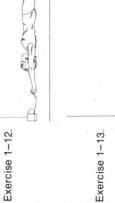 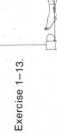 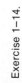   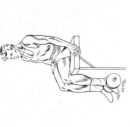 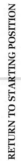 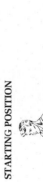

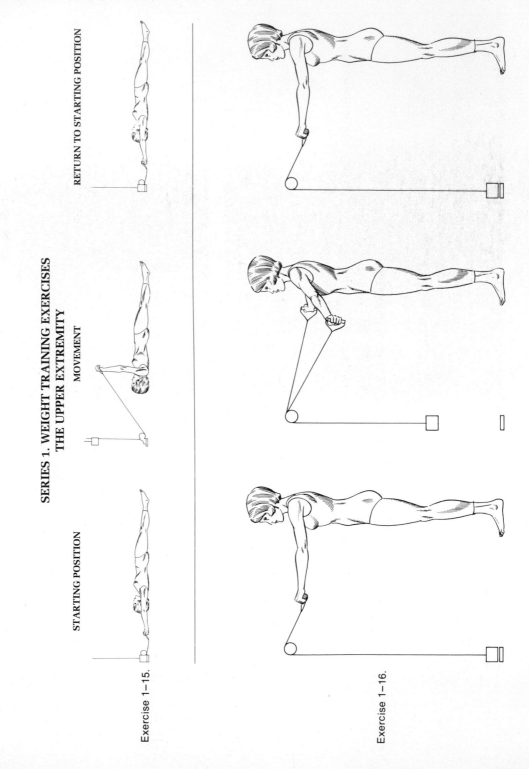

SERIES 1. WEIGHT TRAINING EXERCISES
THE UPPER EXTREMITY

STARTING POSITION

MOVEMENT

RETURN TO STARTING POSITION

Exercise 1–15.

Exercise 1–16.

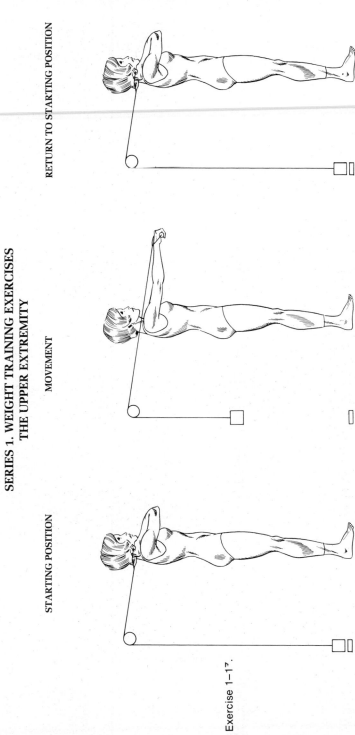

RETURN TO STARTING POSITION

SERIES 1. WEIGHT TRAINING EXERCISES
THE UPPER EXTREMITY

MOVEMENT

STARTING POSITION

Exercise 1–1ᵀ.

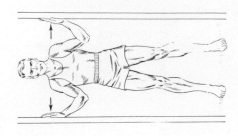

Exercise 2–3.
Push Out

**SERIES 2. ISOMETRIC TENSION EXERCISES
THE UPPER EXTREMITY**

Exercise 2–2.
Pull Up

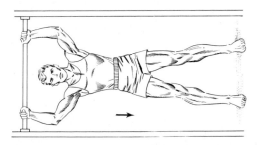

Exercise 2–1.
Pull Down

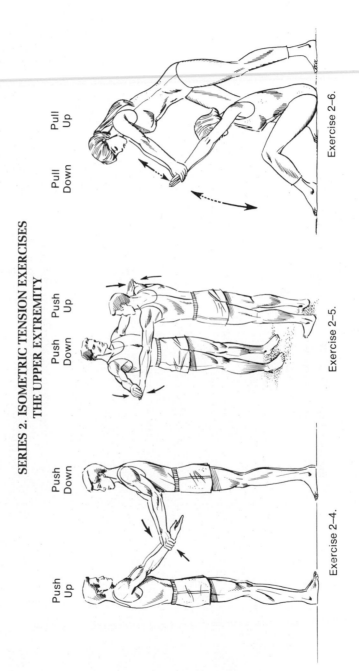

SERIES 2. ISOMETRIC TENSION EXERCISES
THE UPPER EXTREMITY

Push Up   Push Down   Exercise 2–4.

Push Down   Push Up   Exercise 2–5.

Pull Down   Pull Up   Exercise 2–6.

**SERIES 2. ISOMETRIC TENSION EXERCISES
THE LOWER EXTREMITY AND TRUNK**

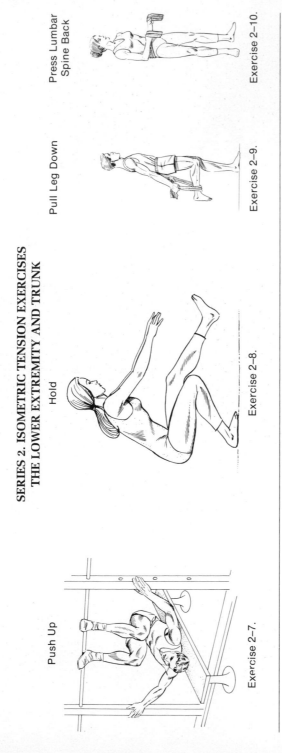

Push Up

Exercise 2–7.

Hold

Exercise 2–8.

Pull Leg Down

Exercise 2–9.

Press Lumbar
Spine Back

Exercise 2–10.

THE TRUNK—HEAD—NECK

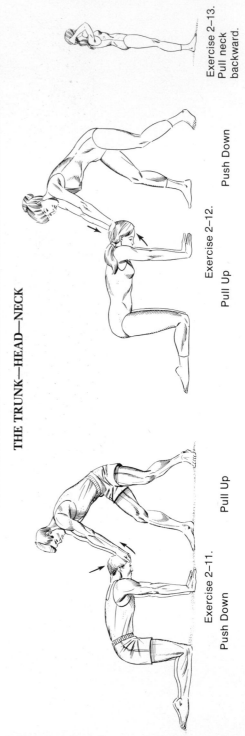

Push Down   Pull Up

Exercise 2–11.

Pull Up   Push Down

Exercise 2–12.

Exercise 2–13.
Pull neck
backward.

SERIES 3. FLEXIBILITY EXERCISES FOR MAJOR JOINTS

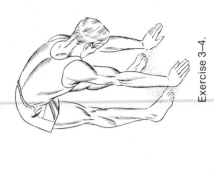

Exercise 3–4.

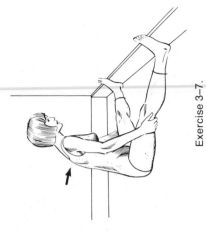

Exercise 3–7.

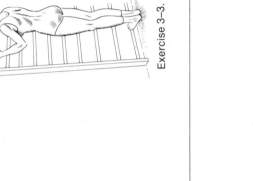

Exercise 3–3.

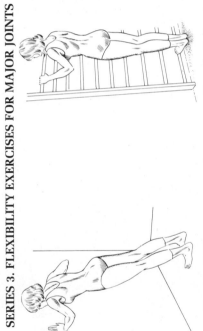

Exercise 3–2.

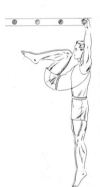

Exercise 3–6.

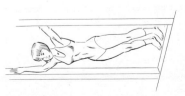

Exercise 3–1.

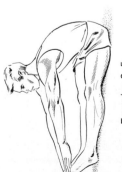

Exercise 3–5.

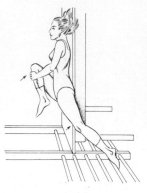

Exercise 3–10.

SERIES 3. FLEXIBILITY EXERCISES FOR MAJOR JOINTS

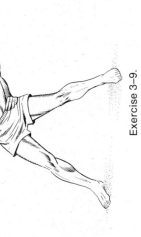

Exercise 3–9.

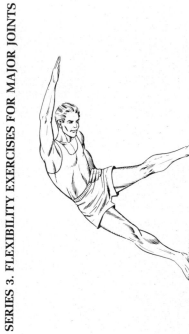

Exercise 3–8.

SERIES 4. POSTURE EXERCISES

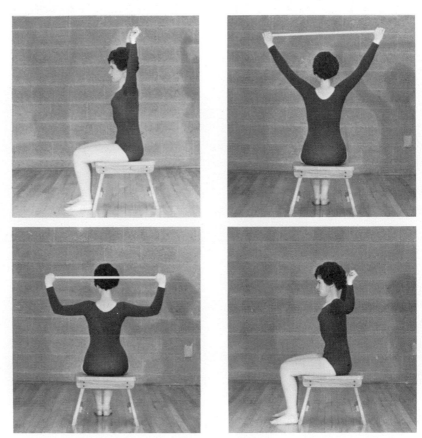

Exercise 4–1.
(Photographs taken from Wells, K. F.: *Posture exercise handbook: a progressive sequence approach.* New York: The Ronald Press Company, 1963.)

SERIES 4. POSTURE EXERCISES

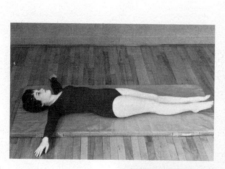
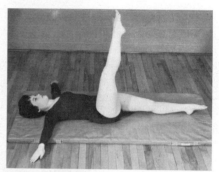
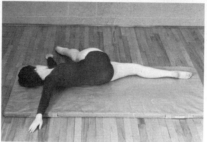

Exercise 4–2.

SERIES 4. POSTURE EXERCISES

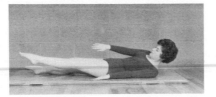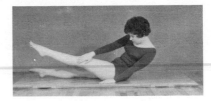

Exercise 4–3.

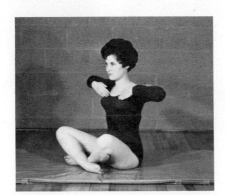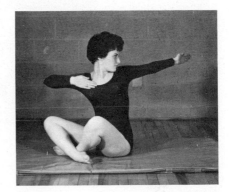

Exercise 4–4.

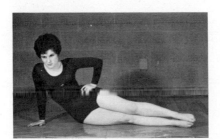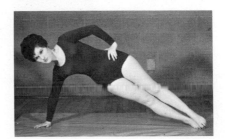

Exercise 4–5.

SERIES 4. POSTURE EXERCISES

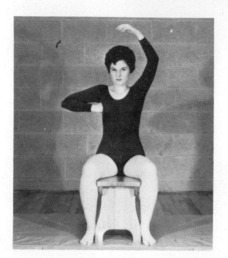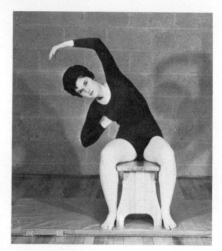

Exercise 4–6.

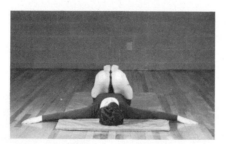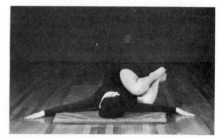

Exercise 4–7.

SERIES 5. SPORTS AND GYMNASTICS TECHNIQUES

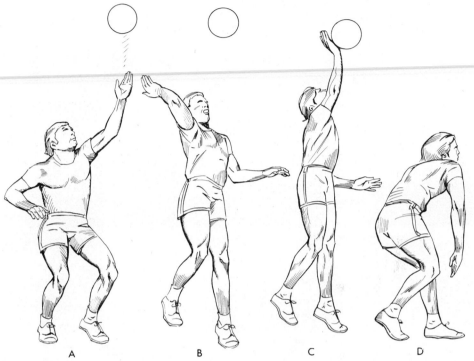

Figure 5–1   Volleyball serve.

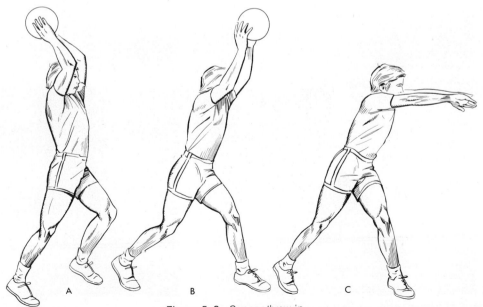

Figure 5–2   Soccer throw-in.

SERIES 5. SPORTS AND GYMNASTICS TECHNIQUES

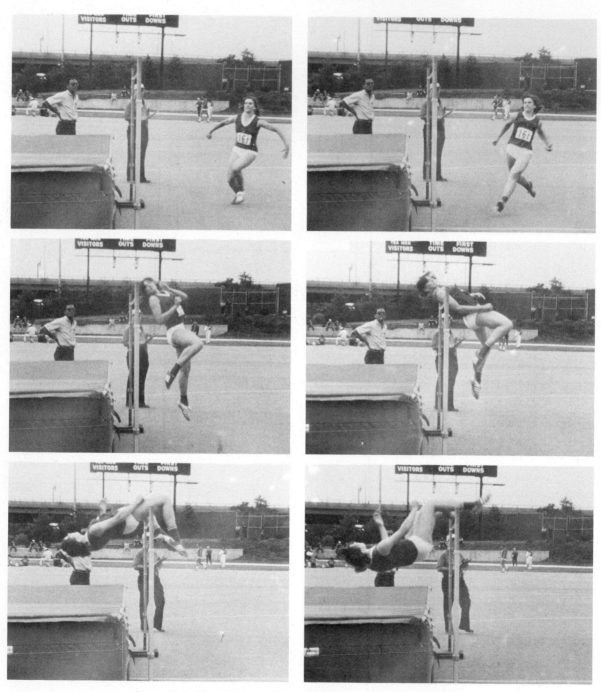

Figure 5–3   The high jump. (Time between each frame is 0.094 sec.)

SERIES 5. SPORTS AND GYMNASTICS TECHNIQUES

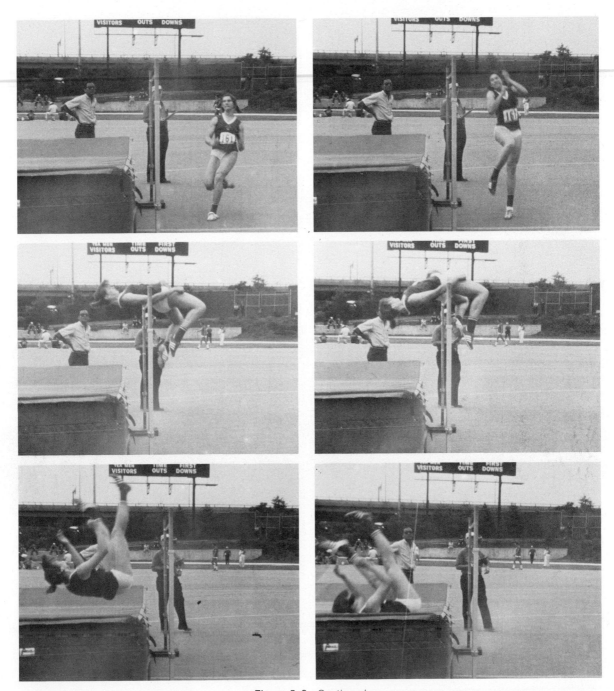

Figure 5–3 *Continued*

SERIES 5. SPORTS AND GYMNASTICS TECHNIQUES

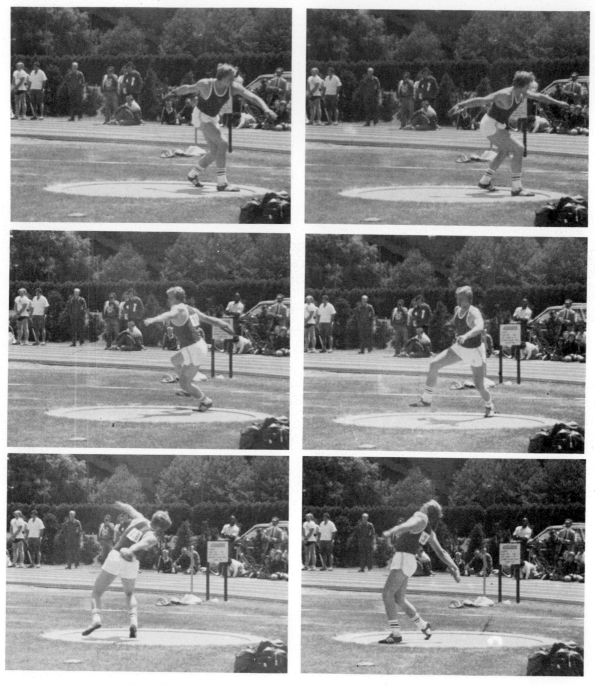

Figure 5–4   The discus throw. (Time between each frame is 0.125 sec.)

SERIES 5. SPORTS AND GYMNASTICS TECHNIQUES

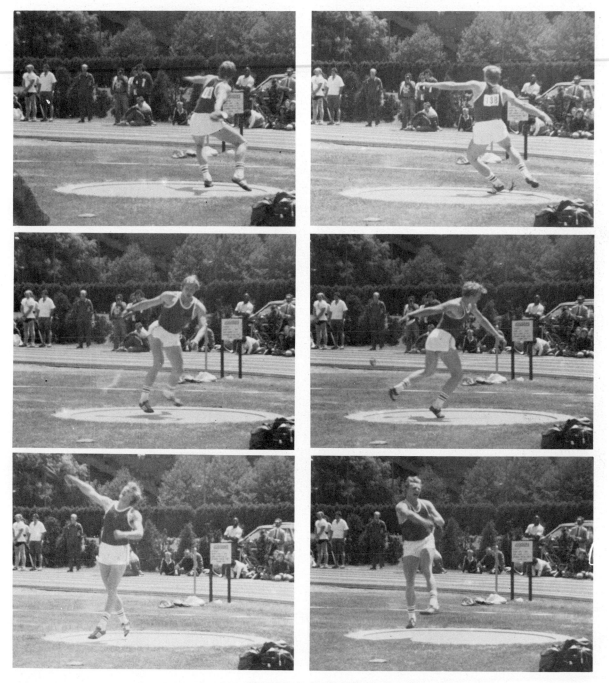

Figure 5–4   *Continued*

SERIES 5. SPORTS AND GYMNASTICS TECHNIQUES

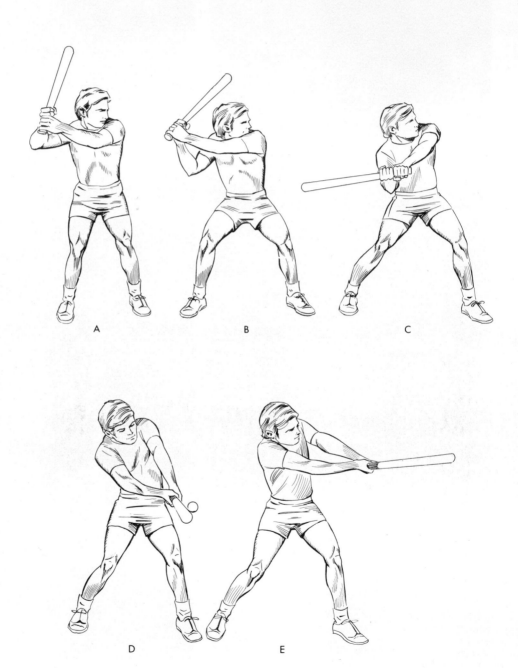

Figure 5–5   Baseball swing.

SERIES 5. SPORTS AND GYMNASTICS TECHNIQUES

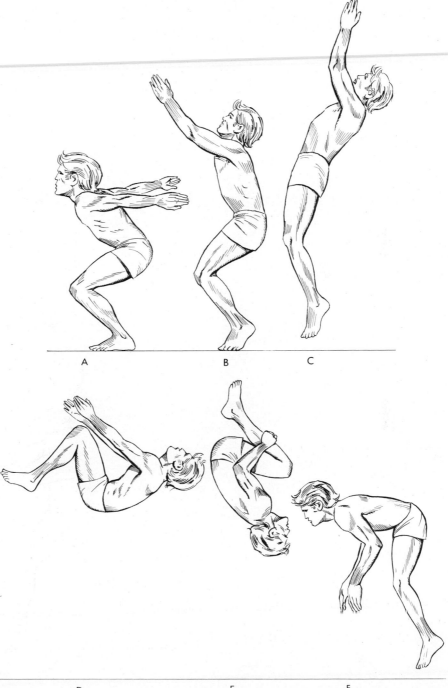

Figure 5–6 Backward somersault.

SERIES 5. SPORTS AND GYMNASTICS TECHNIQUES

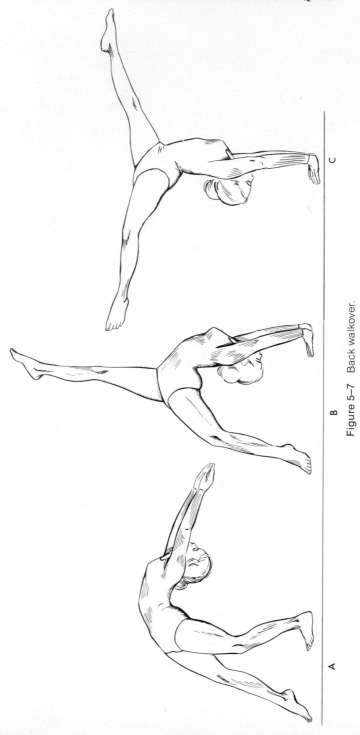

Figure 5–7   Back walkover.

SERIES 5. SPORTS AND GYMNASTICS TECHNIQUES

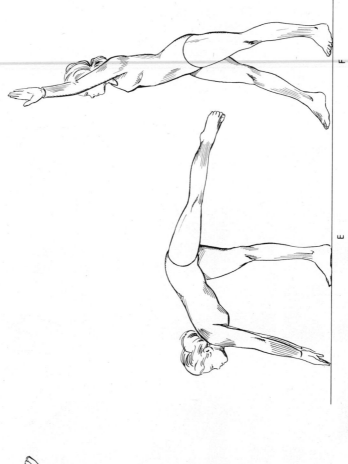

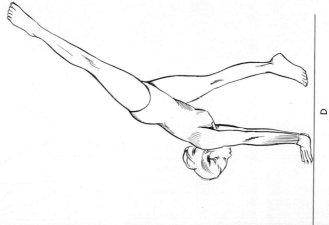

Figure 5-7 Continued

SERIES 5. SPORTS AND GYMNASTICS TECHNIQUES

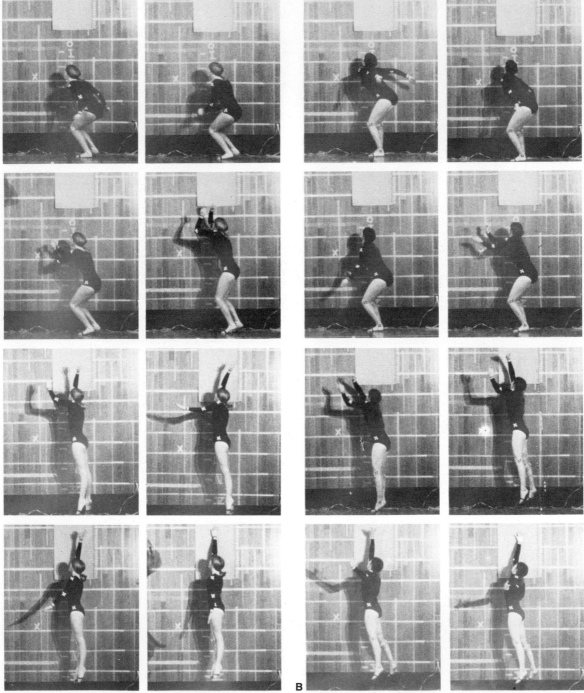

A   B

Figure 5–8   Vertical jump. *A*, Good technique. *B*,Poorer technique.
(Time between each frame is 0.094 sec.)

Index

Note: Page numbers in italics indicate illustrations; those followed by (t) indicate tables.